Publishing Sciences Group, Inc.
Acton, Massachusetts

a subsidiary of CHC Corporation

# Clinical Pharmacy
# Sourcebook

International Standard Book Number: 0-88416-101-3

Library of Congress Catalog Card Number: 75-12030

# Authors

**Philip O. Anderson, Pharm. D.**
Formerly, Chief Pharmacist, U.S.P.H.S. Indian Hospital, Clinton, Oklahoma.

**J. Dennis Andrews, Pharm. D.**
Assistant Clinical Professor of Pharmacy, University of California, San Francisco, California.

**James A. Balmer, B.S.**
Instructor of Clinical Pharmacy, Duquesne University, Pittsburgh, Pennsylvania.

**R. Paul Baumgartner, B.S.**
Director of Pharmaceutical Services, Appalachian Regional Hospitals; and Assistant Clinical Professor, College of Pharmacy, University of Kentucky, Lexington, Kentucky.

**Charles N. Bell, M.S.**
Assistant Professor, Department of Hospital and Clinical Pharmacy, Northeast Louisiana University, Monroe, Louisiana.

**J. Edward Bell, Pharm. D.**
Assistant Director, Clinical Division, Department of Pharmacy, University Hospital, University of Michigan Medical Center, Ann Arbor, Michigan.

**Robert W. Bennett, M.S.**
Assistant Professor of Clinical Pharmacy, Purdue University, Lafayette, Indiana.

**Diane Bernstein, Pharm. D.**
Instructor of Clinical Pharmacy, University of Southern California, Los Angeles, California.

**Norman F. Billups, Ph.D.**
Professor of Pharmacy, University of Kentucky, Lexington, Kentucky.

**Lawrence R. Borgsdorf, Pharm. D.**
Docent Clinical Pharmacist at Kansas City General Hospital and Medical Center; Assistant Professor of Clinical Pharmacy, School of Pharmacy; and Assistant Professor of Medicine, School of Medicine, University of Missouri, Kansas City, Missouri.

**Vincent E. Bouchard, M.S.**
Director, Department of Pharmacy, University Hospital, University of Michigan Medical Center, Ann Arbor, Michigan.

**James R. Boyd, M.S.**
Instructor of Clinical Pharmacy, St. Louis College of Pharmacy, St. Louis, Missouri.

**Gerald G. Briggs, Pharm. D.**
Pediatric Clinical Pharmacist, Memorial Hospital Medical Center, Long Beach, California.

**May E. Briscoe, Ph.D.**
Research Associate, Appalachian Regional Hospitals, Lexington, Kentucky.

**Bobby G. Bryant, Pharm. D.**
Assistant Professor of Hospital Pharmacy, Purdue University, Lafayette, Indiana.

**Larry Cacace, Pharm. D.**
At the time he coauthored a chapter, was Supervisor, Drug Information Service, Memorial Hospital Medical Center, Long Beach California.

**Thomas J. Caldwell, Pharm. D.**
At the time he coauthored a chapter, was Clinical Instructor, State University of New York at Buffalo; and Supervisor, Unit Dose Satellite Pharmacy, Buffalo General Hospital, Buffalo, New York.

**Philip Cole, M.S.**
At the time he coauthored a chapter, was Assistant Director of Pharmaceutical Services, Providence Hospital, Southfield, Michigan.

**James H. Coleman, III, Pharm. D.**
Director of Pharmacy Services, Tennessee Psychiatric Hospital and Institute; and Assistant Professor of Clinical Pharmacy, University of Tennessee, Memphis, Tennessee.

**Wayne F. Conrad, Pharm. D.**
Assistant Professor of Pharmacy, State University of New York at Buffalo; Director of Pharmaceutical Services, E. J. Meyer Memorial Hospital, Buffalo, New York.

**Ray Cook**
At the time he coauthored a chapter, was a Staff Pharmacist at Memorial Hospital Medical Center, Long Beach, California.

**Clyde R. Cooper, Pharm. D.**
At the time he coauthored a chapter, was a Staff Pharmacist at Charles F. Kettering Memorial Hospital, Kettering, Ohio.

**Lawrence A. Corbin, B.S.**
At the time he coauthored a chapter, was a Pharmacy Resident, Mercy Hospital, and candidate for the Doctor of Pharmacy degree, Duquesne University, Pittsburgh, Pennsylvania.

**R. Timothy Coussons, M.D.**
At the time he coauthored a chapter, was Director of Medical Service, Veterans Administration Hospital, Oklahoma City, Oklahoma.

**Tim R. Covington, Pharm. D., M.S.**
Assistant Professor of Clinical Pharmacy, College of Pharmacy, University of Oklahoma, Norman, Oklahoma.

**James C. Cradock, M.S.**
With the Clinical Drug Distribution Section, Drug Development Branch, Drug Research and Development, NCI, NIH, Bethesda, Maryland.

**Gary W. Cripps, Pharm. D.**
Associate Professor of Clinical Pharmacy, University of Tennessee, Memphis, Tennessee.

**Carl T. DeMarco, J.D.**
Director, Health Law Center, Aspen Systems Corporation, Rockville, Maryland.

**Sister M. Gonzales Duffy**
Director of Pharmacy Services, Mercy Hospital, Pittsburgh, Pennsylvania.

**Fred M. Eckel, M.S.**
Associate Professor of Hospital Pharmacy, University of North Carolina; and Director of Pharmacy Services, North Carolina Memorial Hospital, Chapel Hill, North Carolina.

**Brian J. Ellinoy, Pharm. D.**
Pharmacist with the PROMIS Laboratory, Medical Center Hospital of Vermont, Burlington, Vermont.

**Sister Emmanuel, D.C., M.S.**
At the time she coauthored a chapter, was Adjunct Associate Professor of Clinical Pharmacy, Wayne State University, Detroit, Michigan.

**R. Lee Evans, Pharm. D.**
Coordinator of Outpatient Pharmacy Services, Memphis, and Shelby County Mental Health Center, and Tennessee Psychiatric Hospital and Institute; and Assistant Professor of Clinical Pharmacy, University of Tennessee, Memphis, Tennessee.

**Susan P. Flinkow, B.S.**
Director of the Bureau of Methadone Rehabilitation, Division of Special Health, State Department of Health, Richmond, Virginia.

**Clarence L. Fortner, M.S.**
Director, Clinical Research Pharmacy Service, Baltimore Cancer Research Center, National Cancer Institute, Division of Cancer Treatment, Baltimore, Maryland.

**William R. Garnett, Pharm. D.**
Instructor in Clinical Pharmacy, University of North Carolina, Chapel Hill, North Carolina.

**Robert H. Gassett, M.S.**
Formerly, Clinical Instructor of Pharmacy, State University of New York at Buffalo; and Assistant Director of Pharmaceutical Services, E. J. Meyer Memorial Hospital, Buffalo, New York.

**Margaret C. Gebhardt, B.S.**
Clinical Pharmacy Specialist, North Carolina Memorial Hospital, Chapel Hill, North Carolina.

**Philip P. Gerbino, Pharm. D.**
Assistant Professor of Clinical Pharmacy, Philadelphia College of Pharmacy and Science, Philadelphia, Pennsylvania.

**R. Allan Gilliam, Pharm. D.**
Assistant Clinical Professor of Pharmaceutics, University of Tennessee, Memphis, Tennessee.

**Lyle M. Glascock, B.S.**
Chief Pharmacist, Wise Appalachian Regional Hospital, Wise, Virginia.

**Shirley A. Glascock, B.S.**
Staff Pharmacist, Wise Appalachian Regional Hospital, Wise, Virginia.

**Frank J. Goicoechea, Pharm. D.**
School of Medicine, University of California, San Francisco, California.

**Daniel A. Goupil, B.S.**
At the time he coauthored a chapter, was Supervising Pharmacist, E. J. Meyer Memorial Hospital, Buffalo, New York.

**Gary E. Griner, Pharm. D.**
At the time he coauthored a chapter, was a second-year Pharmacy Resident, Veterans Administration Hospital, Cincinnati, Ohio.

**Paul E. Hafner**
At the time he coauthored a chapter, was Clinical Pharmacist, Department of Pharmacy, The Ohio State University Hospitals, Columbus, Ohio.

**Philip D. Hansten, Pharm. D.**
Assistant Professor of Clinical Pharmacy, Washington State University College of Pharmacy, Pullman, Washington.

**Earl C. Harrison, M.D.**
At the time he coauthored a chapter, was Assistant Professor of Medicine, University of Southern California, Los Angeles, California.

**Willard L. Harrison, M.S.**
Director, Department of Pharmacy Services, and Project Director, Drug Treatment Program, Medical College of Virginia Hospitals; Associate Professor of Hospital Pharmacy, Virginia Commonwealth University, Richmond, Virginia.

**Marilyn Heins, M.D.**
At the time she coauthored a chapter, was Associate Professor of Pediatrics and Assistant Dean for Student Affairs, Wayne State University School of Medicine, Detroit, Michigan.

**Freya Hermann, B.S.**
Assistant Professor of Pharmaceutical Science, School of Pharmacy, Oregon State University, Corvallis, Oregon.

**J. Heyward Hull, III, M.S.**
Instructor of Clinical Pharmacy, University of North Carolina; and Clinical Pharmacy Specialist, North Carolina Memorial Hospital, Chapel Hill, North Carolina.

**Marianne F. Ivey, B.S.**
Assistant Professor of Clinical Pharmacy, University of Washington, Seattle, Washington.

**Eric A. Jackson, Pharm. D.**
Assistant Director of Pharmacy for Clinical Services, University of Connecticut Health Center, Farmington, Connecticut.

**Roger W. Jelliffe, M.D.**
Associate Professor of Medicine, School of Medicine, University of Southern California and Los Angeles County-USC Medical Center, Los Angeles, California.

**Martin Jinks, Pharm. D.**
Associate Professor of Clinical Pharmacy, College of Pharmacy, University of Minnesota, Minneapolis, Minnesota.

**Hugh F. Kabat, Ph.D.**
Professor and Head, Department of Clinical Pharmacy, University of Minnesota, Minneapolis, Minnesota.

**Allan L. Kelly, M.S.**
At the time he coauthored a chapter, was Assistant Professor of Clinical Pharmacy, Purdue University, West Lafayette, Indiana.

**Donald T. Kishi, Pharm. D.**
Assistant Clinical Professor of Pharmacy, University of California, San Francisco Medical Center, San Francisco, California.

**René H. Levy, Ph.D.**
Associate Professor of Pharmacy, University of Washington, Seattle, Washington.

**Philip Liberman, Pharm. D.**
At the time he coauthored a chapter, was Staff Pharmacist, City of Hope National Medical Center, Duarte, California.

**Arthur G. Lipman, Pharm. D.**
Drug Information Director and Associate Director of Pharmacy Services, Yale-New Haven Hospital, New Haven, Connecticut; Assistant Professor, School of Pharmacy, University of Connecticut, Storrs, Connecticut.

**V. A. Lomonte, Jr.**
At the time he coauthored a chapter, was a graduate student, Department of Hospital and Clinical Pharmacy, Northeast Louisiana University, Monroe, Louisiana.

**Richard L. Lucarotti**
At the time he coauthored a chapter, was Clinical Pharmacist, Department of Pharmacy, The Ohio State University Hospitals, Columbus, Ohio.

**Anthony S. Manoguerra, Pharm. D.**
Assistant Professor of Clinical Pharmacy, University of Minnesota, Minneapolis, Minnesota.

**Domingo R. Martinez, Pharm. D.**
Associate Professor of Clinical Pharmacy, University of Tennessee, Memphis, Tennessee.

**Thomas J. Mattei, Pharm. D.**
Associate Director, Pharmacy Services and Education, Mercy Hospital; and Assistant Professor of Clinical Pharmacy, Duquesne University, Pittsburgh, Pennsylvania.

**John F. Mays, B.S.**
At the time he coauthored a chapter, was Chief Pharmacist at the Shiprock Indian Health Service Hospital, Shiprock, New Mexico.

**Margaret M. McCarron, M.D.**
Assistant Professor of Medicine, University of Southern California, Los Angeles, California.

**Don C. McLeod, M.S.**
Assistant Professor of Pharmacy, State University of New York at Buffalo; and Director, Pharmacy Services, Buffalo General Hospital, Buffalo, New York.

**Paul V. McSherry, B.S.**
At the time he coauthored a chapter, was a Staff Pharmacist at the Shiprock Indian Health Service Hospital, Shiprock, New Mexico.

**James W. Menzie, Ph.D.**
At the time he coauthored a chapter, was a Staff Pharmacist, Patient Care Pharmacy Service, Baltimore Cancer Research Center, Balitmore, Maryland.

**William A. Miller, Pharm. D.**
Director of Pharmacy Affairs, City of Memphis Hospital, and Associate Professor of Clinical Pharmacy, University of Tennessee, Memphis, Tennessee.

**Robert S. Mosser, M.D.**
At the time he coauthored a chapter, was Senior Docent and Professor of Medicine, School of Medicine, University of Missouri-Kansas City, Kansas City, Missouri.

**Paul J. Munzenberger, Pharm. D.**
Assistant Professor of Clinical Pharmacy, Wayne State University, Detroit, Michigan.

**Paul J. Niebergall, Ph.D.**
Director of Corporate Product Development, Marion Laboratories, Kansas City, Missouri.

**Eric Owyang, B.S.**
Associate Clinical Professor of Hospital Pharmacy, School of Pharmacy, and Chief Pharmacist, University Hospitals, University of California, San Francisco, California.

**Frederick G. Pfeiffer, B.S.**
At the time he coauthored a chapter, was Staff Pharmacist, Clinical Center, National Institutes of Health, Bethesda, Maryland.

**Harold M. Prisco, M.S.**
At the time he coauthored a chapter, was Clinical Pharmacist, Department of Pharmacy, The Ohio State University Hospitals, Columbus, Ohio.

**Jane D. Pruett, R.N.**
At the time she coauthored a chapter, was Project Director, St. Elizabeth Hospital, Lafayette, Indiana.

**Charles C. Pulliam, M.S.**
Assistant Professor of Clinical Pharmacy, University of North Carolina, Chapel Hill, North Carolina.

**M. A. Riddiough, Pharm. D.**
Assistant Clinical Professor of Pharmacy, University of California, San Francisco, California.

**Sidney A. Rosenbluth, Ph.D.**
Professor and Assistant Dean for Clinical Affairs, College of Pharmacy, University of Tennessee, Memphis, Tennessee.

**Lawrence C. Rosenthal, B.S.**
At the time he coauthored a chapter, was a Staff Pharmacist at the Shiprock Indian Health Service Hospital, Shiprock, New Mexico.

**John S. Ruggiero, Ph.D.**
Assistant Vice President for Scientific and Professional Relations, and Director of Pharmacy Relations, Pharmaceutical Manufacturers Association, Washington, D.C.

**Roger L. Schnaare, Ph.D.**
Associate Professor of Pharmacy, Philadelphia College of Pharmacy and Science, Philadelphia, Pennsylvania.

**G. E. Schumacher, Pharm. D., Ph.D.**
Director of Clinical Education and Research Programs, Faculty of Pharmacy, College of Pharmacy and Allied Health Professions, Wayne State University, Detroit, Michigan.

**Larry K. Shoup, M.S.**
Director of Pharmacy, Henry Ford Hospital, Detroit, Michigan.

**Harold M. Silverman, Pharm. D.**
Assistant Director of Pharmacy Services, Lenox Hill Hospital, New York, New York.

**Gilbert I. Simon, M.S.**
Director of Pharmacy Services, Lenox Hill Hospital, New York, New York.

**Gary H. Smith, Pharm. D.**
Assistant Professor of Clinical Pharmacy and Director of Drug Information Service, Department of Pharmacy Practice, School of Pharmacy, University of Washington, Seattle, Washington.

**William E. Smith, Jr., Pharm. D.**
Director of Pharmacy and Central Services, Memorial Hospital Medical Center, Long Beach, California.

**David K. Solomon, Pharm. D.**
Assistant Director for Clinical Services and Education, Appalachian Regional Hospitals, South Williamson, Kentucky.

**Donald L. Sorby, Ph.D.**
Dean and Professor of Pharmacy, School of Pharmacy, University of Missouri, Kansas City, Missouri.

**John C. South**
At the time he coauthored a chapter, was Professor, School of Business and Administration, Duquesne University, Pittsburgh, Pennsylvania.

**Walter F. Stanaszek, Ph.D.**
Assistant Professor of Pharmacy, University of Oklahoma, Norman, Oklahoma.

**Edwin T. Sugita, Ph.D.**
Professor of Pharmacy, Philadelphia College of Pharmacy and Science, Philadelphia, Pennsylvania.

**Margo Swanson, B.S.**
Staff Pharmacist, Memorial Hospital Medical Center, Long Beach, California.

**Allan J. Swartz, Pharm. D.**
Director of Pharmacy, City of Hope National Medical Center, Duarte, California.

**Jon J. Tanja, M.S.**
Associate Professor of Clinical Pharmacy and Hospital Pharmacy, Auburn University, Auburn, Alabama.

**David A. Taryle, M.D.**
At the time he coauthored a chapter, was a Resident in the Department of Medicine, University of Colorado Medical Center, Denver, Colorado.

**David S. Tatro, Pharm. D.**
Research Pharmacist, Division of Clinical Pharmacology, Stanford University School of Medicine; and Assistant Clinical Professor of Pharmacy, University of California, San Francisco, California.

**Thomas S. Thielke, M.S.**
Assistant Director, Department of Pharmacy and Central Services, University of Wisconsin Medical Center, Madison, Wisconsin.

**Melvin Thomason, M.S.**
Assistant Professor of Clinical Pharmacy, Temple University School of Pharmacy, Philadelphia, Pennsylvania.

**Arthur S. Watanabe, Pharm. D.**
Associate Director, Drug Information Service, The Intermountain Regional Poison Control Center, Salt Lake City, Utah.

**J. Weiner, B.S.**
At the time he coauthored a chapter, was a Pharm. D. Candidate, College of Pharmacy, Wayne State University, Detroit, Michigan.

**Gary R. Whitfield**
At the time he coauthored a chapter, was a Staff Phar-

macist at the Veterans Administration Hospital, Martinez, California.

**Roger S. Wilson, M.S.**
At the time he coauthored a chapter, was Pharmacist-in-Charge of Training and Education at the Veterans Administration Hospital, Ann Arbor, Michigan.

**Ronald A. Young, Pharm. D.**
At the time he coauthored a chapter, was Assistant Professor, Department of Hospital and Clinical Pharmacy, Northeast Louisiana University, Monroe, Louisiana.

**Ronald A. Young, Pharm. D.**
At the time he coauthored a chapter, was Assistant Professor, Department of Hospital and Clinical Pharmacy, Northeast Louisiana University, Monroe, Louisiana.

**W. Wayne Young, Pharm. D.**
Associate Director of Clinical Pharmacy Services, University Hospital, and Assistant Professor of Clinical Pharmacy, College of Pharmacy, University of Nebraska Medical Center, Omaha, Nebraska.

# Contents

xi

# Foreword

Although clinical pharmacy practice is clearly not restricted to the hospital setting, much of the work in developing this exciting area of pharmacy has taken place in hospitals and related health care institutions. The hospital—with "captive" patients and the ready availability of physicians, nurses, and other health professionals—has been a fertile environment for the development and growth of clinical pharmacy. Thus, it is not surprising that numerous reports related to clinical pharmacy practice have appeared in the journal of the association representing hospital pharmacists. That association, the American Society of Hospital Pharmacists, is pleased to cooperate with Publishing Sciences Group in producing this collection of key articles on clinical pharmacy practice from its official journal, the *American Journal of Hospital Pharmacy*.

For whom is this book intended? We believe it will be useful to anyone who is interested in reviewing a selective sample of the literature on clinical pharmacy practice. Pharmacists in institutional settings will find the book to be a helpful summary of what others have accomplished in clinical practice, and it may serve as a guide for their own clinical efforts. Community pharmacists will be particularly interested in several of the chapters on clinical services for ambulatory patients. Other health care workers—including physicians, nurses, and administrators—may read the book to gain an understanding of the significance of the clinical component of pharmacy. As a text for pharmacy students, the book may be used to illustrate practice models, and it will serve as an important reference source on practical applications of biopharmaceutic and pharmacokinetic principles.

The keynote chapter by Don McLeod was especially

solicited for this book and is published here for the first time. McLeod puts clinical pharmacy in historical perspective and traces the origins of this area of practice. In addition, he reviews the current scope of clinical pharmacy practice and discusses controversial issues in clinical pharmacy practice and education. As chairman of the ASHP Council on Clinical Pharmacy and Therapeutics, McLeod is particularly qualified to discuss the "past, present, and future" of clinical pharmacy.

The section on implementation and administration of clinical pharmacy services is rather slim, reflecting the relative lack of material that has been published in this area. True, administration is administration, and the same basic principles apply whether drug distribution services or clinical services are being managed. Nevertheless, the chapters in this section provide insights into the unique problems (and possible solutions) associated with implementing and managing clinical services in institutional settings.

A large sample of chapters on clinical pharmacy services for hospitalized patients is included in the next section. In addition to examples of specific services (educating inpatients, obtaining drug histories, monitoring pediatric drug therapy), this section presents the basis for a structured approach to clinical pharmacy practice. Three mechanisms for adding structure to clinical services are presented: problem-oriented medical records, pharmacy care plans, and criteria for selective patient monitoring. Also discussed are a clinically oriented hospital pharmacy intern-resident program and clinical pharmacy services in a small hospital.

With the trend toward more institution-based services for ambulatory patients, hospital pharmacists have been developing a greater number of services for such patients. It is not surprising, therefore, to find 16 chapters in the section on clinical pharmacy services for ambulatory patients. Several of these chapters discuss clinical services for patients with chronic illnesses (e.g., hypertension and mental disorders). Extensive pharmacist involvement (including patient evaluation, selection of therapy, and patient monitoring) is demonstrated in some of the chapters. The value of medication profiles, both in monitoring therapy and in detecting potential therapeutic problems, is discussed. Patient noncompliance with prescribed regimens, a health care problem receiving increasing attention, is reviewed in relation to the impact a pharmacist may have on improving compliance. In this regard, the significance of patient-pharmacist consultations is emphasized.

The majority of the chapters in the section on therapeutic considerations were originally published in the *American Journal of Hospital Pharmacy*'s Clinical Forum column. Under the editorship of Charles Pulliam, this column has taken a systematic approach toward outlining the basis for pharmacist involvement in making therapeutic judgments and in evaluating therapeutic accomplishments. Therapeutic problems discussed include secondary failure to oral hypoglycemic agents, digitalis glycoside intoxication, drug therapy in terminally ill patients, and drug-altered laboratory test values. These chapters are perhaps more important for the thought processes they demonstrate than for the specific therapies they present.

Biopharmaceutics and pharmacokinetics are areas of clinical pharmacy practice that have received extensive coverage in the *American Journal of Hospital Pharmacy*. Gerald Schumacher edits a *Journal* column on these subjects and he has been successful in translating complex pharmacokinetic concepts into terms that may be understood and readily applied by practicing pharmacists. Through work such as Schumacher's, a scientific basis is being built for clinical pharmacy practice. Topics in this book's section on biopharmaceutics and pharmacokinetics include dosage regimen calculations, dosing of drugs in renal-impaired patients, and use of bioavailability data in clinical practice.

While clinical pharmacy services have not been thoroughly evaluated, the profession is in the process of doing so, as demonstrated by the chapters in the last section of this book. Evaluations of pharmacists as drug therapy advisors and as drug history interviewers are included. Also presented are: (1) detailed procedures for the selection, training and evaluation of clinical pharmacists, and (2) subjective physician evaluations of clinical pharmacists.

While the emphasis of the chapters in this book is on clinical pharmacy practice rather than education, the bibliography of additional readings contains citations on both practice and education. The bibliography should be useful in suggesting additional literature that readers may wish to pursue.

As a final statement regarding the content of this book, the special features of the index should be mentioned. This detailed index was computer-generated from the data base of the *International Pharmaceutical Abstracts Information System*, an abstracting and indexing service of the American Society of Hospital Pharmacists. Each index entry is a "mini-abstract" and will help readers to be efficient in searching for specific information related to clinical pharmacy.

Special acknowledgement is given to the many authors of chapters in this book. Their dedication in developing patient-oriented pharmaceutical services is an inspiration to all those concerned with improving patient care through effective participation of pharmacists in the drug therapy process.

William A. Zellmer, Editor
*American Journal of Hospital Pharmacy*

# 1 Clinical Pharmacy: The Past, Present, and Future

Don C. McLeod

## Historical Perspective

The essence of clinical pharmacy practice is the application of the pharmaceutical sciences on behalf of the patient, considering all aspects of the patient's medical condition and need to understand his own therapy. This implies *de facto* a close association of the pharmacist with the patient, the patient's physician, and others providing medical care services. There are several historical precedents for the intimate involvement of the pharmacist with the patient and physician, and perhaps mention of these will be of interest to those following the clinical pharmacy movement.

In the Catholic countries of Europe, the patron saints of pharmacy and medicine are Damian and Cosmas, twin brothers of Arabic descent. About the year 300 A.D. the brothers were practicing jointly, Damian serving as the pharmacist and Cosmas as the physician. Their healing powers and philanthropy were known throughout Asia Minor. Their intimate practice, embodying separate roles but a common concern for the patient, certainly embraces the best possible concept for modern clinical pharmacy. Bender[1] relates that in 303 A.D., the brothers, who were Christians, were put to death by Roman persecutors. They were buried in Syria and their relics were later moved to Rome. Physicians and pharmacists throughout Catholic Europe celebrated their memory for centuries after their death. Among the many great artists and sculptors recording miracles and scenes from the lives of Damian and Cosmas are the masters Botticelli, Michelangelo, Tintoretto, and Titian.

The early history of organized pharmacy in Britain is intertwined with the history of medical practice. The members of the Society of Apothecaries, which was founded in 1617, not only dispensed for the physicians, but themselves recommended and prescribed medicines. Despite protests from the physicians, the apothecaries' legal right to give medical advice was upheld in a House of Lords' judgment in 1703 and, under the Apothecaries Act of 1815, they were allowed to charge for advice as well as for the medicines they dispensed. Parallel with this development of the apothecaries as a separate body of medical practitioners, a class of persons known as "chemists and druggists" arose who prepared and sold medicines to the public and competed with the apothecaries in dispensing. The apothecaries progressively assumed the role of general medical practitioners.[2]

In early 1700 in Italy, the doctors and apothecaries were united in a common guild. The famous Board of the Guild of Physicians and Apothecaries in Florence, of which Dante was a member, did much to further the collaboration between the students of both professions. Koup has pointed out the close relationship between the physician, pharmacist, and patient during this period, and its analogy to current clinical pharmacy practice.[3]

There are several early American examples of "clinical" pharmacy practice. In the charter of The New York Hospital issued by King George III in 1771, the apothecary is listed as one of the four salaried positions essential to the conduct of the hospital. One duty spelled out for the apothecary-in-chief in the early days of The New York Hospital was that he should accompany the physicians on rounds each day.

1

William Proctor, Jr., the Father of American Pharmacy, exemplified the practitioner-teacher-researcher model now being developed by leading schools of pharmacy. Proctor graduated from the Philadelphia College of Pharmacy in 1837. He was active in national pharmacy affairs; was a writer, editor, and researcher; and held for 20 years the position of Chairman of Pharmacy at the Philadelphia College of Pharmacy. Concurrent with these varied accomplishments he successfully maintained a pharmacy practice in Philadelphia.[1] It seems that this career serves as a useful model for current clinical pharmacy educators, with perhaps the exception that his practice was not formally associated with physicians in an organized health care setting.

An unexpected occurrence of a clinical pharmacy practice is documented in the writings of the great American short story writer, O. Henry (William Sidney Porter). O. Henry was trained as a pharmacist apprentice in North Carolina long before his career as a writer began. He was later accused of embezzling funds from an Austin, Texas bank and sentenced to the Federal Penitentiary in Columbus, Ohio. Upon entering the prison in 1848, he was assigned as head pharmacist. In a letter to a friend, O. Henry wrote as follows:

> I am a night druggist in the hospital, and as far as work is concerned it is light enough, and all the men stationed in the hospital live a hundred per cent better than the rest of the 2500 men here. There are four doctors and about twenty-five other men in the hospital force. The hospital is a separate building and is one of the finest equipped institutions in the country. It is large and finely furnished and has every appliance of medicine and surgery . . . the work is about the same as in any drug store, filling prescriptions, etc., and is pretty lively up until about ten o'clock. At 7 PM, I take a medicine case and go the rounds with the night physician to see the ones over in the main building who have become sick during the day. The doctor goes to bed about ten o'clock and from then on during the night I prescribe for the patients myself and go out and attend calls that come in. If I find anyone seriously ill I have them brought over to the hospital and attended by the doctor . . . the hospital wards have from 100 to 200 patients in them all of the time. They have all kinds of diseases — at present typhus fever and measles are the fashion. Consumption here is more common than bad colds at home.[4]

While these anecdotes are interesting, they were isolated cases and did not substantially influence the evolution of pharmacy practice in America. They also occurred while the practice of medicine was little more than a combination of witchcraft, folk medicine, and placebo effect. Even as late as 1860, Dr. Oliver Wendell Holmes gave the waggish opinion that if the whole of the *materia medica* then in use could have been sunk to the bottom of the sea, it would have been the better for mankind and all the worse for the fishes.

## Origin of Clinical Pharmacy Practice

When surveying the literature of pharmacy, it is evident that the clinical pharmacy movement has budded and blossomed within the past decade. The germs of clinical pharmacy have existed for several decades in the better hospital pharmacy departments in the country. The motivation and philosophy which led hospital pharmacists to activate pharmacy and therapeutics committees, to push and struggle for formularies of the best pharmaceuticals, and to identify and eliminate causes of medication errors is close akin to the philosophy sustaining the clinical pharmacy movement. The hospital is an organized health care setting in which, under common administrative guidelines, medical care professionals have come together to provide medical care. It is not surprising that those pharmacists trained in this environment are the ones today providing leadership in clinical pharmacy practice, both in hospitals and organized health care settings outside of the hospital.

Francke has shed some light on this germination of clinical pharmacy as follows:

> Using the term clinical in a very broad sense, formal training for clinical practice in hospital pharmacy developed quite apart from the colleges of pharmacy. Whitney at Michigan in the 1930's and Clarke at The New York Hospital in the 1940's were pioneers in this field. I recall the great frustration and disappointment expressed by Mr. Whitney because he could not interest either the dean or the faculty of the college in the prospect of using the tremendous interdisciplinary teaching facilities of a great university hospital for the education and training of undergraduate pharmacy students. This situation began to change in the late 1940's when Flack at Jefferson Hospital in Philadelphia, Purdum at Johns Hopkins and myself at Michigan developed programs which combined residencies and advanced degrees. However, these programs affected only a few graduate students and had almost no effect on the instruction of undergraduate students.[5]

An abortive attempt at "clinical" pharmacy education was begun at the University of Washington during World War II. In an editorial in 1969 announcing a change in title of the journal *Drug Intelligence* to *Drug Intelligence and Clinical Pharmacy*, Francke has described this effort as follows:

> One of the most dramatic events of recent years is the emergence of the concept of clinical pharmacy and its belated adoption by colleges of pharmacy as an educational tool. It is sad to have to say, however, that it was the narrow provincialism of pharmaceutical educators themselves which held back the development of the concept of clinical pharmacy for more than a quarter of a century. Clinical pharmacy as an educational tool was begun by Professor L. Wait Rising of the University of Washington in 1944 but was disapproved by resolution by both the American Association of Colleges of Pharmacy and the

American Council on Pharmaceutical Education in 1946. This action abruptly terminated an imaginative research program in teaching methods without even giving the professor who originated it, the students taking the course, or the pharmacists participating in it an opportunity to be heard. The value of the clinical pharmacy experiment at the University of Washington was again brought to the attention of pharmaceutical educators in 1953 by Professor H. W. Youngken, Jr., then at the University of Washington, but the idea lay dormant for many years until recently resurrected.[6]

The doomed efforts of Professor Rising were aimed at community pharmacy practice, and it is not known if his concept of clinical pharmacy would coincide with the more advanced concepts of today.

In an article entitled "Evolvement of Clinical Pharmacy," Gloria Francke[7] has carefully chronicled the use of the term "clinical pharmacy." It is beyond the scope of this chapter to highlight all events, but it seems clear that certain early uses (in the 1960's) did not connote clinical pharmacy as it is intensely practiced by some today. It appears to me that the flowering of clinical pharmacy closely paralleled two events in hospital pharmacy practice. One was the development of unit dose drug distribution systems in many hospitals in the late 1960's. Another activity associated with the clinical pharmacy movement was the development of the drug information center concept in the early 1960's. Drug information, along with radiopharmacy, were the first easily identified specialty areas in pharmacy practice.

I vividly remember attending the sessions of the ASHP at the APhA Annual Convention in Las Vegas in 1967. I had just obtained the B.S. degree in pharmacy and had entered a hospital pharmacy residency under H.A.K. Whitney, Jr. Prior to the residency, even though I had worked two summers in a university teaching hospital, I had never heard of clinical pharmacy, of Pharm. D. programs, or any "exciting new roles" for the hospital pharmacist. At the Las Vegas meeting, young pharmacists charged with implementing unit dose drug distribution systems were talking about the sort of problems and experiences they were undergoing, and many talked about making rounds with physicians as a part of their daily routine. I also became aware of Pharm. D. programs such as the ones at the University of Kentucky and the University of California at San Francisco. While the elder statesmen of hospital pharmacy inspired awe in me at that time, it was this evolving "clinical pharmacy" as practiced by some younger pharmacists that captured my imagination in the coming months and years. I believe that there are hundreds of hospital pharmacists who can relate similar stories.

Since the early clinical pharmacists were predominantly found in (or associated with) advanced residency and graduate (Pharm. D. and M. Sc.) programs

in university teaching hospitals, it was natural that the schools of pharmacy soon became a ground of contention. It took about one morning of medical rounds or the presentation of the patient data at grand rounds to convince even the most astute hospital pharmacy resident that most of his curriculum had been for naught. The depression that resulted is not described in psychiatric texts. In the more hearty, the German concept of "angst" probably best described the feeling pervading those first few formative years. It was evident that pharmacy school curricula had to be drastically changed, hospital pharmacy practice had to undergo a revolution, and residency training in most hospitals had to be upgraded.

Given the tremendous clinical handicaps resulting from inadequate pharmacy education, it is surprising how rapidly the clinical pharmacy movement has advanced. Responsive chords in many students and young practitioners were clearly struck, and the federal government, through capitation grants to schools of pharmacy, gave considerable support to clinical pharmacy education and practice at a critical time. Many of the things that were merely dreams to young, clinically aspiring pharmacists less than a decade ago are now a reality in many locations. There are still the skeptics in academia and in practice, and the uninitiated in the other health professions, but solid accomplishments are rather commonplace in many hospitals and clinics.

## Current Scope of Clinical Pharmacy Practice

When one surveys major advances in medical practice, it is obvious that most of them occur in university teaching hospitals. The origin and early development of clinical pharmacy practice has likewise taken place in the academic medical care institution. Today a large portion of the clinically trained pharmacists still practice, and often teach, in the major teaching hospitals. On the contrary, there are still many university teaching hospitals where pharmacy is relatively undeveloped.

Thus far, the exodus of the clinically trained pharmacist into non-university settings has been rather small when the vast number of hospitals, health care institutions, and organized health care programs are considered. It seems that schools of pharmacy will soon be somewhat saturated with clinical faculty, and that more clinically trained graduates will be going into community hospitals and other nonacademic settings. This is a necessary development if clinical pharmacy is to be truly an important development in medical care. At this time, only a relatively few community hospitals are actively recruiting clinical pharmacists to function as specialists within the pharmacy department. When "clinical pharmacists" are sought, the director of pharmacy frequently does not envision high-level clinical pharmacy practice.

The most common clinical pharmacy practice model encountered in the teaching hospital is that of a clinical pharmacist (often on the school of pharmacy faculty) providing intensive services to a small group (12-30) of patients on a medical or pediatric teaching service. This pharmacist makes rounds with the medical staff, follows closely the diagnostic proceedings and therapy of patients on the service, and teaches students and residents about cases encountered. This is the only model of clinical practice many students encounter, and there is considerable difficulty relating to this role model since there are only a few ongoing practice responsibilities and the day is spent largely with academic matters. This role model has some personal rewards for the practitioner-educator, but it alone cannot suffice in the majority of hospitals. This is the practice model currently in vogue in many university teaching hospitals.

A variation of this model is the docent program at the University of Missouri in Kansas City. Here the clinical pharmacist is separated from the traditional pharmacy department. The clinical pharmacy practitioner-educator serves as faculty for medical and nurssing students as well as pharmacy students. In the Kansas City program, the docent team provides continuing services, both inpatient and ambulatory, to a defined group of patients. A shortcoming in this model is the continued existence of a traditional pharmacy department largely separated from the clinical activities.

Another clinical pharmacy practice model is that associated with unit dose drug distribution services provided from a decentralized pharmacy in the patient care area. Unit dose systems have been the impetus to clinical pharmacy evolvement in many teaching hospitals as well as community hospitals. Unit dose was an entree into the patient care area which spared the pharmacist the trauma of announcing he was there for clinical reasons. It allowed him to sharpen slowly his clinical abilities and to begin making inroads gradually with the medical staff. Unit dose systems forced the pharmacist to become intimately involved with the nurse, the physician, the medical chart and, to some degree, the patient. It was this arena that spurred many of the younger and more ambitious pharmacists to pursue clinical pharmacy practice.

While unit dose systems forced the pharmacist into the patient care area, it has proven difficult for a pharmacist to work in the satellite pharmacy and maintain a close clinical involvement with patient drug therapy. The magnitude of technical and supervisory activities tends to consume the time and energy of the pharmacy staff, unless there are a great many pharmacists or ample technical staff. Even with adequate supportive personnel, a clinical program of quality is not easy in the presence of a unit dose drug distribution system as operated in most hospitals having the system. Only through wise management, proper recruitment of clinical staff, and much hard work will the clinical program have a large impact on rational drug therapy. Safer handling and administration of drugs will ensue but often with little meaningful clinical involvement with the physician and the therapeutic decision-making process.

The hospital outpatient clinics have been the grounds for a logical extension of the clinical pharmacy concept. Proper choice of drug therapy, and patient education and compliance, are properly a concern of the pharmacist, and many articles have described activities directed toward these matters. As pharmacists began taking medical school courses in many of the Pharm. D. programs and gaining acceptance for their expertise in drug therapy, it was not suprising that a few began managing the chronic drug therapy of selected patients. This is being done in some U.S. Public Health Service Indian Hospitals and in other organized health care settings providing comprehensive services. Common diseases managed by the pharmacist have been hypertension, diabetes, and tuberculosis. If clinical pharmacy is going to make its maximal input into improving rational drug therapy, a significant involvement in ambulatory and community medicine must be developed. If this occurs it will be an outgrowth of the hospital clinical pharmacy programs, not a development within the drugstore establishment.

There are now several easily identified clinical pharmacy specialties developing. The drug information specialist was an important precursor to the clinical pharmacist, and he is probably the most entrenched specialist in most comprehensive clinical pharmacy programs. The drug information center is a sanctuary removed from direct clinical activities, and many drug information specialists have no ongoing clinical responsbilities. In a few hospitals, a competent drug information specialist may exist without a direct clinical pharmacy program. In other hospitals, the drug information specialist is an integral part of the clinical pharmacy team, and provides an important support service to enhance the overall quality of pharmacy programs. Some drug information centers provide services on a regional basis, to both the medical and the pharmaceutical communities.

Pediatrics is a natural area for pharmacy specialization, and the pediatric pharmacist was probably the first identifiable clinical pharmacy specialist. There are now at least a few dozen pediatric clinical pharmacists who have gained acceptance by their colleagues in pediatrics. One factor contributing to the rather rapid entree of the clinical pharmacist into pediatrics has been the generally cordial welcome extended by pediatricians. Of the various medical specialists, the pediatrician has been very supportive of a team approach to medical care, and generally has not acted in a threatened or condescending way toward the clinical pharmacist. This is the only "break" the well-prepared and ambitious clinical pharmacist needs.

Psychiatric clinical pharmacy has become a viable practice in several locations around the country. Again this is an easily identified specialty area in medicine, and community mental health centers have developed all over the country in response to the mental health needs of the community. The best examples of clinical psychiatric pharmacy are in the mental health centers. One of the hallmarks of the community health center is well-organized, interdisciplinary teamwork. There is also a shortage of psychiatrists in many places to deal traditionally with all the patients. Medication is the main therapy afforded most mental patients, and this therapy is often poorly controlled. The forte of the clinical psychiatric pharmacist is drug therapy control and patient assessment. In some community mental health centers, the clinical pharmacist conducts clinics (e.g., lithium and fluphenazine maintenance) and schedules patients back to the pharmacy clinic for reassessment and medication maintenance. The pharmacist, working under policies of the community health center and backup of psychiatrists, may discontinue or alter doses of drugs, initiate new therapy, or refer the patient to the psychiatrist. This is wise use of a long-established health professional in an area where the number of new job descriptions of various counselors, aides, therapists, etc., is almost astounding.

Another specialty area being developed in clinical pharmacy is clinical pharmacokinetics. Clinical pharmacokinetics is a tool, like pharmacology, of which every clinical pharmacist should have a basic understanding and familiarity so that well-established knowledge can be applied to every patient. Clinical pharmacokinetics is also a very complex science that is in every way as difficult to master as cardiology, for example. Every physician should know basic cardiology, but not every physician is a cardiologist (or clinical pharmacokineticist). The Department of Pharmaceutics of the School of Pharmacy at the State University of New York at Buffalo has established the first post-Pharm. D. specialty training program in clinical pharmacokinetics. Levy[8] and Gibaldi[9] have described the philosophy of this concept. To function competently in clinical pharmacokinetics, specialized training in the pharmacokinetic laboratory is definitely indicated. Also, considerable clinical medicine experience is needed if the specialist in clinical pharmacokinetics is to advise and work with the physician in clinical matters. The Pharm. D. graduates at Buffalo (and some other programs) have the clinical medicine experience, and with intensive training in the laboratory, it is felt that selected Pharm. D. graduates should be competent in clinical pharmacokinetics. Quite a few clinical pharmacists are now applying pharmacokinetic concepts, often with computer aid, but this alone is not enough to make them specialists in clinical pharmacokinetics. The scientific arm of the pharmacokinetics laboratory is needed as well.

In the long run, clinical pharmacy must prove to be a viable practice outside of the hospital and its clinics. For a meaningful clinical pharmacy practice to develop in the community, pharmacists trained clinically in the organized health care setting (largely hospitals) must spread their practice concepts outside the health care institution. The ferment will not come from community pharmacies, nor will the thrust of clinical pharmacy programs be aimed at the solo medical practitioner and his patients. Particularly favorable settings should be the group family practices now forming throughout the country. At least one article has described a clinical pharmacy practice as a part of a group family practice in Iowa.[10] This is an exciting possibility and could be the largest specialty practice of clinical pharmacy in the future. If this development takes place, the family practitioner of clinical pharmacy will provide needed nourishment to the health care system and to the clinical pharmacy movement. This clinical pharmacist should be a versatile person capable of providing good drug information, managing the drug therapy of many patients, and serving as a drug therapy educator to the patient and health care team. Many clinical pharmacists should prefer this role to that of the clinical pharmacist in the hospital.

There are many aspects of clinical pharmacy practice that have been described in the literature. Many of these activities are common to all clinical pharmacy practices, or serve as subspecialty activities for a few clinical pharmacists. The advent of total parenteral nutrition (TPN) a few years ago proved to be a clinical entree for many hospital pharmacists. Since the technique was new and involved considerable sterile compounding, many pharmacists quickly became part of the decision-making process for the prescribing and monitoring of TPN therapy. Many of the traditional elements of pharmaceutical compounding were at once combined with the clinical assessment of the patient.

Antibiotic usage studies have been an avenue for the pharmacist to develop ongoing clinical activities in the hospital. Several pharmacy-initiated programs have been described, and the results of these programs have advanced the cause for clinical pharmacy and have improved rational drug therapy.

Adverse drug reaction detection and reporting has been another route for the involvement of the pharmacist in clinical matters. Early articles in the pharmacy literature brought attention, as did medication error studies, to the need for persons knowledgeable and primarily concerned about drugs to become more involved with the drug use process. This sort of need was manifested a few years later by the tremendous attention brought to drug interactions. Although the sudden interest in drug interactions now seems shallow, since many of the interactions were beneficial and almost all are predictable if the pharmaceutical sciences are known, the publicity was beneficial toward increasing sensitivity to drug therapy problems.

Many pharmacists now serve as an integral part of the cardio-pulmonary resuscitation (CPR) team in hospitals. This involvement can be merely technical (supplying drugs ready-to-administer and recording drug usage) or can involve the pharmacist as an initiator of therapy and a therapeutic advisor throughout the procedure. This is the sort of "blood and guts" activity that vividly dramatizes the clinical involvement of the pharmacist, but alone is not a sufficient practice base.

There are several activities that pharmacists frequently undertake in order to insure appropriate drug therapy. One of these is the taking of medication histories from selected patients upon admission to the hospital or prior to clinic treatment. Nonlegend as well as prescription drugs may be the source of drug-induced diseases or abnormal physical and laboratory findings. Another activity is drug therapy counseling at discharge from the hospital or after initiation of therapy in the clinic. Patient medication compliance, prevention of adverse reactions and toxicity, and general patient enlightenment are reasons for medication counseling.

In some hospitals, clinical pharmacists are deeply involved with rather narrow clinical programs, e.g., monitoring of anticoagulant therapy. Probably the most publicity yet garnered for clinical pharmacy in the lay press dealt with the case of Richard Nixon. The following account from the *New York Times* on November 5, 1974 documents well one activity of the clinical pharmacy program at Long Beach Memorial Hospital and the application of clinical pharmacokinetics:

**The *New York Times*, Tuesday, November 5, 1974**

**Latest Bulletin on Nixon**

Long Beach, Calif., Nov 4 — Following is the text of a bulletin issued at 9:15 A.M. today by Dr. John C. Lungren, personal physician to former President Richard M. Nixon, at Memorial Hospital Medical Center, on his patients condition:

Special to the *New York Times*

Former President Nixon still continues to show gradual improvement. His vital signs are stable.

We will attempt careful ambulation today in his room with help. During this activity he will be closely monitored.

We're still concerned that the minor effusion still persists in the left lung (effusion means presence of a minor amount of fluid in the lung which is probably secondary to irritation of the diaphragm from the hematoma).

We're still working with hematologists in the department of pathology to rule out any abnormality in his blood analysis to account for the platelet deficiency.

He remains under sub-intensive care.

Upon Mr. Nixon's rehospitalization, I asked Dr. William Smith, director of pharmacy services at Memorial Hospital Medical Center and an assistant clinical professor, U.S.C. School of Pharmacy, to use the best scientific method to determine how Mr. Nixon handles the anticoagulant drug Coumadin. This request was made on Thursday morning, Oct. 24.

Dr. Smith on that day assigned two pharmacists of his staff who have specialized in anticoagulant drugs the task of analyzing the previous anticoagulation program of Mr. Nixon.

In addition, he telephoned a colleague, Dr. William Barr, professor and chairman, department of pharmacy and pharmaceutics, Medical College of Virginia, to see if the special computer systems they have been developing could be used to determine the parameters of how Mr. Nixon handles the drug.

Since that time, our Dr. Smith, Dr. Barr and a staff of their pharmacokinetics laboratory have completed and tested several computer programs using both digital and analog computers.

Last week, I received an initial computer generated plot of Mr. Nixon's anticoagulation program through Oct. 27, which has proven very useful.

The computer programs will assist us in deciding the importance of such parameters as: absorption rate, blood level drug concentrations and relationships to laboratory tests, and elimination rate of the drugs, all specific to Mr. Nixon. These parameters now have been tentatively determined but require verification by actual drug blood level studies. Blood samples have been drawn and will be sent to Virginia early this week for assay. With this data, the computer will provide us with several drug dosing curves from which we can select the best anticoagulation program specific for Mr. Nixon.

I would like to add, Dr. Smith informs me that the analog computer programs for anticoagulant drugs and several other drugs will soon be available on site at Memorial Hospital Medical Center for future patients. Every patient from here on out who gets admitted on anticoagulation therapy will have this new service available to them.

The pharmacy staff and drug information service at Memorial Hospital continues to assist with reviewing all drugs for Mr. Nixon for possible reactions and interactions and serving as resources for drug-related questions.

Additional perspective on the specific functions of clinical pharmacists may be gained by reviewing the report of the Task Force on the Pharmacist's Clinical Role (Appendix A).

**Issues in Clinical Pharmacy Practice**

**Existence and Definition of Clinical Pharmacy**

In an editorial in July 1972, Whitney asked if the masses of American pharmacy were suffering from the "Ostrich syndrome" (otherwise known as "head-in-sanditis") or if the masses were simply being responsive to inept leadership.[11] This satire was prompted by the report of the Task Force on the Definition of Clinical Pharmacy, Institutional Pharmacy and Group Practice which was adopted by the American Pharmaceutical Association House of Delegates in 1972. This report contained in part the following now infamous statement: ". . . . pharmacy should not be identified as 'clinical pharmacy,' and pharmacists should not be identified as 'clinical pharmacists.' "[12] In reaction to the same report, Provost has written:

Although I agree philosophically with the Task Force statement and the APhA's official position, I recognize that it is a good example of organized pharmacy spitting in the wind. And the wind being created by clinical pharmacy is the briskest that has ever swept the profession. Since we have textbooks and journals with "clinical pharmacy" in their titles, departments and professors of clinical pharmacy in schools of pharmacy, and clinical pharmacist job titles in actual practice, it doesn't make much sense to try to reverse or deter the use of an established term. The situation is reminiscent of resolutions of past years against outpatient dispensing.[13]

From cloistered vantage points, some have questioned the seriousness and intent of the clinical pharmacy movement. At the same time others have engaged in polemics. During this while, several hundred pharmacists, largely based in health care institutions, have brought about an entire new direction to pharmacy practice and a whole new dimension to pharmacy education. The existence of clinical pharmacy is not an issue to the hundreds now practicing it intensively.

There likewise has been considerable speculation and debate over a definition of clinical pharmacy. Those now practicing an advanced kind of clinical pharmacy and continually experimenting with new practice concepts can be eternally grateful that organized pharmacy largely twiddled its pestles and did not straight-jacket the concept with a definition in its infancy. A definition worthy of the movement will probably come in time, but at the present it is sufficient to be merely "in love" without trying to reduce all the emotions, feeling, and acts to a definition of 25 words or less.

Brodie has conceptualized the role of the clinical pharmacist as follows:

> The pharmacist is available in the patient care area on a 24-hour basis. He takes the patient's drug history on admission and instructs him in the home use of medication on dismissal; he maintains a complete pharmaceutical service record, monitors drug therapy and relates it to clinical laboratory tests and adverse drug reactions; he is available to the physician when he plans the drug regimen and assists the nurse in managing the drug portion of patient care plans for which she is responsible. In addition, he becomes a continually available source of drug information, usually reinforced by an organized drug information service. The pharmacist is responsible for analysis and confirmation of drug orders for patients and for the filling of orders by qualified technicians, and is available to the nurse prior to the time of administration of medications. The pharmacist does not assume an independent role in the planning of drug therapy, but coordinates his efforts with those of the nurse and his physician.[14]

There are parts of this conceptualization which some would wish to expand, clarify, or modify, but it largely covers the roles most clinical pharmacists now perform.

## Clinical Pharmacy — Specialty or General Direction?

In a 1972 article still relevant today, Provost has questioned whether clinical pharmacy is a specialty practice or a general direction in pharmacy.[13] At the present, some pharmacists are full-time clinical pharmacists while others are only marginally involved or not involved at all. Some have tried to equate clinical pharmacy with hospital pharmacy, but all leaders in hospital pharmacy have gone out of their way to emphasize that clinical pharmacy practice should transcend any environmental barrier. Those leading clinical pharmacy practitioners have no thoughts of trying to limit the clinical pharmacy movement to the hospital or its clinics. Those hospital pharmacists performing only dispensing functions must know that they are not clinical pharmacists if they have read recent issues of the *American Journal of Hospital Pharmacy* or *Drug Intelligence and Clinical Pharmacy*.

If proper leadership existed in most hospital pharmacies, clinical pharmacy could be a general direction for all of hosital pharmacy (this would not exclude other segments of organized pharmacy from becoming more clinical). In very few hospitals has every pharmacist been expected and required to be a clinical practitioner. Most hospitals with clinical pharmacy services still have some phamacists who merely dispense or perform relatively low level administrative services. The existence of the traditional pharmacist in the face of trained clinical pharmacists with an advanced degree (usually Pharm. D. or M. Sc.) tends to create a caste system in pharmacy. While both are pharmacists, there often exists much misunderstanding between the two. The basic problem in this dilemma is inadequate leadership on the part of directors of pharmacy. It seems that the profession and the clinical pharmacy movement would be better off if all pharmacists were either practicing clinically or performing high-level management functions. There should be no friction between these two pharmacists, since each complements the other. If this does not come about, a sizeable number of clinical pharmacists in the hospital may be employed outside of the pharmacy department in the future. This will tend to dilute the pharmacy image of the clinical pharmacist and insure the continued stagnation of many pharmacy departments.

## Clinical Pharmacy Versus Clinical Pharmacology

Provost has pointed out the close similarity between clinical pharmacy and clinical pharmacology by noting quotations taken from a WHO publication entitled "Clinical Pharmacology: Scope, Organization and Training." This article states:

> The clinical pharmacologist may be concerned with research on the monitoring of adverse effects. . . . The

clinical pharmacologist is also concerned with monitoring the therapeutic use of drugs and the pattern of drug prescribing, including indications, contraindications and suitability. His interests may also involve research in . . . errors by patients in following directions for taking drugs and dispensing errors. . . .

Clinical pharmacologists should play an active part in planning the provision and dissemination of information about drugs.

The analysis of drug levels in body fluids has been shown to be important for the care of individual patients. The clinical pharmacologist has an essential role to play in the practical application of pharmacokinetic data.

Clinical pharmacologists can fulfill an important service by surveying prescribing patterns and the incidence of adverse reactions. His general pharmacological interests and experience make him the most suitable person to coordinate the detection and quantification of adverse reactions to drugs in hospitals.[13]

Provost goes on to say that one could substitute the word "pharmacist" for "pharmacologist" in all of the preceding quotations and the publication from which they were taken could easily become a treatise on clinical pharmacy.

A clinical pharmacologist is usally a physician with an additional training of about two years' duration in clinical pharmacology which prepares him for the scientific study of drugs in man. In an editorial, Francke[15] has stated that there are only about 40 clinical pharmacologists in the U.S. who have both the M.D. and Ph.D. degrees. Francke says that a clinical pharmacist could adequately do 90% of the functions of the clinical pharmacologist, and that if the two work together they would be able to perform even better than they now can.

Charles Walton, one of the most respected pharmacy educators giving sustenance to the clinical pharmacy movement, has written an article entitled "Clinical Pharmacology and Clinical Pharmacy: A Necessary Alliance for Practical Advances in Rational Drug Therapy."[16] Walton suggests that the two groups should work together for mutual benefits, with the clinical pharmacologists serving as strategists and the clinical pharmacists as tacticians in the advancement of rational drug therapy. In this article, Walton states the case for the need of the American College of Clinical Pharmacology to open its membership to selected clinical pharmacists. This undoubtedly has caused anxiety among many M.D. pharmacologists and some pharmacy leaders, but it seems to be a wise strategy to promote closer teamwork between the two groups.

### The Pharmacist As a Primary Practitioner: Will a Search for Relevance Lead to Subservience?

Some clinical pharmacists have begun providing primary health care in a variety of clinic and ambulatory settings. This is quite common in the USPHS Indian hospitals. Pharmacists are now providing continuing care to patients with hypertension, diabetes, mental illness, tuberculosis, and other chronic conditions primarily managed pharmacologically. While this activity by pharmacists is new and exciting, it is not necessarily strengthening to the pharmacy profession. Nurse practitioners and physician's assistants also perform these activities under the auspices of the physician.

Most pharmacists, even those with the Pharm. D. degree, are not well-trained in physicial diagnosis and patient assessment techniques. If the pharmacist is to be a provider of primary health care, he should be educated and trained for this activity, and the patient population should be well-chosen so that the provision of primary health care blends well with the foremost goal of insuring safe and rational drug therapy for a broad base of patients. If this foremost goal is abandoned, clinical pharmacy will lose its identity in an amorphous conglomeration of assistant and allied health practitioners.

### Justification of Clinical Pharmacy Services

If clinical pharmacy is to be a continuing movement and sustaining force in pharmacy practice, the patient and his fiscal representatives must be convinced that the benefit is worth the cost. The clinical pharmacist or his employer should be able to gain reimbursement directly for his services (outside the dispensing process and drug cost). While some data have been generated which document the cost benefit of the clinical pharmacist, more data are needed.

It has been encouraging to learn that in a few areas of the country third party payers are reimbursing specifically for clinical pharmacy services unrelated to the dispensing of drug products. Hopefully, detailed reports will soon be published, thereby promoting widespread acceptance of this practice.

Along with adequate reimbursement mechanisms, a legal basis for clinical pharmacy practice needs to be developed in each state. If clinical pharmacy is to be truly important, it must have a responsibility to the patient and health care system which, if unfulfilled, results in legal action against the practitioner and the health care institution.

If the legal basis of practice is developed and reimbursement mechanisms accepted, the next step is for licensing and accrediting bodies to require certain standards of clinical pharmacy practice, particularly the presence of qualified practitioners as a minimum. Qualifications are probably best determined through a self-imposed certification process for the clinical pharmacy specialists and generalists.

### Issues in Clinical Pharmacy Education

There are currently several smoldering issues confronting clinical pharmacy education. One is the faculty status of practitioner-educators. If practitioners are going to serve as faculty members they should have academic credentials and be deserving of equal voice with the basic scientists in pharmacy education. Some clinical pharmacists should eventually rise to be full professors, without qualifying titles, and some should become deans of schools of pharmacy, just as physician-educators become professors of medicine and deans of the schools of medicine.

Another issue in pharmacy education is whether or not every pharmacist should be trained clinically. If clinical training is to be of a good quality, several prerequisites must be met. The academic capabilities of the student must be quite high, students must be indoctrinated with a clinical practice philosophy early in their education, and a large number of clinical faculty members must exist who can precept the student, often one faculty member for one or two students. These prerequisites are not generally being met, and many B.S. graduates have not had adequate clinical training for the present health care system, let alone systems of the future. Schools of pharmacy do not have adequate faculties to train all students well clinically. Many are hardly giving proper attention to a few Pharm. D. students in a post B.S. program.

The curricula of schools of pharmacy are in need of considerable innovation. Clinically oriented courses are generally being added in the last year or two of the curriculum, but by this time many students are stone-deaf toward clinical pharmacy and professionalism in general. The course titles in the school catalog look rather appropriate, but the parts have not been assembled in a synchronous fashion and quality is often lacking. Pharmacology, medicinal chemistry, and pharmaceutics have been taught in isolation from each other and from the clinical situation.

Another issue in pharmacy education is the adequacy of the role models portrayed by clinical pharmacy faculty. Schools of pharmacy have placed clinical faculty in hospitals so that model clinical practices could be developed, around which the faculty would teach students and residents. Many of these "clinical services" have been eight-hour, five-day-a-week programs which halt completely during vacations and holidays. The faculty activities have usually not been well-integrated with the pharmacy department. There has often been no real responsibility to the pharmacy department, the medical staff, the hospital, or the patient. Pierpaoli has expressed concern about this situation in a recent editorial entitled "The Rise and Fall of Clinical Pharmacy Education."[17] It is of utmost importance that realistic role models be implemented in all teaching programs. It seems rather naive to believe that someone right out of a struggling Pharm. D. program can immediately set himself up as a therapeutic consultant to medical specialists who have been in training for almost a decade. A thorough search for the most qualified and experienced clinical pharmacists must be undertaken. A goal should be for the clinical

pharmacy faculty to be considered as peers and colleagues of the clinical medicine faculty.

## The Quest for Quality in Clinical Pharmacy Practice

There are many critical factors along the pathway to quality in clinical pharmacy practice. For the continued growth and maturation of clinical pharmacy, schools of pharmacy and their affiliated hospitals hold the key to excellence. Practice, in general, will be no better than the educational process of the schools of pharmacy and the training programs of the teaching hospitals. In an invited lecture at the 1975 annual meeting of the American Association for the Advancement of Science, Dean Michael Schwartz outlined the following characteristics necessary for quality in pharmacy education:

1. All schools of pharmacy should be components of academic health science centers, which should include at least schools of medicine and nursing.
2. Each school of pharmacy should have strong basic science teaching and research programs in at least its major disciplines, i.e., pharmacology, medicinal chemistry, and pharmaceutics.
3. Within each academic health science center there need be only one department of pharmacology with its primary base in the school of pharmacy, but serving the teaching needs of all professions.
4. Schools of pharmacy should undertake responsibility for supervising the entire continuum of education and training of all pharmacists and supportive personnel.
5. The full-time clinical faculty should be subject to the same standards of scholarship and expertise by which their counterparts in academic clinical medicine are judged.
6. Each school of pharmacy should have one or more faculty member taking part in the research efforts of the academic health science center in socioeconomic aspects of health care delivery.[18]

Schwartz further suggested that the single most powerful tool available to build an educational structure based on excellence is accreditation. He stated the need for a high level of minimum standards so that weak schools could not continue. Other suggestions were that scholarly effort by clinical faculty must be supported and rewarded, that a system of certification of specialties should incorporate the highest standards and judgments by peers, and that the certification be carried out in a rigorous manner.

The American Association of Colleges of Pharmacy and the American Council on Pharmaceutical Education should give immediate attention to establishing rigorous standards for the Pharm. D. programs in existence. These programs are supplying much of the clinical pharmacy manpower, but the quality of graduates varies tremendously. Some programs have strong clinical pharmacokinetics and medical school components, while others are void in these courses. Some have extensive residency or clerkship requirements, while others do not.

Residency training in clinical pharmacy needs to undergo considerable evolution over the next few years. It seems that clinical pharmacy residencies should be confined largely to progressive teaching hospitals and the ambulatory programs of these hospitals. Furthermore, many believe that clinical pharmacy residencies should take place in those pharmacy departments offering high quality comprehensive pharmacy services in which the total services are well-integrated into a continuum of service. Very few departments currently meet this criterion. As a result, many residents fail to appreciate the enormous teamwork and talents needed for total services. A critical matter in those hospitals with pharmacy residencies is to elevate the level of practice of *all* pharmacists so that residents are being trained to practice as the entire staff is practicing. The dichotomy between what residents are being taught and what they see practiced must cease if true quality is to be obtained.

A matter of considerable importance is the development and eventual certification of clinical pharmacy specialties. Currently, drug information, pediatric clinical pharmacy, psychiatric clinical pharmacy, family clinical pharmacy, clinical pharmacokinetics, and radiopharmacy are logical specialty areas in which practitioners are identified. The impetus and planning of the certification process should come from those pharmacists functioning as specialists. The specialty examining board should be composed of roughly the following persons: several clinical pharmacists nationally recognized in the specialty, at least two prominent physicians closely allied to the specialty, a pharmacy educator of national prominence, and a health care administrator or planner. Except in unusual circumstances, a candidate for certification should have completed a Pharm. D. or clinically oriented M. Sc. program and should have completed a clinical residency or fellowship in the specialty. This initial certification should not be controlled by any pharmacy organization.

Clinical pharmacy must develop into a challenging and rewarding practice if it is to succeed. My own view is that the scope and depth of knowledge and skills in the domain of clinical pharmacy are of such a magnitude that many years of intensive learning are required to master the field. There are no overnight successes. Intellectually, there is no dead end to clinical pharmacy unless imagination and ambition are lacking. It is imperative that many excellent practitioners remain in the clinical arena for a lifetime. Only then will the practice truly advance and become established. I have heard many young clinical pharmacists remark that they can not visualize themselves in their practice when they turn 35 to 40 years of age. The reason for this uncertainty is the lack of a colleague and peer relationship with the physician and the absence of a substantial scientific practice base. It is important that the substance of clinical pharmacy practice sustain the qualified pharmacist through a career of clinical pharmacy practice, often in a specialty area.

In order for clinical pharmacy practice to grow and become established, a new breed of hospital pharmacy department head is required. If clinical pharmacy is to become the practice standard and its practitioners rewarded and encouraged, directors of pharmacy in large part need to have been trained clinically. They must realize the planning, sacrifices, and hard work necessary to developed a comprehensive pharmacy program that is clinically based. They must support well, both professionally and financially, those who achieve clinically as well as administratively.

In the long run, the success of clinical pharmacy will be proportional to its contribution to patient care and public welfare. It must have the consent of other health care practitioners, health care administrators, third-party insurance firms, the government, and the public. There are many determinants of quality, and a concerted effort by practitioners, educators, and department heads is needed to advance clinical pharmacy practice.

## References

1. Bender, G. A.: *Great Moments in Pharmacy*, Northwood Institute Press, 1966.
2. *The Pharmacist in Society*, Office of Health Economics, 62 Brompton Rd., London S.W. 3, (Nov.) 1964.
3. Koup, J. R.: *Deja Vu:* We Have All Been Here Before, *Drug Intel. Clin. Pharm. 7*:191 (Apr.) 1973.
4. Brown, C. T.: O. Henry the Pharmacist, *Amer. J. Hosp. Pharm. 25*:190 (Apr.) 1968.
5. Francke, D. E.: The Importance of an Historical Perspective, *Drug Intel. Clin. Pharm. 8*:55 (Feb.) 1974.
6. Francke, D. E.: Drug Intelligence and Clinical Pharmacy, *Drug Intel. 3*:157 (June) 1969.
7. Francke, G. N.: Evolvement of Clinical Pharmacy, *Drug Intel. Clin. Pharm. 3*:348 (Dec.) 1969.
8. Levy, G.: An Orientation to Clinical Pharmacokinetics, *Clinical Pharmacokinetics*, American Pharmaceutical Association (Academy of Pharmaceutical Sciences) p. 1 (Oct.) 1974.
9. Gibaldi, M.: The Clinical Pharmacokinetics Laboratory of the School of Pharmacy of the State University of New York, *Clinical Pharmacokinetics*, American Pharmaceutical Association (Academy of Pharmaceutical Sciences) p. 11 (Oct.) 1974.
10. Juhl, R. P., et al: The Family Practitioner — Clinical Pharmacist Group Practice, *Drug Intel. Clin. Pharm. 8*:572 (Oct.) 1974.
11. Whitney, H. A. K., Jr.: The Ostrich Syndrome in American Pharmacy, *Drug Intel. Clin. Pharm. 6*:245 (July) 1972.
12. Report of the Task Force on the Definition of Clinical Pharmacy, Institutional Pharmacy and Group Practice, *J. Amer. Pharm. Ass. NS 12*:306 (June) 1972.
13. Provost, G.: Clinical Pharmacy: Specialty or General Direction? *Drug Intel. Clin. Pharm. 6*:285 (Aug.) 1972.
14. Brodie, D. C.: Drug Utilization and Drug Utilization Review and Control, National Center for Health Services Research and Development, p. 41 (Apr.) 1970.
15. Francke, D. E.: The Clinical Pharmacist and the Clinical Pharmacologist, *Drug Intel. Clin. Pharm. 6*:207 (June) 1972.

16. Walton, C. A.: Clinical Pharmacology and Clinical Pharmacy — A Necessary Alliance for Practical Advances in Rational Drug Therapy, *J. Clin. Pharmacol.* *14*:1 (Jan.) 1974.

17. Pierpaoli, P.: The Rise and Fall of Clinical Pharmacy Education, *Drug Intel. Clin. Pharm.* *9*:97 (Feb.) 1975.

18. Schwartz, M.: Educational Needs for Pharmacy Practice in the Year 2000, Presented at the 141st Meeting, American Association for the Advancement of Science, New York City, (Jan. 28) 1975.

## APPENDIX A
### Report of Task Force on the Pharmacist's Clinical Role

The pharmacist is a health resource whose potential contribution to patient care and public health is grossly underdeveloped and which, thereby, is used ineffectively. In order to initiate an appraisal of potential and emerging roles for the pharmacist, the University of California School of Pharmacy and the National Center for Health Services Research and Development co-sponsored an interdisciplinary Conference on Pharmacy Manpower in September 1970. A "clinical" role prompted the greatest apparent interest and enthusiasm among the participants, although this role, as yet, lacks precise definition. Included in the results of the Conference were three mandates calling for: (1) the development of a set of working criteria for a clinical role, (2) a demonstration of role-effectiveness, and (3) a determination of cost effectiveness.

In response to the first of these mandates the National Center convened an interdisciplinary Task Force to draft a set of criteria. It was agreed that an assessment should be made on the basis of "functions" — those now being performed or likely to be performed during the next five years. It was assumed that the "procurement and distribution" and "management" functions traditionally performed by pharmacists would be performed by non-pharmacists. This would occur except in cases where pharmacists might perform a supervisory function, including the supervision of allied health personnel. The Task Force decided, therefore, to concern itself *only* with professional functions.

An arbitrary classification was used in arranging those functions that a pharmacist would perform in a clinical role:

A.  Prescribing Drugs
B.  Dispensing and Administering Drugs
C.  Documenting Professional Activities
D.  Direct Patient Involvement
E.  Reviewing Drug Utilization
F.  Education
G.  Consultation

The Task Force found that existing laws prohibit some possibly useful changes. For example, when the role of the pharmacist is extended to include the treatment of minor illnesses, there is an immediate legal challenge because existing laws restrict the diagnosis and prescription of treatment to the physician or other clinician. The same problem is encountered when the pharmacist's role in the hospital includes the administration of drugs, a function which in many states is assigned legally to the nurse. The Task Force attempted to avoid suggesting that the pharmacist perform functions that were obviously in direct conflict with existing laws. On the other hand, it attempted to point the way to functions that would be reasonable in light of the pharmacist's training and present day health care needs.

The Task Force continually found a clinical role for the pharmacist to be compatible with the health team concept. It identified him as an active participant on the patient care team with his unique contribution coming from his expert knowledge in the field of drug use. Although the report only occasionally refers to his relationship to the health team, the Task Force intended that the pharmacist would function through the health team effort.

The work of the Task Force has been completed, and its report will become a working reference document for the Drug-Related Studies Program of the National Center. The report will be made available to the profession of pharmacy as a guideline for the further development of a clinical role for the pharmacist.

### A. Prescribing Drugs

The physician determines if drug therapy is indicated and usually chooses the drug to be used as part of his overall therapy. Under certain circumstances the pharmacist does assist in planning drug therapy, and at times may prescribe medications at the request of the physician.

1.  Pharmacists, in reissuing prescriptions designated to be refilled at the request of the patient (p.r.n.), may be regarded as performing a prescribing function.
2.  Pharmacists, in complying with "standing orders" of the physician, may be performing an independent prescribing function. "Standing orders" refers to a prearranged plan or understanding between the physician and the pharmacist which permits the latter to dispense medications under certain circumstances without the immediate concurrence of the physician.
3.  Pharmacists and pharmacy residents often help medical students to plan drug regimens.
4.  Physicians may share responsibility for prescribing with the pharmacist when the latter has demonstrated competence. This may include the selection of drugs, the dosage forms, and frequency of use, based upon the physician's diagnosis.
5.  Pharmacists prescribe over-the-counter (OTC) drugs. Also, by recommending against the purchase and/or use of OTC drugs, they enter into the prescribing function.

6. Pharmacists prescribe medications in emergency situations when it appears to be in the best interest of the patient.
7. Pharmacists, after consultation with the prescriber, may select and dispense a drug other than the one prescribed by the physician, when they practice under the authority of the drug formulary system.
8. Pharmacists may be considered to be performing a prescribing function when they reply to inquiries from patients about continued use of medications previously prescribed.

## B. Dispensing and Administering Drugs

The responsibility for dispensing medication upon an order from a physician rests with the pharmacist and his staff. The physician has a legal right to dispense, although in general he does not do so. Exceptions are found in rural communities where a pharmacist is not available and in those few cases where the physician chooses to dispense. When the pharmacist performs the dispensing function, it is assumed that he has drugs available by both brand and established (generic) names in products which are of known and acceptable quality. Furthermore, it is assumed that he has the knowledge to exert a discriminating judgment in selecting a drug product when several products of the same therapeutic class are available that meet the needs of the patient. When generic-name drugs are dispensed, it is assumed that if there is a potential savings the patient will benefit.

1. The pharmacist receives and interprets the drug order and either supervises the dispensing function or performs it himself.
2. The pharmacist should consult with the physician when the latter prescribes products of suspected or known low quality, or when a question arises as to the appropriateness of a drug or drug product in light of the patient's condition.
3. The pharmacist has a responsibility for personally dispensing or supervising the filling of orders that require technical knowledge and skill, such as preparing and dispensing intravenous fluids, radiopharmaceuticals, compounded prescriptions, etc.
4. The pharmacist's dispensing function in the hospital overlaps with the administration of drugs, an act performed traditionally by the nurse. This is manifest today or will be in the future through (a) administration of medicine by the pharmacist, (b) administration by a technician who works under the supervision of the pharmacist, or (c) administration by a nurse who is responsible for this act. In addition to the pharmacist's potential responsibility for administration of bedside medication, his responsibilities could include the starting of as well as sharing in the assessment of intravenous therapy, and administering drugs in special programs, i.e., cancer chemotherapy.
5. The pharmacist, wherever he practices, may administer biological products for immunizations, i.e., polio (oral or injectable) and smallpox vaccines.
6. The pharmacist's function in preparing the dispensing and medication extends logically to inclusion of the function of administering drugs.

Combining these functions provides for improved drug-use control. The nurse realizes that her traditional role in administering drugs is one delegated by the physician, but she appears amenable to the transfer of this role to the pharmacist. If this transfer takes place, the pharmacist's function would include responsibility for administering drugs; and his decision may determine who performs individual tasks. There are ethical, legal, and economic problems today that provide barriers to this transfer of function, but model state health legislation may eliminate some of them. In addition, the pharmacist will require special training if he is to service such an expanded role.

## C. Documenting Professional Activities

The pharmacist is required to keep certain records of his activities in order to meet legal requirements. These are largely operational in nature and pertain to the acquisition and dispensing of narcotics, dangerous drugs, and appliances. In addition to keeping legally-required records, the pharmacist should keep records to document his activities related to patient care. The following are reasonable functions for the pharmacist to perform:

1. The pharmacist should obtain a drug history by recording medications currently used (prescription and OTC) and idiosyncrasies to specific drugs. He notes the past history of drug and/or chemical intoxication and present exposure to industrial, domestic and/or environmental chemicals, etc. The pharmacist may be able to obtain a detailed drug history by using check off forms. This history becomes the medication part of the patient profile record developed by the health care team. In the community the pharmacist may use a system designed to meet the limitations of both his and the patient's time. This may include the use of a self-administered questionnaire and of automated equipment to provide record linkage with other health care providers used by the patient.
2. The pharmacist should have a meeting with the patient for purposes of reviewing instructions and counseling for home use of medications (a) at time of discharge from the hospital or (b) at time of delivery of medication to him at his community pharmacy. These instructions include mode of administration, conditions of storage, time of renewal, and signs of untoward reactions. The patient is advised in the event of an unanticipated drug reaction to contact the physician or, if the physician is unavailable, the pharmacist.
3. The pharmacist in the hospital or other health care facility has access to the patient's chart and has the obligation to notify the physician when real or potential drug problems arise, such as development of an adverse drug reaction. He also checks charts to determine if changes in drug therapy are properly recorded. In outpatient clinics, the pharmacist may dispense or administer medication directly from instructions in the chart order.
4. The pharmacist, among others, makes proper reporting of adverse drug reactions (ADR) to those collecting ADR data.

5. The pharmacist's records in the community indicate when patients should renew their prescriptions; and if they fail to do so, the pharmacist should contact them in order to assure continuity of care. This is a follow-up function, primarily applicable to, but not limited to, the chronically ill patient.

6. The pharmacist prepares adequate records to assure himself of a documented source of expanding clinical experience which enhances his services as a drug specialist and consultant. The pharmacist in the hospital should make rounds with the physician and others on the health care team, or independently as appropriate. In the community setting, his direct contact with patients and physicians permits him to acquire a body of experience through which he becomes a useful clinician in the total care of patients.

7. The pharmacist's function in reviewing chart orders and other documents is to focus on four questions: (a) Is use of these drugs or this drug necessary? (b) Are they the drugs of choice (best drugs for need)? (c) Is the monitoring effort directed to the desired effects? (d) Is the monitoring effort designed to identify adverse drug reactions?

8. The pharmacist in the community setting does not have, in all cases, the equivalent of the patient's hospital chart. He may have no data on the patient's diagnosis or condition; in fact, he may not know whether the physician is treating symptoms or a specifically diagnosed disease. The pharmacist's record, therefore, becomes the historical record of drug utilization, which in time defines the pattern of prescribing of the physician and the pattern (rate, cost, etc.) of utilization by the patient. This permits a periodic review and control function by the pharmacist. The record permits him to monitor therapy for both under- and over-utilization and to identify patients procuring drugs from multiple sources unknown to the physician(s). It also provides an opportunity to acquire information upon which rates of clinical response to individual drugs can be determined by epidemiologic techniques. These data, in correlation with other health records, provide a basis for judgments in which a benfit/risk ratio can be established or, expressed otherwise, an index for predicting likely drug effectiveness.

## D. Direct Patient Involvement

The pharmacist should have a direct contact with the patient when he enters or leaves either the hospital system or the community (non-hospital) system. The objective of this contact in either case is the same, but implementation is adapted to fulfill local needs. The pharmacist should be capable of performing the following functions:

1. Conduct an admission interview, or equivalent, to obtain the drug history.
2. Conduct a discharge interview, or equivalent, to review instructions and provide counsel for home use of medications.
3. Provide patient education in personal health matters, i.e., smoking, drug abuse, need for annual health checkup, and other preventive measures.
4. Provide patient education and referral when patients are continually using laxatives, antacids, analgesics, etc., or when patients describe symptoms such as one of the cardinal signs of cancer.

5. Screen patients and direct them to sources of appropriate services — a triage function based on the pharmacist's knowledge of community resources and services and means for obtaining access to them.
6. Provide instructions for home use of medications: how and when to take, how to store, cautions in use, when to reorder, expiration date, when to see the physician.
7. Provide instructions in the use of appliances such as inhalers, colostomy bags, trusses, etc. Anatomical models and other demonstration equipment are useful. Special facilities to insure privacy are desirable.
8. Interpret physician's instructions as they relate to drug therapy as well as the total treatment regimen.
9. Conduct rounds in the hospital and develop a system in the community for following a patient's progress when under drug treatment. The monitoring of patients should determine if patients are taking their medicines.
10. Acquaint patients with the name of their pharmacist and how he can be reached. A pharmacist should make arrangements with other pharmacists to provide for the special needs of his patients when he is not available.

## E. Reviewing Drug Utilization

Some functions in this section have been noted, in part, previously.

1. Demonstrating concern for the need for organized programs to review and control drug utilization.
2. Developing and/or promoting planned drug utilization review programs.
3. Developing techniques that will lead to identification of drug prescribing patterns by physicians and drug use patterns by patients.
4. Disseminating accurate information concerning the use of drugs to physicians, other members of the health care team, and the public.
5. Implementing a local formulary system of drug-use control in the hospital and in the community.

## F. Education

Education refers to those ongoing activities that are designed to influence the prescribing, the dispensing, and the use of drugs. The pharmacist's goal as a member of the health care team is to improve patient care by improving the use of drugs and lessening the degree of misuse. Specific functions include:

1. Participation in continuing education through self-directed study and other methods.
2. Organization of inservice and continuing education programs — seminars, lectures, etc.; for hospital staffs, group medical practices, and professional societies.
3. Participation in the health education of the patient.
4. Participation in public information programs to promote respect for drugs as agents of good health.
5. Participation in the activity of the Pharmacy and Therapeutics Committee or its equivalent organization.
6. Organization of drug information service for physicians and other clinicians.

7. Participation in special programs in the hospital, such as grand rounds, teaching rounds, nursing conferences, medical staff meetings, etc.

## G. Consultation

The pharmacist should exert a consultative function by being available to the physician and other clinicians and to the patient for advice and guidance. Although his role as consultant is based primarily on his role as a drug specialist, it is based also on his knowledge of personal and public health matters, community health resources, the treatment of minor illnesses, etc. The pharmacist exerts an *active* role when performing as a consultant. Particular consultations are carried out with the physician and patient concerning:

1. The screening process. For example, the pharmacist might perform certain screening procedures, i.e., determine blood pressure, and in consultation with a physician at some remote point decide what measures should be taken. This is part of the triage function.
2. The selection of drugs and monitoring of drug therapy.
3. The refusal to furnish medication when the best evidence supports this position.
4. The referral of patients to sources of competent medical care.

## Summary

The pharmacist's usefulness as a specialist in his own field can be enhanced by his assuming an attitude that will lead to an active concern for direct patient welfare. In addition, the pharmacist's usefulness as a professional health worker will likewise be enhanced through active participation in patient care with other health professionals. The present clinical role of the pharmacist is associated more easily today with hospital than non-hospital practice. However, the opportunity for clinical experience in the care of ambulant patients does exist. One difficulty at the present time is the fragmentation of the out-of-hospital delivery system. The role will become more uniform as the medical care delivery system is standardized in group medical practice, health education centers, and other systems. Furthermore, much of community pharmacy practice remains rooted in traditional patterns in which the pharmacist appears to be more or less apathetic to direct patient care needs. When pharmacists become identified actively with group medical practice or perhaps modify their own traditional practice arrangements, the true clinical nature of community pharmacy practice will emerge.

Drug-Related Studies Program
National Center for Health Services Research and Development
Health Services and Mental Health Administration
Rockville, Maryland 20852
May 1971

**Task Force
To Develop Criteria for a
Clinical Role for the Pharmacist**

Mrs. Mary Louise Anderson
Community Pharmacist
613 Faulkstone Road
Wilmington, Delaware 19803

Mr. W. James Bicket
Community Pharmacist
2700 Sheridan Road
Zion, Illinois 60099

Charles W. Bliven, Ph.D.
Executive Secretary
Amer. Assoc. of Colleges of Pharmacy
850 Sligo Avenue
Silver Spring, Maryland 20810

Mr. Vincent E. Bouchard
Coordinator, Hospital Pharmacy Program
Mercy Hospital
Pride and Locust Streets
Pittsburgh, Pennsylvania 15219

Mr. Allen J. Brands
Pharmacy Liaison Rep. for PHS
5A-27 Parklawn Building
5600 Fishers Lane
Rockville, Maryland 20852

Mr. Herbert S. Carlin
Associate Professor and Director of
  Hospital Pharmacy Services
Univ. of Illinois Medical Center
Post Office Box 6998
Chicago, Illinois 60680

Virginia Cleland, Ph.D.
Professor of Nursing, College of Nursing
Wayne State University
Detroit, Michigan 48202

James W. Freston, M.D.
Chairman, Div. of Gastroenterology
University of Utah Medical Center
Salt Lake City, Utah 84122

Clyde C. Greene, Jr., M.D.
General Medical Director
Pacific Telephone Company
140 New Montgomery Street
San Francisco, California 94105

Paul Lofholm, Pharm.D.
Community Pharmacist
Ross Valley Medical Center
1350 South Eliseo Drive
Greenbrae, California 94904

Margaret M. McCarron, M.D.
School of Medicine
University of Southern California
2025 Zonal Avenue
Los Angeles, California 90033

Mr. Eric Owyang
Chief Pharmacist
University of California Hospitals
San Francisco, California 94122

Mr. Raymond L. Sattler
Pres., Student Amer. Pharm. Assn.
3867 Walnut Avenue
Concord, California 94520

Lawrence Weaver, Ph.D.
Dean, School of Pharmacy
University of Minnesota
Minneapolis, Minnesota 66566

Mr. Jack Weiblen
Vice President
Memorial Hospital Medical Center
2801 Atlantic Avenue
Long Beach, California 90801

**NATIONAL CENTER FOR
HEALTH SERVICES RESEARCH AND DEVELOPMENT**

Donald C. Brodie, Ph.D., Director, Drug-Related
Services
Joe B. Graber, M.P.H., Special Assistant to the
Director

Reprinted from *HSRD Briefs* (No. 4, Spring 1971), National Center for Health Services Research and Development, Health Services and Mental Health Administration, Rockville, Maryland.

# 2 Implementing Clinical Pharmacy Services — A Roundtable Discussion

Lawrence R. Borgsdorf, Don C. McLeod, William E. Smith, Jr., and David S. Tatro

Various aspects of implementing clinical pharmacy services in institutional settings are discussed.

Specific clinical pharmacy functions are identified, and the progression that might be followed in implementing these services is discussed. Other topics include the influence of the present level of pharmacy service on the ability to implement clinical services, the relationship of clinical functions to drug distribution functions, and staffing considerations relative to clinical pharmacy services.

*The following roundtable discussion was recorded at the American Society of Hospital Pharmacists Institute on Clinical Pharmacy Services in San Francisco, California, March 4-7, 1973. Participants were given an outline of points to be covered beforehand, but the actual discussion was completely spontaneous and unrehearsed. William A. Zellmer, Associate Editor of* American Journal of Hospital Pharmacy, *served as moderator.*

*Zellmer:* Before we get into some of the problems and techniques of implementing clinical pharmacy services, we should identify exactly what we mean by the term. What kinds of functions are we talking about when we speak of clinical pharmacy services? Larry, do you want to give us your comments?

*Borgsdorf:* It became evident to me at this Institute that there is a huge disparity among many people in what they consider to be clinical pharmacy services. I get the impression that we should set definite limitations on the term, perhaps just arbitrarily. For example, I prefer to say that distributive functions are not clinically oriented—it's a cold statement and it needs some interpretation, but I don't think I ought to do that right now.

Basically, I think the functions that have evolved in the last four or five years relating to pharmacist monitoring and interviewing of patients seem to be generally accepted as aspects of clinical pharmacy services. Another activity we are getting into very definitely now is patient education, not the traditional thing of "take one three times a day"—repeating what it said on the label —but going into depth about why patients are getting certain therapy—what's the importance of this antidiabetic drug or this thyroid drug or this drug for the heart or blood pressure; the importance of taking it; what can happen in the long run if the drug isn't taken; and even explaining what kind of side effects can be expected, whether they are serious or not, what to do if they start to occur, etc. I think that's really an important aspect of clinical pharmacy right now.

*McLeod:* Maybe a good white paper is needed on this subject. In many ways, I have trouble differentiating between what some people call clinical service and others call drug information services. Drug information is a component of clinical pharmacy practice, I think; not in the sense that you sit behind a desk and wait for a phone call, but there is a certain amount of material you may already have organized along with the basic reference sources and the ability to use these materials wisely in a patient care situation. I think that merges well with clinical pharmacy.

There are many clinical things some pharmacists have done well for years. It appears to me that much of the thinking and the activity that go into establishing a good formulary system—deciding which of the many tetracyclines you really need, which anticholinergics you really need for ulcer therapy, etc.—is the kind of thinking and activity we are talking about now with clinical pharmacy. I think the difference is that, before, these activities applied to the whole hospital and affected the general care of all patients in the hospital. These functions weren't clinical in the sense that they were services performed at a particular patient's bedside or for a patient who appeared at the outpatient window, but they were clinical nevertheless. That kind of information and knowledge is what makes up much of our basic tools today in clinical pharmacy practice, I think. We have added some other basic tools too—biopharmaceutics, a much better appreciation of laboratory values, of pathology, anatomy, and many of the traditional courses taught in medical schools. So some of the old skills have become combined with the new medically oriented things and we're somehow getting at this thing we call clinical pharmacy services.

There are many ways to apply this knowledge about the safe and appropriate use of drugs and still call it clinical. As Larry pointed out, it might be merely good instruction to the patient. We've overlooked some of the things that we can actually do with a patient because of the emphasis on how to influence and change what the doctor does; no matter what he does, there are still many things we can do with patients in various settings.

*Smith:* My frame of reference is that of a pharmacy director in a community hospital trying to establish a goal or purpose. Somehow, we have to have safe and effective drug therapy for patients. Clinical pharmacy to me is a composite of many different functions, all directed toward that basic goal. I don't see how you can eliminate a safe and effective drug distribution system from that basic goal. I just don't agree (looking at it from a community hospital's viewpoint) that you can separate the drug distribution system component from the drug information component. The two are intertwined because of manpower and cost considerations. That doesn't mean the pharmacist has to do the distribution, but it's a part of clinical pharmacy. Then all of the other things —the rounds, interviews, patient education, drug information, cardiac arrest involvement—are the specific clinical tasks that the pharmacist does in providing clinical pharmacy service.

Now another thing I want to comment on is that, depending on the facility and its goals, clinical pharmacy service in hospital A will be different from that in hospital B which might be different than that in hospital C. So the people who throw brickbats and say "this is a clinical program and this one isn't," or "if you don't do patient interviews, you don't have a clinical program," are really not making sense.

*Zellmer:* Bill, something you said relates to Don's remarks about clinical pharmacy services having a great deal to do with drug information. Is there really much difference between what we mean by clinical pharmacy services and what we mean by drug information services?

*Smith:* Well, drug information has two aspects. One is a formalized, structured staff drug information service which requires in-depth analysis of the patient problem to answer questions. The other aspect of drug information can be provided by the pharmacist in the patient care area. He can answer certain questions from his own experience or from available references and does not

have to dig into the medical literature. But drug information is only one component of clinical pharmacy service. Rounds, per se, can be an important part of clinical service without having drug information as part of the rounds; the same for patient interviews. It depends on how broad a definition we want for drug information.

*Zellmer:* But if there isn't some transaction involving drug information, I don't see how you can say it's part of clinical services.

*Smith:* All right, let me back up and say that drug information can go to physicians, nurses, patients or to a pharmacist. But I think most people look at drug information as a pharmacist-physician transaction.

*Zellmer:* Dave, you're primarily involved in drug information services. Do you have any comments on what clinical pharmacy services are, particularly in relation to drug information?

*Tatro:* One thing that concerns me is "fragmentation" of the patient—dividing him up between different areas, and possibly even doing that through clinical pharmacy service. I like to think that one function of drug information and of clinical pharmacy is coordinating a total concept of patient care and working with different departments, not just the physician, nurse or pharmacist. What I'm thinking of here is other departments such as laboratory, dietary, and in some instances, medical records, but primarily a department like dietary where drug knowledge and expertise can have a great effect on patient care.

*Zellmer:* Are you talking about the pharmacist as the manager of the patient's drug therapy and then interacting with these various departments?

*Tatro:* No, maybe just troubleshooting or finding specific problem areas and helping to overcome these.

*McLeod:* Do you have an example?

*Tatro:* Yes, while dieticians may be going to great lengths to keep a patient on a low-sodium diet, the pharmacist may know that the patient is receiving a significant amount of sodium from his drugs which is something the dietary department may not know.

*McLeod:* Another twist on that is all these potassium supplements people are buying which ought to be provided in a dietary approach. Just to get 40–50 mEq of potassium a day on prescription at the drugstore costs the patient eight or ten dollars a month. This amount of potassium can be picked up in elemental foods like beans and certain fruit juices.

*Tatro:* Also, besides patient interviews, other patient consultations can be provided. These might entail sitting down and talking with the patient about aspects of his drugs as they relate to his disease state and answering questions, rather than just asking questions for a drug profile.

Getting back to the drug information area, I see it as only one aspect of clinical pharmacy and as something which can aid the pharmacist in other areas. There are other areas in the hospital, the community hospital in particular, where drug information can function, such as inservice education, special programs, patient monitoring, etc.

## Physician Acceptance

*Smith:* Can I throw out the topic of this pharmacist-patient interaction combined with a third party—the physician? Look at it from the viewpoint of a private practice physician and what he sees as the physician-patient relationship and what he will or will not allow in terms of somebody else interjecting himself into this relationship. I think that the vast majority of physicians at this time will not be receptive to much pharmacist input on their own in patient histories, patient interviews, independent patient drug rounds, observing the patient for adverse reactions and everything else.

*McLeod:* Are you speaking from personal experience in a community hospital?

*Smith:* I sure am. It's an impingement or interference with the physician and the patient relationship, and he's not going to want somebody coming in there and telling the patient "drug *x* is going to do this and these are the problems you have to anticipate."

*Zellmer:* You can perhaps build up to that, but you're saying initially physicians are not going to want that?

*Smith:* This day, right now, in 1973, the vast majority of physicians in community hospitals are not going to accept that kind of pharmacy involvement.

*Tatro:* How about the patients of specific physicians who wouldn't mind?

*Smith:* I'm saying the majority of the physicians are not going to want these services as part of a structured, formal clinical program for the patient masses.

*Borgsdorf:* I think much of this problem centers in the way it's approached, because we have had just the opposite experience. Everybody has a different way of getting started, and for us it was through the physician making demands on the pharmacist. We've had pharmacists who had no intention of becoming involved clinically, other than in the teaching aspects, but have been essentially pulled out of the pharmacy by the medical staff. The administrators cleared the way for them.

*Smith:* Are you in a university-based center?

*Borgsdorf:* No, we're not. We're in a general, city hospital, but I'm talking about pharmacists in outlying private hospitals with whom we've worked through education programs. Our emphasis was to use these facilities and pharmacists to teach clinical pharmacy, and the offshoot has been that the physicians were impressed with the pharmacists' abilities and the concepts of the clinical work they were doing.

*Smith:* Well, my response is related to our involvement with our medical staff—questioning their prescribing and everything else.

*Borgsdorf:* From day one?

*Smith:* Yes. The private physicians in my area don't want anything that smells of a hospital telling them how to practice medicine, and we're part of the establishment; we're part of the administration.

*Tatro:* There are certain problem areas that can be identified, approached and solved by pharmacists without necessarily being an infringement on physicians. I'm thinking, for example, of something to do with antibiotic usage and microbial resistance in the hospital where you could compile information and present it to the medical staff. This information could be valuable and at the same time you could be introducing physicians to a service you can offer. They could decide if the service is good or not, but the chances are they are going to appreciate it and find it useful and maybe think about other things the pharmacist can do.

## Progression of Clinical Services

*Zellmer:* What do you see as the recommended progression of moving into clinical pharmacy services? Where does a person start?

*Smith:* You start by an assessment of the opportunities you have in your own facilities, and once you have determined that, then you will know where to start. In one facility you might start with a monitoring service, in another place you might be able to start with rounds. You have to be able to assess the environment of the facility you are in and determine what will be successful and what will not, and once you decide that, you don't push something which will get you into trouble. It depends upon the facility.

*McLeod:* There are really several variables here. One is your own staff. You might have somebody who fits very well in a certain area and may have a keen interest in, say hyperalimentation, and get very good at that, and suddenly that's a meaningful clinical program influencing patient care. You may have someone who's very good in antibiotics and infectious diseases who makes the proper inroads with the key people there, and suddenly you have a meaningful clinical program. You should decide who you can influence and who will buy what you are saying. For example, if the chairman of the department of pediatrics is very open to pharmacists coming in and doing something, and the chairman of another department is not, then it's obvious where you're going to start.

*Smith:* I think the P & T committee is a possible group to start with. If you have a P & T committee that is receptive to these things, then you can run studies just with them. You're going to hit somebody in every discipline.

If you don't have a P & T committee, then you have to sort out the physicians who historically have had a good relationship with the pharmacy department and those who made demands on the pharmacy department. If you find only one on the whole staff, that's where you start. If you have 50, then you go with 50.

Don's right, you have to be able to evaluate the capability of your staff. It's one thing to say, "Okay, we're going to do all these grand and glorious things" and get physician support, but if you don't have the horses on your staff to do it, man, you're dead.

*McLeod:* Another thing here, looking at it administratively, there may be somebody on your staff who really wants to do a particular thing and he may be able to do a reasonably good job at it, but that project may not be a very high priority item compared to some of the basic things you ought to do first in the hospital. So you have to have a rein on what tends to pop up and start going on.

*Zellmer:* So what you're saying is, to get started with a clinical program, take the road of least resistance.

*Smith:* You take the road that has the least roadblocks in it, yes. You take the road which you believe will produce the greatest payoff. You should know where you're going; you've got to know where you want to end up. If the pharmacy director doesn't know what he wants to do, there is no way that the administrator, the nursing director or the medical staff can know where you want to end up.

*Zellmer:* What about looking at it from the opposite point of view and determining what patient care needs can be fulfilled by a clinical pharmacy service, rather than taking the road of least resistance?

*Smith:* I think you have to know what the patient care needs are and present your program in a way so that it's well received by the people who are going to make the decision to cooperate or not. If you have physicians who do not want pharmacists to interview patients, you don't cram that down their throats. Back off, go some other way, and then when you have a good experience, you expand to some other area.

*Borgsdorf:* I think there is another important point, and that is when you are developing clinical services, you should not just take the straight, steady line and push until you get resistance. Instead, you should keep your ears open because you're going to hear comments about the program. I think it's important that these comments be followed up. Now maybe this will take you off your initial track, but in the long run, it will develop a stronger relationship between the medical staff and the pharmacy staff.

*Smith:* If a member of the medical staff comes in and asks you to do something, you do it, because if you don't do it, he'll never come back again.

*McLeod:* I think it's important to establish a record in your hospital of being receptive to ideas in solving problems, whether they involve a clinical pharmacy problem or not. For example, in our own hospital we had the problem of physicians receiving mail samples at the hospital and not knowing what to do with them. So the pharmacy put in a box with a hole in the top where physicians could deposit the samples and get them out of their pockets. Quick action on a problem like that creates a good image.

## Character of Clinical Functions

*Zellmer:* Should clinical pharmacy services consist of functions that other health care workers are presently doing but not doing well, or should these functions be things that no one is doing now?

*Smith:* You have to realize that the clinical pharmacy movement is a reaction and response to defects in the traditional way of taking care of patients. It's because of medication errors, inappropriate prescribing, a lack of basic drug information, the lack of physician monitoring of patients—clinical pharmacy is responding to these things.

*Borgsdorf:* Something we didn't cover when we were talking about clinical pharmacy services relates to a role that isn't being performed now, and this is predicting or evaluating the potential for adverse reactions, but in addition to that, anticipating what can be done if they do occur.

*Tatro:* Yes, the important thing is the earliest possible detection. In some cases, even though you know an adverse reaction can occur, you still have to go ahead with the drug.

*Borgsdorf:* Sure, you can't predict when an adverse drug reaction is going to happen. It's not going to be in seven out of 100 patients; it could be 50 out of 100 and then nothing for several years. We are only realizing this now as pharmacists are getting more sophisticated and more involved in direct patient care.

*McLeod:* Also, certain characteristics of patients which can be easily determined through the chart are going to enable you to predict who may or may not have an adverse reaction.

*Smith:* Historically, and from my own personal experience, the profession by and large reacts to situations and we are all trying to catch up. So let's look ahead to the next decade at the kinds of drug information or new technology or new areas related to drugs or to patient care which are going to evolve. It seems to me that we are going to have a better understanding of drug interactions and they are going to become a bigger problem than they are now. We are going to have drugs that will be very specific and very toxic and will be used in very selected circumstances. We are going to be involved with drugs that are going to require blood level studies to monitor their use. This gets into the whole area of kinetics and blood levels. I don't see how the traditional practice of physicians or the traditional practice of pharmacists is going to be able to cope with that kind of information requirement and sophistication in patient care. It's going to be a necessity from the patient's viewpoint to have the input of pharmacists. We need to make the assumption this is going to happen and gear ourselves for it.

## Level of Pharmacy Service

*Zellmer:* Let's shift gears slightly and focus our attention on perhaps a more immediate problem. One of the things that's striking about this Institute is the large number of registrants who are practicing in hospitals with relatively low-level pharmacy services. Is it realistic for these pharmacists to be thinking of clinical services? Do you need to have a certain minimum level of basic pharmaceutical services before you can implement clinical services?

*McLeod:* A good example of this is the people associated with schools of pharmacy who are going into the hospitals trying to teach clinical pharmacy practice to students when the basic level of pharmacy services in the hospitals is not up to par. Pharmacy services are woefully inadequate in many of these hospitals and yet you have people coming and teaching clinical pharmacy, pharmacy students are running around the wards taking interviews and talking to nurses about drugs and making rounds. That's a real farce if you're training students to be good pharmacy practitioners, whether clinical or not.

*Borgsdorf:* I don't agree with that because with the emphasis being changed to try to make the pharmacist more productive and more patient-oriented, I think it's a crime to hold students back when there is a teaching situation even if there isn't a good drug distribution system in the hospital.

*McLeod:* I sympathize with that thought, but I'm afraid what's going to happen is that schools of pharmacy will keep these clinical teaching projects going and when spring vacation comes, the hospital will be totally vacated of students and no one will be performing those clinical functions. In some cases, the dean of the school of pharmacy and the clinical faculty don't have any basic service responsibility to the hospital. They're in there doing things, but the doctors probably wouldn't miss them if they didn't show up one day. This is an unhealthy situation. Granted, you have to get teaching going. But the schools must give serious consideration to improving the basic pharmacy services in these hospitals. You can't just bring in the student in the senior year and put him on the ward. If that's his only understanding of pharmacy services, we're educating people for something for which there is no overwhelming demand.

*Borgsdorf:* I'm not sure whether students are taken into a hospital like that without being informed ahead of time that this is not an ideal situation.

*Smith:* Going back to your last question, Bill, if you're talking about a hospital with a certain level of pharmacy services at point *a* and having to leapfrog all the way to point *x* to get a clinical program, that's a big jump. How far it wants to jump in the first step depends on how much it thinks it can get done.

I can't get away from the thought that you have to assess your environment and decide how much you can accomplish how soon.

*Zellmer:* I think the kind of question we're attempting to answer here is, if you're trying to get from point *a* (your present level of pharmacy service) to point *x* where you're providing clinical services, what are the steps in between? It depends on what point *a* is, doesn't it? If point *a* is a ward stock system, the steps involved would seem to be different than if it's a unit dose system.

*Smith:* If you're asking if you can jump from a ward stock system to a clinical program, I must say that I feel that unit dose is a vehicle to get to clinical service. I can't think of any other way to give pharmacists time to do clinical activities.

*Tatro:* Some aspects of drug distribution are still clinical pharmacy. While the filling of unit dose carts is not clinical pharmacy, if a patient profile is associated with it and you're monitoring therapy, then that aspect of the distribution system is clinical. The screening of i.v. orders can be an aspect of clinical pharmacy whereas the mere dispensing of the i.v. isn't.

*Smith:* If you want to look at this by itself, there isn't anybody who can come up with a logical reason why a hospital should not have a unit dose system in this day and age. There is no logical explanation to come up with that is going to permit a hospital not to have a pharmacy-controlled i.v. admixture system.

You can look at a unit dose system and an i.v. admixture service as examples of pharmacy trying to get closer to patients. The thing to be very careful about is that the unit dose and i.v. admixture systems are structured in a way that will allow time to do clinical functions later on. For example, if you are going to run a unit dose system by providing doses four times a day, with pharmacists checking doses four times a day, you are going to have to change that before you can do clinical things. I know of a hospital pharmacy right now that was advised not to send up its doses more than once a day, but it's doing so four times a day. The system is now half way through the hospital and the pharmacy wants more people but the administrator says no; all the pharmacy had to do in the beginning was to limit the number of times a day it sent doses to the floors and it wouldn't be in this problem.

*Zellmer:* Are you saying, Bill, that if a pharmacist is thinking of implementing a unit dose system he should have clinical services in mind as an objective for some later date?

*Smith:* If he can do that from day one, he is going to save many headaches, much time and the need to regear everything later on. Likewise, if somebody's running a manual distribution system, he should try to figure out how that system is going to be adaptable to a computer system, so, when that day comes, the conversion will be easier.

*Borgsdorf:* Again, I'll disagree to some extent. I think there has to be a vehicle to get pharmacists on the floor to interact with the medical and nursing staffs, but I think the vehicle does not have to be the drug distribution system. We've had several hospitals where students were the vehicle. While we were not planning on the pharmacist being asked to stay on the floor after the students left, this is what happened.

*Smith:* But if you don't have students what's the vehicle then? There are only two ways; one is to manhandle the distribution system and the other is to get prior acceptance from the medical staff for proposed clinical activities.

### Barriers Against Clinical Services

*Zellmer:* If we think in terms of barriers against implementing clinical pharmacy services, it seems from some of the things that have been said here, one of the barriers is faulty thinking on the part of pharmacists who are talking about implementing clinical services but are not taking the right steps to get to that objective.

*Smith:* It has been my experience that pharmacists spend more time thinking of all the reasons why they shouldn't implement change than they spend trying to figure out why they ought to do it. Another problem is the automatic assumption by everybody that it's going to cost more money, which just isn't true.

If we could achieve acceptance for clinical services now from medical practitioners and hospital administrators, I doubt very seriously that the pharmacy profession could provide the services because I do not believe most chief pharmacists have the management ability to implement these changes. I think it's eventually going to boil down to two basic problems, and they are the facilities that the pharmacy departments have now, and the one-time change-over costs of going from an old service to a new service. There is a change-over cost—an investment in equipment and people—before the trade offs come from some other department at some other time. As hospitals continue to experience economic constraints, it's going to be more difficult to get seed money; making changes is going to be much more difficult than in the past.

*Tatro:* I don't think you can think of the barriers without considering attitudes. There are fears from people in other departments, such as nursing service, that when you start implementing clinical pharmacy service you are going to affect their position and their job. Now, even if these fears are not founded in fact, they exist and act as a block against you.

The economy of the country was mentioned, and I think that you also have to apply this to the university setting. Traditionally, we have looked to the universities for new ideas and new concepts and now they are being held back because of the cutback in funding for regional medical programs, as well as other projects. So there could conceivably be a switch in the source of new ideas and innovations, and possibly the community hospital is going to be a source.

*McLeod:* Going back to this matter of attitudes, I think we'd be surprised what could be accomplished if pharmacists had the right positive attitude toward clinical services. In many hospitals, there are already enough pharmacists, and what's needed is proper organization and management. At this Institute, I've heard of 500-bed hospitals which have 25 pharmacists and are unable to implement clinical services. Many of the pharmacists on the staff don't want to become involved clinically, and the inadequate use of technicians and clumsy distribution systems may also be factors.

*Borgsdorf:* Another problem is the time commitment that goes with the personalized services required in clinical rotation. You just can't conduct clinical services on a 40-hour week. Even if you could, you can't prepare yourself to keep up on a 40-hour week. It requires a greater commitment if you want to practice clinical pharmacy correctly. Most pharmacists are not willing to make this kind of commitment. We have to do what we can with what we have.

*McLeod:* I would disagree mildly with what you said. A couple of years ago a sizeable part of the staff of one large teaching hospital just didn't want to exert any influence on the physician and talk to him about drugs or challenge his choice of product. New policies and administrative decisions forced these pharmacists into an interface with physicians. As President Truman used to say, "If you can't stand the heat, get out of the kitchen." Some of these pharmacists got out of the kitchen and they are doing quite well working in chain drug stores. We now have contemporary people in this hospital and nobody was forced to leave.

*Borgsdorf:* There's another major problem that has to be mentioned and that is that many pharmacists don't have the necessary self-confidence for clinical involvement. They are reluctant to get themselves involved in clinical situations because they don't really feel they are prepared for it and they are afraid. They are in the patient care areas and making mistakes and getting stepped on. As we move into clinical services, we have to at the same time move into some sort of continuing education so we are continually improving or "retreading," as some people call it, the abilities of these pharmacists to make them more functional.

*Smith:* Along the same line, one of the things that must be overcome is society's attitudes, administrators' attitudes and the medical staff's attitudes about pharmacists. For the last 25 years, pharmacy has been going down the wrong paths. People basically feel that pharmacists cost too much money and all they do is take drugs from one bottle and put them in another. So we have to fight history. Physicians have been burned many times by pharmacists saying the wrong things to their patients, or physicians may have asked for information from pharmacists and didn't get anything back.

*Borgsdorf:* It requires pharmacists to get up to the patient areas and become involved with the whole patient care system. It requires an individual selling job.

*Smith:* Something that has really upset me in the last half dozen years is the many schools running all of their students through some kind of clinical clerkship program as training to become clinical practitioners. Somewhere, sometime, somehow, there's going to have to be a number of those people trained as managers of clinical services. I don't see how a school can take 100 or 150 students and train them to be clinical pharmacists without training some of these people to manage a program. It doesn't make any sense. This might be left to the residency programs, and maybe we are going to have to have several different kinds of residencies. I do not believe that the profession has ever turned out people with management skills, and what we are basically facing is a management problem—how do you engineer changes in pharmacy practice in 7,000 hospitals?

*Zellmer:* Within pharmacy we can identify a great number of barriers to clinical services. It would seem as though you need some sort of organized effort to overcome these barriers. Can you be more specific as to what we need to make these changes in the profession?

*Smith:* Chief pharmacists are going to have to be able to understand what's in the literature. They need to be able to ask a series of questions—how much nursing time is involved in medication activities, how many medication errors are committed, etc. All of these things are in the literature. Then they need to put together some kind of macroscopic view of these problems in their own facility and write a document for the administrative structure justifying clinical services. Most administrators don't have any idea of what's happening relative to drug therapy in their own facilities.

Once you put the whole picture together, how are you going to change? The ASHP is going to have to look at some specialized institutes aimed at pharmacy directors—a clinical pharmacy institute aimed specifically at pharmacy directors, covering the problems in patient care, the documentation of these problems, writing reports. You might also need a specialized institute aimed at staff pharmacists. We're going to have to figure out a way to lead pharmacists from step one at least to the point where they have the opportunity to implement clinical services on their own.

*Tatro:* When talking to administrators about clinical services, you have to evaluate the purpose you are serving. What impact are you having on patient care? How do you measure what you are doing in an area of clinical pharmacy? I haven't seen any way to measure this, but I think somewhere along the line you have to objectively evaluate the impact you are having.

### Cost-Benefit Analysis

*Smith:* Cost-benefit analysis is one of the magic terms in health care today. To me, this means doing a cost analysis of the traditional service to establish a baseline cost. Then you implement a clinical program. And it has to be hospitalwide in a community hospital for two reasons. One, the marketplace—meaning the majority of hospitals—will not accept studies done in university centers. Two, the medication involvement differs by patient type. You cannot do a study of medical patients and extrapolate that to OB patients or to pediatric patients.

To implement a clinical service on a hospitalwide basis is a multiyear project. So on the one hand you are faced with a baseline, multiyear project, and on the other hand you are going to come back at some later time and study the incidence of adverse reactions, length of hospital stay and everything else. And during this time in which you are measuring the pharmacist's input, you are going to have to hold variables—like changing nursing care, advances in drug therapy, new surgical procedures—all constant just to measure pharmacy input. I don't think that can be done.

The other approach is to look at it from a systems viewpoint—who's doing what, what it is costing—and come up with an economical change in the system and still have clinical programs. You then take each clinical function and determine how many patients benefited from that function. Now the question is, what is significant? Is it 10%, 20%, 50% or 80% of the patients? It all depends on what is acceptable in that given circumstance.

*Zellmer:* Bill, you said "benefited." What exactly do you mean? How did you measure benefit?

*Smith:* What is beneficial to patients is determined by the decisions made on the local level. It's a subjective evaluation. There's no way out of it. And to try and scientifically say we are going to reduce hospital stay by half a day, I don't think is practical. I don't think it's feasible. And so, if you can say these are the clinical functions that pharmacists are going to provide, and these are the reasons, then you have a way of coming up with whether or not the actual provision of the services resulted in any benefit. And if your intervention affects 20 patients out of 100, that's significant to those 20 patients.

*Tatro:* The lack of this "performance" data is acting as a barrier right now.

*Smith:* I agree. For example, consider patient interviews. There's a facility not too far from here that has been doing patient interviews for six to seven years. Now, how many of the thousands of patients interviewed think those interviews have ever been significant? A great deal of time and money has been spent; what's been the payoff? Nobody knows.

You can come up with your own data collection forms for *x* number of patients and come up with an answer. And that's really all you have to do in your own facility. You don't have to have one of those fantastic, complicated Public Health Service grants to do a cost-benefit analysis study.

*McLeod:* I think that is very true, and again, it goes back to this defeatest attitude of so many pharmacists which may result in part from lack of substantiation or lack of figures or facts to prove the value of clinical services. But there are many things which could be achieved by adjusting staffing if the directors of pharmacy organized things properly.

*Smith:* I would be willing to bet that a majority of the hospital administrators, physicians and nurses will agree that there are patient drug therapy problems in any facility. There's no argument on that. So all we need to do is to figure out a way to get acceptance to put a pharmacist in the patient care area, and assuming he can do a reasonably good job, he's going to minimize these problems. And when he puts facts and figures on this accomplishment, that's all administrators want to know. Now, you can't do it at one time, you have to do it every year or every two years—you have to keep updating the data—but you don't need a million-dollar government study to do this kind of thing.

*Zellmer:* So you're saying that if you are confronted

with a barrier against clinical services in your individual practice setting, whether it is a barrier from physicians, administrators or nurses, first of all get everyone to agree that drug therapy problems exist and then demonstrate how pharmacists can alleviate these problems.

*Smith:* You have to show that drug therapy problems exist and that they exist in your facility. You can do this very easily through medication incidence reports.

*Tatro:* The problem also extends to teaching institutions. Schools aren't all pulling in the same direction. In some instances, they haven't accepted the commitment to clinical pharmacy and students are coming out without the tools and the background needed to function in the clinical area. There has to be total commitment within pharmacy, especially at the education level, so we can work toward the same goal.

*Borgsdorf:* There are a couple of other things that pharmacists in particular claim to be barriers against clinical pharmacy which I don't think are significant. One of these is patients. I don't think this is one of our problems. Patients in general are interested in anyone who can contribute to their health care.

The other barrier which I think is overrated is the lack of acceptance by the medical staff. If they are properly oriented, they will accept some clinical activity by pharmacists. Of course, they will not accept a pharmacist who's there one day, two days, or even three days a week. Pharmacists must be there in the patient care area whenever there are problems. This attitude, "I'll see you Monday after the weekend," has got to go. Physicians won't accept that.

*Smith:* In other words, what we are saying is that you cannot provide professional service on a part-time basis. You have to commit yourself.

*Borgsdorf:* One person can commit himself; it doesn't require three pharmacists during the day. As long as a person is willing to accept phone calls at night and is willing to come in and see a patient, the acceptance by the medical staff is strong.

**Responsibilities for Drug Distribution**

*Zellmer:* Going back to the provision of clinical services—in your opinion, should clinical pharmacy services operate independently of the drug distribution function of the pharmacy department?

*McLeod:* I think we are talking about one and the same thing. We're talking about safe, appropriate and rational use of drugs. That involves basic compounding sometimes; it involves getting the right drug to the patient once a good course of therapy has been chosen; it involves making sure that appropriate and good therapy has been chosen initially; it involves making sure that whoever is giving drugs is doing it correctly. At Duke, for example, diazepam is frequently used to treat status epilepticus. The medical literature indicates that this is probably the drug of choice, but we've observed that just by giving this drug too fast intravenously (and nurses are

giving it slow compared to the way they give many drugs) we are getting respiratory arrest. No matter what you do in reaching a conclusion that diazepam is the drug of choice, if somebody administers that drug the wrong way, it's not the drug of choice. So I don't see how you can separate out drug administration, not the simple act of giving it, but the responsibility and the follow-through to make sure its being done properly. I don't see how you can separate out some of the compounding problems, like with intravenous admixtures, and the selection of the appropriate source of the drug from many suppliers. All this bears directly on the patient, and it's all part of one spectrum. You can have certain individuals in a given hospital who are specialized in certain functions, such as the classical case of the drug information specialist. I think you can have certain people who don't have anything to do with drug distribution, but the basic idea of good pharmacy services is safe and rational use of drugs and it involves distribution, compounding, administration, selection of drugs, monitoring for adverse reactions and patient response to drug therapy. I don't think you can separate any of these components from the total pharmacy service.

*Zellmer:* Any disagreement?

*Borgsdorf:* I am kind of a maverick on this point. I agree with Don to a great extent, but I think that if a pharmacist is going to practice clinically, he should be separated from the distribution function, and perhaps even from the pharmacy department.

*McLeod:* What do you mean by distribution function?

*Borgsdorf:* If a pharmacist is going to practice clinically, he should be allowed to develop his role without being tied to drug distribution, and that also excludes troubleshooting unit dose errors or interpretation of orders. It takes away from his involvement on the floor. I've seen too many instances where troubleshooting, even though it's not intimately involved in distribution on a full-time basis, has pulled a clinical practitioner out of many situations where he should have been actively participating as a consultant.

*Smith:* But I don't think we have the luxury of unlimited manpower. I'm looking at the total picture—every hospital.

*McLeod:* Also, don't just think of the teaching hospital where you've got teaching duties, but think about the community hospital. I know of a few individuals who do all of these things I was talking about pretty effectively in terms of the total pharmacy system in the hospital.

*Borgsdorf:* Sure, there are always going to be isolated instances. But I think overall, the effectiveness of a clinical operation is going to be decreased by distribution functions. Maybe we are in a growing stage where it will take time to evolve to the point I'm talking about.

*Smith:* If I were to look at things strictly from a staff pharmacist's viewpoint in a clinical practice, I would try to arrange my practice so that I would be involved in the nice parts of clinical functions, and to heck with the drug distribution! I don't think that this is in the best interest of the patient, and I don't think we have the luxury to have one staff for clinical functions and another staff for drug distribution. I also believe that we are in serious trouble as a profession if we ever reach the point when it is beneath the pharmacist's responsibility to make sure that patients get their drugs.

*Borgsdorf:* I don't think anyone is saying that.

*Smith:* What I am saying is that the pharmacist should oversee the distribution system and get the system working so that it takes the least amount of his time. I don't think that we have the luxury, as much as I would like to see it, of completely separating distribution and clinical functions. We are going to have to compromise in order to get a majority of the work day, which may mean 75 to 80%, to do clinical things. If we can accomplish that, we have really accomplished something.

Now I will agree with you, Larry, that one of the real problems we have is that as pharmacists become more involved clinically, the medical staff makes more demands. This is a nice problem to have. We get down to the constraints of time, and because of personal interests, the distribution system becomes secondary and eventually can become a pain in the neck. That's a management problem, because that segment of the day devoted to distribution can't be put any place else. It's just as important as the clinical activity of the day. I recognize the problem, but looking at it from a very pragmatic viewpoint, you cannot separate the two functions.

*Zellmer:* It seems to me, though, that the thing Larry is talking about is going to happen because of the specialization that is taking place.

*Smith:* The pharmacy profession needs to hang on to some of the traditional things, even though they become secondary. This is the compromise we have to make in order to implement clinical services in the 7,000 hospitals in this country.

*Borgsdorf:* I agree that at this point in time we have some real problems. But we have to keep an open mind. For example, it's entirely conceivable that a clinical pharmacist on a floor with a ward stock distribution system might have a more significant effect in improving drug therapy than the implementation of a unit dose system. No study has ever been done on this. While pharmacists are still tied intimately to the drug product, there's no reason why this relationship couldn't be less intimate but yet more effective in terms of promoting rational therapy.

*Smith:* Let's look at an example based on my experience. We centralized our system at one time—left the pharmacists on the floor while centralizing the distribution system. What has happened to the pharmacists who are left on the floor? There are so many problems that nurses continually come to them. While you could tell the nurses that they have to communicate directly with the central pharmacy, I don't think you can practice in a vacuum like that.

*Borgsdorf:* I'm doing it now, and my cohorts are doing it.

*McLeod:* You're hired largely for teaching functions, though.

*Borgsdorf:* Well, it actually turns out to be a majority service. You know, service and teaching go hand in hand. We haven't been faced with all these medication problems, and in reality, we've decreased the problems because we decreased the utilization of drugs. It has been reduced from eight or nine to maybe two or three drugs per patient. I'm not sure that we could have accomplished this any other way. We just don't have the problem of being pulled off by distribution functions. In fact, our problem is having enough time in the day to do those activities that physicians want us to do. We wouldn't be able to do that if we were tied in with distribution.

*Smith:* But you have a dual pharmacy staff taking care of the patient. You've got the pharmacists in the clinical area taking care of one part of the patient and you have other pharmacists in another area of the hospital taking care of the distribution problems.

*Borgsdorf:* You centralized the unit dose system and you had exactly the same thing if you left pharmacists in the satellite areas.

*Smith:* Getting a distribution system without a pharmacist running the central area, that's the trick.

Larry, do you think that kind of staffing arrangement can be implemented in 7,000 hospitals?

*Borgsdorf:* I'm not sure it can be. How many pharmacy students are going into medicine, dentistry or podiatry because they are not satisfied? At least the upper 10% of every class. So we are losing the best part of the class. These people want to do something with their lives and their education. And they realize they don't like drug distribution but love the idea of applying knowledge, and they don't get that opportunity through traditional systems. Even unit dose does not give it to them.

*McLeod:* In terms of the majority of the general hospitals in this country which may have 150 beds or less, there is no way in the forseeable future that we are going to have one pharmacist in these hospitals running a good distribution system and another doing a good job with clinical services. The hospitals will be lucky if they each get one pharmacist who can administer a reasonably safe drug distribution system.

## Staffing Considerations

*Zellmer:* If we make the assumption that a pharmacy department is ready for clinical services in that it already has progressive distribution services, what are the staffing considerations? Do new pharmacists trained in clinical pharmacy have to be hired or can the present staff be "retreaded," so to speak?

*Smith:* It depends on where you start. As a general rule, almost every pharmacy would have to increase its staff, including both professional and technical persons, because it's starting so low to begin with. It really depends on what you need to get the job done. Most of the time you're going to need more people, which means you're going to have to justify them.

*Zellmer:* One question I would like to explore relates to the need to remove the pharmacist from many of the details involved in drug distribution systems to free him for clinical pharmacy. Of the clinical activities in which pharmacists are involved today in hospitals, aren't there a great deal of technical, routine tasks that perhaps could be performed by a supportive person of some sort?

*Smith:* I think you can look at any person at any level of performance and find things that lower-trained people can do. But there isn't always somebody one step down the ladder to do it. There isn't a bottomless pit of people and money to do things.

*Zellmer:* My point is, if you are trying to expand clinical services, might this be an area to look at?

*McLeod:* I think there are some aids we could use here. For example, some pharmacists, in order to make rounds, need to have a card on each patient with the patient's name, the drugs he is getting, basic diagnosis of the patient, etc. Perhaps these cards could be put together by a supportive person. Of course, a good computer system could give it to you too. This would save time by pharmacists not having to physically write so many things down, but they would still have to look at charts and pull all the data together.

Much effort devoted to making rounds is not very productive, in my opinion. When I look at the fact that I have been on teaching rounds for two hours, and we talked about two or three patients, I may have learned something personally, but I didn't really make much impact on patient care in that hospital in those two hours. I'm not saying we shouldn't go on teaching rounds, but that inefficient use of time bothers me. I think everybody must have these feelings sometimes.

*Tatro:* Relating to a specific area such as mine where we are dealing primarily with drug information, there are many areas where supportive persons could be utilized—for example, screening questions and retrieving the information which you are eventually going to use. You hope to use the information in a judgmental way and don't want to spend all of your time retrieving the information. Anyone can do that. I don't know what level of training is needed for this, but it certainly doesn't require a pharmacist.

## Staff Promotion

*Zellmer:* Let's look for a moment at the present organizational structure of hospital pharmacy departments. Some clinical practitioners have claimed that they are stifled because they need to assume administrative responsibilities in order to advance within the department. Is this true?

*Smith:* At the present time the answer is very definitely yes. If you want to get ahead financially you have to go the route of management.

*McLeod:* Is that true in your hospital?

*Smith:* No, it's not true in my hospital. It's true if you want to get to the same level of compensation as a director, but if you want to get to the same level as most of the managers, the answer is no. I think that it will always be that way. I don't think somebody in clinical pharmacy can match or be greater in position than the person who has the responsibility for the whole operation.

We've gone the route of having the top level of our clinical staff equivalent to other department supervisors so they don't have to go to the management level to get a few more bucks.

*McLeod:* Bill, would you feel threatened if you were the administrative director of pharmacy services and there was another pharmacist as director of clinical services and the two of you had to get together to make decisions?

*Smith:* I don't think you can run a total pharmacy service as a partnership. One person has to be responsible. I would not feel threatened by that, but it just doesn't make any sense. You can't run a department by a committee. One person has to make the final decisions.

*McLeod:* Maybe what you do could be done by somebody we now call a hospital administrator. I can think of two or three people I would like to get together within a medical center to manage a pharmacy service. You might have one pharmacist as director of drug information, another as director of clinical services, and an administrative director. As a team, you would get things done.

*Zellmer:* Without getting hung up on that particular issue, are we agreed that you need a separate system for promoting and advancing clinical practitioners in the pharmacy department?

*McLeod:* I think they advance for different reasons, for different abilities, and their performance has to be evaluated.

*Borgsdorf:* How do you evaluate clinical performance?

*McLeod:* You set standards, just like with anything else.

*Borgsdorf:* The administrator sets standards or the clinical group sets the standards?

*Smith:* In our particular case, we run it as a management team, it's not a one-man rule.

*McLeod:* Do you have somebody to call on to tell you how individual pharmacists are doing?

*Smith:* We have a monitoring committee of our staff to do this. But basically, whoever is responsible for the allocation of dollars determines what the standards are in his department. You can't have an organization running in several directions. There are certain objectives for the department, and the objectives have to be achieved by the people in the department. If a pharmacist decides he wants to go in one direction and the objectives of the department are in another direction, there has to be a parting of ways.

*Zellmer:* Gentlemen, I'm sure we could go on for several hours, but we have covered the points we agreed to discuss and the time is getting late. You've dealt with some important issues in contemporary pharmacy practice, and I'm sure many will be interested in your remarks and will find them useful in confronting the decisions they must make with regard to implementing clinical services.

# 3 The Legal Basis for Clinical Pharmacy Practice

Carl T. DeMarco

The legal basis for various clinical pharmacy activities is discussed.

The activities covered are drug history taking, maintaining medication profiles, drug monitoring, drug administration, drug prescribing, and patient consultation.

It is concluded that the law is not clear on all aspects of clinical pharmacy practice, but because of historical precedent, national or local standards of practice, and some state pharmacy acts, pharmacists may proceed cautiously with clinical functions.

In dealing with the legal implications of clinical pharmacy, it is virtually meaningless to speak in terms of "clinical pharmacy" per se. Even a casual perusal of the literature reveals wide disparity of what is meant by the term and what activities it includes. Additionally, there is virtually nothing in the law that speaks of clinical pharmacy. Therefore, this chapter will examine the legality of certain specific functions performed by pharmacists that relate directly to patients.

This subject can be divided into two major questions. First, what clinical activities are legal, and second, what new liabilities might be encountered? This chapter will concentrate on the first question and merely raise some legal issues arising under the second.

It is important to note at the outset that most of the legal issues faced today by pharmacists engaging in clinical activities will be determined in accordance with state practice acts. To the extent possible, but not exclusively, this chapter refers to New York law. Also of importance are such national standards as those of the federal Food, Drug and Cosmetic Act, the Joint Commission on Accreditation of Hospitals, Medicare regulations and the like.

## Drug History Taking

A logical place to start is the point at which the patient enters the hospital. We find that increasing numbers of pharmacists are taking patient medication histories. In fact, a recent study compared pharmacist-acquired drug histories with physician-acquired medication histories from the same patients. One of the conclusions of the study was:

In comparing physician-acquired data with pharmacist-acquired data, several things were obvious. Physicians did not generally obtain a comprehensive medication history. The pharmacist was more proficient in acquiring comprehensive medication histories. Much of the information obtained in the pharmacist-acquired medication history revealed that a significant percentage of patients were poorly informed about many aspects of drug therapy.[1]

This study confirmed the findings of a previous study.[2]

Now that we find pharmacists doing such a good job at it, it's almost an afterthought to ask whether this is a permissible clinical activity under law. Be that as it may, the question has been raised and requires attention.

While state laws, New York included, do not speak specifically about patient medication histories, pharmacists have for decades obtained patient information. Sometimes the pharmacist needed to know how to spell a patient's name or needed his address or telephone number. On a higher plane, the pharmacist, in order to properly interpret a prescription order, may ask a patient about his disease state or about medications previously received. Such information may also be important when the patient orders nonprescription medications. In any event, it seems well established that pharmacists have traditionally sought and utilized patient histories in relation to the compounding or dispensing function despite the apparent lack of specific statutory authorization. What pharmacists are doing in clinical settings today may differ in a quantitative sense but does not necessarily differ qualitatively, although it may, for the goal is to obtain sufficient information concerning a patient's drug history upon which to make reasonable judgments concerning present or prospective drug therapy.

## Medication Profiles

Recently, New Jersey has taken steps to require all pharmacists, including hospital pharmacists, to obtain and maintain certain information in the form of patient profile records. The record must include: (1) the family name and the first name of the person for whom medication is dispensed (the patient); (2) the complete address of the patient; (3) the patient's birthdate; (4) all known allergies and idiosyncrasies of the patient and chronic conditions which may relate to drug utilization; (5) the original date the medication is dispensed pursuant to the receipt of a physician's prescription order—in dispensing medication as a renewal (refill) of a new prescription, the date(s) of renewal (refilling) must be entered; (6) the number assigned the prescription; (7) the prescriber's name; (8) the name, strength and quantity of the drug dispensed; and (9) the initials of the dispensing pharmacist. Under other regulations specifically applicable to hospitals which are also being considered by the New Jersey Board of Pharmacy, these records will have to be made available to the hospital pharmacy and therapeutics committee for drug utilization review studies. The patient profile record regulation was contested in court litigation but was upheld on appeal.[3] It would not be surprising if other states follow with similar legislative or regulatory actions.

## Drug Monitoring

Drug monitoring can take place in at least two ways. First, the surveillance can occur between the time of prescribing and dispensing or administering any drugs. Secondly, it could occur as an in-process control after the patient is receiving medication. Often the two will overlap. Regardless of when the action takes place, the legal considerations are substantially the same. As with patient medication profiles, drug monitoring is specifically mentioned in few, if any, pharmacy laws. Again, New York is no exception. However, the *Guidelines for Pharmaceutical Services for Proprietary Nursing Homes in New York City,* as prepared by the New York City Department of Health and dated July 1972, in section II(d) (iii), place the following duty upon pharmacists:

> II(d) (iii). Check adverse reaction medication error forms and charts to prevent these from occurring.

Under Section II(d) (viii), the pharmacist must spot check:

> b. Patient charts against drug receipt book to see if medication was properly ordered, received and administered
> c. Check for proper utilization of the medication by comparing the physical count in the medication container against the amount received from the pharmacy and the number of doses administered to the patient as shown on the medication chart . . .

Admittedly, this regulation applies only to pharmaceutical services in proprietary nursing homes. But it does set a legal precedent and it's hard to believe that anyone would argue that patients in hospitals or community pharmacies should be denied as high a level of care and surveillance as patients in proprietary nursing homes.

## Drug Administration

In increasing numbers, hospitals are developing, under the direction and supervision of their pharmacy departments, drug administration programs. By doing so, hospitals centralize in one department full responsibility for drugs from the time they enter the hospital until they are administered or dispensed to patients.

Under present New York law, there is no provision that has a direct bearing on drug administration—except for one word—"dispensing." As might be expected, the definition of the practice of pharmacy includes ". . . the dispensing of drugs, medicines and therapeutic devices . . ."[4] Dispensing itself is not defined in the law but has been considered to be the issuance of one or more doses of a drug in a properly labeled container for use by a patient. Now, if a pharmacist can issue multiple doses of a medication to a patient with instructions as to how the patient shall take the medication, why can't the same pharmacist give the patient one dose of the medication each time the drug is to be taken and instruct the patient to take the medication at that point in time? If the pharmacist is reliable enough to properly entrust the patient with multiple doses of prescription medications for self-administration, is he not equally as trustworthy to have a patient take one dose at a time? Administration seems to be a discreet subdivision of dispensing. And it's probably safer than dispensing, from a drug security point of view and, more importantly, through minimization of patient medication errors.

It may be true that pharmacists, generally, would need some additional training to administer injectables, but such training is insignificant when compared to his total education in relation to drugs. Since the law authorizes dispensing, it is plausible to argue that this subsumes administration of medications.

This extrapolation of the pharmacy law in relation to drug administration would have to be balanced against any prohibitions contained in the medical and nursing practice acts to determine if pharmacist administration is permissible.

Other standards are also important. The Joint Commission on Accreditation of Hospitals states that:

> . . . Written policies and procedures that govern the safe administration of drugs shall be developed by the medical staff in cooperation with the pharmacist and with representatives of other disciplines, as necessary. . . .[5]

It goes on to say:

... All medications shall be administered by appropriately licensed personnel in accordance with any laws and regulations governing such acts ...

These statements and their interpretation leave the door wide open for a pharmacist to administer drugs if permitted by state law. In any event, he has responsibility for cooperating with the medical staff in preparing policies and procedures that govern administration of drugs.

A significant characteristic of pharmacy-based drug administration programs to keep in mind is that such programs are generally the product of the combined efforts of pharmacists, nurses and physicians and are only one facet of a total hospital medication system. Even if pharmacist administration is not permissible under the state pharmacy law, this joint effort by hospital professionals somehow sanctifies such programs in the minds of government officials.

Concerning these last two points—drug monitoring and drug administration—the New York pharmacy law seems to be going in the wrong direction. The pharmacy law, Article 137, as set forth in handbook 11, has been replaced by a new Article 137, which has not yet been printed and distributed by state authorities. Some aspects of the pharmacy law have been changed that are of significance and possibly detrimental to the practice of pharmacy. The old law stated:

Other unlicensed assistants may be employed in registered pharmacies and drug stores for other purposes *than the practice of pharmacology* and the dispensing, compounding or retailing of drugs, prescriptions, or poisons.[6] (Emphasis added.)

From this language, it can be assumed that acts that could not be performed by unlicensed assistants had been reserved for licensed pharmacists. One phrase, "the practice of pharmacology," is especially interesting for the old law defined "pharmacology" as:

... the science that treats of drugs and medicines, their nature, preparation, *administration* and *effect*.[7] (Emphasis added.)

Now doesn't that sound like what clinical pharmacists are talking about? Why was that verbiage not carried over into the revised law? Did the legislature, or its advisors, i.e., the board of pharmacy, intend to remove those functions from the practice of pharmacy? Only by examining whatever legislative history may exist could we shed any light on this question. Hopefully, this was not the intent of these omissions.

**Drug Prescribing**

In considering clinical activities, it's appropriate to also take a look at what some consider to be the ultimate in drug therapy, i.e., prescribing. In his inaugural address in 1972, ASHP President Hill stated:

I suggest that the physician and the pharmacist review their respective roles in rational drug therapy. The physician could decide on measurable therapeutic goals. The pharmacist could decide upon the choice of drugs, dose, route, frequency, etc., and the physician could measure the results achieved by the pharmacist. Such a model for care would have two advantages. The patient could benefit from the therapeutic expertise of the pharmacist and from the quality control function which would be introduced into the system.[8]

In fact, this is being done to some extent. In hypertension clinics and in some other areas pharmacists are initiating drug therapy, ordering lab tests, adjusting dosages, changing drug orders or withdrawing medications, etc., all within established boundaries while working closely with physicians.[9,10]

But what is there in the law that bears on this undertaking? To put it simply, not much! We do know, however, that in the past, under laws not radically different and in some cases the same, pharmacists did perform like duties. President Hill also traced this history in the same address:

During the nineteenth century the community pharmacist, or druggist, or apothecary, was considered an important professional in health care delivery. He provided first aid and triage services for a variety of ailments. He was one of the few learned citizens of the community and was used by the public to solve a variety of homely problems. He was the primary source for all drugs, medicines and pharmaceuticals, including home remedies which so many grandmothers, aunts and mothers skillfully administered. Most of these services gradually drifted away from pharmacy during the first half of this century.

The pharmacist gave up counterprescribing as unethical; he elected instead to rely upon the prescribing habits of physicians to determine the quantity and scope of drug therapy services to be rendered. He even gave up and eventually lost the right to refill authentic prescriptions without the prior authorization of the original prescriber. The typical pharmacist retreated from patient contact in order to increase his prescription productivity and in doing so, he lost his role as community counselor. When pharmacists recognized their untenable position, they reacted— those who elected to stay—by placing greater emphasis on merchandising of nonprescription items and later, nondrug items.[8]

If we thus use historical precedent and analogy with prior pharmacy laws, we can agree that pharmacists, to some extent, always had the right to tell patients what drugs to take.

In addition to the changes cited by Dr. Hill, the federal Food, Drug and Cosmetic Act, specifically the Durham-Humphrey Amendments of 1951, established a prescription class of drugs which could be dispensed only pursuant to the prescription order of a practitioner authorized by law to administer drugs.[11] Note carefully the word *administer,* not prescribe. Earlier we took a look at the legal basis upon which it could be argued that pharmacists have a right to administer drugs. Can we then say that pharmacists, derivatively, can write lawful prescriptions? A point to ponder.

Perhaps the easiest approach to the question of prescribing is to invoke principles of agency. It is a general principle of agency law that one person can authorize another to act on his behalf. The authorized agent can then exercise the rights of the principal in manner consistent with, and within the scope of, the authority granted.

Of course there are limitations imposed by law on certain powers and duties that cannot be delegated. For example, a lawyer cannot authorize a nonlawyer to argue a case in court. A surgeon cannot authorize a nurse to perform heart surgery. But the courts have generally been pretty liberal in allowing physicians to delegate a variety of duties to others. The question in our case is whether physicians can delegate their prescribing authority to pharmacists. Pharmacists are certainly well educated in the use of drugs, their effects, dosages, side effects, etc.

Assuming that this authorization is permissible,[a] we must still recognize that this approach has some shortcomings. The authority would apply only to that physician's patients. The right would be limited in accordance with the scope of authorization which might extend only to certain types of drugs or to certain disease states. It would also render the pharmacist a subprofessional vis-a-vis the physician and could ultimately destroy his status as an independent professional.

The best solution to the problem would be to amend the pharmacy laws to specifically include prescribing, based upon the diagnosis of a physician.

### Patient Consultation

The last aspect of clinical pharmacy that shall be considered is patient consultation either during the patient's stay in the hospital, at the time of discharge or in the outpatient clinic or home care programs. *Drug Intelligence and Clinical Pharmacy*[12] presented three case studies of this activity. As in the other areas we've been looking at, the New York Law is a poor specimen for gathering samples of legal authority in this area. The law does state the pharmacist's responsibility for properly labeling prescription containers, but it limits this to "... directions for the use of the drug by the patient *as given upon the prescription.*"[13] (Emphasis added.) Board regulations[14] might be interpreted to expand this authority, but that's going a bit far.

As a point of reference, other state laws do contain language that applies to the patient consultation area of pharmacy practice. For example, the definition of the practice of pharmacy in the Maryland Pharmacy Law contains the following language:

> ... the practice that is concerned with ... the responsibility of providing information, as required, concerning such

drugs and medicines and their therapeutic values and uses in the treatment and prevention of disease ...[15]

Other state pharmacy laws have similar provisions.[16,17]

Some state boards of pharmacy have rules bearing on the subject. For example, the California Board of Pharmacy regulations contain the following language:

> No pharmacist shall exhibit, discuss, or reveal the contents of any prescription, nor shall he discuss the therapeutic effect thereof, or the nature, extent, or degree of illness suffered by any patient served by him, *with any person other than the patient or his authorized representative,* the prescriber or other licensed practitioner then caring for the patient, another licensed pharmacist serving the patient, or a person duly authorized by law to receive such information.[18] (Emphasis added.)

The Minnesota Board of Pharmacy has a similar regulation.[19]

As you might expect, we sometimes find language to the contrary. For example, the Maine Pharmaceutical Association's code of ethics states:

> The Pharmacist shall make no attempt to prescribe or treat diseases and he should refrain from any practice which might be construed as trespassing into the field of Practicing Medicine ...[20]

Sometimes we're our own worst enemies.

### Liability

Clinical functions must be performed with the same diligence and due care that is used in the performance of traditional duties. Other factors that need consideration include: the reasonable man concept to determine whether we have a new point of reference against which to measure these new functions, i.e., the reasonable and prudent "clinical" pharmacist; whether the new levels of service will be adopted by courts as the legal duty of care owed to patients, the breach of which might result in negligence; and the effect of the presence or absence of specific statutory or regulatory authorization on determining negligence.

### Conclusion

In conclusion, it seems safe to say that the law is not at all clear on all aspects of clinical pharmacy.[21] But there's enough in historical precedent, present national or local community standards of practice, and even pharmacy acts, to enable pharmacists to proceed along these lines with caution. We must remember that laws and regulations cannot cover all the specifics of professional practice, especially in relation to emerging trends. That is why laws charge specific persons, the practitioners themselves, with the appropriate authority to practice the profession after long and careful education and training and examination. Professionals must then discharge their public trust to best serve the interest of the public, and this includes the duty to develop new tech-

---

[a] But cf., e.g., opinion of the Attorney General of Oregon, No. 6992, July 5, 1973, which holds that Oregon law does not permit blanket authorization from a physician to a pharmacist to substitute an "equivalent product" for specific brand-named products in a prescription based upon the rationale that this would constitute the "practice of medicine." If such substitution is not lawful, *a fortiori*, prior authorization to prescribe would be unlawful.

niques and methods that improve their service.[22] After all, if the professionals don't do it, who can?

## References

1. Covington, T. R. and Pfeiffer, F. A.: The Pharmacist-Acquired Medication History (Clinical Forum), *Amer. J. Hosp. Pharm. 29*:692–695 (Aug.) 1973.

2. Wilson, R. S. and Kabat, H. F.: Pharmacist Initiated Drug Histories, *Amer. J. Hosp. Pharm. 28*:49–53. (Jan.) 1971.

3. *Rite Aid of New Jersey vs. Board of Pharmacy of New Jersey,* Superior Court of New Jersey, Appellate Division, No. A-19966-71, May 8, 1973.

5. Accreditation Manual for Hospitals, Joint Commission on Accreditation of Hospitals, Pharmaceutical Services, Standard V, Looseleaf Edition, July 1972.

6. New York Pharmacy Law, Article 137, § 6806 (4), repealed.

7. Ibid., § 6801 (12), repealed.

8. Hill, W. T., Jr.: A Broader Perspective for the ASHP, *Amer. J. Hosp. Pharm. 29*:597–599 (July) 1972.

9. Ellinoy, B. J., Mays, J. F., McSherry, P. V. and Rosenthal, L. C.: A Pharmacy Outpatient Monitoring Program Providing Primary Medical Care to Selected Patients, *Amer. J. Hosp. Pharm. 30*:593–598 (July) 1973.

10. Mattei, T. J., Balmer, J. A., Corbin, L. A. and Sister M. Gonzales Duffy: Hypertension: A Model for Pharmacy Involvement, *Amer. J. Hosp. Pharm. 30*:683–686 (Aug.) 1973.

11. Food, Drug and Cosmetic Act, § 503 (b)(2); 21 U.S.C. 353 (b)(2).

12. Wertheimer, A., Shefter, E. and Cooper, T.: The Pharmacist as a Drug Consultant—Three Case Studies, *Drug Intel. Clin. Pharm. 7*:58–61 (Feb.) 1973.

13. New York Pharmacy Law, Article 137, § 6810 (1971).

14. Regulations of the New York Board of Pharmacy, § 257.18.

15. 43 Md. Ann. Code, § 250 (a)(1971).

16. Fla. Stat. Ann., § 465.031 (4) (1965).

17. Pa. Stat. Ann. § 390-2 (11)(1968).

18. 16 Cal. Admin. Code § 1764 (1969).

19. Regulations of the Minnesota Board of Pharmacy, § 36.

20. Maine Pharmaceutical Association Code of Ethics, Chapter 2(5).

21. Barker, K. and Valentino, J.: On a Political and Legal Foundation for Clinical Pharmacy Practice, *J. Amer. Pharm. Ass. NS 12*:202–206, 237 (May) 1972.

22. Steeves, R. and Patterson F.: Legal Responsibilities of the Hospital Pharmacist for Rational Drug Therapy, *Amer. J. Hosp. Pharm. 26:*404–407 (July) 1969.

# 4 Clinical Pharmacy Services — Management by Objectives

William E. Smith

Successful implementation of clinical pharmacy services in a hospital requires goals to be achieved, teamwork of hospital personnel, programming of work to be performed, measuring accomplishments, cost controls and the development of the abilities of all pharmacy personnel. The management style of "management by objectives" has been used since 1968 and is a major reason why the implementation of clinical pharmacy services has been successful at Memorial Hospital Medical Center of Long Beach, California. Objectives among the Director of Pharmacy and Central Services and (1) hospital administration, (2) department supervisors, (3) personnel of each satellite pharmacy, and (4) each pharmacist have been identified and are being used to measure accomplishments. Examples of objectives are presented. Department personnel know their functions and the goals of the department; this results in excellent department morale. Management by objectives has proven to be a good method to establish individual performance appraisal for each pharmacist practicing in the patient care areas.

Clinical pharmacy is capturing the interest and imagination of pharmacists, pharmacy educators, nurses, hospital administrators, physicians and government agencies.[1] At the present time, however, very few hospitals have implemented a hospitalwide clinical pharmacy service. Successful implementation of a clinical pharmacy service requires a management approach which will define and implement services, achieve desired results and patient care benefits, and at the same time keep all personnel moving in the direction of the change in pharmacy services. It is no small task to change a hospital medication system and alter the drug therapy responsibilities of the physician, pharmacists and nurse to achieve working harmony and improved patient care.

Memorial Hospital Medical Center of Long Beach implemented a hospitalwide clinical pharmacy service in 1968.[2] Since that time refinements in systems and services have been made and new programs have been added. Much of our success is attributed to the implementation of a management by objectives system approach to pharmacy management. A definition for the word "objective," from Webster's Intercollegiate Dictionary, is "an aim or end of action: point to be hit, reached, etc." In its briefest form, management by objectives, as described by Odiorne,[3] is "a managerial method whereby the superior and the subordinate managers in an organization identify areas of responsibility in which the man will work, set some standards for good—or bad—performance and the measurement of results against those standards."

The major premises of management by objectives can be stated as follows:[3]

A. Business management takes place within an economic system that provides the environmental situation for the individual firm. This environment, which has changed drastically over the past 30 years, imposes new requirements on companies and on individual managers.

B. Management by objectives is a way of managing aimed at meeting these new requirements. It presumes that the first step in management is to identify, by one means or another, the goals of the organization. All other management methods and subsystems follow this preliminary step.

C. Once organizational goals have been identified, orderly procedures for distributing responsibilities among individual managers are set up in such a way that their combined efforts are directed toward achieving those goals.

D. Management by objectives assumes that managerial behavior is more important than manager personality, and that this behavior should be defined in terms of results measured against established goals, rather than in terms of common goals for all managers, or common methods of managing.

E. It also presumes that while participation is highly desirable in goal-setting and decision-making, its principal merit lies in its social and political values rather than its effects on production, though even here it may have a favorable impact, and in any case seldom hurts.

F. It regards the successful manager as a manager of situations, most of which are best defined by identifying the purpose of the organization and the managerial behavior best calculated to achieve that purpose. This means that there is no one best pattern of management, since all management behavior is discriminatory, being related to specific goals and shaped by the larger economic system within which it operates.

Successful implementation of clinical pharmacy services requires definition of areas of responsibility for the pharmacy department in the institution as well as responsibilities of the physician, nurse and pharmacist in patient care. Standards for quality services must be developed, and performance and results of both the services provided and the pharmacist's clinical practice must be measured against the established standards.

## Goals and Standards for Clinical Pharmacy Services

The guiding principle of goal-setting is:[3]

High performance goals are needed in every area of responsibility and every position where performance and results directly and vitally affect the contribution of the man to the organization.

Figure 1 is an abstract representation of pharmacy services at Memorial Hospital Medical Center. The pharmacy department has been represented abstractly by the region within the circle. The interaction between the pharmacy department and other groups within Memorial Hospital is represented by the arrows which also depict the flow of information and/or materials.

*Figure 1. The interactions of the pharmacy department and other departments*

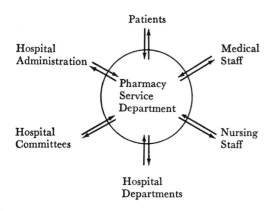

Clinical pharmacy services require objectives or goals for each group identified. Examples of some pharmacy service goals in relation to the different groups in Figure 1 are listed below:

*Patients*
1. To provide safe and effective drug therapy at the lowest possible cost
2. To provide a safe and efficient drug distribution system for all patients treated

*Medical Staff*
1. To provide quality drug information as needed and when needed
2. To work cooperatively with the medical staff to provide safe and effective drug therapy for all patients

*Nursing Staff*
1. To provide drugs in unit doses accurately and on time
2. To provide quality drug information as needed and when needed

*Hospital Administration*
1. To provide department services in a quality manner and at the least cost
2. To keep administration informed of objectives, programs, successes, failures, future plans and needs, costs and savings generated

*Hospital Committees*[a]
1. To refine and define the pharmaceutical needs of patients
2. To integrate clinical pharmacy services into overall hospital planning
3. To assist in the planning and implementation of systems and procedures to improve patient care

*Hospital Departments*
1. To provide drug products accurately and as needed
2. To provide information on drugs, chemicals and related subjects as needed

To achieve these goals of service, the pharmacy department at Memorial Hospital Medical Center believes:

1. Pharmacists should practice in patient care areas.
2. A unit dose drug distribution system is essential.
3. Pharmacy technicians should perform technical tasks.
4. Pharmacists should perform tasks that require professional judgment.
5. Services must be provided to physicians and nurses in a cooperative manner.
6. The reference point for all services and for making changes when disagreement exists has to be "what is best for the patient."

These six items illustrate the complexity of implementing clinical pharmacy service.

## Management of the Department of Pharmacy and Central Services

To implement clinical pharmacy services and achieve department service goals, a department management team has been developed. Figure 2 is an organizational chart of department management and pharmacist areas of practice. A management by objectives system has been developed in the past three years among the Director of Pharmacy and Central Services and:

1. Hospital administration
2. Department supervisors
3. Personnel of each satellite pharmacy
4. Each pharmacist

Objectives have been identified and are now being used to measure accomplishments.

The Supervisor of the Drug Information Service is responsible for department drug information services. The Supervisor of Inpatient Services is responsible for the technicians and their job responsibilities. The Supervisor of Pharmacy Technology is responsible for unit dose drug packaging. The Assistant Director is responsible for the coordination of the work of these three areas.

---

[a]Examples of hospital committees where a pharmacy representative is a member are: Patient Care; Epidemiology; Intensive Care; and Pharmacy, Diagnostic and Therapeutic Services.

*Figure 2. Organization chart of Memorial Hospital Medical Center Department of Pharmacy and Central Services*

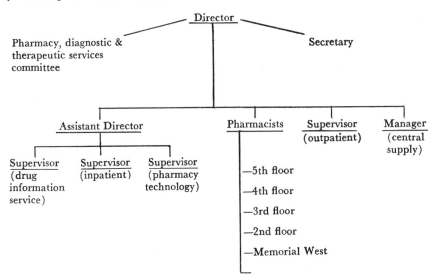

Each department manager is responsible for developing a list of annual objectives for his area of responsibility. The objectives are reviewed and modified as necessary by the Assistant Director and Director. The net result is agreement with department priorities to meet service objectives for the year.

To illustrate types of objectives established for fiscal year 1971, some examples will be given. A specific date is established for each objective which is the time the objective is to be completed.

> Objective for Director of Pharmacy and
> Central Services and Hospital Administration
> *Pharmacist's Clinical Practice (December 1970)*
> Prepare report to identify problem areas and approaches to improve the pharmacist's clinical practice, capability and performance. Report will set objectives for the next two to three years for further development of the pharmacist's clinical practice such as: relationship with the nurse, physician and patient. These relationships are to be departmental and individual, such as: drug information needs and services; patient rounds and admission interviews; drug educational conferences for the medical staff.

The purpose of the above objective is to recognize the dynamic changes that are taking place, and should be in the pharmacist's clinical practice. Also, the pharmacist's clinical practice still requires a great deal of attention, planning and development to achieve goals of service.

> Objective for Inpatient Services Supervisor
> *Pharmacy Assistants (April 1971)*
> Prepare report giving a profile of the assistant's work load activity. Report will compare actual to the theoretical technician task list. Report will also assess the status of Phases I, II and III of training. Successes and problems will be presented. Proposals to continue the successes, solve the problem areas and for future training programs if needed will be included in the report.

The Inpatient Services Supervisor has been developing a training program for assistants. It is valuable to periodically assess the progress and the deficiencies of programs and propose plans for future implementation. The success of clinical pharmacy services depends a great deal on the ability and performance of the technicians. The purpose of the above objective, therefore, is to assess the status of assistant development.

> Objectives for Supervisor, Pharmacy
> Technology Laboratory
> *Unit Dose Packaging (May 1970)*
> Develop monthly reporting system measuring production by dosage form. Establish acceptable daily production figures. Determine costs of unit dose packaging. Prepare report for Director on costs and monthly reporting system.
>
> *Unit Dose Packaging (May 1971)*
> Prepare report outlining proposals to increase packaging efficiency and reduce packaging costs. Monthly work production reports are to be related to maximum output potential.

Single unit packaged drugs are a basic requirement for implementing clinical pharmacy services. Until the pharmaceutical industry meets its responsibility to provide unit packaged drugs, hospital personnel will have to package drugs. The above objective then is to complete a review of packaging costs and to propose ways to reduce the costs of packaging.

The decentralized pharmacy service provides unique opportunities to individualize services by patient areas. This part of department management has only recently been implemented. Each pharmacist was asked to submit individually a list of:

1. Services with which he is pleased
2. Services in need of attention
3. Top three priorities that need attention.

The pharmacist staff per pharmacy unit, with the Director, will begin to program and make changes to improve services.

One of the significant advantages of clinical pharmacy services is the opportunity to implement an individualized development program for each pharmacist. The pharmacist's performance and, therefore, performance appraisals, should be based on clinical practice expertise. Up to recently, a "good pharmacist" has been one who could type fast, dispense many prescriptions, and know something about drugs.

The department management approach of management by objectives is now being extended to the performance appraisal of each pharmacist. Each pharmacist is submitting to the Director his/her own list of self-educational objectives for the next year. Some examples of objectives submitted are:

1. Complete teratology report
2. Perform utilization study on cephalosporins and present findings to the Pharmacy, Diagnostic and Therapeutic Services Committee
3. Study antibiotics in depth and present a department conference on the subject area selected.

In each of the examples, the emphasis is on action; e.g., prepare a report, conduct a conference, propose new areas to be studied.

## Key Management Problems

Management by objectives relates to key management problems as listed below:[3]

1. *Knowing what is expected in terms of objectives.* Employees, including managers, like to know what is expected of their performance.
2. *Obtaining teamwork by identifying common goals.* Teamwork both within and outside the pharmacy department is an absolute necessity to successfully implement clinical pharmacy services.
3. *Programming work by setting terminal dates.* Work has to be completed and in a logical sequence. Dates to complete tasks helps to get the work completed.
4. *Recognizing progress through agreement between goals and accomplishments.* Progress usually leads to more progress and success.
5. *Salary administration; how should increases be allocated?* This is an important and oftentimes difficult part of management. The strain on health care systems and the cost of clinical pharmacy services will require more definitive and exacting ways to give salary increases to pharmacists.
6. *Assessing promotability by identifying potential for it.* Every pharmacist should be encouraged to perform to his maximum capability and his potential for greater responsibility should be periodically identified.

The advantages of management by objectives are in terms of better results, lower costs, improved performance, more motivated people, improved quality of service, more businesslike management of salaries and the development of each employee's best abilities.

The limitations of management by objectives as outlined by Odiorne are:[3]

1. It cannot appraise and completely identify potential. The system deals only with performance on the present job. Appraisal of potential must be done separately.
2. The system presumes that the man and his boss will together establish suitable standards that will serve the company well.
3. It implies that the boss understands the strict limitations on what he is supposed to do, and will refrain from playing bad.
4. In action, it often aggravates a problem that appraisal should help to solve. It stresses results alone and doesn't provide for methods of achieving them.

## Experiences With Management by Objectives for Clinical Pharmacy Services

For this management system to be effective, follow-through is required on each objective. Was the report completed? Was the department reorganized? Did the pharmacist's clinical abilities really improve? Was the pharmacist's project completed with quality or completed just to meet an assignment? Time is required to follow up each objective, but it is time well spent.

The objectives established for each year should not be easy to achieve. Some pressure must be self-imposed to complete objectives. Yet not too many objectives should be established because the result will be quantity instead of quality.

The first year of applying management by objectives will most likely see too many objectives established, so the first year is essentially a year for learning and gaining experience. It is important to incorporate into each objective a statement which will allow for the measure of the objective being completed.

A general personal feeling about this management approach is reflected in the following quote:[3]

Most good work in management aims at accomplishing some specific end - achieving a particular goal, solving a particular problem, or reaching some fixed terminal point. The definition of these objectives for the whole organization, for all its subordinate organizations, and for the individuals in them is the logical starting place for management improvement because:

—If you don't have a goal, you have no idea whether you are on the right road or not.

—You can't assess results without some prior expectations against which to measure them.

—You don't know when things are drifting if you aren't clear what goal would comprise "non-drifting" or "purposive action."

—People can't perform with maximum effectiveness if they don't know what goals the organization is seeking (and why), or how well they are doing in relation to these goals.

A basic concept of management by objectives is to measure results. How can the results of management of clinical pharmacy services by objectives at Memorial Hospital Medical Center be measured? A hospitalwide clinical pharmacy service has been implemented and justified in costs and benefits to patients. Objectives have been set to continue to improve and refine services and to reduce costs and pharmacist personnel requirements. Department morale is excellent as shown by a very low personnel turnover rate in all job categories. Each pharmacist is challenged by his daily practice. The medical staff is steadily increasing its utilization of the pharmacist for drug information. The involvement of department personnel in hospital operations, committee programs, etc., continues to increase.

## Conclusion

The successes the Department of Pharmacy and Central Services has had at Memorial Hospital Medical Center has been a direct result of the management by objectives system utilized in department management.

A multitude of objectives have been created from implementing a clinical service and a unit dose drug distribution system. These objectives exist at every level—hospital administration, pharmacy and central service management, and staff pharmacists. Each department manager and pharmacist knows what the department objectives are and determines for himself, with approval by the Director, what contributions he can make in achieving department service objectives.

## References

1. Report of Task Force On the Pharmacist's Clinical Role, National Center for Health Services Research and Development, HSRD Briefs, No. 4 (Spring) 1971.
2. Smith, W. E. et al.: Clinical Pharmacy: General Hospital, *Hospitals 44*:88 (Nov. 1) 1970.
3. Odiorne, G. S.: Management By Objectives, Pitman Publishing Corporation, New York, New York, 1965.

# 5 A Service-integrated Approach to Clinical Pharmacy Practice through a Hyperalimentation Program

Wayne F. Conrad, Robert H. Gassett, and Daniel A. Goupil

Two different approaches toward implementing clinical pharmacy services and an example of the application of one of these approaches are discussed.

In one approach, basic pharmacy services form the foundation for clinical practice. The second approach is to develop clinical pharmacy services independent of other pharmacy services. The authors favor the former method and illustrate how they initiated clinical services through involvement in a parenteral hyperalimentation program.

Pharmacists must analyze the needs and opportunities in their institutions to determine how they may best become involved in clinical services.

The objective of this chapter is to support a general direction for pharmacy by which clinical services may be achieved in most hospitals.

## Administrative Approaches to Clinical Pharmacy Practice

Two distinct administrative approaches are part of the clinical pharmacy movement. In one approach, basic pharmacy services form the foundation for clinical practice. Clinical services result from the extension of these established services and their ultimate integration with clinical functions. An alternate approach is to develop a clinical pharmacy program independent of other pharmacy services. This has frequently resulted in the formation of a second group of pharmacists separated by location and function. The major concern of the latter group is the therapeutic manipulation of the patient, while the original group's concern is drug distribution. A major advantage associated with this second approach toward clinical practice is expediency. A program may be quickly implemented since it depends mainly on the initiative and aggressiveness of the participants.

The service-integrated approach to clinical practice is founded on a firm base of fundamental services. The total pharmacy service may be viewed as a pyramid with clinical pharmacy, as perhaps the ultimate pharmacy program, at the apex. The apex is supported by numerous building blocks of nonclinical programs, e.g., sound pharmacy administration, an active and effective pharmacy and therapeutics committee, pharmaceutical tech-

nology, a progressive drug distribution system, drug information services, etc. The potential and logical extension of these services are clinical functions ranging from increased physician-pharmacist interaction to provision of patient-specific therapeutic information and pharmacokinetic evaluations such as serum drug level studies.

The service-integrated approach to clinical pharmacy practice may appear less dramatic and more painstaking. It is generally achieved over a rather lengthy period of time. However, it offers several advantages such as comprehensiveness of service, operation from a point of recognized expertise, efficient utilization of available resources and economic justification.

The service-integrated approach identifies the pharmacist—to the patient, the nurse and the physician—with the responsibility for all of the pharmacy's services. The clinical pharmacist may, at times, be of invaluable assistance through his monitoring of the patient, but just as frequently, his major contribution may be in solving a drug distribution problem, identifying an i.v. incompatibility or formulating a special dosage form. It is the pharmacist acting in this comprehensive capacity that offers the maximum support to the health care team.

Although clinical ability is an essential tool required for physician-pharmacist interaction, acceptance of the pharmacist by the physician and realization of his potential contribution are just as necessary. As a result of building a firm foundation of nonclinical services, the pharmacist becomes recognized and respected for his pharmaceutical ability. This is a significant advantage in the development of a clinical program in that it removes some of the pressures associated with separation from basic services, in which case the pharmacist is expected to know the "right answers" and be instrumental in solving therapeutic management problems.

An important element to the widespread acceptance and implementation of pharmacy services in hospitals is economic justification. Documentation of the value of pharmacist involvement in the clinical setting is desperately needed. Realizing that the pharmacist is of value in isolated situations is quite different from hiring one or more pharmacists whose sole responsibilities are taking patient histories, monitoring drug therapy, advising patients on discharge, etc. We can all justify these things to each other, but can we justify them to hospital administration? In lieu of quantification of the value of clinical programs, justification of clinical service function in terms of the extension of, and the integration with, already recognized basic service functions can be very helpful. Almost without exception, clinical functions separated from basic services in the hospital have been at least partially, and many times completely, funded by schools of pharmacy with clinical education as the prime interest. A serious credibility gap will arise if we can only justify clinical practice in terms of teaching students whose major justification for existence, in turn, will be to teach more students.

### Pharmacy Involvement

The essential element to implementing a clinical service program through the service-integrated approach is *involvement*. The pharmacist must be significantly involved in patient-specific, drug-related activities so that he knows what the therapeutic problems are in his hospital. The pharmacy must make the transition from being on the periphery of patient care to being an integral part of it.

At several institutions around the country, refinement of drug distribution via implementation of a unit dose system has provided the means for this transition.[1,2] Successful unit dose dispensing requires substantial pharmacy involvement. The pharmacist must concern himself with the distribution of each dose for each patient, and in addition, assume the primary responsibility for the preparation of doses for administration. Extensive communication is required, not only concerning the medication order, but for all the other information needed to get the right drug to the right patient at the right time. Consequently, the pharmacist's sphere of influence expands to include more direct patient care. Pharmacist involvement in this way is naturally conducive to further extension to include clinical functions.

While a unit dose system has been a useful vehicle for expansion to clinical functions, it is not essential. It may not even be practical in some hospital situations. The essential element of involvement may be achieved using other functional programs.

### Hyperalimentation and the Service-integrated Approach

Hyperalimentation represents an emerging era of recognition for hospital pharmacists. From the initial efforts of Dudrick and Flack,[3] it has been an example of physicians seeking the assistance of the pharmacy because of recognition of pharmacy expertise in product formulation and sterile production or aseptic transfer. However, this specific area of practice may also afford the pharmacist an opportunity to move from the periphery of patient care into the center, in a way analogous to a unit dose system.

Hyperalimentation at E. J. Meyer Memorial Hospital began like it has at many other institutions. A physician became interested in trying a new form of nutritional therapy. Initially, members of the medical and nursing staffs were preparing the solutions on the nursing unit. The pharmacy became involved when the department suggested, that due to the complexities of formulation and preparation, as well as the high potential for contamination, these fluids should be prepared in the pharmacy.

From this initial involvement, the role of the pharmacy continued to expand. In cooperation with the surgical department, several specific hyperalimentation formulas were devised. A basic formula was designed to provide the ideal ratio of protein fragments to exogenous calories in the form of carbohydrates with an appropriate replacement of necessary electrolytes and vitamins. Alcohol-free, low electrolyte and essential amino acid formulas were designed to meet specific patient requirements. A wet method of preparation using a closed, sterile, transfer technique was initiated.

The pharmacy also became involved in the administration of hyperalimentation solutions. It was felt that administration of hyperalimentation fluid requires a constant infusion pump. Therefore, the pharmacist developed an assembly technique which was compatible with the infusion pump and allowed the once-daily assembly of a 24-hour volume of solution for administration. If more than one liter of solution is required for a 24-hour period, additional bottles are connected in a series to minimize the potential for contamination associated with frequent changing of bottles.

As an outgrowth of his participation in administration and assembly techniques, the pharmacist became the focal point for the resolution of problems concerning the set-up and use of hyperalimentation solutions. The pharmacy began a program to check each assembly on a daily basis to insure that the proper administration technique was being followed.

Up to this point, pharmacy input was primarily through basic service functions. However, as the involvement and recognition of the pharmacist increased, the role of the pharmacist expanded to include clinical functions.

As hyperalimentation therapy became an accepted and more frequently used clinical tool, the number of physicians requesting hyperalimentation solutions increased. Because of a concern for the proper utilization of hyperalimentation solutions, the pharmacy suggested guidelines under which these fluids should be used. A mechanism was devised whereby all requests for hyperalimentation were evaluated by the pharmacy before therapy was initiated. This screening was designed to answer three questions: Was the physician ordering hyperalimentation knowledgeable in the use of hyperalimentation solutions? Was the patient an appropriate candidate to receive the solutions? And, to what extent would hyperalimentation modify the patient's other therapy? Physicians not having prior experience with hyperalimentation therapy were supplied this information by the pharmacy. If, through a review of the patient's chart, the pharmacist suspected that the patient should not be maintained on this form of therapy, the physician was contacted. This meeting allowed the physician and the pharmacist to review the patient's care and discuss alternatives.

The clinical involvement of the pharmacist also included monitoring the clinical response of the patient. Once a patient was placed on hyperalimentation therapy, the pharmacist used the patient's chart to obtain basic information to initiate a patient profile. This included the patient's name, age, sex, diagnosis, a brief summary of his present clinical situation and a list of his medications. Pertinent laboratory data, such as blood glucose, creatinine, blood urea nitrogen, total protein, sodium, potassium, chloride and blood gases were recorded. Then, on a daily basis, the pharmacist monitored these laboratory values plus other data such as the patient's weight, temperature, fluid input and output, urine sugars, bacteriological data, and the physician's progress notes. The pharmacist also saw the patient regularly as he monitored the assembly equipment. The overall objective was to monitor the clinical response of the patient while receiving hyperalimentation therapy in an attempt to provide consultation to the physician concerning the safe and proper utilization of these fluids. This type of monitoring has frequently resulted in alterations in primary solution formula and in electrolyte concentration, as well as infusion rate changes and cessation of therapy.

Acting as a primary resource to nurses concerning hyperalimentation therapy has been another area of involvement for the pharmacist. He not only resolves the equipment problems but attempts to minimize their occurrence by providing lecture presentations and demonstrations on hyperalimentation therapy and equipment assembly. Video tape presentations have been prepared to further extend the availability and utilization of these presentations to the nursing staff.

While monitoring the hyperalimentation patient, the pharmacist has frequently become involved in monitoring other types of therapy, especially in areas closely associated with parenteral nutrition, such as trauma, burn therapy and oral nutrition. In addition, the pharmacy has used the service-integrated approach to establish comprehensive services in other areas. For example, concern over irrigation solutions has led to implementation of more rigid controls over this form of therapy, pharmacy involvement in techniques for deep wound irrigation, and consultations concerning the therapeutic management of patients requiring various types of irrigation therapy.

### Summary

At Meyer Hospital, hyperalimentation has been used as the catalyst for clinical pharmacy services. The basic pharmacy service functions of formulation and preparation were readily accepted by the pharmacy and expanded to include responsibility for developing and monitoring fluid administration. This physically moved the pharmacist from the periphery into a more integral part of patient care activity. Once on the nursing unit, he had access to detailed, patient-specific information, giving him the opportunity to monitor the patient's response. Demonstrated competence in formulation and preparation of hyperalimentation solution and in daily monitoring of the patient and administration assembly earned the pharmacist acceptance by the medical and nursing staffs. As a result, the pharmacist became further involved in hyperalimentation therapy and similarly involved in other types of therapy.

However, hyperalimentation services do not necessarily denote a clinical pharmacy program. Likewise, a unit dose system does not assure clinical involvement. Rather, these programs are examples of how a pharmacy department can utilize basic service programs as building blocks to achieve clinical practice as part of comprehensive pharmacy services. The essential element is involvement. It is up to each individual pharmacy department to analyze the needs and opportunities of its particular institution in order to determine how this involvement can best be achieved.

### References

1. Smith, W. E.: Clinical Pharmacy Services in a Community Hospital, DHEW Pub. No. HSM 72-3019, Washington, D.C., 1972.

2. Durant, W. J. and Zilz, D. A.: Wisconsin Information Service and Medication Distribution, *Amer. J. Hosp. Pharm.* 24:625–631 (Nov.) 1967.

3. Flack H. L., Gans, J. A., Serlick, S. E. and Dudrick, S. J.: The Current Status of Parenteral Hyperalimentation, *Amer. J. Hosp. Pharm. 28:*326–335 (May) 1971.

# 6 Clinical Pharmacy and the Pharmaceutical Industry

John S. Ruggiero

The relationship of emerging clinical pharmacy practice to the pharmaceutical industry is discussed with reference to the professional image which pharmacists present to others, acceptance of the pharmacist as an individual providing health-related services, and the need for communication of the changes in pharmacy practice.

The development of the pharmaceutical industry is discussed as an outgrowth from the profession of pharmacy, along with the problems presented by acceptance of changing roles. A number of comments are reported from industry executives as they view the effect of clinical pharmacy on the pharmaceutical industry.

Although the term clinical pharmacy has been used quite regularly during the past five years or so, there does exist (whether we want to believe it or not) considerable confusion in the minds of many as to wnat the term means. There is confusion even to the point of the term being stricken from identification with a particular or special type of pharmacy practice—as witness the report of the American Pharmaceutical Association task force to define certain terms among which was "clinical pharmacy."[1] The recommendation, which was adopted by APhA, recognized the need for clinical involvement and the need for increased patient-oriented pharmacy services, but concluded that the clinical functions of pharmacy do not constitute a specialty. If there is confusion among the practitioners as to what clinical pharmacy is, you may imagine the vagueness and lack of comprehension on the part of others. Thus, it is difficult to assess the impact of this uncertain entity on a complex and dynamic industry.

Nevertheless, as a former educator accustomed to playing the role of prognosticator and crystal ball gazer, and as the proverbial fool, I shall rush in where angels fear to tread. In doing so, however, let me first at least, not altogether foolhardy, attempt to establish certain premises upon which an evaluation may be made.

## The Health Care System

First, although it is probably becoming a cliché, it is not any less true that society is increasingly questioning the current system of health care. It is questioning the quality or lack of quality of health care, the availability or lack of availability of health care and the cost of health care delivery. As more and more people become involved in the questioning and more and more become dissatisfied, they increasingly turn to local, state and federal agencies for answers and solutions. That health expenditures from governmental sources approach 38% of all health expenditures should be no surprise to those who are aware of the increased involvement along these lines.[2] Before the passage of Medicare legislation in 1966, government involvement was around 25%.[3] If (or perhaps more correctly, when) national health insurance legislation is passed, it is not difficult to envision the government picking up the tab for 75–80% of all health expenditures in a relatively short period of time. Of course, we are talking about an increasing dollar figure in addition, one which has grown from 42.1 billion dollars in 1966 to 75 billion dollars.[3] The Congress and the President have declared that one of our principal national goals is to promote and assure the highest level of health care attainable for every person.

In attempts to find the answers to our country's health manpower problems, many task forces, advisory commissions and committees have been appointed to study the issue and provide recommendations. The National Advisory Commission on Health Manpower found that although the number of health practitioners is important, it is secondary to the manner or system of coordinated utilization of the resources available. The Commission warned that the educational system should be so constructed as to be able to keep abreast of scientific and social changes and to anticipate the demands of the next 25 years.[4]

Toward this end, many recent meetings, conferences

and symposia have been devoted toward interdisciplinary sessions involving physicians, pharmacists, nurses, educators, health planners, dentists, public health officials, government bureaucrats, etc. A comment made by Wilson helps to put these meetings into perspective and causes one to stop and reflect on where we are going. Dr. Wilson said at an invitational conference on pharmacy manpower in 1970, "Thus far, it seems to me that our interdisciplinary conferences have suffered from two shortcomings. First, everyone calls for the creation and promulgation of the health team or a 'teamwork' approach to health. By contrast with the volume of lip service paid to this important concept, however, it is still very difficult to find a real health team in action outside of the institutional setting. Second, one very important participant in the health care process is being left out. He is not invited to our interdisciplinary deliberations, nor is he given due consideration in the health team concept. I refer, of course, to the patient."[5]

Dr. Wilson continues, "Any number of reasons can be adduced to explain the gulf between lip service and reality in the health team concept and our neglect of the patient as an active participant in his own health care. To me, one of the most convincing is what Robert Ardrey has called the 'Territorial Imperative.' In his book by that title, Ardrey eloquently demonstrates that winning and protecting a given territory is among the fundamental drives of animals from the warbler to the warthog. He suggests that this animal heritage may explain a good deal of human behavior as well."

I am inclined to agree with Mr. Ardrey and Dr. Wilson, having observed the phenomenon myself in university faculty meetings and in certain industrial sessions. It takes a relatively short leap of the imagination to see "territorial imperative" at work in the formation or nonformation of functional health teams. Each profession is all for teamwork so long as it does not involve surrender of a hard won "turf."

## Pharmacy's Role

As far as pharmacy is concerned, the profession is anxiously seeking change as a result of pressure from within. There is a need to develop new roles or activities for the pharmacist to replace those lost as a result of the changing emphasis from his former involvement in the compounding and manufacturing of pharmaceuticals to that of distributor and dispenser. However, an acceptance of role change is conditioned by the willingness of others to perceive and place a value on the need and the urgency for a redefinition of roles and responsibilities. Presently, perception of what a pharmacist is and what he can do is confused by what he actually does. The physician and the pharmacist *should be* working together and mutually concerned with patient care. But let's face it. For the most part, it just isn't so today. There are still many pharmacists who do not understand or refuse to accept their responsibility to serve as a source of professional guidance to the public. As emphasized by Ebert in an address before the APhA in Montreal, "The busy physician consults less with the pharmacist than he does with the detailman. At a time when the physician is inundated with new and potent pharmaceutical agents and with drugs which often cause serious side effects, he is more remote from the source of expert knowledge than in the past. Outside of the hospital, the physician rarely consults with the pharmacist."[6]

In a recent appearance before the American Association of Colleges of Pharmacy in Houston, The Honorable Paul G. Rogers, Chairman of the Subcommittee on Public Health and Environment of the U.S. House of Representatives, commented that "Pharmacists are the most *improperly* used health asset in this country. The lack of primary care involvement of today's pharmacist as a first contact or entry into the health delivery system is evident. As you know, clinical pharmacy became a required subject for all pharmacy schools with the passage of the Health Manpower Act. What we in the Congress were stressing was that your students should assume a more direct relationship with the patient with regard to drug misuse, abuse and nonprescription advice. However, pharmacists and schools of pharmacy have been reluctant to utilize their potential abilities. For the most part, they have been reluctant to meet head on the problems of the country in the health field."[7] Congressman Rogers went on to cite the missed opportunity for the pharmacist to play a meaningful role in monitoring methadone prescribing, which ultimately led to action by the Food and Drug Administration to remove methadone from retail pharmacies. The placing of paregoric on prescription-only status is another example where the public felt the need for stricter control over an item which pharmacy obviously could not handle.

Although I think that we all will agree that the challenge exists for the pharmacist to develop roles, which meet the needs of society, the services must, of course, be needed and must represent significant contributions to health care. It seems that a considerable part of the problem of role identification is that many of the functions which the pharmacist seeks to perform are now being performed by others. Brodie has said, for example, "The pharmacist must demonstrate either that he can perform a given role more effectively than others, or that *he* is the preferred person to perform the role."[8]

Each person in the current health professional scheme is searching for ways wherein *his* background or expertise can be utilized to the fullest. Derzon characterizes this phenomenon as a need for "trading up" of functions. He says that "Much of this started with the enlightened and overworked physician, who began to realize that with an allied health team around him he can in effect 'trade down' in order to increase his own professionalism while others on the team 'trade up' for the same reasons. This trading causes certain problems though, since most health professionals, having been conditioned by personal experience and exposure, are now competing in overlapping ways to improve their own contribution to patient care services. In essence, pharmacists will not broaden their roles successfully within and around the hospital or in the community unless physicians, in particular, want a change, nurses actively seek clinical advice and counsel, consumers see the value, and administrators are willing to invest in the necessary extras."[9]

In this regard, how effective has pharmacy been in communicating to physicians, nurses, and other health professionals concerning their service-oriented outlook and increased patient orientation? For that matter, how effective has pharmacy been in communicating the message among practitioners of pharmacy and its related industries? The biggest error made in communication is assuming that it has been accomplished. This error is most likely to occur in close relationships where people take things for granted.

### Relationship Between Pharmacy and Industry

Let me then briefly recall for you the relationship which exists between pharmacy and the industry, and hopefully, develop some understanding of the job pharmacy has or has not done in communicating its "clinical pharmacy" role (or for that matter, an appreciation of what industry has heard or wants to hear).

I need not go into much detail to establish for this audience the relationship which exists between pharmacy and the pharmaceutical industry. The industry, afterall, is an outgrowth of the profession and the product of the profession's concern for the development of standardized products, which could be made available via mass production techniques.

Early in the twentieth century, when chemotherapy and preventive medicine emerged as the cornerstones of medical practice, the ability to alter biochemical, physiological and pathological processes by the use of standardized and potent medications became an accomplished fact. The facilities, equipment and personnel required to manufacture products such as synthetic organic compounds, antitoxins and standardized plant and animal extracts soon exceeded the scope and capability of the traditional practice of pharmacy. These specific and potent products could only be produced in the highly sophisticated and complex environment of an industrial plant or laboratory. Except for a small number of preparations, primarily ophthalmics and dermatologicals, industrial laboratories today supply the greatest proportion of all prescription items used.

The emergence of this new technology at the manufacturing level had an important impact on the role of the pharmacist. The mortar and pestle yielded to the production efficiency of precision equipment and machines, and a partnership developed between the industry and the profession which has persisted and flourished. Together their talents and genius for research development and manufacturing skill have produced the innovative drugs which have revolutionized health care in the world. The cooperation which brought this about will continue to be essential for the emerging health care system of the future.

Those of us who are keenly aware of the practical aspects necessary for maintenance of this success will point to the not insignificant economic progress which has attended this partnership of pharmacy and the industry. In 1970, the American public spent 5.2 billion dollars for prescription medications, more than a three billion dollar increase from that spent in 1960. During that same period, the numbers of prescriptions dispensed in pharmacies rose from 743 million to 1.43 billion.[10] These figures will continue to rise according to all projections by industrial, government and private marketing experts.

In the light of what has been recorded as economic, professional and scientific progress on the one hand, and the confused appearance (as already discussed) of the merchant, semiprofessional but economically successful pharmacist seeking new roles for professional identification on the other hand, one might be excused for being slightly confused, somewhat bewildered, or perhaps at best, vaguely interested.

It should go without saying that in a relationship such as exists between the profession of pharmacy and the pharmaceutical industry, any serious activity on the part of one creates interest, curiosity and concern in the other. The activity and involvement in clinical activities on the part of the pharmacist is no exception. The industry has been aware that it is going on, watching its development, participating in and aiding with experimental and pilot projects, and generally making individual company assessments of where the movement is, what it will develop to be and how the company should prepare for it, if in fact, it should prepare for it. This evaluation is being made by companies with large and diversified interests as well as those with limited but specific involvement in one or two types of products, as well as by all of the types in between. The evaluation is being made by companies with hospital products only, those which deal exclusively with products handled in the community, those which deal directly with the pharmacist only and those which rely completely on wholesale distribution of their products. The company assessment is being made by people who are basically research-oriented, by those concerned with product development and design and those concerned with production as well as those involved in marketing, sales and distribution. This composite assessment will ultimately determine the company's policy — which, of course, will be different from that of any other company.

While we are reflecting about evaluating changes in systems and new roles for people, it is important for us also to remember that although we have witnessed many significant changes in our lifetime because of major breakthroughs in technology and science, there are still a few basic facts which temper change. First, remember that the practitioners, scientists, market analysts and others who are responsible for the current methods of practice in the profession and in the industry are themselves the products of the system. Their ideas and concepts which have resulted in considerable success are strongly ingrained. Remember also that the size and complexity of organization structures and the tendency for current successful operations to avoid risk are additional barriers to change. Why change when things are going well? Certain top management people are dedicated to resisting change because, for one thing, it is costly and, of course, there is the uncertain risk involved.

These points should be taken into consideration when evaluating the acceptance of pharmacy's new roles and their effect on the industry.

## Survey of Pharmaceutical Companies

In preparation for providing an industry-wide view of the effect of clinical pharmacy on the pharmaceutical industry, I wrote to about 30 companies and asked for reactions on this subject from people who are involved in research, development, marketing, sales and professional relations. Some of their comments are presented below.

1. "Clinical pharmacy requires a broad knowledge of reported clinical experience on specific products. Pharmacists will need more input on educational material of this type from industry, in order to have full and easy access to all significant clinical data. Industry should prepare to keep pharmacists in clinical pharmacy as well informed as it does the physician."
2. "Hospital and clinical pharmacies represent a growing market, especially with the advent of health maintenance organizations. Many HMO's have pharmacies associated with them, right on the premises. We recognize the growth which will occur in the pharmacy directly affiliated with a health care institution."
3. "We foresee a clinical pharmacist being an expert on drug dosage effects, toxicity and the like. The pharmaceutical industry will have to be concerned with providing this *pharmacist specialist* with information such as bioavailability, stability, adverse reactions, side effects, etc. The clinical pharmacist can then disseminate this information to the medical practitioner who would come to him as an expert on drugs. Consequently, since the clinical pharmacist is really meant to play a part in the health care system and will be very intimately connected with the physician and nurse, technical information dispensed by industry will have to take this into account."
4. "Managers and directors in various areas of the company criticize pharmacists as a group for their inability to work well with others as well as their inability to communicate effectively. Since clinical pharmacy is intended to motivate pharmacists to a more viable relationship with patients, physicians and other members of the health team, courses in clinical pharmacy will tend to improve the social lubrication of pharmacists."
5. "There are too many peculiarities and exaggerations in the thinking of some pharmacists regarding their proper role for the present and the future. Too many hospital pharmacists today are not satisfied with dispensing medications and devising improved systems for drug product delivery, but instead are setting themselves up as carping critics of the physician—pointing to overuse of drugs, irrational use, etc. They enjoy the position of the Monday morning quarterback, who has no responsibility for calling the plays, but enjoys picking apart the decision made by the coach during the heat of battle."
6. "Our company feels that the clinical pharmacist will develop as a specialist in pharmacy practice separate from the individual, who will maintain the dispensing or distributive function. We are spending a lot more time and money with pharmacists and with colleges of pharmacy trying to keep an eye on the developments."
7. "We have created special categories of personnel whose chief responsibilities are to maintain liaison with colleges of pharmacy and students who are receiving this patient-oriented training in hospitals associated with the colleges. Increasing time is being spent in our sales managers' meetings to acquaint our detailmen with the new programs."
8. "The new role of clinical pharmacy will involve the pharmacist in intensive study of the patient's requirements and the available drugs for his treatment, with all of their strengths and limitations. For example, drug complaints provide a riddle for most of the pharmaceutical industry. No one made it his business to know the details of the schedule of doses and their interplay with other medications. Hence, an untoward response appears from almost a void. The manufacturer must record the complaint as it arrives in his office, determine if it is of such a magnitude as to be reported to the FDA, and always hold his files open for inspection. His most diligent efforts to gain further information are usually fruitless, for mistakes are often suspected and usually impossible to confirm. The very presence of a clinical pharmacist will add scientific credibility in significant measure. Industry will really welcome this development."
9. "The term clinical pharmacy means different things to different people. It can be practiced at the community pharmacy level as well as in the hospital environment. The pharmaceutical industry, of course, is interested and concerned with improving patient care and the professional services required to accomplish this.

   "As I view it, drug interaction is closely related to clinical pharmacy, and herein lies great opportunity for pharmacists to serve their patients or customers—but how many are performing this function? Pharmacy associations, educators, some pharmacists and a few industry people talk about it, but I see very little done in actual practice."
10. "Clinical pharmacy has already had several implications for the pharmaceutical industry. Among the earliest was the unit-dose concept, which has in many respects, revolutionized pharmaceutical packaging, reduced medication errors, and given nurses more time for nursing care. Clinical pharmacy also brought to the pharmaceutical industry the concept of centralized intravenous additive programs and has greatly enhanced investigations of drug incompatibilities and interactions. The industry has worked closely with clinical pharmacists in active practice and, in addition, a number of firms have pharmacists oriented to clinical pharmacy on their own staffs."
11. "I'm afraid that the pharmacy schools are training their students for something which the students will have little opportunity to practice in most retail outlets. I think this is particularly true as the trend to more and more chain-type operations progresses. In addition, widespread acceptance by the medical profession is very far in the future. I liken this situation somewhat to the selling done by the pharmacy schools to get pharmaceutical industry to hire pharmaceutical chemists. This has been perpetuated for many years, and the pharmacy schools continue to turn out pharmaceutical chemists who find that the only place they can be employed is in another pharmacy school or that they must return to their basic pharmacy training and become product development oriented. Likewise, I am concerned that the emphasis now being placed on clinical pharmacy will produce a lot of young pharmacists, who are frustrated because they cannot perform in the manner in which they think they are qualified to perform."
12. "It is difficult to describe my concerns over the clinical

pharmacy program, but it is only when you consider that we have a number of pharmacists-scientists on our staff who have devoted their entire professional career to studying the biopharmaceutics of only a few drug products that you realize how unqualified an individual B.S. level pharmacist is to make these decisions and comparisons. I have seen numerous questionnaires from hospital pharmacists who ask a tremendous number of questions, and in essence, want a complete NDA sent to them so that they can determine whether the FDA has made a good or bad decision. I also gather from the construction of some of their questions that they have no idea which questions are really important and which ones are not. In order for the clinical pharmacist to function, he will have to have at his disposal the clinical data regarding the efficiency of the dosage form of each particular supplier. Whether or not this information will be made available during the next decade is perhaps questionable."

13. "An influence of clinical pharmacy is readily seen in the increased number of adverse drug reaction reports which we receive from pharmacists who are directors of drug information centers. I have been told that I practice 'clinical pharmacy' here with my company. If so, here is a description of my duties. When reports of adverse effects are received, my first objective is to determine what experience has been observed in this respect in the past. When this knowledge has been collected, I contact the attending physician, if possible, to provide him with our knowledge on the subject and to learn any clinical details which he may have observed. Once the investigatory phase is completed, we report the event to the FDA. These reports frequently provide recommendations for possible package insert changes. I am often involved in the medical liaison portion of defense preparation for product liability by providing answers relevant to a product at the time of an alleged incident. The fulfillment of my job is very dependent upon my pharmacy background and my experience with the company."

other hand, the movement isn't currently viewed as something which will sweep the country by storm. The greatest number of practitioners of pharmacy do not, cannot or will not provide the types of service inferred in clinical practice, and seemingly, are content with their current role. The image which these pharmacists portray represents pharmacy to the consumer, governmental agencies, other members of the health professions and the pharmaceutical industry. These pharmacists who perform the necessary and important functions of controlling and distributing medications to people who need medicine will be with us for a long time, and they will continue to have a significant influence on the drug industry.

The involvement of pharmacists in services related to health care will depend considerably upon the future direction and emphasis on health care created by new government programs and consumer pressures and the resultant methods of reimbursement associated with these services. To the extent that these pharmaceutical services are accepted and utilized, there will be a concomitant effort on the part of the industry to assist in their development. It would be unrealistic to believe, however, that the industry would support efforts which are viewed as mere shifting of professional responsibilities within the health team without attendant significant advantages for the patient.

## Conclusion

Although these represent but a handful of opinions and expressions, I do believe that I see a message coming through as it relates to the question of the effect of clinical pharmacy on the pharmaceutical industry. It is clear to me that although there is confusion as to what matter, shape, or form clinical pharmacy is or will be, there is a greater involvement among certain pharmacists, particularly those practicing in the hospital environment, to perform drug-related services beyond the distribution function. Companies are aware of this activity and have become increasingly involved to a varying degree depending upon the nature of their product mix. More and more industry attention is being focused on the pharmacists in the university and hospital setting where this clinical activity is greatest. This increased attention has also spilled over into the retail area as evidenced by changed detailing patterns and advertising which is geared more to the pharmacist's understanding of drugs rather than solely on profit incentives. On the

## References

1. Anon.: Report of the Reference Committee on Professional Affairs, *J. Amer. Pharm. Ass. NS 12:* 306–312 (June) 1972.
2. 1972 Reference Data of Health, Center for Health Services Research and Development, American Medical Association, Chicago, Illinois, p. 82.
3. Ibid., p. 126.
4. Report of National Advisory Commission on Health Manpower, Vol. I and II, Government Printing Office, Washington, D.C., November 1967.
5. Wilson, V. E.: Pharmacy and the Health Care Enterprise, *In* Graber, J. B. and Brodie, D. C. (eds.): Challenge to Pharmacy in the 70's, DHEW Publication No. (HSM) 72-3000, National Center for Health Services Research and Development, Rockville, Maryland, pp. 113-117.
6. Ebert, R. H.: Changes in the Health System, *J. Amer. Pharm. Ass. NS 9:* 402–404 (Aug.) 1969.
7. Rogers, P. G.: Increased Responsibility for Pharmacists, *Amer. J. Pharm. Educ. 36:* 367–371 (Aug.) 1972.
8. Brodie, D. C.: *Action in Pharmacy 4:* (Jan.) 1972.
9. Derzon, R. A.: Should the Pharmacists' Role be Redefined, *In* Graber, J. B. and Brodie, D. C. (eds.): Challenge to Pharmacy in the 70's, DHEW Publication No. (HSM) 72-3000, National Center for Health Services Research and Development, Rockville, Maryland, pp. 12-17.
10. Leibson, R. A.: *Drug Trade News:* (Mar. 8) 1971.

# 7 The Problem-oriented Medical Record: An Ideal System for Pharmacist Involvement in Comprehensive Patient Care

Lawrence R. Borgsdorf and Robert S. Mosser

The problem-oriented medical record (POMR), rapidly gaining prominence, has been shown to improve patient care and the education of health professionals who work with it. However, few reports have appeared in the literature with respect to the pharmacist's involvement with the POMR. A few pharmacists involved in comprehensive patient care have had the opportunity to work with the problem-oriented system, and this chapter discusses the results of this active involvement.

The design and organization of the POMR, its usefulness in the inpatient to outpatient comprehensive care flow pattern, and the feasibility of the system for interprofessional communication, teaching and peer evaluation, with special emphasis on the pharmacist's emerging clinical role, are discussed. In addition, guidelines for the pharmacist's participation with the system are presented to aid those who have not yet become involved with the concept of the POMR.

The problem-oriented medical record (POMR) is a logical method of documenting patient care in our complex health care system. It provides a systematic method of integrating the principles of the basic health sciences with the everyday activities of actual medical practice. Use of the problem-oriented system allows each member of the health care team to contribute toward the solving of patients' problems.[1]

The purpose of this chapter is to comment on the integration of the pharmacist into the health care team by skillful, informative use of the POMR.

## Components of the POMR

A review of the components of the POMR will serve as a base for further discussion. The POMR is organized into four major sections, each designed to promote the development of pertinent, patient-specific information in a logical, systematic way (Figure 1).

The foundation of the problem-oriented record is the data base. This base is a collection of patient-centered medical facts built from sources such as the medical history, physical examination, X-ray and other laboratory reports.

The next component is the problem list which serves as the coordinating or indexing element of the record. A problem is defined as anything which concerns the patient or requires management. The problem list is developed from the facts established in the data base, with each problem being assigned a number and a descriptive title which serve to identify the problem. The list is dynamic, i.e., problems are added or modified as new problems are identified and as old problems are clarified or resolved.

The third component is the plan, a logical sequence of problem-oriented orders which outline the rationale of diagnostic procedures, drug usage and other therapeutic measures. Each segment of the plan is identified by the appropriate problem number and title. The degree of care with which each plan is developed will determine the outcome of the problem.

The final component is the progress notes. The uniqueness of the problem-oriented progress notes is twofold. First, each entry is numbered and titled according to the specific problem to which it refers. Secondly, the progress notes are written in a manner which encourages and reflects logical, progressive thinking. Each note is developed as a series of successive steps, with each building upon the preceding step so that a logical conclusion, based on the data available for the particular problem, is reached. The acronym SOAP serves as a guide for developing the notes. A basic description of elements of the "SOAPed" progress note follows:

S—*subjective*—observations or statements made by the patient.

O—*objective*—data which are referable to, and useful in, evaluating the problem.

A—*assessment*—analysis of the subjective and objective data.

P—*plan*—steps to be followed as a result of the assessment reached in the preceding step.

An important feature of this system is the amount of "feedback" made possible. As data are accumulated, more sophisticated assessments are made. Subsequently, the problem list is refined and new plans are developed from the "feedback" generated by these assessments (as noted by wavy arrows in Figure 1).

*Figure 1. Components of the problem-oriented medical record*

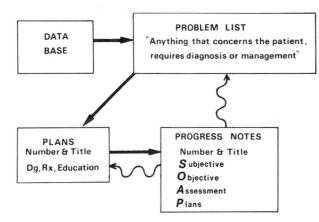

### Contribution to the POMR by the Pharmacist

Until recently, the POMR has been utilized primarily by physicians and nurses. Not long ago, our docent team pharmacists, who are involved in direct patient care activities at Kansas City General Hospital and Medical Center, began contributing to the system. While the full extent of their contributions has not yet been realized, the following areas of involvement have been clearly delineated.

The pharmacist can utilize each of the major components of the POMR for patient-oriented contributions which augment those of the other health team members.

Such data as a medication history and profile, and information on allergies and adverse reactions to drugs contribute significantly to the completeness of the data base. On occasion, potentially significant drug-related problems are identified and are added to the problem list.

The problem-oriented progress notes are an important component of the record with respect to the pharmacist's direct contribution in a problem-oriented format. By analyzing the subjective and objective data, a solid base is provided from which comments and recommendations concerning therapy may be made. The pharmacist can notate information such as a drug-of-choice for the particular problem, expected therapeutic results, possible side effects, recommended laboratory tests and other parameters to follow in evaluating therapy. Problem-oriented flow sheets, correlating medications with

therapeutic results, provide a means for developing objective data useful for evaluating therapy. The progress notes thus provide the pharmacist with a forum for directly contributing to improved drug therapy.

In addition, the pharmacist, by following the problem list, can predict and notate in the progress notes classes of drugs which should not be used in conjunction with a particular disease state listed as a problem.

### Use of the POMR by the Pharmacist

Although the pharmacist can contribute directly to the POMR, the record itself may assist the pharmacist in many activities. The problem-oriented system is organized so that each of the components can be utilized by the pharmacist not only for patient care, but for teaching and other activities.

Because drugs used for one disease may be contraindicated in other diseases, scanning of the problem list may help the pharmacist prevent the use of a contraindicated drug.

The problem-oriented orders provide a rapid screening device for determining if a drug is being used properly. It is a simple procedure to review the medications ordered and compare them to the problem for which they were ordered. Thus, the pharmacist may determine if a particular drug is being used rationally for a given problem.

Because all professionals dealing with the patient are encouraged to maintain the progress notes, the pharmacist, by following the notes prepared by other professionals involved in patient management, may often pick up clues of developing drug-related problems that are not initially recognized as being associated with drug therapy.

The role of the pharmacist as a clinical consultant may be readily visualized in the operating problem-oriented record system. By preparing problem-oriented progress notes, the pharmacist can document in a logical manner recommendations for therapy, alternative therapy and modifications of therapy. In addition, problem-orientation allows the pharmacist to direct his recommendations toward a specific goal.

### Use of the POMR in Comprehensive Inpatient-Outpatient Care

In many institutions, especially those used for teaching, professional staffs frequently rotate with a resulting lack of continuity in comprehensive patient care. This is often seen in many clinic settings where patients lament, "Oh no, another doctor. What happened to my old one?" Not only does this situation distress the patient, but the physician finds these circumstances annoying. In these cases, the physician usually has to start from the beginning with the patient by attempting to develop his own ideas of the patient's problems and, at the same time, by attempting to reconstruct previous therapy.

The POMR eliminates many of these frustrations. A current problem list and completed data base provide more than adequate patient information. By using the problem list as an index, the physician can go back in the record and evaluate previous notes made on a specific problem to see how the problem evolved and was assessed. For example, a·physician may readily evaluate a patient's hypertensive disease by going back into the record and chronologically reviewing each note with the specific problem number and title referable to hypertension. The POMR offers the same advantages for a pharmacist who is attempting to evaluate therapy for a particular problem or series of problems.

An additional advantage of a properly maintained POMR is its ability to help smooth the flow of inpatient-to-outpatient comprehensive care. During the initial hospitalization, a properly prepared problem-oriented plan is developed which outlines the anticipated therapeutic results and well defined end-points and parameters with which to evaluate therapy. The plan also contains suggestions for alternative therapy which may be utilized in the event primary therapy fails. In this way, a physician or pharmacist seeing a patient for the first time can get a well-defined idea of the patient's disease state and treatment program. Because the therapy and the goals of therapy are defined and can be easily followed, comprehensive care can be delivered with a minimum of confusion and a maximum of rationality.

The pharmacist may also contribute to comprehensive care by developing carefully prepared plans for drug therapy. If these plans include a summary of what is currently being used as well as alternative therapy, it will be much easier for a rational therapeutic program to be followed. This is particularly valuable in institutions where a pharmacist is available only for inpatient activities. If a patient being discharged from the hospital is to be followed in a clinic, the pharmacist can develop a therapeutic program on discharge which will help assure continuity of drug therapy outside the hospital.

Although primary emphasis so far has been with respect to patient care, the POMR also provides a mechanism for developing other activities such as interprofessional communication, teaching and peer evaluation.[2]

## Interprofessional Communication

The POMR, in addition to promoting the development of rational and logical thinking, promotes written and verbal communication among professionals. The problem orientation allows each professional to utilize his own special talents and knowledge as a contribution toward solving the patient's problems. Because the problems are identified and well-organized as opposed to traditional record-keeping systems, the pharmacist is afforded an opportunity to respond to particular problems. This response is not always one-way. Indeed, the POMR encourages communication between the pharmacist and other health professionals in an attempt to develop the most rational approach for solving a problem.

## Teaching

The problem-oriented progress notes also facilitate efficient and effective teaching. "SOAPing" of the progress notes, by outlining in each entry the basis of reasoning, integrates the basic principles of the academic health sciences with the daily activities of patient care or clinical sciences. Each member of the health care team has a unique contribution to make toward the education of students as well as other members of the team. For example, the input by the pharmacist on a given problem provides visibility for the thoughts, concepts and data specific to the pharmacist's expertise. Professionals from other specialty areas can then follow the notes and expand their own education with respect to the pharmacist's view.

Teaching is accomplished by providing specific objective data and then analyzing the data with respect to a particular problem. Properly prepared and maintained flow sheets correlating drug administration with therapeutic parameters add significantly to the assessment of therapeutic results. It is this assessment of the available data and their relationship to a specific patient which provides the basic teaching mechanism.

The progress notes provide a forum for the pharmacist to express to everyone involved in the care of the patient any concerns regarding important drug actions which should be watched. Warnings or alerts as to expected side effects, signs of toxicity and monitoring of specific parameters provide important educational material for students and all members of the health care team.

## Peer Evaluation

The POMR encourages peer evaluation. The emphasis on evaluation is placed on the progress notes because the system requires that professional abilities and thought processes be organized. An audit of the progress notes will allow for an evaluation of a given individual's clinical competency. The evaluation is not for physicians only; it is for each person who utilizes the POMR—the pharmacist, nurse, dietician and others.[3]

Peer evaluation is not a threat but, rather, a method whereby weaknesses in our abilities or knowledge can be identified and evaluated for the purpose of improving our performance. Our goal is to encourage education to increase capabilities or knowledge in areas determined to be deficient.

## Suggestions for Use of the POMR by the Pharmacist

The function and design of the POMR and some of the areas in which a pharmacist may become involved as an integral member of the health care team have been discussed. Use of the POMR opens the door to active, direct participation by the pharmacist at several levels of practice: medication history, consultation, evaluation of therapy and teaching. However, the pharmacist can be as useful only as his participation allows; therefore, optimal use of the POMR is essential. To maximize participation by the pharmacist, the following recommendations should be considered when utilizing the POMR:

1. Limit comments to the progress notes.
2. Always use the "SOAP" format for notes.
   S—obtain the subjective data yourself; contact with the patient is important.
   O—accumulate and notate the objective data so that they are applicable to the problem being discussed.
   A—assess the problem from a therapeutic or drug standpoint.
   P—limit comments to "suggestions," i.e. always allow room for discussion and further evaluation, being aware of the medical-legal implications of comments.
3. When asked a question about a particular problem, also notate your response in the progress notes for others to see and learn.
4. Develop flow sheets which will allow rapid and easy evaluation of the effectiveness of a given therapeutic regimen.
5. Follow through on recommended therapy—evaluate as to effectiveness, side effects and other pertinent points. Also point out interesting and valuable observations, providing an explanation whenever possible.
6. Carefully follow progress notes written by other members of the health care team. These often give clues to developing drug problems or therapeutic misadventures.

## References

1. Weed, L. L.: Medical Records, Medical Education, and Patient Care: The Problem-Oriented Record as a Basic Tool, The Press of Case Western Reserve University, Cleveland, Ohio, 1969.

2. Hurst, J. W.: Ten Reasons Why Lawrence Weed is Right, *N. Engl. J. Med. 284*:51–52 (Jan. 7) 1971.

3. Ellinoy, B. J., Schuster, J. S., Yatsco, J. C. and Rosenthal, L. C.: Pharmacy Audit of Patient Health Records—Feasibility and Usefulness of a Drug Surveillance System, *Amer. J. Hosp. Pharm. 29*:749–754 (Sept.) 1972.

# 8 Development of a Pharmacy Care Plan

Robert W. Bennett, Bobby G. Bryant, Allan L. Kelly, and
Jane D. Pruett

The concept of a pharmacy care plan, as developed on a pilot basis for patients in one nursing unit, is discussed.

The purpose of a pharmacy care plan is to promote systematic evaluation of the pharmacy-related needs of patients. There are five parts to pharmacy care plans: (1) initial assessment of the patients, (2) formulation of a plan by a pharmacist, (3) daily review and assessment, (4) medication counseling at discharge, and (5) postdischarge follow-up.

It is concluded that pharmacy care plans permit the pharmacist to make more efficient use of his time and permit him to document the results of his patient care activities.

The important role that a clinical pharmacist can play on the health team is a topic receiving considerable attention. Experience has shown us that a pharmacist is a valuable health team member if a well-defined and organized approach toward providing patient-oriented pharmacy services is used. Clinically-oriented pharmacy services in the hospital are often provided in a fragmented fashion, with some of the patients receiving most of the services while others get little or none. The real health care value of clinical pharmacy practice lies in providing these services to every patient in a manner which can be easily coordinated with the plans of all health team members. It is for these reasons that we developed a pharmacy care plan.

This plan was implemented in St. Elizabeth Hospital, a 380-bed nonteaching, private hospital in Lafayette, Indiana. A pilot program was conducted for a four-month period on one nursing unit. The pharmacist was stationed on the unit for 20 hours per week. The patient census of the unit varied from 23 to 33 patients during the study, and a total of 325 patients was involved.

## Rationale for Developing the Plan

Most other health care professionals already utilize written plans of patient care. Such plans identify all of the problems of each patient and the best approaches to solving these problems.

For example, when a physician admits a patient to the hospital, he formulates a medical care plan for that patient. The traditional medical record consists of an unintegrated conglomeration of information that the physician has hurriedly placed in the chart. This information may or may not be complete depending on the physician and the time he has to devote to the record. A clear idea of the patient's health problems and the plans for handling them is extremely difficult to obtain from this system of charting.

A valuable solution to this record-keeping dilemma, which is beginning to gain wide acceptance, is the problem-oriented medical record.[1] This approach to the organization and content of medical records clearly identifies the individual patient's problems and encourages systematic planning to resolve them. This problem-oriented system allows the physician to categorize the patient's problems and record them in separate areas of the chart. The physician then enters his plans for the patient and the patient's progress under that section of the problem-oriented chart which deals with that problem only. This written, categorized plan on the patient's problems allows both students and practitioners to easily determine specific goals for the patient, and is a valuable tool for effective treatment of patients as well as for the education of health professionals.

The nurse also formulates a plan of care for meeting the needs of the patient. The Joint Commission on Accreditation of Hospitals requires that a brief, written nursing care plan be prepared for each patient.[2] The basic purpose of the nursing care plan is to facilitate comprehensive, individualized nursing care. The nursing care plan outlines the nursing problems of a patient and the nursing procedures to be used to meet the patient's needs.

The nursing care plan is initiated at the time of admission when the nurse makes a written assessment of the patient using the physician's plan of care, the nursing history interview and the input from other health team members, such as pharmacists. A necessary adjunct to the planning is the daily care conference where the professional knowledge and experience of all members of the nursing team and other health team members can be utilized to appraise the success of, and make modifications in, the plan of care. It is important to note that the plan is continually evaluated and revised according to the changing needs of the patient.

### The Pharmacy Care Plan

In a similar manner, we initiated a pilot pharmacy care plan designed to more systematically evaluate pharmacy-related needs of patients. The pharmacy care plan devised for use in our hospital consists of five major parts:

1. Initial assessment of the patient,
2. Formulation of a plan by the pharmacist,
3. Daily review and reassessment,
4. Medication counseling at discharge,
5. Postdischarge follow-up.

### Initial Assessment of the Patient

Each patient admitted to the study unit was interviewed by the pharmacist as soon as practical. Before the interview, the pharmacist reviewed the patient's chart to determine the diagnosis, preexisting disease states and any other pertinent data. The interview usually began with a brief medical, family and social history to help the pharmacist gain an understanding of the patient. This initial discussion facilitated the next step, obtaining a thorough drug history, the importance of which has been demonstrated.[3,4] Information was sought on any prescription and nonprescription drugs administered during at least a month period prior to admission. During the interview, the pharmacist was able to acquire an understanding of the patient's feelings and fears in regard to his disease state and resultant hospitalization. He also gained insight into the patient's attitude toward drugs, drug therapy and his drug usage patterns. A further objective of the interview was to establish a rapport with the patient which would increase his confidence in the pharmacist.

The average interview time was about fifteen minutes. The information gathered in this interview and from the patient's chart was recorded in the patient's pharmacy record as the data base for the plan. From this data base, the patient's pharmacy-related needs could be determined. The identified needs might simply involve patient instruction or advice on a currently used medication, or they might require a systematic educational program on the relationship of drug therapy to the patient's disease condition.

An example of these two extremes of patient needs may help to illustrate the point. The first example involved a 55-year-old male patient admitted to the hospital with a fractured ankle. During the pharmacist's initial interview, the patient reported that he suffered from nasal stuffiness which he treated with decongestant nose drops prescribed by his physician. Over the past two months the nose drops had failed to relieve the patient's symptoms at the prescribed dose, so he had increased the amount and frequency of dosing. The patient was also continuing to use the drops at his bedside while in the hospital. The pharmacist explained to the patient that the abuse of his nose drops could lead to rebound vasodilatation and induce a chronic rhinitis. The patient agreed to discontinue the use of his drops for a while. When he was discharged from the hospital a few days later, he was relatively symptom-free and had decided to use his drops judiciously in the future. This was the only pharmacy-related problem found in this patient and it required less than five minutes for the pharmacist to advise him. The only other time devoted to this patient, besides the initial interview, was the monitoring of his drug therapy which consisted only of pain relievers.

The other extreme of pharmacy involvement is exemplified by a 20-year-old male admitted to the hospital in diabetic coma. Past history on the patient showed that he had been a known diabetic since age nine with repeated hospitalizations because of poor control. The clinical signs and symptoms at the time of this admission were typical for diabetic acidosis. The laboratory test results confirmed the diagnosis, showing extreme hyperglycemia and glycosuria, positive serum and urine ketones and badly deranged electrolytes. After the patient was under control, the pharmacist interviewed him to assess his current knowledge of diabetes and to determine what his needs were. It was found that the patient did not accept the fact that he had diabetes and felt that the disease drastically impaired his enjoyment of life. The pharmacist found that the patient's understanding of what causes diabetes was very poor. The young man did not understand why he had to take insulin, the signs and symptoms of diabetic coma and hypoglycemic reactions, or how certain external influences (e.g., infections) could affect his disease. Also, the patient neglected testing his urine for sugar and acetone, did not rotate his insulin injection sites and had difficulty reading the calibrations on his insulin syringe because of severe diabetic retinopathy. The patient's fiancee knew nothing about diabetes and marriage plans were in the near future. It took the pharmacist about 20 minutes to conduct this interview.

### Formulation of a Plan

After the pharmacy-related needs of each patient were determined, the pharmacist formulated a plan to meet those needs. Again using the diabetic patient as an example, planning indicated that all health team members should talk with the patient to impress upon him that properly controlled diabetes would not impair his life style. The patient was then given, and told to read, a diabetic teaching pamphlet. The pharmacist then outlined on his planning sheet the approach he planned to take toward teaching this patient about his disease (Figure 1). It took about ten minutes to write out these plans. For most patients the planning was not this extensive and required only two or three minutes to formulate.

In this hospital, the team nurse is responsible for gathering the various plans for the patient and coordinating their implementation. This makes it possible for all team members to quickly learn all of the plans for the patient, and the scheduling of discussions with the patient prevents overloading him with too many details at once.

*Figure 1. Pharmacy care plan for a diabetic patient*

| Patient's Name: | Room No.: |
|---|---|
| **Problems and Plans** | **Remarks** PPF-10 |

1) Acceptance of disease; to be discussed by all team members. Emphasize that many famous and active people have diabetes and it changes their life very little if at all. A diabetic can hold most any kind of job, marry, have children, play sports, do most anything he wants. Emphasize that the key to success is his willingness to follow the rules that will be set down for him.

1) 10/1/72 - The patient was very interested, asked many questions.

2) Discussion of what causes diabetes, why insulin must be taken. Patient should have read pamphlets before this discussion. Review the symptoms of diabetes.

2) 10/2/72 - Patient seemed to understand what he was being told but then was unable to repeat the information when asked questions. Needs reinforcement.

3) Review the symptoms of diabetic coma and insulin shock. Supplement the discussion with the charts contained in the pamphlets.

3) 10/3/72 - Patient understood and had experienced most of these symptoms. Will probably need to review them again.

4) Discuss the balance between diet, insulin, and exercise, and how external factors, i.e., infections, can throw the balance off.

4) 10/4/72 - Patient responded well. Needs to talk with nurses and dietician.

5) Reinforce teaching on foot care and good hygiene.

5) 10/5/72 - Patient understands. I only wonder if he will do this. Needs more work.

6) Work with nurses on instruction for giving insulin injections, sterile technique, rotating sites, etc. Obtain a pre-set syringe to show the physician.

6) 10/6/72 - Patient is doing well. We can only hope he will continue to do so at home. Physician decided against pre-set syringe at this time after observing patient drawing up his own insulin.

7) Talk to fiancee about diabetes and giving insulin. Dietician will discuss diet with her. Nurse and physician will also talk to her.

7) 10/5/72 - She understands quite well, and is willing to do whatever is necessary.

8) Review everything with the patient and answer any questions.

8) Patient seems to understand what he has been told and is able to recall it. Has a good attitude and accepts his disease much better.

9) Counsel on discharge medications.

9) Patient discharged only on insulin, no counseling required.

Prepared by: _____

### Daily Review and Reassessment

At the beginning of the day, the pharmacist quickly reviewed each patient's chart to check for new information. The pharmacist would briefly visit with the patient, if necessary, to gain more information or to evaluate a particular response to drug therapy. A few patients with more complex problems sometimes required five or ten minutes for the pharmacist to review them each day. However, most patients required only a quick check.

The patient's drug therapy was monitored, using a drug-rationale-results profile system first used at the University of Maryland[5] (Figure 2). Both objective and subjective parameters of response to drug therapy were followed. Problems involving the patient's drug therapy were discussed with the proper health team member. Most of the problems were identified as a result of following the parameters of patient response. To avoid wasting time, care was taken to follow only those parameters deemed pertinent to the patient. Observations made by the pharmacist were recorded in the patient's pharmacy record.

Next, the pharmacist began teaching the patients for whom he had developed plans. The results were recorded in the remarks section of the planning form. The plan was continually reassessed by the pharmacist according to the needs and response of the patient. This function usually required a total of about 40 minutes of the pharmacist's time per day.

### Medication Counseling at Discharge

Through discharge counseling, the pharmacist and other health team members can help the patient make the difficult transition from the controlled hospital environment to the home situation. First, the pharmacist conducted a brief review of the principles which were important to the patient's continued health and well being. The review was then followed by counseling of the patient on his medication. The value of discharge medication counseling and effective methods to use have been established in previous studies.[6-9] Medication counseling by the pharmacist averaged five minutes per patient receiving counseling. However, many patients did not need this interview because the pharmacist's education program had already included medication counseling.

*Figure 2. Patient profile sheet used for monitoring drug therapy*

| DIAGNOSIS: | Congestive Heart Failure |
|---|---|
| DRUG ALLERGIES: | None |
| Admitted: 8/28/72 | PATIENT ADDRESSOGRAPH DRR-103 |

| Drug and Dose | Rationale | Parameter of Effects |
|---|---|---|
| Digoxin 0.25 mg Stat and q AM. 8/28 | Cardiotonic to increase the force of myocardial contraction. | Pulse rate EKG Improvement of CHF signs Electrolytes esp. K+, renal function GI symptoms (dig. toxicity) |
| Furosemide 40 mg Stat and q AM 8/28 | Diuretic to relieve the edema | Urine output and fluid intake Serum electrolytes esp. K+ Body weight Orthostatic hypotension BUN, Blood glucose, serum uric acid |
| Chloral Hydrate 500 mg HS 8/28 | Hypnotic | Gastric irritation Sleep patterns Hangover |
| Milk of Magnesia 30 cc prn 8/28 | Laxative | Effectiveness Diarrhea Renal function ($Mg^{+2}$ retention) |

### Postdischarge Follow-Up

Postdischarge follow-up of the patient by the pharmacist is not a common practice today and it was not a required function of the pharmacist in this program. However, the role of the pharmacist continues to grow and this practice should become a necessary function of the pharmacist. The purpose of the follow-up is to prevent the occurrence of problems in the patient's drug regimen. The pharmacist could talk with the patient when he returns for outpatient visits. If the patient is not scheduled for outpatient visits, the pharmacist could either make arrangements to talk with him at designated intervals or discuss the patient with his community pharmacist to arrange for continuing service. Many community pharmacists already perform this service quite well, and it should become the duty of the hospital-based pharmacist to supply them with the patient information they need. A written record of the postdischarge follow-up should be maintained.

For example, the diabetic patient was followed for three weeks postdischarge. The patient called the pharmacist every three days to discuss his insulin dosage, urine tests and general feelings. Following this period, the patient was told to check with his community pharmacist who was then detailed on the patient. The patient has not had to be readmitted to the hospital and has been well-controlled.

### Conclusion

Our experience in the pilot program demonstrated that the pharmacy care plan is a valuable tool for the pharmacist to allow him to better distribute his efforts to areas where they can do the most good. It forced the pharmacist to develop objectives and set goals for each patient. Recording the plans that were made for the patient insured that no plans were overlooked. Since every patient on the unit was included in the planning, there was greater continuity in the clinical services offered by the pharmacist. Patients for whom no pharmacy-related needs were identified required very little attention by the pharmacist.

The pharmacy care plan also strengthened the pharmacist's professional stature. Since the plan was written, the other health team members had an opportunity to read and become acquainted with what services the pharmacist was providing to the patient. In addition, when the pharmacist used the pharmacy care plan, benefits to the patient were documented and the pharmacist's presence in the patient care area was more easily justified.

The pharmacy care plan has been implemented as an on-going program on the original nursing unit, and pilot projects are currently in progress on two additional units. Since the plan is not yet hospitalwide, we have not been able to evaluate it on a large-scale basis. However, the excellent rapport that we have been able to establish with patients, pharmacists, physicians and nurses makes us feel confident the plan works well.

### References

1. Weed, L. L.: The Problem-Oriented Medical Record, First Edition, Dempco Reproduction Service, Cleveland, Ohio, 1969.

2. Accreditation Manual for Hospitals, Hospital Accreditation Committee, Joint Commission on Accreditation of Hospitals, Chicago, Illinois, p. 52, Standard V, December 1970.

3. McHale, M. K. and Canada, A. T.: The Use of a Pharmacist in Obtaining Medication Histories, *Drug Intel. Clin. Pharm.* 3:115–119 (Apr.) 1969.

4. Wilson, R. S. and Kabat, H. F.: Pharmacist Initiated Patient Drug Histories, In *Clinical Pharmacy Sourcebook*, pp. 346-350.

5. Fletcher, H. P., Department of Clinical Pharmacy Services, University of Maryland Hospitals, Baltimore, Maryland, personal communication.

6. Greiner, G. E.: The Pharmacist's Role in Patient Discharge Planning, In *Clinical Pharmacy Sourcebook*, pp. 163-167.

7. Latiolais, C. J. and Berry, C. C.: Misuse of Prescription Medications by Outpatients, *Drug Intel. Clin. Pharm.* 3:270–277 (Oct.) 1969.

8. Melahy, B.: The Effect of Instruction and Labeling on the Number of Medication Errors Made by Patients at Home, *Amer. J. Hosp. Pharm.* 23:282–292 (June) 1966.

9. Maddock, R. K.: Patient Cooperation in Taking Medicine, *J. Amer. Med. Ass.* 199:169–172 (Jan.) 1967.

# 9 Clinical Pharmacy Services: Prognostic Criteria for Selective Patient Monitoring

W. Wayne Young, J. Edward Bell, Vincent E. Bouchard, and Sister M. Gonzales Duffy

Reported are the results of a study designed to formulate an equation for use in selecting patients who should be monitored by pharmacists.

In formulating a predictive mathematical equation for selective patient monitoring, chi-square tests and Mann-Whitney U tests were employed to test 48 separate patient variables. Multiple regression analysis and discriminant functions were employed to test groups of significant variables. The discriminant function finally formulated contained the following variables: the number of abnormal laboratory test results; the number of drugs in the pharmacist drug history; the type of admission; the patient's admission temperature; the physician's estimate of the patient's initial status; and the number of different diagnoses at the time of admission. The discriminant function correctly classified 78% of the "contribution" patients and 86% of the "no contribution" patients in a retrospective study of 150 patients. Any written communications to the physician were operationally defined as contributions to patient care. The equation was very accurate (79% to 87%) for orthopedic surgical and medical patients retrospectively.

The discriminant function was less accurate for the prospective study. It was found that 61% of the "contribution" patients and 54% of the "no contribution" patients were classified correctly. The equation was very accurate for predicting orthopedic surgical and medical "contribution" patients.

The discriminant function decision score can be adjusted to select a variable number of patients dependent upon the desired patient load for a clinical pharmacist (i.e., a lowering of the decision score includes more patients). The equation was used to predict a clinical pharmacy staffing pattern for the entire hospital in which the study was conducted.

In a previous report the methodology of a research project to formulate a mathematical function for selective patient monitoring was described.[1] The study was done in three parts: (1) a retrospective study to formulate a discriminant function was performed and 48 patient-related variables were screened for their individual and combined discriminant ability; (2) a prospective study was performed to test two discriminant functions; and (3) a study was made in order to project a staffing pattern for the hospital in which the study was performed.

The discriminant function, a mathematical linear function, was selected to be used because of its usefulness in delineating groups. In this study, contributions to patient care were defined as written communications by the pharmacist to the physician in the patient's chart. Patients were separated into "contribution" and "no contribution" groups.

## Retrospective Study Results

The types of statistical analyses of variables in the retrospective study are summarized in Table 1. Some variables proved to have little or no discriminant ability at all. Thirty-two variables had significant discriminant ability. These variables are listed in Table 2 with their $z$ scores and associated $p$ values (in descending order). This list was used to select variables for discriminant analyses and the stepwise multiple regression analyses. Inspection of Table 2 revealed that certain variable groups were able to differentiate the "contribution" and "no contribution" groups. These general variable groups are listed in Table 3.

Multiple correlation and stepwise regression analyses were performed on combinations of significant variables for screening purposes. This analysis was also applied to the variables entering the final discriminant function (the results of the first four preliminary regression analyses are not presented in this publication and the reader is referred to the entire research report). The results of these analyses were used to formulate discriminant functions. Variables included in the four regression equations had the greatest potential predictive ability and for that reason were tried in the discriminant function program.

Any variable which entered a regression equation and

## Table 1. Statistical Tests Utilized in the Analysis of Variables in the Retrospective Study

| STATISTICAL TEST | GENERAL CATEGORY OF VARIABLE |
|---|---|
| Chi-square test | Sex |
| | Race |
| | Physician estimate of initial status |
| | Type of admission |
| Mann-Whitney U test | Age |
| | Previous admissions |
| | Drugs prior to admission per physician history |
| | Drugs prior to admission per pharmacist history |
| | Different diagnoses |
| | Drugs administered |
| | Laboratory tests performed |
| | Written consultation requests |
| | Specialty services utilized |
| | Nursing directives |
| | Abnormal laboratory test results |
| | Nursing information units |
| | Physician visits |
| | Temperature and pulse |

## Table 2. P Values, Z Scores and Variables with Discriminant Ability

| TEST | | VARIABLES |
|---|---|---|
| Mann-Whitney U | | |
| $p<$ | $z$ | |
| 0.00003 | −6.64 | Total number of abnormal laboratory results |
| 0.00003 | −5.82 | Abnormal laboratory results—first 24 hours |
| 0.00003 | −5.49 | Drugs prior to admission: pharmacist history |
| 0.00003 | −5.21 | Total number of laboratory tests performed |
| 0.00003 | −4.93 | Total number of different diagnoses |
| 0.00003 | −4.74 | Abnormal laboratory results—second 24 hours |
| 0.00003 | −4.60 | Laboratory tests performed—first 24 hours |
| 0.00006 | −4.34 | Different diagnoses—first 24 hours |
| 0.00006 | −4.22 | Nursing information units—first 24 hours |
| 0.00006 | −4.04 | Total temperature |
| 0.00007 | −3.99 | Total number of nursing information units |
| 0.00007 | −3.97 | Laboratory tests performed—second 24 hours |
| 0.00009 | −3.89 | Drugs prior to admission: physician history |
| 0.0001 | −3.81 | Total number of drugs administered |
| 0.0001 | −3.73 | Drugs administered—second 24 hours |
| 0.0002 | −3.55 | Total number of physician visits |
| 0.0006 | −3.26 | Drugs administered—first 24 hours |
| 0.0006 | −3.26 | Admission temperature |
| 0.0015 | −2.96 | Physician visits—first 24 hours |
| 0.0018 | −2.91 | Total pulse |
| 0.0021 | −2.86 | Nursing information units—second 24 hours |
| 0.0023 | −2.83 | Temperature at 24 hours |
| 0.0052 | −2.56 | Physician visits—second 24 hours |
| 0.0075 | −2.43 | Total number of specialty services used |
| 0.0143 | −2.19 | Admission pulse |
| 0.0150 | −2.17 | Specialty services used—first 24 hours |
| 0.0207 | −2.04 | Pulse at 24 hours |
| 0.0222 | −2.01 | Temperature at 48 hours |
| 0.0274 | −1.92 | Pulse at 48 hours |
| 0.0287 | −1.90 | Specialty services used second 24 hours |
| Chi-square | | |
| $p<$ | $x^2$ | |
| 0.0005 | 19.128 | Type of admission |
| 0.005 | 8.938 | Physician estimate of initial status |

also had a significant $p$ value was used in discriminant functions for the 24-hour time period and the 48-hour time period. In the original retrospective data collection the pharmacist history was not always available. It was found that both the pharmacist and physician histories were significant discriminators between the "contribution" and "no contribution" groups and, therefore, entered the regression equations. For this reason each discriminant function was tried with either one or the other of the two drug history variables. This was of practical importance since it was desirable to have a discriminant function which was reasonably accurate at the end of the first 24 hours of the patient's stay. In addition, it was hoped that a function could be derived that did not utilize data generated from the pharmacist history since the pharmacist could then evaluate the patient more rapidly.

Twelve discriminant functions were analyzed for their predictive ability. The accuracy of these functions ranged from 67% to 80% for the "contribution" group of patients and 79% to 88% for the "no contribution" group of patients. The discriminant function variables tested were derived from regression equations. Twenty-four-hour values were tested and compared to 48-hour values. Each function was tested with data generated from either the physician drug history or pharmacist drug history. Discriminant functions were tried with variables from regression equations using data from both drug histories and variables fom both time periods. Two discriminant functions tested contained transgenerated variables (i.e., summation variables for the entire 48-hour time period). Transgenerated variables which proved significant in a regression equation were tested in a discriminant function.

The tenth discriminant function tested was derived from the final multiple linear regression equation. This particular discriminant function classified the two pa-

## Table 3. Significant General Variables

| GENERAL VARIABLE |
|---|
| Abnormal laboratory test results |
| Drugs prior to admission: pharmacist history |
| Drugs prior to admission: physician history |
| Laboratory tests performed |
| Different diagnoses |
| Nursing information units |
| Temperatures |
| Drug doses and intravenous fluids administered |
| Physician visits |
| Pulses |
| Specialty services utilized |
| Type of admission |
| Physician estimate of initial status |

tient groups studied as accurately—with fewer variables —as any of the other discriminant functions. It was noted that all of the variables in the tenth discriminant function except one (cumulative diagnoses) could be obtained within 24 hours of the patient's hospital stay. Since the correlation of 24-hour different diagnoses and cumulative different diagnoses was high (0.9565), it was decided to use a discriminant function (discriminant function eleven) derived from the tenth discriminant function using 24-hour diagnoses. This was the final and best discriminant function.

It was also necessary to derive a discriminant function (number twelve) using the same variables as discriminant function eleven and substituting the physician drug history for the pharmacist drug history as a variable in order to perform the projected staffing pattern study.

### The Discriminant Function

The discriminant function is a combination of ratios between the variables, hence, it may be multiplied by any convenient constant without altering its accuracy.[2] For ease of use of the function, the coefficients of the variables were multiplied by a constant in order that the coefficient of the first variable would be unity. Table 4 lists the actual coefficient estimates and the final coefficients used after the estimates were multiplied by 1/0.004.

In order to adjust the discriminant function to a midpoint of zero, the average discriminant score, 64.85 (obtained by using the average values of the variables), was subtracted as a constant in the discriminant function

equation. This adjusted the linear scale in such a way that any "contribution" classification was a positive discriminant score and any "no contribution" classification was a negative discriminant score. Zero was the discriminant decision score.

The final discriminant function equation was:

$$X_1 + 0.4076872X_2 + 0.2847117X_3 + 0.6224251X_4 - 1.731900X_5 + 1.753979X_6 - 64.85127 = D(I)$$

where:
- $X_1$ = number of drugs in pharmacist history
- $X_2$ = number of 24-hour different diagnoses
- $X_3$ = number of abnormal laboratory test results reported at the end of the first 24 hours
- $X_4$ = admission temperature in Fahrenheit degrees
- $X_5$ = type of admission—emergency = 1, elective = 2
- $X_6$ = physician estimate of status—no distress = 1, some distress = 2
- $D(I)$ = discriminant score.

This discriminant function equation was derived from a regression equation. The correlation coefficients and results of the regression analyses of the variables of the final discriminant function are presented in Tables 5 and 6. R is the coefficient of multiple correlation and $R^2$ indicates the proportion of variance that can be explained by all the variables at that point in the regression equation. The F score and $p$ value associated with each step of the regression are given.

As more variables entered the regression equation, the amount of explained variance increased from 0.401 to 0.498. The predictive ability of the discriminant function (and of the regression equation) was 77.5% for the "contribution" group and 85.5% for the "no contribution" group. The predictive ability of the regression equation, when 14 variables had entered the equation (0.498 explained variance), was 84% for the "contribution" group and 87% for the "no contribution" group. The inclusion of the extra variables beyond the first six adds very little power to the regression equation and cannot justify the increased amount of time it would require for the pharmacist to collect the data. These six variables were found to be sufficient in their predictive ability and would be expected to be practical for actual use.

Table 7 lists the variables of the final discriminant function in the order in which they entered the regression equation (from which the function was derived) and the average values for each variable in the "no contribu-

#### Table 4. Coefficient Estimates and Adjusted Coefficients of the Final Discriminant Function

| VARIABLE | ESTIMATE | FINAL COEFFICIENT |
|---|---|---|
| Pharmacist drug history | 0.004281599 | 1.0000000 |
| Different diagnoses—first 24 hours | 0.001745553 | 0.4076872 |
| Abnormal laboratory test results—first 24 hours | 0.001219021 | 0.2847117 |
| Admission temperature | 0.002664974 | 0.6224251 |
| Type of admission | −0.007415301 | −1.731900 |
| Physician estimate of initial status | 0.007509833 | 1.753979 |

#### Table 5. Correlation Coefficients of Variables of the Discriminant Function

| VARIABLE ENTERING EQUATION | | $X_1$ | $X_2$ | $X_3$ | $X_4$ | $X_5$ | $X_6$ | $X_7$ |
|---|---|---|---|---|---|---|---|---|
| Abnormal laboratory results | $X_1$ | 1.0000 | | | | | | |
| Pharmacist drug history | $X_2$ | −0.0867 | 1.0000 | | | | | |
| Type of admission | $X_3$ | −0.3736 | −0.0020 | 1.0000 | | | | |
| Admission temperature | $X_4$ | 0.1401 | 0.0284 | −0.2162 | 1.0000 | | | |
| Physician estimate of status | $X_5$ | 0.3718 | −0.1994 | −0.4077 | 0.2426 | 1.0000 | | |
| Different diagnoses | $X_6$ | 0.3454 | 0.2150 | −0.2656 | 0.1858 | 0.0497 | 1.0000 | |
| Pharmacist contribution | $X_7$ | 0.3760 | 0.3529 | −0.3708 | 0.2878 | 0.2604 | 0.3573 | 1.0000 |

**Table 6. Results of Regression Analysis of Variables of the Discriminant Function**

| STEP | VARIABLE | R | R² | F | p< |
|---|---|---|---|---|---|
| 1 | Abnormal laboratory test results | 0.376 | 0.141 | 24.37 | 0.001 |
| 2 | Pharmacist drug history | 0.539 | 0.291 | 31.04 | 0.001 |
| 3 | Type of admission | 0.588 | 0.345 | 12.23 | 0.001 |
| 4 | Admission temperature | 0.616 | 0.379 | 7.84 | 0.001 |
| 5 | Physician estimate of status | 0.624 | 0.390 | 2.57 | — |
| 6 | Different diagnoses | 0.633 | 0.401 | 2.60 | — |

**Table 7. Average Values of the Variables of the Final Discriminant Function**

| | AVERAGE | | |
|---|---|---|---|
| VARIABLE | NO GROUP | YES GROUP | BOTH GROUPS |
| Abnormal laboratory test results—first 24 hours | 1.1867 | 4.4000 | 2.7933 |
| Pharmacist drug history | 1.0267 | 2.3867 | 1.7067 |
| Type of admission | 1.5600 | 1.2000 | 1.3800 |
| Admission temperature | 98.3920 | 99.1333 | 98.3707 |
| Physician estimate of initial status | 1.1067 | 1.3200 | 1.2133 |
| Different diagnoses—first 24 hours | 2.2533 | 3.3333 | 2.7933 |

tion" group, the "contribution" group and the combined groups.

The six variables were used in five "stepwise" discriminant functions using the first two variables which entered the regression equation, adding one at a time. The percent accuracy obtained after each addition was recorded. The results of these five analyses are given in Table 8. These results show that as the number of variables increased—the linear distance ($D^2$) between the two groups generally increased—the F statistic decreased although the level of significance remained the same. Each variable improved the predictive ability of the discriminant function.

The average discriminant score for the "no contribution" group was −2.08713 and for the "contribution" group was 2.08713. Mahalanobis' D-square, the linear distance between the groups, was 4.17426. The F statistic was 25.210 with six and 143 degrees of freedom which was significant ($p < 0.001$).

The discriminant scores of all 150 patients were plotted in histograms. Figure 1 shows the total distribution of the discriminant scores. Figure 2 shows both distributions ("contribution" and "no contribution" groups) superimposed. The discriminant scores ranged from −5.65368 to 9.67833. The range of scores of the "contribution" group was greater than the range of scores of the "no contribution" group. This might reflect that there is a wider variety of patients for whom the pharmacist makes a contribution. The majority of the "contribu-

**Table 8. Stepwise Discriminant Function Analysis of the Six Variables of the Final Discriminant Function**

| | | | | % ACCURACY | |
|---|---|---|---|---|---|
| NUMBER OF VARIABLES | D² | F | p< | CONTRI-BUTION | NO CONTRI-BUTION |
| 2 | 2.888847 | 53.80448 | 0.001 | 71.0 | 83.0 |
| 3 | 3.511909 | 43.30933 | 0.001 | 76.0 | 81.5 |
| 4 | 3.919329 | 36.00198 | 0.001 | 77.5 | 81.5 |
| 5 | 3.800941 | 27.73896 | 0.001 | 77.5 | 83.0 |
| 6 | 4.174266 | 25.20992 | 0.001 | 77.5 | 85.5 |

tion" patients had discriminant scores which ranged from −3.50 to 6.0 (a range of 9.50). The majority of the "no contribution" patients had discriminant scores which ranged from −5.50 to 0.00 (a range of 5.50). This reflected the predictive ability of the discriminant function for each of the two groups.

It was possible that the actual "contribution" patients were misclassified by the discriminant function as "no contribution" patients if: the patient had a discriminant score typical of a "no contribution" patient; some aspect of the patient's therapy or disease influenced the pharmacist to write a communication; the pharmacist wrote

*Figure 1. Discriminant scores of all patients in the retrospective study*

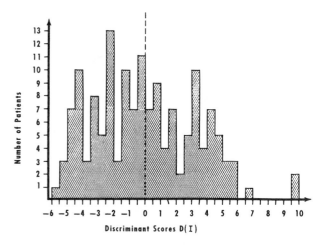

*Figure 2. Discriminant scores of all patients in the retrospective study ("contribution" and "no contribution" groups superimposed)*

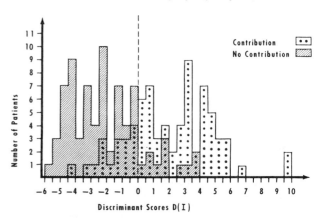

a note which was of questionable therapeutic importance; or the discriminant function was in error. It was also possible that actual "no contribution" patients were mis-classified by the discriminant function as "contribution" patients if: the pharmacist was unaware of a contribution he might have made or was unavailable at critical times when he might have written a communication; the patient had unusually high values for any of the four numerical variables in the discriminant function inconsistent with his clinical status; or the discriminant function was in error.

If the discriminant function equation itself is in error, it is possible that the error can be attributed to some unmeasured or unmeasurable quality of the patient. In the 12 discriminant functions that were tested, 356 scores out of 1,800 were misclassifications. Sixty-five patients were misclassified at least once. Six patients were never classified correctly. The same 15 patients (10% of the total) were misclassified in 75% of the discriminant functions. It is possible that these 15 patients had some unknown qualities about them which were not measured. These patients accounted for 9 of the 17 misclassifications in the "contribution" group and 6 of the 11 misclassifications in the "no contribution" group. It is possible that for these patients there were no measurable prognostic variables which could be incorporated into a predictive mathematical equation, and only human judgment seasoned with clinical experience could be the deciding factor. As the expertise of the clinical pharmacist increases, it is hoped that a sharper delineation between the two groups might evolve.

**Type of Illness**

The type of illness of the patient was not given a numerical score nor analyzed by discriminant function techniques. The numbers of patients in each of the seven general illness categories included in the study are given in Table 9. The types of illness were grouped into a 2 × 2 contingency table for chi-square analysis (see Table 10). The results of this analysis showed that there is a significant relationship between the major categories of

illness and the pharmacist's ability to contribute to patient care.

The results of the retrospective study for patients in each illness category are presented in Table 11. Only the orthopedic surgical and medical groups contained sufficient numbers of patients for any pattern to be established.

Figure 3 shows the discriminant scores of the orthopedic surgical patients in the retrospective study. Seven of the 45 patients (15%) were misclassified. Sixty-nine percent of the orthopedic surgical patients were in the "no contribution" group. These 31 patients represented over 41% of the "no contribution" patient population in the retrospective study. The results indicate that over two-thirds of the orthopedic surgical patients studied were "no contribution" patients and 87% of these pa-

**Table 9. Type of Illness Related to Pharmacist Contribution (Ungrouped Contingency Table)**

| TYPE OF ILLNESS | TOTAL | CONTRI-BUTION | NO CONTRI-BUTION |
|---|---|---|---|
| Orthopedic surgical | 45 | 14 | 31 |
| Orthopedic medical | 6 | 2 | 4 |
| Medical | 67 | 40 | 27 |
| Medical surgical | 8 | 5 | 3 |
| Neurosurgical | 3 | 2 | 1 |
| Neurosurgical medical | 10 | 8 | 2 |
| General surgery | 11 | 4 | 7 |

**Table 10. Type of Illness Related to Pharmacist Contribution (Grouped Contingency Table)**

| TYPE OF ILLNESS | CONTRI-BUTION YES | NO | RESULTS |
|---|---|---|---|
| Surgical patients: Medical surgical Orthopedic surgical Neurosurgical General surgery | 25 | 42 | $X^2 = 8.0$ $C = 0.22$ $0.02 > p > 0.01$ |
| Medical patients | 40 | 27 | |
| Mixed: Orthopedic medical Neurosurgical medical | 10 | 6 | |

**Table 11. Accuracy of the Final Discriminant Function Related to Major Type of Illness of Patients in the Retrospective Study**

| TYPE OF ILLNESS | CONTRIBUTION GROUP NO. OF PATIENTS | NO. CLASSIFIED CORRECTLY | % CLASSIFIED CORRECTLY | NO CONTRIBUTION GROUP NO. OF PATIENTS | NO. CLASSIFIED CORRECTLY | % CLASSIFIED CORRECTLY |
|---|---|---|---|---|---|---|
| Orthopedic surgical | 14 | 11 | 79 | 31 | 27 | 87 |
| Medical | 40 | 33 | 83 | 27 | 22 | 81 |
| Orthopedic medical | 2 | 2 | 100 | 4 | 3 | 75 |
| Medical surgical | 5 | 4 | 80 | 3 | 3 | 100 |
| Neurosurgical | 2 | 1 | 50 | 1 | 0 | 0 |
| Neurosurgical medical | 8 | 5 | 63 | 2 | 2 | 100 |
| General surgery | 4 | 2 | 50 | 7 | 7 | 100 |
| Total | 75 | 58 | 78 | 75 | 64 | 86 |

Figure 3. Discriminant scores of the orthopedic surgical patients in the retrospective study

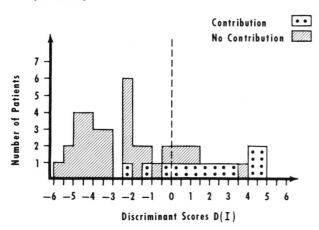

Figure 4. Discriminant scores of the medical patients in the retrospective study

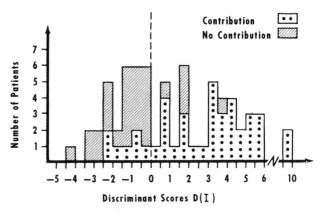

tients were calssified correctly. In the orthopedic surgical category, 79% of the "contribution" patients were classified correctly, however, these patients represented only 19% of the "contribution" patients in the retrospective study.

Forty-five percent of the patients in the retrospective study were medical patients. Of these 67 patients, 40 were in the "contribution" group. Eighty-three percent of the "contribution" patients and 81% of the "no contribution" patients were classified correctly. Figure 4 shows that the majority of the "no contribution" medical patients had discriminant scores of 0.0 to −1.5 and the "contribution" patients had a wider variety of discriminant scores with the majority of scores between 3.0 and 6.0.

The final discriminant function was very accurate (between 79% and 87%) for the two largest categories, orthopedic surgical and medical, which accounted for 75% of the patients or 112 of 150. The number of patients in the remaining categories was too small for any conclusions to be drawn on the accuracy of the discriminant function equation.

**Prospective Study Results**

The patients included in the prospective study were selected from the two units in the hospital covered by clinical pharmacy services. One unit was the teaching unit of the hospital from which patients were selected who had unusual disease states or interesting therapeutic or diagnostic problems. The majority of the patients on this unit naturally have more communications written in their charts by the pharmacists than would be expected on a normal medical unit. The other unit consists mainly of orthopedic patients. Since June 1, 1971, one of the two clinical pharmacists assigned to this unit had been selectively monitoring the patients using his own judgment as to his potential for patient care contributions. In order to test the final discriminant function it was necessary to select patients currently being moni-

tored and, as stated the majority of the patients were expected to be "contribution" group patients.

Seventy patients were randomly chosen for this study. Forty-two of the 70 patients chosen were readmissions. The data needed for discriminant functions eleven and twelve were collected on each patient and discriminant scores for each patient were calculated. The actual classification of each patient was determined by reviewing the patient's medical record daily until discharge to check for a written communication. The predictive discriminant scores were compared to the actual classification results in order to determine the accuracy of each of the discriminant functions.

The results of the prospective study showed that 57 of the 70 patients were actually in the "contribution" group. Since the final discriminant function was less accurate for the "contribution" group in the retrospective study, it was expected that the results of the prospective study would reflect this lower degree of accuracy. The results of discriminant function eleven showed that 46 of the 70 patients were correctly classified prospectively; 68.5% of the "contribution" patients and 54% of the "no contribution" patients were classified correctly. Thus, the discriminant function was less accurate for the prospective study.

Figure 5 is a histogram of the discriminant scores of the 70 patients in the prospective study calculated from

Figure 5. Discriminant scores of patients in the prospective study

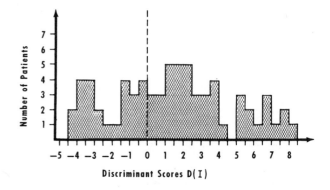

discriminant function eleven. The scores are within the same range as in the retrospective study. This is an indication of the validity of the discriminant function. The majority of the scores were between −4.50 and +4.50. Figure 6 shows the discriminant scores of the "contribution" and "no contribution" groups superimposed. As in the retrospective study, the "contribution" group had a wider range of scores whereas the "no contribution" group covered a smaller range.

*Figure 6. Discriminant scores of patients in the prospective study ("contribution" and "no contribution" groups superimposed)*

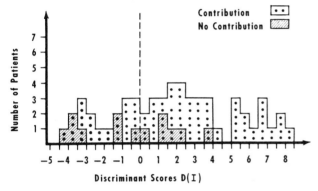

Many of the patients in the "contribution" group who were misclassified had scores between −2.0 and 0.0. The scores of the "contribution" group ranged from −4.5 to +8.5. The "no contribution" patient scores were between −4.5 and +4.0. Since there were only 13 patients in the "no contribution" group, the results may be unrepresentative of the accuracy of the "no contribution" predictive ability of the discriminant equation.

Figure 7 shows the discriminant scores of the medical patients in the prospective study. This was the largest group in the prospective study accounting for 41 of the 70 patients. The discriminant function correctly classified 35 of the 41 patients (85.5%). In the retrospective study, 82.5% of the "contribution" medical patients and 81.5% of the "no contribution" medical patients were correctly classified compared to 87.5% of the "contribution" medical patients and 33% of the "no contribution" medical patients in the prospective study. The discriminant function appears to be quite accurate for the "contribution" group of the medical patients prospectively.

*Figure 7. Discriminant scores of medical patients in the prospective study*

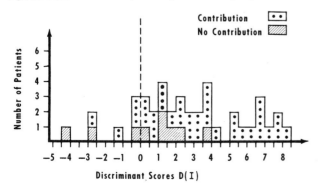

Figure 8 shows the discriminant scores of the orthopedic surgical patients in the prospective study. Eight of the 13 "contribution" patients were classified correctly. The one "no contribution" patient was classified correctly. Prospectively, the function had fair ability to classify the orthopedic surgical patients.

Chi-square analysis was performed on the accuracy of predictions for "contribution" patients in the retrospective and prospective studies (Table 12). A chi-square value of 0.90 was calculated indicating that the null hypothesis (no difference between the prospective and retrospective predictive ability of the discriminant function for "contribution" patients) can be accepted ($.5 < p < .3$).

The retrospective and prospective results compared favorably, especially for the "contribution" group patients. The percent accuracy obtained in both studies using the best discriminant function (number eleven) is shown in Table 13. As previously explained, a decreased accuracy was expected for the prospective patients because of the unusually high number of "contribution" patients in the prospective study; 77.5% of the "contribution" patients in the retrospective study and 68.5% of the "contribution" patients in the prospective study were classified correctly.

The difference in accuracy of the two discriminant function studies can be accounted for by many different factors. The error inherent in variable measuring and subsequent derivation of the discriminant function might account for some difference. The change in clinical personnel and the advance in clinical expertise of the remaining personnel during the time period between the studies might account for a greater number and variety of patients benefitting from clinical pharmacy

*Figure 8. Discriminant scores of orthopedic surgical patients in the prospective study*

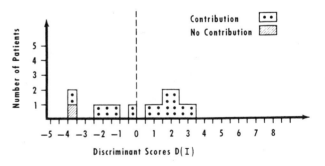

**Table 12. Analysis of the Predictive Ability of the Discriminant Function for "Contribution" Patients in the Retrospective and Prospective Studies**

| STUDY | PREDICTIONS FOR "CONTRIBUTION" PATIENTS | | RESULTS |
| | RIGHT | WRONG | |
| --- | --- | --- | --- |
| Retrospective | 58 | 17 | $X^2 = 0.90$ |
| Prospective | 39 | 18 | $0.5 > p > 0.3$ |

**Table 13. Results of Retrospective and Prospective Studies**

| | NO. OF PATIENTS | | % CORRECTLY CLASSIFIED | | | | | |
| | | | CONTRIBUTION | | NO CONTRIBUTION | | ALL PATIENTS | |
| TYPE OF ILLNESS | A[a] | B[b] | A | B | A | B | A | B |
|---|---|---|---|---|---|---|---|---|
| Medical | 67 | 41 | 82.5 | 87.5 | 81.5 | 33.3 | 82.0 | 85.5 |
| Orthopedic medical | 6 | 4 | 100.0 | 0 | 75.0 | — | 83.5 | 0 |
| Orthopedic surgical | 36 | 14 | 78.5 | 61.5 | 87.0 | 100.0 | 84.5 | 64.0 |
| Medical surgical | 8 | 2 | 80.0 | 50.0 | 100.0 | — | 87.5 | 50.0 |
| Neurosurgical | 3 | 1 | 50.0 | 100.0 | 0 | — | 33.3 | 100.0 |
| Neurosurgical medical | 10 | 0 | 62.5 | — | 100.0 | — | 70.0 | — |
| General surgery | 11 | 8 | 50.0 | 20.0 | 100.0 | 100.0 | 82.0 | 50.0 |
| Total | 150 | 70 | 77.5 | 68.5 | 85.5 | 54.0 | 81.5 | 66.0 |

[a] Retrospective study.
[b] Prospective study.

services. Spurious correlations in the retrospective variable analysis could have caused the importance of any variable to be over- or under-estimated.

### The Discriminant Score

Zero was defined as the discriminating score between the "contribution" and "no contribution" groups in the retrospective and prospective studies because it was the midpoint between the linear array of the two groups. In practice, any value on the scale can be chosen to be the discriminant decision score. If a clinical staff is small, it may be desirable to use a higher (+2.0 or +3.0) discriminant score as a decision point to selectively monitor the few patients who have the greatest potential for pharmacist contribution. With a larger clinical staff a lower discriminant score (−1.0 or −2.0) may be the most useful decision point.

A lower discriminant decision score will definitely predict a greater number of "contribution" patients, however, some of these patients will be misclassified. The risk of misclassifying the "no contribution" patients is not significant because the risk involved in monitoring these patients is only the loss of a pharmacist's time, and that may be minimal since the patient is a "no contribution" patient. On the other hand, there may be a risk involved in not monitoring a potential "contribution" patient because of a misclassification. In general, the majority of the misclassifications occurred between −2.0 and +2.0. This region may be thought of as a "doubtful" region where the difference between "contribution" and "no contribution" patients is nebulous.

As stated previously, a greater degree of accuracy in classifying the "contribution" patients can be obtained by defining −2.0 as the discriminant decision score. The accuracy of the best discriminant function (number eleven) in classifying "contribution" patients with discriminant decision scores of 0.0 and −2.0 is presented in Table 14. The increase in predictive ability of the discriminant function was 15.5 percentage points for all "contribution" patients. The decrease in predictive ability of the discriminant function was from 54% to 31% for the "no contribution" patients. However, the total accuracy increased from 66.0% to 74.5% when the discriminant decision score was lowered to −2.0. Increases in the predictive ability of the discriminant function occurred in the medical, orthopedic surgical and orthopedic medical categories.

### Discriminant Function Twelve

The pharmacist drug history was one of the variables included in discriminant function eleven. In order to perform the clinical staffing pattern study, the discriminant function had to be applied to patients from units of the hospital not covered by clinical pharmacy services. Therefore, it was necessary to derive a discriminant function of comparable accuracy using the physician drug history. The accuracy of discriminant functions eleven and twelve, with both discriminant decision scores, is presented in Table 15. These results support

**Table 14. Accuracy of Discriminant Function Eleven in Correctly Classifying "Contribution" Patients Using Discriminant Decision Scores of 0.0 and −2.0**

| GROUP | NO. OF PATIENTS | DISCRIMINANT SCORE 0.0 | | DISCRIMINANT SCORE −2.0 | |
| | | NO. CORRECT | % CORRECT | NO. CORRECT | % CORRECT |
|---|---|---|---|---|---|
| Medical | 32 | 28 | 87.5 | 31 | 97.0 |
| Orthopedic surgical | 13 | 8 | 61.5 | 11 | 85.0 |
| Orthopedic medical | 4 | 0 | 0 | 3 | 75.0 |
| General surgery | 5 | 1 | 20.0 | 1 | 20.0 |
| Medical surgical | 2 | 1 | 50.0 | 1 | 50.0 |
| Neurosurgical | 1 | 1 | 100.0 | 1 | 100.0 |
| Total | 57 | 39 | 68.5 | 48 | 84.0 |

## Table 15. Accuracy of Discriminant Functions Eleven and Twelve Using 0.0 and —2.0 Discriminant Decision Scores

| | % CORRECTLY CLASSIFIED | | | |
|---|---|---|---|---|
| | DISCRIMINANT SCORE 0.0 | | DISCRIMINANT SCORE —2.0 | |
| GROUP | FUNCTION ELEVEN | FUNCTION TWELVE | FUNCTION ELEVEN | FUNCTION TWELVE |
| Medical | 85.5 | 73.0 | 83.0 | 80.5 |
| Orthopedic surgical | 64.0 | 54.0 | 84.5 | 86.0 |
| Orthopedic medical | 0 | 0 | 75.0 | 75.0 |
| General surgical | 50.0 | 25.0 | 25.0 | 62.5 |
| Medical surgical | 50.0 | 50.0 | 50.0 | 50.0 |
| Neurosurgical | 100.0 | 100.0 | 100.0 | 100.0 |
| Overall % | 66.0 | 61.5 | 74.5 | 76.0 |

the use of the discriminant function with the physician history to estimate the results of the discriminant function with the pharmacist history.

### Clinical Staffing Pattern Study

In order to determine the projected "total patient load" for an expanded clinical pharmacy service in the institution studied, a representative random sample of patients from nursing units not covered by clinical pharmacy services was selected. The sample was taken from 351 hospital beds with each unit being sampled for 25% of the beds on that unit. The data needed for discriminant function twelve with the physician drug history were collected on each patient, and each patient's discriminant score was calculated. The individual discriminant scores for those 90 patients are plotted in Figure 9.

Forty of the 90 patients (44.4%) sampled had positive discriminant scores. Based on that percentage, it is expected that 156 patients out of 351 beds would have positive discriminant scores. A correction factor of +5% was applied to approximate the number of patients discriminant function eleven would have predicted if it had been used. The corrected projection was 173 patients.

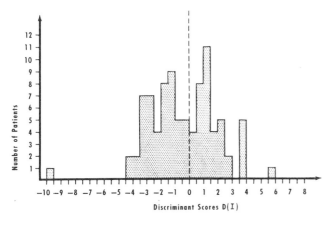

*Figure 9. Discriminant scores of patients in the clinical staffing pattern study and not in the prospective study*

The projected "total patient load" would be 269 patients which also includes the patients in the burn unit, intensive care unit and cardiovascular recovery. However, since the patient census of the hospital is normally 90% of the bed capacity, this figure would then become 242 patients or approximately 50% of the patients in the hospital excluding obstetric, gynecology, pediatric and nursery patients. To adequately monitor 242 patients, eight full-time equivalent pharmacists would be required based on the current 30 patients per pharmacist workload.

The projection of eight pharmacists was made utilizing a discriminant decision score of zero. If the discriminant decision score is decreased or increased, staffing requirements also decrease or increase. Table 16 shows the number of full-time equivalent pharmacists required and the "total patient load" when the discriminant decision score is —2.0, 0.0 and +2.0.

## Table 16. Staffing Requirements for Projected Patient Loads Based on Various Discriminant Decision Scores

| DISCRIMINANT DECISION SCORE | PROJECTED TOTAL PATIENT LOAD | NO. OF FULL TIME EQUIVALENT PHARMACISTS REQUIRED |
|---|---|---|
| +2.0 | 117 | 4 |
| 0.0 | 242 | 8 |
| —2.0 | 323 | 11 |

### Summary and Conclusions

A discriminant function was derived from a retrospective study of 150 patients monitored by clinical pharmacists at Mercy Hospital in Pittsburgh. The 150 patients were operationally defined as "contribution" or "no contribution" patients on the basis of whether or not the pharmacist wrote a communication on the drug information communication sheet. The discriminant function was used to calculate a score for each patient, and based on the value of that score, the patient was predicted to be a member of one of the two patient groups. The discriminant function retained good discriminating ability with a minimum number of variables and the data needed for the function could be collected 24 hours after the patient's hospital admission. The variables included in this discriminant function were: the patient's admission temperature in Fahrenheit degrees; the number of different diagnoses; the number of abnormal laboratory test results; the physician's estimate of the patient's initial status; the type of hospital admission; and the number of drugs being taken prior to admission as recorded by the pharmacist. The function correctly predicted 82% of the 150 patients when a discriminant decision score of 0.0 was used.

The discriminant function was cross-validated in a prospective study of 70 patients. Again based on discriminant scores, patients were predicted to be members of either of two patient groups. The results showed that by using a discriminant decision score of 0.0, the function correctly classified 66% of the 70 patients. When the discriminant decision score was lowered to −2.0 the function correctly classified 74.5% of the 70 patients. The function was particularly accurate for medical patients in the prospective study and generally had acceptable predictive ability.

Although the primary intent of the research was to develop a discriminant function for selective patient monitoring, the function was also used to estimate a "total patient load" for the clinical pharmacy service in the hospital. Using this estimate, it was possible to predict the number of full-time equivalent pharmacists required for a hospitalwide service.

The function can be readily used on hospital units. Assuming a medication history is an automatic procedure performed by the clinical pharmacist, the time required to collect the data and calculate the discriminant score for one patient is estimated at less than five minutes. Adjusting the discriminant score allows for variation in selection of patients for monitoring. By this selective process the pharmacist can effectively concentrate his activities on those patients who have the greatest potential for benefit from his clinical services.

### References

1. Young, W. W. et al.: Clinical Pharmacy Services: Prognostic Criteria for Selective Patient Monitoring, *Amer. J. Hosp. Pharm. 31*: 562–568 (June) 1974.

2. Rao, C. R.: Advanced Statistical Methods in Biometric Research, John Wiley and Sons, Inc., New York, 1951, p. 237–258, 286–338.

# 10 Techniques for the Selection and Monitoring of Patients by Pharmacists

Clyde R. Cooper

Specific guidelines for monitoring patients by pharmacists and the criteria necessary to avoid wasted man-hours in uncomplicated cases are presented.

A macroscopic patient review is discussed. This includes evaluating the patient's location in the hospital, age, allergies, laboratory tests, diet, diagnosis, and drug therapy. This preliminary review combined with the patient interview and patient rounds with the medical staff are the means proposed to determine whom to monitor. Those patients with the greatest need are then followed microscopically utilizing a patient profile form. The patient's therapy, drugs, laboratory tests, and nonlaboratory parameters are recorded on this form.

A detailed discussion and examples of the microscopic review and use of the patient profile form are included. Methods are suggested on how to communicate pharmaceutical judgments to the medical and nursing staff.

Clinical pharmacy has been aptly defined by many recognized leaders in patient-care oriented programs.[1-6] However, implementation of the defined concepts is handicapped, generally, by unawareness of the necessary procedures and techniques for practicing the clinical concepts. Some clinical pharmacy pioneers have proposed drug monitoring forms called pharmaceutical service records or drug profile sheets.[6] But specific guidelines as to how the clinical pharmacist can determine which patients to monitor, the criteria necessary to avoid wasted effort and man-hours in uncomplicated cases, and the monitoring techniques necessary have been generally neglected.

To establish a common understanding of clinical pharmacy, the concept must be redefined. Clinical pharmacy means a closer alliance of the pharmacist with the physician and nurse—an alliance whose goal is to provide specific drug-patient information to the medical and nursing staffs and a critical eye for possible oversights in the prescribed drug therapy. Monitoring techniques refer to those procedures used to observe, record or detect information necessary for clinical pharmaceutical judgments. To make these judgments and to function effectively, the clinical pharmacist must be knowledgeable about drug therapy and be familiar with, and read regularly, the medical and pharmaceutical journals. In addition, he needs to throw away the shackles of the old attitudes of servitude—he must approach the physician with confidence, leaving his temerity behind.

What does the clinical pharmacist hope to accomplish through monitoring patient therapy? This is a very important, recurring question. The clinical pharmacist hopes to improve drug prescribing practices by promoting safe and efficacious drug usage. His purpose is to:

1. Act as a resource person for drug therapy

2. Detect and prevent potential drug interactions and adverse reactions

3. Detect and prevent possible drug-induced diseases

4. Detect and prevent potential drug toxicities[7]

His goal is to provide better patient care by offering pharmaceutical service beyond the traditional verification of seemingly inappropriate dosages and clarification of ambiguous orders.[8] He hopes to offer more than the traditional storage and distribution of drugs.

Presupposing the existence of a Kardex, the pharmacist in the clinical environment needs to review on a macroscopic level the patient's drug regimen. In-depth analysis of every patient and complete drug histories are not possible, unfortunately, as the pharmacist is often simultaneously responsible for drug distribution for 80-130 patients, supervision of pharmacy technicians and clinical monitoring activities. If, however, the technicians have had an in-hospital

63

training program and are capable of transcribing drug orders and dispensing first doses as needed, the pharmacist can function more independently and effectively.

## The Macroscopic Review

The macroscopic review, or overview, entails reviewing the patient's location within the hospital and his age, allergies, laboratory tests, diet, diagnosis and drug therapy. Any of these items of information may indicate  problem areas warranting closer monitoring.

### Patient's Location

Patients in the intensive care areas of the hospital should be monitored routinely. These patients are the most critically ill and the most apt to develop complications from what otherwise might be tolerable omissions or commissions in drug therapy. The intensive care patients are more likely to be receiving cardiac glycosides, diuretics and oto-hepatotoxic antibiotics. Their electrolyte balance and acid-base levels are often more unstable.

### Patient's Age

The older and debilitated patient, like the intensive care patient, is more susceptible to disease processes. The geriatric patient is often treated for cardiac difficulties, delayed wound healing, decubitus ulcers and orthostatic complications. The pediatric patient and the neonate, too, pose special problems. For example, tetracycline may cause increased intracranial pressure with bulging of the fontanelle in the neonate, while the one- to three-year-old child may develop permanent molar discoloration and enamel hypoplasia.[9] In the prenatal state, tetracycline may cause inhibition of bone growth with delayed formation.[10] Another example would be the greater incidence of hemophilus influenza in children under three and the specific indication, therefore, for ampicillin rather than penicillin G.[11]

### Allergies

If the history is obtained and interpreted accurately, allergies are significant indicators in monitoring the patient, as they reveal potential drug complications. Patients who are subject to allergic conditions, such as asthma, pollinosis and food allergies, are more apt to experience adverse reactions to drug therapy than those without a history of allergy.[12] Patients allergic to ampicillin may be sensitive to cephalothlin or dicloxacillin.

Emphasis must be placed on accurate allergy data. Often normal drug side effects (such as diarrhea with ampicillin) may be reported as an allergy, or a patient's fears (for example, toward narcotics and "sleeping pills") may be reported as an allergy. For interpretation as a drug allergy, the clinical pharmacist must determine the symptomatology of the allergic response, the time of occurrence, its relation to the method of administration and the source of the information.

### Laboratory Data

Problems associated with drug-laboratory test interactions have been reported.[13] If the pharmacist is aware of potential difficulties in this area, unreliable results and needless expense can be avoided. Further discussion of laboratory tests and their significance to the clinical pharmacist will follow under the discussion of the microscopic review.

### Diet

Dietary restrictions are important considerations as well. The sodium content of medicinals is important when sodium is restricted in the diet. The amount of potassium is also important if hyperkalemia exists. The use of the Michigan Regional Drug Information Network articles on sodium and potassium content of selected medicinals is highly recommended.[14-15] Even the time of administration of the drug, whether with or without food, may influence drug absorption and effectiveness.

### Diagnosis

The diagnosis is one of the most important determinants in selecting patients to be monitored. Obstetrical patients are in the hospital for what is usually an uncomplicated, normal and healthy experience. If, however, an obstetrical patient develops toxemia, this would warrant monitoring attention. In coronary care patients admitted for myocardial infarctions, problems of hypoprothrombinemia and drug interactions due to oral anticoagulant therapy exist. When correlated with the patient's drug therapy, the diagnosis may reveal the extent of possible drug problems.

### Drug Therapy

The drug therapy is the major determinant in monitoring patients. For example, if the patient is on digitalis and diuretics, the pharmacist should monitor the potassium level. The meaning of potassium levels and normal variations associated with acid-base levels must be known. Ability to calculate the recommended maintenance digoxin dosage based on creatinine clearance according to Jelliffe's formula is essential.[16] For patients on antibiotic therapy the pharmacist should ask if the dose prescribed is within the range recommended for the infecting organism. Is the antibiotic the best choice in view of the patient's BUN, creatinine clearance and culture and sensitivity? If the drug selected is not so indicated, what drug and what dosage will provide an adequate minimum inhibitory concentration to irradicate the infection? Antinauseant medication is not always selected thoughtfully. Diphenhydramine, while good for inhibiting some types of nausea, is inadequate for others. Trimethobenzamide, while good for morning sickness, is not reliable for the nausea associated with post-x-ray or cytotoxic cancer therapy. In patients being treated with cancer chemotherapeutic agents and hematopoietic toxic compounds, one must watch for the complication of leukopenia. If the patient experiences leukopenia, should the drug be withheld or prophylactic antibiotic therapy started? Treatment with drugs possessing nephrotoxic or hepatotoxic properties are an indication to watch the patient's creatinine and SGOT and SGPT levels.

## Patient Interviews

An additional method of determining whom to monitor is interviewing every new patient upon admission to the hospital. While inquiring about drugs taken prior to admission, past drug complications and pertinent familial history, the clinical pharmacist can correlate the information with the probability for drug interactions and monitoring needs.

## Patient Rounds

Still another approach is patient rounds with the medical staff. The pharmacist is perhaps of greatest use here because suggestions can often be made prior to determining therapy. In addition, the pharmacist can better correlate drug therapy from personal contact on rounds with the medical staff than he can by reading their progress reports. Additional medical knowledge gained here is often transferrable to other patients as well.

## The Microscopic Review

Once the macroscopic review is completed and the selection of patients to be monitored has been made, these patients should then be reviewed microscopically or in greater detail.

The microscopic review should include recording on a patient profile form all the data necessary for a reliable, critical drug-patient analysis. General areas to be included on the patient profile form are laboratory tests (chemistry, hematology, urinalysis, coagulation data, culture and sensitivity), diagnostic tests (EKG, EEG), fluid balance, vital signs, drug allergies, history, diagnosis and surgical procedures, medications prior to admission, medications administered within the hospital, as well as progress notes, nurses' and pharmacists' notes. Not every parameter on the form should necessarily be recorded. Only those factors pertinent to each individual patient's care should be recorded. The diagnosis, age, sex, weight and attending physician are basic items of information.

## Patient's Drugs

Knowledge of the patient's drugs, both current and discontinued, is essential for the possible influence they may have on subsequent therapy. Was the patient on a MAO inhibitor within the last seven days? Has the patient proved to be refractory to some preceding therapy that would alter the choice of current drug therapy? Is the patient taking diphenylhydantoin with a tricyclic antidepressant or a phenothiazine? If these drugs are taken concurrently, the pharmacist should check the nurses' notes for a decrease in the patient's seizure threshold and occurrence of dizzy spells. Tricyclic antidepressants and guanethidine given simultaneously should make the pharmacist check for nullification of the effect of the guanethidine by the tricyclic antidepressant. The potassium levels of patients receiving cardiac glycosides and diuretics should be checked routinely as potassium depletion may increase the sensitivity of the heart to the toxic effects of the cardiac glycosides. Examples of drug interactions deserving of the pharmacist's attention may be found in Hartshorn's *Handbook on Drug Interactions*[17] and other similar publications.

## Laboratory Data

The laboratory data are of paramount importance. The CBC may indicate dehydration, allergic responses, cytopenic responses and infections. Chloramphenicol, phenylbutazone and other drugs can cause blood dyscrasias; therefore, periodic CBC's should be performed and watched on patients receiving these drugs. The urine is checked for bacteria count, WBC's and RBC's to determine urinary tract infections and renal damage. Knowledge of the urinary $p$H is essential for accurate and successful drug therapy with sulfonamides, methenamine and many other drugs dependent on the proper urinary $pH$ for effectiveness or excretion percentages. Glucose levels, fasting or postprandial, are important if correlated with diuretic or steroid therapy. Awareness of organic and inorganic iodides in preparations administered to patients will help to eliminate invalid PBI results. Probenecid administered with the combination product of propoxyphene and aspirin-phenacetin-caffeine or chlorthalidone would suggest checking for increased uric acid levels. Mefenamic acid in peptic ulcer patients would indicate checking for occult blood. Each drug suggests checking for different laboratory values.

### Nonlaboratory Data

Nonlaboratory determinations—the impressions of the clinician, the patient's chief complaints, past medical history, temperature, pulse, respiration and blood pressure are also factors to be noted. The electroencephalogram, electrocardiogram, lung scan, brain scan and intravenous pyelogram can all be important determinants in patient monitoring. Any complications that develop such as rashes, convulsions, cardiac or respiratory arrests or sudden changes in the patient's condition should be noted.

### Case Studies

The following are taken from experiences at Kettering Memorial Hospital. By routinely monitoring intensive care patients, the pharmacist discovered a woman seventy years of age with elevated temperature and first to third degree burns around the neck and throat being treated for *Proteus miralbis* in the burn area with cephalexin 250 mg qid. The culture and sensitivity data showed the microorganisms to be resistant to cephalosporins. After correlating this with the pharmacology of cephalexin and the probability of development of *Pseudomonas* in burns, the pharmacist suggested administration of gentamycin topical cream and substitution of ampicillin in place of the cephalexin. The patient generally improved and attained a normal body temperature.

Diagnosis was considered to be an important determinant in the macroscopic review. While reviewing one patient's Kardex, it was noted that the patient was admitted for gastroenteritis and dehydration. Further investigation revealed that prior to hospital admission, and also currently, the patient was receiving a combination product of reserpine and chlorthalidone for hypertension. The diuretic component of this combination was recognized by the pharmacist as a possible contributor to the dehydration. This information was pointed out to the physician who subsequently modified the patient's drug therapy.

Allergies are obvious pertinent factors. Patients have reported allergies to propantheline because of dry mouth or diphenhydramine because of drowsiness. One patient admitted to the hospital for tachycardia and heart palpitations secondary to an allergic response to an "antihistamine" revealed something else: The patient took, without his physician's knowledge, two "diet pills" along with one "cold capsule." What developed was a summation in response from the two amphetamine tablets and the ephedrine in the cold capsule. The pharmacist, by identifying the medications, and as a result of his conversations with the patient, expedited an accurate diagnosis and discharge.

The progress note on one patient revealed that the physician was about to discontinue as ineffective the antiparkinson drug, levodopa. The patient profile showed that the patient was on methyldopa concurrently. When the actions of both drugs—one blocking the formation of dopamine and the other being a precursor to dopamine—was explained, the methyldopa was discontinued. The patient was discharged shortly after with his parkinsonism controlled.

Another patient, admitted for acute thrombophlebitis and uncontrolled diabetes while being treated with diethylstilbesterol 5 mg qd, hydrochlorothiazide 25 mg qd and chlorpropamide 250 mg qd, showed a fasting blood sugar of 178 mg/100 ml, 188 mg/100 ml, 211 mg/100 ml (Folin and Wu) on successive days. The patient's physician was advised of the hyperglycemic effect of the diuretic and the steroid. There was a need for the steroid since the patient had a history of prostatic cancer. In discussions with the physician, primary emphasis was placed on the hyperglycemic effect of the diuretic. The value of furosemide and ethacrynic acid in causing less hyperglycemia was considered. The pharmacist made a library check to verify information and to supply documentation.

In many cases, the pharmacist is a silent figure in patient care. He may monitor the patient's condition without comment while having doubts about the appropriateness of some aspect of care until his doubts are either proven or documented. The patient's need may, as in the above steroid-hyperglycemia example, overshadow the potential contraindications. The pharmacist in these cases will take no action. At other times he may advise the nurse. When the patient is on long-acting sulfonamides he may advise her to push fluids, providing fluid intake is not limited. Or, he may silently observe the patient's condition such as when he monitors the $pH$ of the urine with methenamine mandalate therapy. The clinical pharmacist's action varies according to the situation and needs of the patient. Some cases will demand prompt action and direct physician confrontation while others can best be dealt with through short concise notes.

## Summary

It would be highly desirable if every patient in the hospital could be monitored by a pharmacist at least once during his hospital stay. This, however, is not always possible. Accordingly, every attempt must be made to determine those patients most likely to benefit from the clinical pharmacist's services. The macroscopic review, the direct patient interview and patient rounds with the physician are tools in making this determination. Once a need is recognized, the microscopic review and patient profile form are the techniques used to assist the pharmacist in effective monitoring and communication of information. Findings must then be offered in a competent manner to the physician based on an accurate and detailed profile compiled in the general manner proposed.

## References

1. Bell, J. E., Grimes, B. J., Bouchard, V. E. and Duffy, Sr. M. F.: A New Approach to Delivering Drug Information to the Physician Through a Pharmacy Consultation Program, *Am. J. Hosp. Pharm. 27*:29-37 (Jan.) 1970.

2. Bouchard, V. E.: Toward A Clinical Practice of Pharmacy, *Drug Intel. Clin. Pharm. 3*:342-347 (Dec.) 1969.

3. Godwin, H. N.: Developing a Clinical Role for the Hospital Pharmacist, *Drug Intel. Clin. Pharm. 2*:152-157 (June) 1968.

4. Smith, W. E., O'Malley, C. D. and Weiblen, J. W.: Clinical Pharmacy: General Hospital, *Hospitals 44*:88-99 (Nov. 1) 1970.

5. Sperandio, G. J. and Belcastro, P. F.: The Clinical Pharmacist: Adviser, Teacher, Consultant, *Mod. Hosp. 22*:100-101 (Jan.) 1968.

6. Smith, W. E.: Role of a Pharmacist in Improving Rational Drug Therapy as Part of The Patient Care Team, *Drug Intelligence 1*:244-249 (Aug.) 1967.

7. Goldman, L.: The Pharmacist's Role in Monitoring Drug Therapy, *Hosp. Pharm. 6*:5-13 (June) 1971.

8. Cacace, L. G.: How Patient-Drug Profiles Help Clinical Pharmacists, *Hosp. Topics 47*:534 (Aug.) 1969.

9. Mull, M. M.: Seminar: The Tetracyclines, A Clinical Reappraisal, *Am. J. Dis. Children 112*:483-491 (Nov.) 1966.

10. Cohlan, S. W. et al.: Fetal and Neonatal Hazards from Drugs Administered During Pregnancy, *N.Y. State J. Med. 64*:493-499 (Feb. 15) 1964.

11. Kagan, B. M.: Antimicrobial Therapy, W. B. Saunders Co., Philadelphia, Pennsylvania, 1970, pp. 18, 139-140.

12. Block, L. H.: Drug Interaction Crisis, presented at Fourth Annual ASHP Midyear Clinical Meeting, Washington, D.C., Dec. 14-15, 1969.

13. Elking, Sr. M. P. and Kabat, H. F.: Drug-Induced Modifications of Laboratory Test Values, *Am. J. Hosp. Pharm. 25*:485-519 (Sept.) 1968.

14. Fish, K. H., Jr. and Pearson, R. E.: Sodium Content of Selected Medicines, *Hosp. Pharm. 5*:5-32 (July) 1970.

15. Pearson, R. E. and Fish, K. H., Jr.: Potassium Content of Selected Medicines, Foods and Salt Substitutes, *Hosp. Pharm. 6*:6-9 (Sept.) 1971.

16. Jelliffe, R. W.: An Improved Method of Digoxin Therapy, *Ann. Internal Med. 279*:703 (Oct.) 1968.

17. Hartshorn, E.: Handbook on Drug Interactions, Donald E. Francke, Cincinnati, Ohio, 1970.

# 11 Postadmission Drug and Allergy Histories Recorded by a Pharmacist

James C. Cradock, Gary R. Whitfield, James W. Menzie, and Clarence L. Fortner

A system whereby pharmacists conduct drug and allergy history interviews on all patients admitted to a 50-bed cancer research unit is described.

Some findings from the first 142 interviews are discussed.

A case study of a 54-year-old white male with malignant melanoma and severe renal impairment is presented. The patient's laboratory values and drug therapy are discussed in relation to his renal impairment.

The authors conclude that patient drug and allergy history interviews conducted by a pharmacist are superior to having a patient complete a prepared questionnaire.

In attempting to provide more complete and more patient-oriented pharmacy services, the pharmacist may frequently find that implementation of certain programs (e.g., unit dose dispensing, intravenous additive services) may result in increased expenditures for personnel, equipment, supplies and the need for increased space. In an era of spiraling hospital costs, programs that result in expanded pharmacy service with minimal increase in expenditures would appear to be of particular merit. Patient interviews by the pharmacist to obtain drug and allergy history information and/or patient counselling about the use of drugs by the pharmacist require no capital fund outlay for equipment, minimal cost increase for supplies and little or no increase in personnel costs if the pharmacist is already located in the patient care area. In addition, the pharmacist is provided with patient contact and the opportunity to utilize his knowledge of drugs and drug products to contribute to patient care. In the area of drug and allergy histories the pharmacist's knowledge of the drug's appearance and of the composition of drug products is superior to that of other health professionals questioning the patient about his drug and allergy history.

Two years ago a survey of 20 randomly sampled hospital charts at the Baltimore Cancer Research Center (BCRC) was conducted to determine the completeness of the drug and allergy information recorded by the physician. A positive or negative history of prescription drug usage and allergy was usually, but not always, indicated in the charts. The recording of nonprescription drug usage was considerably less fre-

quent. Subsequently, a pharmacist began the current procedure of interviewing all newly admitted patients to the BCRC to record their drug and allergy history utilizing as a guide nine basic questions (Figure 1). Supplemental questions are asked to be certain that the patient understands the question and to determine the frequency and duration of drug use. In addition questions are asked to differentiate as much as possible drug allergies (e.g., rash) from nonallergic drug reactions (e.g., nausea). Regardless of whether the information is interpreted by the pharmacist as representing a true allergic episode or as describing a nonallergic drug reaction, the implicated agent and resulting symptoms are recorded on the drug and allergy history form. The interview techniques used have been described previously.[1] However certain points should be emphasized. Although an effort is made to use terminology generally familiar to the layman, rephrasing questions in more readily understandable terms is necessary in some patient interviews. For example, we found that the interpretation of the words "drug" and "medicine" by several patients was varied. Some patients denied using drugs or medicines, however, they admitted using aspirin or vitamins regularly only when specifically asked in the appropriate case about headache medication or vitamin usage. In addition, certain patients thought the word "drug" denoted only those agents associated with an addiction liability.

Interviews of children and patients with a communication problem (e.g., some degree of aphasia) are conducted with the assistance of an adult family member.

Figure 1. Drug and allergy history form

Standard Form 505
Rev. August 1967
Bureau of the Budget
Circular A—32 (Rev.)

| CLINICAL RECORD | HISTORY—Part 2 |
|---|---|

PAST HISTORY

INSTRUCTIONS.—*Include (1) OCCUPATION (Civilian and military), (2) MILITARY HISTORY (Include geographic locations and dates), (3) HABITS (Alcohol, tobacco, and drugs), (4) FAMILY HISTORY, (5) CHILDHOOD ILLNESSES, (6) ADULT ILLNESSES, (7) OPERATIONS, (8) INJURIES, and (9) DRUG SENSITIVITIES AND ALLERGIC REACTIONS.*

DRUG AND ALLERGY HISTORY

1. What drugs, medicines, or pills are you taking now?

2. Did you bring any medicine to the hospital?

3. What other drugs have you taken in the last year? ( On readmissions, ignore drugs taken while in the PHS hospital here).

   (If drug's name is unkown, for what condition were the drugs prescribed?)

4. What do you use for:
   Constipation:
   Diarrhea:
   Colds:
   Headache:
   Cough:
   Sleep:
   Contraception:
   Vitamins:

5. Are you allergic to anything at all--e.g.: Drugs, Foods, Animals, Clothing or Tape?

   a. . Have you ever had hayfever, asthma, or hives?

6. Did you go to a physician or take anything to counteract this allergic condition?

7. How much do you smoke?                    average per day
8. How much do you drink?                     average per day
9. Have you ever taken narcotics, LSD, marihuana, sniffed glue?

Use other side if necessary          Pharmacist
                    (Continue on re-erse side)

| PATIENT'S IDENTIFICATION (For typed or written entries give: Name—last, first, middle; grade; date: hospital or medical facility) | REGISTER NO. | WARD NO. |
|---|---|---|

HISTORY (Parts 2 and 3)
Standard Form 505
505-105

At the completion of the interview the information obtained is transcribed in duplicate onto the drug and allergy history form. The original is placed in the history section of the patient's hospital chart and the duplicate is attached to the patient's drug profile in the pharmacy. If the pharmacist feels that some of the information should be brought to the physician's attention immediately, it is also communicated verbally. Two instances will illustrate: One patient scheduled to undergo an intravenous pyelogram mentioned a history of allergy to iodine to the pharmacist but not to the physician; another patient reported to the pharmacist a sensitivity to general anesthetics. This information was conveyed to the physician for the first time by the pharmacist.

## Results

Some of the results obtained from the first 142 interviews are summarized in Table 1. All patients interviewed were referred to the BCRC for treatment of a malignancy and other underlying medical problems. Most patients had a history of recent (less than three months) hospitalization prior to admission to the BCRC. All but one patient consented to an interview by a pharmacist. The patient that objected was

Table 1. Some Results from First 142 Patient Interviews Conducted by a Pharmacist

| | |
|---|---|
| Patients taking prescription drugs at time of admission | 75% |
| Patients taking prescription drugs during past year | 90% |
| Patients taking nonprescription drugs within several weeks of admission | 92% |
| Patients reporting a history of allergy | 31% |

also refusing the requests of physicians and nurses. The high percentage of patients taking prescription drugs at the time of admission was probably due to the fact that all patients had a major medical illness (i.e., advanced cancer) and that the patients were under the referring physician's care during the period shortly before admission. Many patients knew the names of the medications that they had received. If the patient did not know the name of the medication, the pharmacist obtained the information from a family member, the patient's physician or the patient's pharmacist. Of the 57 reported allergies the most often mentioned and their frequency were: penicillin (13), sulfonamides (6), iodine-containing compounds (5) and adhesive tape (4). In response to the question regarding smoking and drinking habits, most patients stated that they had recently stopped smoking and that they were only mild social drinkers, if at all. Although a number of the patients stated that they had received narcotics under a physician's direction, none of the patients had used these drugs without such supervision. However, five patients stated that they had experimented with either or both marijuana or lysergic acid diethylamide (LSD). The drug and allergy history, medical history and hospital course of one patient are summarized to illustrate the role of the pharmacist-obtained drug and allergy history information as it relates to patient care.

## Case Presentation

A 54-year-old white male was transferred to the BCRC for evaluation and treatment of malignant melanoma and severe renal impairment. While the patient was hospitalized at the referring facility a serum calcium of 22 mg/100 ml and a BUN of 38 mg/100 ml were reported. Following treatment with prednisone, Amphogel, and 2 liters/day of intravenous fluids containing 88 mEq of sodium bicarbonate per liter, the serum calcium was reduced to 14.8 mg/100 ml.

The medical history and physical examination obtained at the BCRC included the following: The patient was a chronically ill white male with a history of malignant melanoma diagnosed in 1968 and a recent history of fatigue, 10-pound weight loss, hyperuricemia, azotemia, hypercalcemia, hyponatremia and hypokalemia. Some blood chemistry values determined shortly after admission included: a BUN of 90 mg/100 ml, serum sodium of 129 mEq/liter and serum potassium of 4.6 mEq/liter. Subsequent treatment with 2 liters/day of normal saline, oral sodium phosphate solution, prednisone and allopurinol resulted in a decrease in serum calcium to 10-11 mg/100 ml and return of serum sodium concentration to values within the normal range. However, the BUN remained elevated. The patient reported taking an oral calcium preparation, vitamin D capsules, and thiamine chewable tablets to the pharmacist taking the drug and allergy history. In addition the patient reported that he had been receiving ampicillin therapy prior to admission. Other information included: lactose intolerance, moderate drinking habits and moderate smoking habits. Since the patient had taken both calcium and vitamin D preparations for a long period of time and had exhibited an elevated serum calcium, the pharmacist brought this information to the physician's attention. The physician was aware of the history of calcium usage but not of the concurrent use of vitamin D. Since the patient's renal status was not markedly improving and cancer chemotherapy could not be started until the renal impairment was corrected, the patient was presented to the renal consultant. This physician felt that the patient was in the early diuretic phase of renal failure which was due in part to calcium-vitamin D intoxication. The patient's BUN continued to rise to 120 mg/100 ml, and despite supportive treatment his condition continued to deteriorate and the patient expired in his sleep 17 days after admission.

## Discussion

In our experience, pharmacist-recorded drug and allergy histories have resulted in more complete drug and allergy history information. These interviews have provided the pharmacist with patient contact at the time the patient is admitted which has increased the pharmacist's awareness of patient care. In addition the pharmacist has endeavored to see that hospital regulations concerning medications and allergies are complied with. All medications brought to the hospital by the patient are obtained and stored in the pharmacy during the hospitalization period. All medications received by the patient during his hospitaliza-

tion are prescribed by the physician and distributed from the nursing station. Another policy requires that drug reaction information be placed in the nurses' Kardex and in the front of the patient's chart. After the interview the pharmacist checks to see that these procedures have been carried out.

Due to the location of the Patient Care Pharmacy Service within the patient care area and the small patient census (50 beds) of the BCRC, the drug and allergy history program was instituted with no increase in personnel or equipment. These interviews require only an average of ten minutes per patient and this figure is in agreement with the estimate of others.[2] The relatively short period of time required per interview would indicate that a pharmacist operating from a satellite pharmacy or located within a small hospital would likely have time to conduct these interviews without adversely affecting existing pharmacy services. However, a large centralized pharmacy service might encounter difficulty in allocating time for the pharmacist to interview patients. Wilson and Kabat[2] reported that the major problem encountered in interviewing patients is the time spent in locating the patient.

We feel from our experience that the patient should be personally interviewed by the pharmacist. This method seems superior to one in which the patient completes a prepared form in private because some patients will have difficulty in understanding the written terminology regardless of the manner in which it is presented. The art of conducting an interview requires that certain questions be rephrased or approached differently in order to obtain complete information. The purpose of the drug and allergy history interview is to obtain as complete a history of drug usage and allergy as possible. The limiting factor should be the recall ability of the patient and not their ability to correctly understand the question. Lastly, these interviews have demonstrated that the pharmacist is interested in patient care and that he can provide an additional useful service.

## References

1. Fortner, C. L.: Approaching the Patient and the Techniques Involved in Patient Drug and Allergy Interviews by a Pharmacist, *Voices–12/60 1*:12:20-24:00, side 1 (Apr.) 1971.
2. Wilson, R. S. and Kabat, H. F.: Pharmacist Initiated Patient Drug Histories, In *Clinical Pharmacy Sourcebook*, pp. 346-350.

# 12 Pharmacist-coordinated Self-administration Medication Program on an Obstetrical Service

Richard L. Lucarotti, Harold M. Prisco, Paul E. Hafner, and Larry K. Shoup

A pharmacist-coordinated self-administration medication program developed for an obstetric service is described.

The pharmacist is responsible for coordinating all medication activities; his duties include verifying and reviewing all medication orders, assigning patients to the self-administration program, instructing the patient about her medications (including the use of a patient medication brochure), monitoring patients who have been instructed, and performing the discharge medication consultation.

The distribution function, including the medications used in the program, and how they are packaged and dispensed, is also discussed.

Data showing pharmacist time involvement in performing these activities are presented.

Drug distribution systems in many hospitals have evolved from ward stock into a modern unit dose drug distribution system. Unit dose systems were primarily developed to reduce medication errors. Although unit dose drug distribution systems have reduced inpatient medication errors, they have had little effect on the patient's compliance rate after discharge from the hospital.

The self-administration medication concept redirects the emphasis from a pharmacy-oriented drug distribution system to a patient-oriented drug distribution system. A self-administration medication program improves patient care by increasing the benefits which the patient derives from the medication therapy. The properly instructed patient not only receives the benefit of the medication but also obtains an increased understanding of the medication therapy and how to correctly take his medication after discharge. The pharmacist can readily and effectively provide this component of the patient's total medication therapy in addition to the proper distribution of the medications.

In the case of the postpartem patient whose course of medication therapy is short and relatively uncomplicated, it was felt that the patient would benefit from the medication information and develop and follow good self-administration habits while under supervision in the hospital. In addition, those patients going home on the medications started in the hospital would be much better prepared for proper use of their prescribed drug therapy.

The concepts of unit dose and self-administration were coordinated and instituted in 1970 in the 72-bed Physical Medicine Rehabilitation Center of The Ohio State University Hospitals.[1] This system was modified and extended to the two obstetric nursing units in September 1971. Coordination of this system is the responsibility of a pharmacist who performs the following duties essential to a complete self-administration medication program:

1. Verifying all medication orders
2. Assigning patients to the self-administration medication program
3. Sending the medication orders to the central pharmacy area to be filled
4. Instructing the patient about the medications
5. Monitoring the patient's drug therapy
6. Conducting discharge medication consultation.

### Patient and Medication Order Entry into the System

The pharmacist performs these duties working through this system in the following manner. Medication orders are written on a physician's order form. These written orders are transcribed onto a drug administration form and a carbon copy is placed onto a drug dispensing card by the ward secretary. She completes the information on the drug dispensing card and pages the attending clinical pharmacist. This portion of the system is a modification of the system described elsewhere in the literature.[2]

At the nursing unit the pharmacist performs the first of his responsibilities: verification of the medication orders. He does this by reviewing the physician's order form, drug administration form and drug dispensing card containing these medication orders. During this verification process the pharmacist:

1. Checks for completeness and accuracy of transcription by the ward secretary
2. Schedules the medication for administration
3. Reviews the drug therapy for completeness, appropriateness and possible therapeutic incompatabilities.

Upon completing this verification, the pharmacist countersigns the drug dispensing card and determines if the patient is a good candidate for the self-administration medication program. The pharmacist does this by reviewing the patient's chart, consulting with the nurse or physician and/or communicating with the patient in order to determine patient dependability and help predict compliance to the therapy regimen. This procedure also allows the pharmacist to obtain an awareness of the patient's social background and overall medical situation which will aid him later in instructing the patient about the self-administered medications.

**Filling the Medication Orders**

The pharmacist then sends the drug dispensing card to the central pharmacy where the orders are filled from a supply of prepackaged self-medications (Table 1). The self-medications to be prepackaged, the quantities in each package and the directions for use were determined by physicians, pharmacists and nurses at the onset of the program. The complete prepackaged self-medication unit consists of the medication in unit dose form and a patient medication brochure in a zip-lip container prelabeled with the appropriate directions. In a study of 100 patients over a two-week period, 94.5% of the self-medication orders written were for the prepackaged self-medications. In addition, the patient self administering her medications received an average of 5.3 prescriptions and needed only 0.23 refills. Each self-medication order is given a prescription number, and a short patient identification label is typed and attached to the prepackaged medication (Figure 1). A medication order for non-prepackaged medication will be filled by placing the appropriate amount of unit dose packaged medication into a zip-lip container and preparing the complete prescription label. After filling the self-medication orders, appropriate notations are made on the drug dispensing card. This card is filed accordingly in the central unit dose area. Upon completion of the filling procedure, the medications are sent to the nursing unit to be distributed by the pharmacist.

**Patient Instruction**

On the nursing unit the pharmacist checks the medications against the patient's drug administration form.

### Table 1. Medications Prepackaged for the Obstetrical Self-Medication Program

| MEDICATION | DOSES/ PACKAGE | DIRECTIONS FOR USE |
|---|---|---|
| Tace 72 mg | 4 | Take one capsule twice a day for two days |
| Ferrous gluconate 320 mg | 15 | Take one tablet three times a day with meals |
| Ampicillin 500 mg | 24 | Take one capsule four times a day at 7 a.m., 11 a.m., 4 p.m. and 10 p.m. |
| Darvon Compound-65 | 6 | Take one capsule every three hours as needed for pain |
| Ascodeen-30 | 12 | Take one or two tablets every four hours as needed for pain |
| Secobarbital 100 mg | 3 | Take one capsule at bedtime as needed for sleep; may repeat one time if necessary |
| Pericolace | 5 | Take two capsules at bedtime on the first night and one each night thereafter as needed for bowel movement |
| Fleets Phospho Soda 15 ml | 3 | Take the contents of one bottle on the second postpartem day if you have had no previous bowel movement |
| Oral Varidase | 16 | Take one tablet four times a day for four days |

He also reviews the drug administration form for any doses which the nurse may have given during the night or during the time period when the self-administration orders were being filled. The pharmacist instructs the patient on each medication she is to self-administer. In general, the pharmacist informs her about what the medication is, why she is taking it, when to take it, possible side effects, the importance of taking each dose at the prescribed time, precautions and any other information which the pharmacist feels will aid the patient. She is also informed that she must notify the nurse or pharmacist for refill requests. In addition, the pharmacist points out the medication brochure (Figure 2) contained in the prescription package and the type of information she can derive by reading it. If for various reasons the

*Figure 1. Standard label for one of the nine prepackaged medications and the short identification label needed to dispense the medication to a patient*

**Take one (1) capsule every three (3) hours if needed for pain. Do not exceed one capsule every three hours.**
**Darvon Compound - 65**

NO. 6

**THE OHIO STATE UNIVERSITY HOSPITALS**
Department of Pharmacy, Columbus, Ohio
(614) 422-4921      REG. NO. AM 2281854

MRS. JOHN DOE      P15130
ROOM 500    r1      3.3.72
DR. SMITH

*Figure 2. A patient medication information brochure*

TACE 72 mg. CAPSULES

This medication has been ordered to prevent excessive swelling of your breasts. A certain amount of breast swelling and leakage is to be expected after delivery because of your body's natural production of milk. But, stimulation of the breasts following delivery can cause them to fill and expand rapidly, thus causing excess pressure and pain. To help avoid breast discomfort, here are some suggestions:

1. Take this medication properly. Take the first dose within 8 hours after delivery. After the first dose, take 1 capsule about every 12 hours. For example, take 1 capsule with breakfast (about 9 A.M.) and 1 capsule at bedtime (about 10 P.M.). Be sure to take a total of 4 capsules of this medication.

2. Wear a moderately tight supporting bra.

3. Burp and feed your baby on your knees instead of across your breasts.

4. Avoid any unnecessary stimulation of the breasts, such as that caused by hot showers, wash cloths, or loose clothing.

5. Avoid mechanical stimulation such as massaging or suckling.

6. Avoid excess fluid intake.

patient does not comprehend the language or is totally uncooperative and therefore the pharmacist feels that the patient is not capable of properly self-administering all or some of the medications, he will not leave those medications at the bedside of the patient. If the pharmacist feels the patient is capable of taking her medication but needs further instruction, the patient will be closely monitored. The pharmacist records on the patient's drug administration form that he has given the patient instructions.

## Monitoring the Patient

After the initial instruction is completed, the patient is on her own to administer the medications. A monitoring system must be maintained in order to insure that the patient is properly taking her medications. There is an attempt to see all patients at least once by the pharmacist after their initial instruction. However, those receiving antibiotic therapy or other important medications, or those patients who have had some difficulty with the initial instruction, are given priority for monitoring. In addition, the nurse aids in the monitoring of patient compliance by performing casual checks during her daily interaction with the patients.

## Discharge Consultation

The discharge consultation is a form of monitoring and is the final service which the pharmacist performs

for the patient. After reviewing the patient's drug administration form, the pharmacist meets with the patient and ascertains whether the patient understood her medication therapy and if she fulfilled the instructions which were given to her. In addition, the pharmacist reinforces any instructions about medications the patient has taken in the hospital and any she will continue to take at home. He also gives instruction about all prescriptions written for her at discharge and answers any final questions she may have.

## Pharmacist Work Load Time Study

A time study was conducted over a 16-day period, including 20 work shifts, about five months after the postpartem self-administration medication program was initiated. The average amount of time spent by the pharmacist performing each of the duties directly related to the self-administration medication program was computed (Table 2). The total average time of about 24 minutes for these duties, along with the average time needed to fill a patient's self-medication orders (about ten minutes), may be used as a guideline to determine pharmacist time involvement per patient. However, our experiences have shown other factors contributing to the amount of time required. Table 3 shows the amount of time the pharmacist actually spent during an eight-hour work shift performing duties directly related to the self-administration program and various other pharmaceutical services. During the average eight-hour work shift, approximately 106 minutes are spent on the two obstetric nursing units. About 61 of these minutes (57.5% of the total time) are spent performing the described duties of the self-administration medication program,

**Table 2. Average Time Required Per Patient to Perform Pharmacist's Duties Directly Related to Self-Medication Program**

| DUTIES | AVERAGE TIME/PATIENT (min) |
|---|---|
| Verify medication orders | 1.77 |
| Consult with physician or nurse | 2.50 |
| Review patient's overall situation and compare medications dispensed with those listed on drug. administration form | 1.39 |
| Initial instruction on one or more medications | 8.59[a] |
| Documenting the instruction | 1.26 |
| Monitoring the patient | 2.03 |
| Reinstruction upon refill | 2.48 |
| Discharge consultation | 3.55 |
| Total time | 23.57 |

[a] Patients received an average of 5.3 prescriptions which required 10–12 minutes of initial instruction. Times for instruction on orders of one or two medications are averaged here, making this figure lower than would be anticipated for the average patient.

**Table 3. Average Pharmacist Time Involvement in the Obstetrical Self-Medication Program per Eight-Hour Work Shift**[a]

| CATEGORY | TIME | |
| --- | --- | --- |
| | Minutes | % of total |
| Average time spent performing duties directly related to the self-administration medication program | 61.3 | 57.5 |
| Average time spent performing other pharmaceutical services | 45.4 | 42.5 |
| Average total time involvement | 106.7 | 100.0 |

[a] A total of 84 patients are represented in this study.

and about 45 minutes (42.5% of the total time) are spent performing other pharmaceutical services. It was found that the presence of a pharmacist on the nursing units prompted his involvement with pharmacy duties other than those associated with the self-administration medication system. Questions from nurses about nurse-administered medications and intravenous admixtures, inquiries from the nurseries and labor and delivery area, obtaining *stat* medication and discussion of medications and pharmacy procedures in general comprised the greatest portion of this miscellaneous time.

We have not studied the exact effectiveness of the medication instruction or compliance to therapy regimens before and after discharge. However, there have been no known incidents of gross errors or abuse. In addition there have been less than 5% self-administration errors as determined through our routine monitoring and discharge consultations.

## Conclusions

The patients on the obstetric services admitted to the self-administration medication system have proven themselves to be quite reliable and their medication orders have been basic and routine. These factors have allowed us to establish a clinical program which is relatively uncomplicated. The self-administration medication programs instituted on the obstetric nursing units and at the Physical Medicine Rehabilitation Center have provided experience and an excellent foundation for extention of the self-administration concept to other areas. We have recently expanded the concept to patients on a thoracic surgery unit recovering from heart surgery where the knowledge, proper understanding and proper self-administration of their medications is essential.

The self-administration medication concept can greatly increase the benefits which the patient derives from the medication therapy. An increased knowledge and understanding of the medication therapy and subsequent increased capability of properly self-administering the medications are the two main benefits. However, these additional benefits are totally dependent on the quality and effectiveness of the instruction. This can be most readily and effectively provided by the pharmacist.

## References

1. Roberts, C. J. and Miller, W. A.: Clinical Pharmacy, Self Administration, and Technician Drug Administration, *Drug Intel. Clin. Pharm.* 6:408–415 (Dec.) 1972.
2. Berry, C. C.: A Pharmacy Coordinated Unit Dose Dispensing and Drug Administration System—Description of the System, *Amer. J. Hosp. Pharm.* 27:890–898 (Nov.) 1970.

# 13 The Hospital Pharmacist in an Interdisciplinary Inpatient Teaching Program

Martin Jinks

An education program for coronary care patients is discussed with particular emphasis on pharmacy involvement in the program.

The steps in planning the program are reviewed. Pharmacy involvement centers around direct patient counselling regarding discharge medications and providing patients with a general monograph regarding the use of prescription drugs and monographs on specific drugs the patient is taking. The rationale behind providing specific drug information to the patient is discussed.

"The most important contribution to compliance is the understanding the patient has of the illness, the need for treatment, and the likely consequences of both."[1] This statement in a recent review on patient compliance emphasizes the importance of a comprehensive, disease-oriented approach to drug compliance as opposed to teaching drug facts in isolation from other considerations. Theoretically, a patient who understands the basic disease process, in addition to drug facts, can express his concerns regarding therapy more intelligently and can often participate actively in the decision-making processes concerning the planning of therapeutic regimens for his own care. Active participation is the key to any education/compliance activity because it develops in the patient an attitude of alliance and collaboration with the health professionals caring for him.

One group of patients for whom such an approach would be particularly valuable is the coronary care patient. In no other group of patients are the consequences of noncompliance more dramatic than in the coronary patient who is negligent or unwilling to adhere to a therapeutic plan. In the coronary care unit (CCU) at St. Paul (Minnesota) Ramsey Hospital, the patients display a multitude of determinants indicating that they have a high risk of becoming compliance failures. Several factors promoting noncompliance in these patients are (1) chronic illnesses requiring long-term maintenance, (2) advanced age, (3) lack of continuous follow-up by a single physician and (4) a large number of medications.

Because the special needs of this group of patients are easily identified and because these needs can be met if the expertise and activities of a number of different health disciplines are coordinated, an interdisciplinary teaching program for this limited population seemed feasible and logical. The initial organizational task involved soliciting input from interested health professionals who were involved independently in providing services to CCU patients. Following expressions of interest from several disciplines, a committee of nurses, a pharmacist, a social worker, a dietitian, and a cardiologist was formed to develop a statement of goals and to pursue the establishment of a comprehensive, interdisciplinary patient education program for CCU patients. With the writing of the following goals, the Health Education and Rehabilitation Therapy (HEART) Program was inaugurated:

1. To provide the patient and family with the necessary information to:
   a. Understand and accept an acute cardiac episode
   b. Prevent future cardiac episodes due to avoidable causes
2. To motivate the patient and family to adjust to the illness
3. To assist the patient and family in the utilization of rehabilitative and teaching data
4. To provide continuity of care from the CCU, general medicine, home, outpatient department, and other community resources
5. To develop criteria for evaluating the program.

## Planning the Program

The selection of appropriate teaching content was determined by how important the information would be to the patient in attaining the stated goals. Once the scope of the content was agreed upon by the committee, each section was delegated to the health resource person most qualified to organize it. For example, a section on medications was delegated to the pharmacist who is responsible for developing specific objectives for his teaching activities and determining the best resources and techniques to assure the objectives are met.

The planning committee must have official sanction within the institution to have power to initiate such a program, and at St. Paul-Ramsey Hospital, the content and teaching techniques of the resource persons are subject to review and approval by the cardiac committee, a standing committee of physicians within the institution.

*Scope.* The CCU patient is the common denominator bringing the efforts of the various health professionals together, and his needs must be categorized into related topics which comprise the scope of the teaching. The HEART committee determined the CCU patient's needs to be in the following areas:

1. Basic anatomy and pathophysiology
2. Medications
3. Physical therapy
4. Diet
5. Pacemakers
6. Psychological and social support.

*Objectives.* Once the scope of the teaching was defined in terms of specific topics, the objectives were then stated for each teaching area. The objectives specify precisely what behavior change the patient should exhibit after being exposed to the teaching material. Based on the objectives, the details of the teaching content were selected.

Stating objectives for each subject area was not only helpful in choosing content, resources, and techniques for obtaining the desired results, but was also essential for evaluation and improvement of the program. Presenting objectives to other HEART committee members was also helpful in generating feedback from professionals of other disciplines who have a different perspective on the subject matter. This different perspective often resulted in clarification of the objectives or the writing of additional important objectives which might have otherwise been overlooked.

The objectives written by the pharmacy department were as follows:

1. After discussing the drug handouts with the pharmacist, the HEART patient will know the following information about his medication:
   a. The visual identity of each drug
   b. The name of each drug
   c. How each drug works with respect to the disease being treated
   d. Any special instructions regarding administration where appropriate
   e. Any ancillary information such as storage or expected side effects where appropriate

   f. The common adverse reactions of each drug.
2. Having learned the above information concerning his medications, the HEART patient will comply intelligently with the medication plan provided him.

*Resources and Techniques.* After the objectives were written, the necessary information to meet these objectives was assembled and the techniques which were best suited to present the material were developed. Nurses, pharmacists, dietitians, social workers and physical therapists do the actual teaching and provide the printed teaching material to patients.

An important technique is to establish a favorable patient expectation so that the patient will be involved in the program as an informed participant. To establish this expectation, a folder is presented to the patient upon his initiation to the program. The folder contains an introductory letter explaining the scope of the program with a list of the various health professionals involved in the teaching, the statement of program goals, and the objectives for each related topic. Having this information at the outset, the patient can then anticipate developments in his therapeutic plan and can learn in an organized, premeditated fashion.

The teaching process itself involves a bedside interaction with the patient by the appropriate health professional. During this interaction, the objectives are explained in terms of their significance to the care of the patient, and the information is presented in the context of its relation to meeting the objectives. To enhance the teaching process, a variety of teaching tools are employed. For example, the CCU nurse utilizes a plastic facsimile of a heart to illustrate the points to be made concerning anatomy and pathophysiology. In addition, each resource person has developed appropriate teaching material to use as teaching guides which are given to the patient to be added to the patient folder. Examples of these include a booklet of sodium content of foods compiled by the dietitians and the monographs on the prescription drugs developed by pharmacists. This printed material becomes the patient's property upon discharge and serves as resource material for reinforcement and review by the patient long after the hospital episode.

*Assigning Responsibility.* Initiation of a patient into the HEART Program is the responsibility of the CCU charge nurse who adheres to criteria for admission established by the HEART committee. The HEART Program will accept any patient who may reasonably be expected to benefit directly or indirectly from such a patient teaching program and who is diagnosed as having:[a]

---

[a]The opening qualifying statement allows the omission of patients who are senescent or who may have other conditions preventing benefit from a teaching program but does permit "indirect" benefit derived through teaching relatives or others who might be caring for such individuals.

1. A premyocardial infarction syndrome
2. An acute myocardial infarction
3. Chronic cardiac disease
4. A disease in which a pacemaker will be or is installed.

At the same time, the charge nurse also assigns a primary teaching nurse who is the staff CCU nurse caring for the patient and who then becomes the patient's advocate in the HEART Program with the responsibility of monitoring the patient's learning progress throughout his stay.

Once the patient is placed in the program, it is important to assure a coordinated sequence of learning experiences by providing a step-by-step blocking out of the program in terms of the level and order of the teaching components. Therefore, whatever teaching is to take place has been put in a formal checklist, and the responsibility for seeing that the items on the checklist are covered belongs to the primary teaching nurse. The checklist is the crucial document in providing a continuity of input from those teaching resource persons who are not directly involved at the patient's bedside. The pharmacy, dietary and social services in particular are dependent on the correct utilization of this document for notification in the proper sequence.

### Pharmacist-Patient Interaction

One or two days prior to the patient's expected discharge date, the primary teaching nurse calls the pharmacy department requesting a pharmacist to instruct the medication section. She also supplies a tentative list of the discharge medications which she obtains directly from the physician. With this much advance notification, the pharmacy staff can plan its activities so that a pharmacist can visit the patient at his bedside on or before the date of discharge for the average of 15 to 20 minutes needed to counsel the patient regarding his medications. Pharmacists as well as pharmacy interns and students are involved in the teaching program.

Because the patient population for the program is limited in number, the activity has not imposed an unreasonable burden on the pharmacy department. The number of patients instructed ranges from one to four per week, a workload which is compatible with the otherwise traditional system of providing pharmaceutical services in our institution.

### Drug Monographs

To facilitate the teaching process and to provide printed material for reinforcement and review, a series of drug monographs has been developed by the pharmacy department. The monographs are of two types.

The first type is a statement of general guidelines for the use of prescription medications (see Figure 1). All HEART patients receive this monograph in the patient folder whether they are discharged on medication or not. It serves to review for the patient some seemingly obvious but frequently overlooked principles of drug use and misuse, and it is also an excellent public relations instrument for the pharmacy department.

The second type of monograph is a review of a specific drug entity, and for each drug prescribed the patient receives a separate monograph. Twelve monographs have been produced covering sixteen drugs (Table 1), encompassing approximately 80% of the drugs which are prescribed for HEART patients.

The monograph approach is convenient since the number of cardiac drugs for outpatient use is limited. For example, experience has shown that anywhere from 50-75% of all HEART patients discharged on medications leave with a prescription for one of the digitalis preparations.

*Content and Format.* Based on the objectives of the program, the format of all monographs is uniformly divided into two main sections under which the six basic objectives are covered. A typical monograph illustrating the format is presented in Figure 2.

*Visual Identification.* It is important that the patient appreciate the distinguished physical features of his medication. This helps avoid confusion when multiple prescriptions are being taken simultaneously. Certain drugs present a particular problem in this respect; a good example is sodium warfarin for the patient who must alternate daily doses. The patient may also protect himself from an incorrectly rewritten prescription or an error in the refill of a presciption by recognizing an unexpected change in the physical appearance of the drug and calling this to the attention of the physician or pharmacist.

To produce an awareness of the differences in appearances of prescription medications, each monograph contains a description of the physical characteristics of the product, noting the size, shape, color, and identification number. However, written descriptive terms are often ambiguous to the patient, and therefore the teaching pharmacist routinely takes the filled prescriptions or samples of the specific drugs being discussed to use as teaching tools.

The descriptive terms in the monograph are very specific for a given product dosage form and are dependent on the institution's formulary. Care must be taken to continually revise this part of the monograph when trade-named products change.

*Name of the Drug.* Patients commonly describe their medications in terms of appearance rather than by referring to the drug by name. "My white heart pill" could apply equally to digitoxin, digoxin, nitroglycerin, quinidine, or furosemide. A patient making

*Figure 1. General information regarding prescription drugs for HEART patients.[2]*

---

To assure effectiveness and safety from your prescription medications, please follow these suggested guidelines:

1. *Take your medication as directed.* There is always a reason, sometimes several, for the physician's order. It may be important to take a drug only after meals; in other cases, only before meals. Try to take drugs on time. This will assure a constant level of drug in your system.

2. *Be sure you understand what is intended by the directions.* Instructions to take one tablet "four times daily" could mean either after meals and at bedtime or every six hours including nightime. The correct interpretation depends on the drug being taken. If the directions are unclear, ask the pharmacist or physician to clarify the directions for you.

3. *If you miss some doses:* If you forget two or three doses of a medication in a row, do not try to "catch up" by taking all the missed doses at once. If you are concerned about having missed two or more doses, do not hesitate to call your clinic or the pharmacy department to find out what you should do in this situation.

4. *Take the whole prescription.* Don't stop taking a prescription drug after you begin to feel better unless your physician approves. Often anything less than a full course of treatment may prevent the medicine from completely correcting the condition even though you feel "well." For example, not taking a full course of antibiotics for an infection allows the "bug" to either become resistant to the drug or to grow back, causing a reinfection.

5. *Discard unused medication.* Destroy unused portion of medicines remaining from a prescription which has been discontinued by your physician. Do this by flushing the remainder down the toilet. Many accidental poisonings *of children* have occurred from medications carelessly put aside by adults.

6. *Understand and obey the physician's refill instructions.* There are some prescriptions that are not refillable at all, and a new prescription must be written. Some can be refilled if the physician specifies this on the prescription. The pharmacist must follow his directions, and will tell you if there is a restriction on refills. At St. Paul-Ramsey Hospital, medications are usually dispensed in thirty-day quantities to assure close monitoring of your progress by the physician and pharmacist. As a general rule, a prescription should not be refilled for more than one year without visiting a physician.

7. *If you must take a drug for long periods:* If you are to continue taking a drug, be sure you have enough medication or refills to last between clinic appointments. Should you run out of medication and refills before your next clinic visit, even if only a matter of days before the appointment, do not assume it is alright to go without your medicine for even this short period of time. Call your clinic or the pharmacy department for specific instructions if you run out of medication before your next appointment.

8. *Never share your medication.* Do not share your medication with someone else, and do not take medication prescribed for another person. Your prescription fits you as precisely as good eyeglasses or bridgework. It was written for you on the basis of age, weight, sex and physical condition. Never allow someone else to take your medication, even if his symptoms are similar.

9. *Avoid drug accidents.* Keep medicines out of the reach or sight of children. If a child can see a box or bottle, he will often figure a way to reach it. A safe, useful drug for you can be poison to a child. At home, avoid keeping medications in your pocket or purse since this is a common way children accidentally obtain drugs. Keep in a locked cabinet if possible. Also, avoid taking medicine in front of small children since a child may want to follow your example.

10. *If you don't have a prescription refilled:* Be sure to tell your physician if you choose not to have a prescription refilled or if you don't use the medication after your purchase it. If you don't inform him, the physician might think you are not responding to a particular drug product, and his evaluation of your progress will be made incorrect. Not taking a medicine ordered could be dangerous because it might allow a condition to get worse while the physician assumes it is being treated with drugs.

11. *If you see more than one physician:* Be sure each physician knows all the drugs you are taking. This includes any nonprescription drugs (e.g., antacid liquid or tablets, aspirin or combination pain relievers, cold/hayfever products, laxatives, etc.) that you take routinely. These products frequently contain drugs in low doses which at higher doses are available on prescription only. Nonprescription drugs should be respected. When several medications are used at the same time, interactions between them can produce unwanted effects, so it is important that your physician have a complete list. Also, tell each physician you consult (and dentist too) about any allergies or bad reactions you may have had to any drug.

12. *Store your medication properly.* Do not store any prescription medication under conditions of high temperature, high humidity, or direct sunlight. Make certain that the pharmacist places the drug name on each container, and do not remove the drug from its original labeled container and place it in another container.

13. *Bring all your medication with you when visiting the clinic or your physician.* By allowing someone else to double-check your current medication plan, you can eliminate any confusion or questions about the exact drugs, doses, and frequency of administration of your prescriptions.

---

contact with a physician unfamiliar with his case can facilitate the treatment of drug-related complications by knowing the names of the drugs involved. This is especially true in the acute situation when the prescription or the patient's medical records are not immediately available.

*How the Drug Acts.* Because the patient has learned the basic pathophysiology of his disease early on in the program, he readily understands the usefulness of the drugs when the drug actions are explained. This genuine comprehension of drug therapy as it relates directly to his disease is a capstone in the process of convincing the patient of the importance of faithful compliance.

*Administration and Ancillary Information.* Special instructions regarding drug administration are provided in the monographs to reinforce verbal instructions. Examples of special instructions include emphasizing the sublingual only administration of nitroglycerin, the administration of Dyazide after meals if not tolerated on an empty stomach, and the proper dilution of potassium chloride syrup. Ancillary information regarding storage and expected side effects is also provided for each drug where appropriate.

**Table 1. Drugs for which Monographs Have Been Developed for HEART Patients**

| | |
|---|---|
| Digoxin | Potassium supplement |
| Digitoxin | Quinidine |
| Thiazide diuretics | Procainamide |
| Spironolactone | Allopurinol |
| Dyazide | Propranolol |
| Aldactazide | Aminophylline |
| Furosemide | Warfarin |
| Methyldopa | Nitroglycerin |

*Figure 2. The patient monograph for digoxin.*

Digoxin (Lanoxin)

A. *How it Acts:*
   1. Digoxin (Lanoxin) is a *digitalis preparation*. Digitalis preparations act by:
      a. Increasing the pumping action of the heart.
      b. Slowing the rate of the heart beat.

B. *Other Information and Precautions:*
   1. Digoxin (Lanoxin) tablets exist in two sizes, 0.125 mg and 0.25 mg. The 0.125 mg size is a small, yellow tablet with "Wellcome Y3B" imprinted on it. The 0.25 mg tablet is a small, white tablet with "Wellcome X3A" imprinted on it.
   2. Digoxin differs from many drugs in that it requires a large dose at first (the digitalizing dose) and a lower but steady dose later (the maintenance dose).
   3. The maintenance dose may vary from time to time depend-on your response to the drug, so do not be alarmed if your physician makes occasional dosage adjustments, especially at the beginning of treatment. Dosage adjustments do not mean that you are unusual or that the digoxin is not doing what it should.
   4. Often a diuretic (medication to reduce body water) and a potassium supplement (KCl elixir or syrup) are prescribed with digoxin. While removing extra water from the body, certain diuretics may also remove too much body potassium, and this potassium loss reduces the effectiveness and safety of the digoxin. This is why potassium supplements are prescribed. Therefore, it is very important that you take your potassium supplement faithfully.
   5. *Notify the Doctor if Any of the Following Occurs:*
      a. An unexplained loss of appetite.
      b. Nausea, vomiting, or diarrhea.
      c. Blurred vision, yellowish vision or white halos around dark objects.
      d. An unexplained skin rash.

Patients having multiple prescriptions written for them upon discharge sometimes express confusion over the many sets of directions. In this case, the pharmacist will provide a daily calendar of drug administration to help the patient avoid administration errors during the initial outpatient adjustment period.

*Adverse Reactions.* The potential untoward effects of the medications are discussed in terms of those symptoms which may be observed by the patient, and the pharmacist always prefaces his statements by reassuring the patient that such reactions are rare to avoid unnecessarily alarming him. It is especially important to distinguish between those untoward effects which are frequent and of little consequence and those which merit immediate, serious attention.

Although there are those who would recommend against discussing this aspect of drug therapy with the patient to avoid alarming him, there are two important reasons for discussing untoward effects. First, the credibility of those responsible for the care and education can be severely reduced if a significant drug reaction occurs which is totally unexpected by the patient. All the effort that has gone into building an alliance with the patient to motivate him into informed, collaborative involvement and compliance may be destroyed if this unpleasant but important aspect is omitted and a drug reaction occurs. Secondly, patients given this information may recognize initial symptoms of an adverse reaction and seek medical advice early enough to avert more serious consequences. The value of explaining side effects fully is illustrated by two cases in our experience in which mild digitalis intoxication was detected by patients who, recognizing the early symptoms of toxicity learned in the HEART Program, sought medical help before significant complications developed.

## Conclusion

In the St. Paul-Ramsey Hospital HEART Program, the pharmacy department has been given exclusive responsibility for developing the objectives concerning medications. Because the pharmacist has a perspective and expertise unlike that of any other health professional involved in this area, he is uniquely qualified for the task. Indeed, because the proper compliance with medication regimens is so important for the continued good health of the patient after discharge, the objectives and teaching approaches of the pharmacist should set the example as a prototype for the educational efforts of the other members of the health education team.

### References

1. Blackwell, B.: Drug Therapy — Patient Compliance, *N. Engl. J. Med. 289*:249-252 (Aug. 2) 1973.
2. Cohen, M. R.: From Your Newsletter, *Hosp. Pharm. 8*:93, 96 (Mar.) 1973.

# 14 Heparin Therapy by Continuous Intravenous Infusion

Margo Swanson and Larry Cacace

A protocol for continuous intravenous heparin therapy is presented.

The intramuscular, subcutaneous, and intravenous (intermittent and continuous) modes of heparin administration are compared. It is recommended that activated whole blood clotting time rather than the Lee White test be used to monitor therapy. It is also recommended that heparin be administered by continuous intravenous infusion.

Heparin, the most effective anticoagulant available, is a mucopolysaccharide composed of d-glucosamine and d-glucuronic acid. The content of esterified sulfuric acid is very high, up to 40%, which makes heparin the strongest organic acid occurring within the body. Heparin inhibits in order of increasing effectiveness, thrombin, thromboplastin, factor V, thromboplastin generation, factor IX, factor XI, and factor XII. It also inhibits the aggregation of platelets by thrombin but not ADP.[1]

The anticoagulant effect of heparin is measured by a determination of the clotting time of the blood. Heparin has been shown to be superior to oral anticoagulants in the prevention and propagation of experimentally produced thrombus if the clotting time is maintained above one and one-half times normal.[2-8] It is the purpose of this chapter to present a method of continuous intravenous heparin therapy and the effectiveness of this method in maintaining the clotting time above one and one-half times normal.

## Study of Effectiveness

Heparin is used frequently in the intensive medical care unit for the prevention and treatment of thrombo-embolic phenomenon. The effectiveness of this heparin therapy was monitored in terms of prolongation of the Lee White clotting times in 150 patients at Memorial Hospital Medical Center of Long Beach. All patients received heparin by subcutaneous or intermittent iv injection. Since there were no control Lee White clotting times on most patients, the range of

25 to 45 minutes was considered therapeutic since normal is approximately 6 to 16 minutes. Thirty patients had one or no clotting time determinations during heparin therapy, so the effectiveness of their therapy is unknown. Approximately 80% of the clotting times done were not in the therapeutic range. Even though some were in the therapeutic range, they may not be significant because the clotting time was not done correctly, i.e., within one hour before administration of the next dose. There were also six incidences of severe hemorrhagic complications in this group (Figure 1).

## Plan for Improvement

In an effort to improve the effectiveness of the heparin therapy in our hospital, the literature was reviewed with particular reference to methods of heparin administration and the effectiveness of each method. The effectiveness of each method was determined in terms of prolongation of the clotting time (Figure 2).[9,10] It can be seen from Figure 2 that continuous iv heparin therapy produces the most effective and constant anticoagulant level.

The advantages and disadvantages of each method of administration were considered with particular reference to continuous iv heparin therapy (Table 1).[9-26] Patients in the intensive medical care unit routinely have an intravenous infusion, therefore, this is not a disadvantage at our hospital. To overcome the two major disadvantages of continuous iv heparin

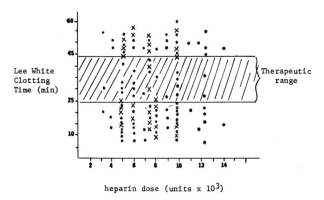

Figure 1. Lee White clotting times of patients before implementation of continuous intravenous infusion of heparin and use of ACT; about 80% of the lab results are outside the therapeutic range (• = subcutaneous doses; x = intermittent iv. doses of heparin)

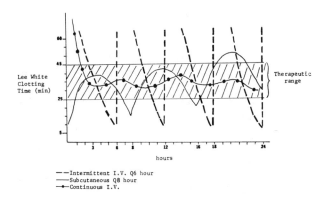

Figure 2. Comparison of the theoretical effect of heparin when given by various routes of administration; continuous intravenous infusion avoids the "valleys and peaks" resulting from subcutaneous and intermittent intravenous injections

therapy, i.e., control of flow rate and fluid volume, the intensive medical care committee was requested to purchase IVAC-500 Infusion Pumps.* With the IVAC-500 pump as little as 50 ml of fluid can be infused accurately over a six-hour period. A Travenol Soluset† is used because it was found to be more accurate in the delivery of fluid than other solution sets.

## Method Used

Table 2 is the method of continuous iv heparin therapy that was proposed by the pharmacy and has now been adopted by the medical staff. It should be emphasized that the doses recommended are for prophylactic anticoagulation only. The doses must be higher if there is a pulmonary embolus or thrombophlebitis present.

---

*IVAC Corporation, 11353 Sorrento Valley Road, San Diego, California.
†Travenol Laboratories, Inc., 4501 Colorado Boulevard, Los Angeles, California.

## Table 1. Comparison of Advantages and Disadvantages of the Routes of Heparin Administration

INTRAMUSCULAR

*Disadvantages*

1. Discomfort, local hematoma and risk of necrosis
2. Delay in reaching a therapeutic level
3. Absorption unpredictable and uncontrollable
4. Large doses required
5. Frequent injections required
6. Clotting times must be done at a certain time
7. Neutralization with protamine sulfate, if necessary, is difficult

*Advantages*

1. Avoidance of indwelling venous catheter or needle

SUBCUTANEOUS

*Disadvantages*

1. Local pain, ecchymosis and hematoma
2. Delay in reaching therapeutic level
3. Absorption unpredictable and uncontrollable
4. Large doses required
5. Frequent injections required
6. Clotting times must be done at a certain time
7. Neutralization with protamine sulfate, if necessary, is difficult
8. Hemorrhagic complications
   a. Hemorrhage into the rectus abdominis muscle
   b. Femoral nerve paralysis secondary to a hematoma in or on the ileacus muscle
   c. Retroperitoneal hemorrhage

*Advantages*

1. Avoidance of indwelling venous catheter or needle

INTERMITTENT INTRAVENEOUS INJECTION

*Disadvantages*

1. Difficult to maintain clotting time in therapeutic range
2. Large doses required
3. Requires frequent intravenous injections
4. Clotting times must be done at certain times

*Advantages*

1. Immediate therapeutic level

CONTINUOUS INTRAVENOUS HEPARIN THERAPY

*Disadvantages*

1. Must have intravenous catheter or needle
2. Large fluid volume required
3. Drip rate difficult to control

*Advantages*

1. Clotting time can be maintained continuously in therapeutic range
2. Neutralization with protamine sulfate, if necessary, is immediate
3. Less heparin required by this method than by any other
4. Clotting times can be done at any time
5. Flexibility in dose adjustment
6. Clotting time returns to normal levels in 1 to 2 hours after drip is stopped

An initial loading dose is given by intravenous push to get an immediate anticoagulant effect. At the same time an iv drip infusion of heparin is begun with a dose for six hours based on the patient's weight. The dose of heparin is divided into four equal doses and each is given in 50 to 100 ml of intravenous fluid every six hours. An IVAC infusion pump is used to control the drip rate and the amount of fluid administered. This method also allows easy dose adjustment at any time. It has been our experience that the required 24-hour dose of heparin by iv infusion is decreased by about 33% when compared to subcutaneous and intermittent iv administration.

The initial loading dose gives an immediate anticoagulant effect. The half-life of the initial dose is approximately one to two hours and varies with the dose.[27] The intravenous drip infusion is effective in approximately two hours and will then maintain a therapeutically effective level continuously. Figure 3 shows the effect of the initial iv dose, the continuous intravenous infusion and the theoretical summation of these two.

As the heparin therapy was being monitored it was noted that the Lee White clotting times were quite variable, while the dose of heparin remained the same. Since this raised doubts about the accuracy of the Lee White clotting times, our pathology department was consulted. The pathology department has now adopted the activated whole blood clotting time (ACT) to determine the effectiveness of heparin therapy. The ACT of whole blood is a quick, easily performed and standardized test. It is inexpensive and is a reliable improvement over the Lee White test as a monitor of heparin therapy. The correlation coefficient is 0.762 for ACT and Lee White in heparinized individuals.[28,29]

Figure 4 shows the effectiveness in terms of prolongation of the clotting times of continuous intravenous heparin therapy with an IVAC infusion pump. It can be seen that the majority are in the effective range.

The clinical effectiveness of continuous intravenous heparin therapy in terms of decreasing the incidence of thrombo-embolic phenomenon for patients in our hospital should be determined in the future. Others have shown continuous iv heparin therapy to be a safe, effective method of decreasing thrombo-embolic phenomenon.[30-33] The acceptance by our medical staff of this method of heparin administration has been excellent. Approximately 95% of the patients anticoagulated with heparin in our hospital now receive it by continuous intravenous infusion.

It is our conclusion that based on prolongation of clotting time, the best method of heparin administration to maintain an effective therapeutic range is by

## Table 2. Protocol for Continuous Intravenous Heparin Therapy

ACTIVATED WHOLE BLOOD CLOTTING TIME (ACT)

Normal Range = 1 min/20 sec to 2 min/10 sec
Therapeutic Range = 3 min to 4 min
(ACT of 3 and 4 min are about equal to Lee White times of 30 and 50 min, respectively)

In order to properly evaluate heparin therapy, a control clotting time should be obtained before starting heparin therapy. The second clotting time should be obtained 6 to 8 hours after starting heparin to check for adequate anticoagulation. The patient's heparin therapy may then be regulated with a daily clotting time when the therapeutic level has been reached.

SUGGESTED HEPARIN DOSES FOR PROPHYLACTIC ANTICOAGULATION

Initial loading dose—5,000 units iv push
10,000 units iv push for pulmonary emboli and thrombophlebitis

Intravenous heparin drip is started at the same time as the iv push dose is given. The dose is ordered according to body weight and given in 50 ml or 100 ml of iv fluid every 6 hours. An IVAC-500 pump should be used to control the rate of flow.

| Weight (lb) | Dose (units in 100 ml every 6 hr) (prophylactic anticoagulation) |
|---|---|
| 100-120 | 3,000 |
| 120-130 | 4,000 |
| 130-140 | 4,500 |
| 140-150 | 5,000 |
| 150-160 | 5,500 |
| 160-170 | 6,000 |
| 170-180 | 6,500 |
| 180-190 | 7,000 |
| 190-200 | 7,500 |
| 200-210 | 8,000 |

SUGGESTED PROCEDURE FOR ORDERING HEPARIN

1. Determine initial dose from diagnosis and weight of patient
2. Order "ACT now," 6 hours after starting heparin and daily
3. Order initial dose of heparin iv push immediately after the *stat* ACT is performed (test done at bedside)
4. Order dose in 100 ml of D5W every 6 hours per Buretrol (soluset) by IVAC-500 pump to begin immediately after iv push dose
5. Check 6 hour ACT and adjust dose if necessary
6. Check daily ACT and adjust dose if necessary
7. Check with nurse and make sure dosage is running in properly and on time
8. Check for hemorrhagic complications (chart, M.D., nurse, patient)

DOSAGE ADJUSTMENTS

| ACT | Adjustment |
|---|---|
| 2 min/30 sec or less | 5,000 units iv push; increase by 2,000 units q 6 h |
| 2 min/30 sec to 2 min/ 55 sec | Increase by 500 or 1,000 units q 6 h |
| 3 min to 4 min | No change |
| 4 min/5 sec to 4 min/20 sec | Decrease by 500 or 1,000 units q 6 h |
| 4 min/30 sec or greater | Decrease by 2,000 units q 6 h |

**(Table 2, cont.)**

NOTES

1. Decreased heparin dosage may be required for:
   a. Patient in CHF
   b. Females over 60 years of age who are more sensitive to heparin (use about 1,000 units less every 6 hours than above recommended dose)
   c. Decreased kidney function
   d. Liver disease

2. Increased heparin dosage may be required for:
   a. Pulmonary emboli (use 2,000 units or more every 6 hours than above recommended dose)
   b. Thrombophlebitis (use 2,000 units or more every 6 hours than above recommended dose)
   c. Disseminated intravascular coagulation
   d. Infection or febrile states
   e. Malignant diseases

3. The following may potentiate the effect of heparin:
   a. Dextran
   b. Bishydroxycoumarin

*Figure 3. Theoretical summation of an intravenous dose and a continuous intravenous infusion of heparin (based on clinical data); a rapid effect is obtained with a continuous therapeutic effect maintained after 2 to 3 hours*

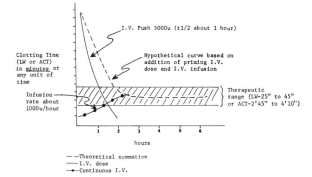

*Figure 4. ACT's of patients on continuous intravenous and subcutaneous heparin therapy; most patients fall within the therapeutic range while on intravenous drip*

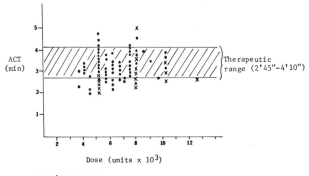

continuous intravenous infusion. The advantages of this method of administration far outweigh any disadvantages.

## References

1. Goodman, A. and Gilman, L.: The Pharmacological Basis of Therapeutics, 4th Ed., The MacMillan Company, London, England, 1970, p. 1446.
2. Wessler, S.: Studies of Intravascular Coagulation II. A Comparison of the Effects of Dicumarol and Heparin on Clot Formation in Isolated Venous Segments, *J. Clin. Invest. 32*:650–654 (July) 1953.
3. Wessler, S.: Studies in Intravascular Coagulation IV. The Effect of Heparin and Dicumarol in Serum-Induced Venous Thrombosis, *Circulation 12*:553-556 (Oct.) 1955.
4. Schwartz, S. I.: Prevention and Production of Thrombosis by Alterations in Electric Environment, *Surg. Gynecol. Obstet. 108*:533-536 (May) 1959.
5. Carey, L. C. and Williams, R. D.: Comparative Effects of Dicumarol Tromexan and Heparin on Thrombus Propagation, *Ann. Surg. 152*:919-922 (Nov.) 1960.
6. Zweufler, A. J.: Standardized Technique for the Study of Thrombus Growth: Effect of Heparin Therapy, *J. Lab. Clin. Med. 60*:254-260 (Aug.) 1962.
7. Hoak, J. C., Commer, W. E. and Warner, E. D.: The Antithrombotic Effects of Sodium Heparin and Sodium Warfarin, *Arch. Internal Med. 117*:25-30 (Jan.) 1966.
8. Wessler, S., Freiman, D. G., Ballon, J. D., Katz, J. H., Wolff, R. and Wolf, E.: Experimental Pulmonary Embolism with Serum-Induced Thrombi, *Am. J. Pathol. 38*:89-101 (Jan.) 1961.
9. Duff, I. F., Linman, J. W. and Birch, R.: The Administration of Heparin, *Surg. Gynecol. Obstet. 93*:343-362 (Sept.) 1951.
10. Rapport, S. I.: Clotting Factor Assays on Plasma from Patients Receiving Intramuscular or Subcutaneous Heparin, *Am. J. Med. Sci. 234*:678-686 (Dec.) 1957.
11. Simon, H. B.: Daggett, W. M. and DeSanctis, R. W.: Hemothorax as a Complication of Anticoagulant Therapy in the Presence of Pulmonary Infarction, *J. Am. Med. Assoc. 208*:1830-1834 (June 9) 1969.
12. Wynn, A. and Goodwin, J. F.: Prolonged Anticoagulant Therapy with Heparin, *Brit. Med. J. 2*:893-896 (Apr. 26) 1952.
13. Handley, A. J.: Heparin Administration by Constant Infusion Pump, *Brit. Med. J. 2*:482-484 (May 20) 1967.
14. Spracklen, F. H. N., Model, D. G. and Besterman, E. M. M.: The Dangers of Intermittent Intravenous Heparin Therapy, *Postgrad. Med. 42*:724-726 (Nov.) 1966.
15. Harden, R.: A Method for Intravenous Administration of Heparin in Myocardial Infarction, *Brit. Med. J. 4*:1106-1107 (Nov. 2) 1963.
16. Carleton, R. A., Sanders, C. A. and Burack, W. R.: Heparin Administration After Acute Myocardial Infarction, *New Engl. J. Med. 263*:1002-1005 (Nov. 17) 1960.
17. Vieweg, W. V. R., Piscatelli, R. L., Houser, J. J. and Proulx, R. A.: Complications of Intravenous Administration of Heparin in Elderly Women, *J. Am. Med. Assoc. 213*:1303-1306 (Aug. 24) 1970.
18. Parker, W. S.: Rupture of the Rectus Abdominis Muscle with Hematoma, *Arch. Surg. 81*:655-659 (Oct.) 1960.
19. Morrison, F. S.: Retroperitoneal Hemorrhage During Heparin Therapy, *Am. J. Card. 13*:329-332 (Mar.) 1964.
20. Roberta, B., Rosato, F. E. and Rosato, E. F.: Heparin—A Cause of Arterial Emboli?, *Surgery 55*:803-808 (June) 1964.
21. Borkovich, K. H.: Acute Anemia and Abdominal Tumor Due to Hemorrhage in Rectus Abdominis Sheath Following Anticoagulation Therapy, *Arch. Internal Med. 117*:103-106 (Jan.) 1966.
22. Musgrove, J. E.: Hematoma of the Rectus Abdominis Muscle During Anticoagulant Therapy, *Can. Med. Assoc. J. 95*:827 (Oct. 15) 1966.
23. Klassen, J. and Murphy, B. E. P.: Survival After Bilateral Adrenal Hemorrhage During Heparin Therapy, *Can. Med. Assoc. J. 97*:1162-1165 (Nov. 4) 1967.
24. Susens, G. P.: Femoral Nerve Entrapment Secondary to a Heparin Hematoma, *Ann. Internal Med. 69*:575-579 (Sept.) 1968.
25. Griffith, G. C. and Boggs, R. P.: The Clinical Usage of Heparin, *Am. J. Cardiol. 14*:39-68 (July) 1964.
26. Jick, H., Slone, D., Borda, I. T. and Shapiro, S.: Efficacy and Toxicity of Heparin in Relation to Age and Sex, *New Engl. J. Med. 279*:284-285 (Aug.) 1968.
27. Estes, J. W.: Kinetics of the Anticoagulant Effect of Heparin. *J. Am. Med. Assoc. 212*:1492-1495 (June 1) 1970.
28. Allison, S. B.: The Activated Clotting Time in the Control of Heparin Therapy, *Bull. Geisinger Med. Ctr. 21*:199-211 (Nov.) 1969.

29. Hattersley, P. B.: Activated Coagulation Time of Whole Blood, *J. Am. Med. Assoc. 196*:150-154 (May 2) 1966.

30. O'Sullivan, E. F., Hirsh, J., McCarthy, R. A. and De Gruchy, G. C.: Heparin in the Treatment of Yenous Thromboembolic Disease: Administration Control and Results, *Med. J. Australia 2*:153-159 (July 27) 1968.

31. Dale, W. A.: et al.: Heparin Control of Venous Thromboembolism, *Arch. Surg. 101*:744-754 (Dec.) 1970.

32. Pombo, J. F. et al.: Heparin Requirements in Patients With Acute Myocardial Infarction, *Arch. Internal Med. 126*:1000-1003 (Dec.) 1970.

33. Martyn, D. T. et al.: Continuous Intravenous Administration of Heparin, *Mayo Clin. Proc. 46*:347-351 (May) 1971.

# 15 Detection of Drug-induced Blood Dyscrasias

Margo Swanson and Ray Cook

Pharmacist involvement in a hospital program to detect drug-induced blood dyscrasias is described.

Pharmacists obtain comprehensive drug histories on all patients subjected to hemograms or bone marrow studies. Included in the drug histories are the specific hematological side effects that have been reported to occur from the drugs ingested by the patients involved. Specific pharmacist involvement is illustrated in three patient cases.

Of 94 drug histories obtained in this program, an association between drugs and blood dyscrasias was demonstrated in 14 patients.

The incidence of drug-induced blood dyscrasias in the hospital is unknown. The hematological toxicity of certain drugs used in the treatment of neoplastic diseases is well known and expected; however, blood dyscrasias produced by other drugs are seldom anticipated or implicated. Case reports in the literature frequently fail to indicate the true magnitude of this problem. Drugs are frequently ignored or may be unrecognized as a cause of blood dyscrasias, and once it has been established that a drug can cause a particular blood dyscrasia, only a small proportion of cases are likely to be reported. Pharmacists in clinical practice at Memorial Hospital Medical Center of Long Beach are involved in the detection of drug-induced blood dyscrasias. The hematology section of the pathology department has requested pharmacists working in the patient care areas to obtain a drug history on every patient for whom a hemogram or bone marrow studies are performed. Included in the pharmacists' reports are the specific hematological side effects that have been reported to occur from the drugs ingested by the patient. The hematologist utilizes this information in the consideration of drugs as etiological agents in blood dyscrasias. This chapter discusses the preparation of these reports and presents several cases which illustrate the value of this service in improving patient care.

## Drug History Reports

The pharmacist receives chart copies of all physicians' orders, and when a hemogram or bone marrow aspiration is ordered, the pharmacist routinely interviews the patient to obtain a drug history. This information must be as accurate and informative as possible because some drug-induced blood dyscrasias are dose- or duration-related. An example of a completed drug history form is shown in Figure 1.

The first section of the drug history is concerned with drugs taken prior to admission (PTA). Specific information on the names of drugs, doses, duration and any previous courses of administration is obtained. The patient is questioned regarding prescription medications, nonprescription medications, injections of medications received at home or in the doctor's office, allergies, alcohol consumption and exposure to toxic chemicals such as benzene and insecticides. If the patient does not know what drugs he has been taking, the pharmacist may obtain the information from other sources, i.e., the patient's family and friends, physician, community pharmacist, records of previous hospital admissions, etc.

The second section of the drug history is concerned with the patient's current medication. An accurate drug history for this section is easily obtained from the patient's chart.

The third section of the drug history report form is for comments by the pharmacist. In this section are listed the drug-induced blood dyscrasias that have been associated with the drugs the patient has ingested. In an attempt to provide accurate, useful information to the hematologist, the literature is researched and a reference card is prepared with pertinent information for each drug. These cards are kept in a file for future use. An example of such a card is shown in Figure 2. References of case reports in the literature are on the reverse side of this card. Although the true incidence of a particular drug-induced blood dyscrasia is rarely available, other

*Figure 1. Drug history, hemogram and bone marrow report for case #1*

Figure 1. Drug history, hemogram and bone marrow report for case #1

```
                        Drug History

DRUGS PTA
   Ovulen 21 for 5 yrs
   ASA occasionally
   Insecticide spray—exposure to Easy Off 1 week ago
   Quinidine—took 200 mg q.i.d. for about a week in July, has taken 1 or
      2 tablets on several other occasions. On 9/3/71 she took 1 tablet at
      10:00 p.m.

CURRENT MEDICATIONS
   Hydrocortisone 100 mg i.m.q. 8 hr for 5 doses
   Aristocort 8 mg q.i.d.
   Maalox 15 ml q.i.d.

COMMENT
   Quinidine:
      Thrombocytopenia: 119 cases have been reported.
                        Dose: Not dose-related. The majority of pa-
                           tients have a history of previous inges-
                           tion. It can occur upon ingestion of only
                           one tablet.
                        Mechanism: Immune thrombocytopenia.
      Hemolytic anemia: 1 case associated with thrombocytopenia.

                   Hemogram Report—Summary

Clinical Problem: Thrombocytopenic purpura

Diagnosis and Comments:
   1. Severe thrombocytopenia (secondary to quinidine). Aside from the
      clinical history, there is strong evidence to suggest that this is
      secondary to quinidine, i.e., once platelet level had reached 50,000,
      the pharmacist mixed patient's blood with quinidine and found it
      would not clot nor contract (vs. saline control which formed good
      clot with retraction).
   2. Low iron, borderline percent saturation.

                  Bone Marrow Report—Summary

Conclusion: Normal numbers of megakaryocytes in face of thrombo-
            cytopenia is compatible with peripheral immune destruction.

Comment: Normocellular marrow.
```

*Figure 2. Example of card file information on drug-induced blood dyscrasias*

```
METHIMAZOLE (TAPAZOLE, THIAMIZOLE, MERCAZOLE)

APLASTIC ANEMIA: 10 cases
                 Dose: 20–60 mg/day × 1–3 months

NEUTROPENIA: 80 cases
             Dose: 10–60 mg/day × 12 days–4 months
             Mechanism: 16–bone marrow depression
                        2–immunological tests suggested the
                           presence of antibodies against the
                           neutrophils

THROMBOCYTOPENIA: 3 cases
                  Dose: 40 mg/day × 5 months
```

valuable information is obtained. Such information includes dose and duration of drug intake at which the dyscrasia occurred and the mechanism by which the blood dyscrasia is produced.

## Case Presentations

The following case presentations are some examples from Memorial Hospital Medical Center of Long Beach which document the value of this service in improving patient care.

*Case #1.* This 40-year-old white female patient was admitted on 9/4/71 with purpura and extensive bruising. A complete blood count (CBC) on admission showed a severe thrombocytopenia with a platelet count of 2,000/mm³. When a hemogram and bone marrow aspiration were ordered to determine the etiology of the thrombocytopenia, the pharmacist obtained a drug history (Figure 1). The patient had taken quinidine sporadically during the two months preceeding admission for "heart palpitations." On the day prior to admission she had taken one tablet at 10:00 p.m. and developed chills, fever and purpura.

Since quinidine was the most likely etiological agent for this patient's thrombocytopenia, the pharmacist performed an in vitro test, as described by Weintraub[1] in an attempt to confirm this possibility. Two milliliters of freshly drawn blood were added directly to one test tube containing 0.2 mg of quinidine (60 µg/ml) and to one test tube containing 0.2 ml of normal saline. The same procedure was followed using blood from a control subject who had no known history of quinidine thrombocytopenia. In the test tube containing the patient's blood sample and quinidine, there was no clot formation or retraction. Clot formation and retraction occurred in the saline tube containing the patient's blood sample and in both samples from the control subject. These results are consistent with quinidine-induced peripheral immune destruction of platelets in this patient.

The summary of the hemogram and bone marrow report from the hematologist for this patient is shown in Figure 1. The bone marrow showed normal numbers of megakaryocytes which would also suggest that peripheral immune destruction was occurring.

The patient was discharged six days later with a normal platelet count, and she was given specific instructions to avoid the use of quinidine. In this case the pharmacist made a significant contribution in the diagnosis and confirmation of the etiological agent.

Thrombocytopenic purpura as a manifestation of hypersensitivity to quinidine has been frequently reported in the literature.[2,3] The incidence of this particular hematologic effect of quinidine is probably much higher than the literature would indicate. This is a well-known side effect of quinidine and since it has been frequently described, many cases are not reported.

*Case #2.* This 70-year-old male was admitted because of weakness and anemia. The admitting CBC showed a white blood cell count (WBC) of 3,700/mm³, hemoglobin (Hgb) 8.6 g/100 ml and a platelet count of 82,000/mm³. A hemogram and bone marrow aspiration were ordered, and the pharmacist obtained the drug history shown in Figure 3. The patient had a normal CBC during his last hospital admission in 1969. The only hematologically toxic agent he had been exposed to since that time was tolbutamide. Bone marrow depression related to tolbu-

Figure 3. *Drug history, hemogram and bone marrow report for case #2*

```
                    Drug History

DRUGS PTA
   Orinase 500 mg t.i.d. for 2 yrs
   Peritrate 10 mg t.i.d. for 2 yrs

CURRENT DRUGS
   Orinase 500 mg b.i.d.
   Allbee W/C t.i.d.
   Tylenol prn
   Doriden 500 mg hs

COMMENT
   Orinase:
      Aplastic anemia: 12 cases
                 Dose: 500 mg to 2 g/day for 7 wks to 7 yrs
                 Neutropenia: 7 cases, 3 fatal
                 Thrombocytopenia: 5 cases
                 Dose: ? few wks to few months

            Hemogram Report—Summary

Clinical Problem: 70-yr-old male with diabetes and previous history of
             subtotal gastrectomy for ulcer. Anemia.

Diagnosis and Comments: Neutropenia, normochromic, normocytic
                 anemia. Thrombocytopenia, elevated serum
                 iron.

            Bone Marrow Report—Summary

Conclusion: Hypoplastic marrow.

Comments: In about 50% of cases no cause can be found for this prob-
          lem. In the other 50%, toxic exposure, most commonly to
          drugs, is implicated. In this man's case, the pharmacist has
          suggested that the most likely culprit is Orinase.
          The elevated iron may be due to decreased utilization by the
          red cells.
```

Figure 4. *Drug history, hemogram and bone marrow report for case #3*

```
                    Drug History

DRUGS PTA
   Has been taking multiple medications since at least 1962
   During his most recent admission, 1/19/72 to 3/1/72, he received the
      following drugs: B-12 1 mg/day, Titralac 6/day, Robaxin, Talwin,
      Placidyl, Valium, Indocin, Lomotil, Aldoril, Demerol, Dramamine,
      Sparine, Roniacol, Percodan (ASA 224 mg, acetophenetedin, caf-
      feine), Percogesic (acetaminophen), Soma Compound (aceto-
      phenetedin, caffeine), Zactrin Compound (ASA 227 mg, phenacetin
      162 mg, caffeine), Darvon Compound (ASA, phenacetin, caffeine)
   Since his discharge in March: ECC½ 2 tabs every 4 hrs, Demerol 50
      mg every 4 hrs, Darvon Compound prn (4 to 8/day), Titralac (cal-
      cium carbonate 420 mg) 2–6/day, Lomotil prn, Noludar 300 mg hs

CURRENT DRUGS
   Thorazine 250 mg/day
   Dilantin 200 mg/day
   KCl 40 mEq/day
   Amytal 200 mg hs
   Phenobarbital 130 mg hs
   Talwin, Demerol prn
   Percodan prn (6 to 8/day)

COMMENT
   Analgesic Abuse Syndrome:
      Usually occurs from doses of analgesics of 3 to 50 tablets/day for 3
      to 20 yrs. It includes the following symptoms:
            Analgesic nephropathy: Renal papillary necrosis with interstitial
                             nephritis. Increased serum creatinine
                             and decreased creatinine clearance.
      Gastritis, G.I. bleeding, ulcers.
      Hypertension, headache, psychiatric disorders, musculoskeletal
      complaints.
      Anemia: Due to renal disease.
             Chronic hemolytic anemia (phenacetin, G6PD deficiency).
             Iron deficiency.
             Sulfhemoglobin, methemoglobin, Heinz bodies.
   Milk Alkali Syndrome:
      Titralac: Hypercalcemia has resulted from the ingestion of calcium
                carbonate.
      Milk: Patient states he is a "big milk drinker" (several quarts or more
            a day).

            Hemogram Report—Summary

Clinical Problem: 63-year-old white male with high serum calcium.
                 ? multiple myeloma, ? hyperparathyroidism.

Diagnosis and Comments:
   1. Mild normochromic, normocytic anemia without reticulocyte re-
      sponse. The cause for this is not apparent but could be related to
      renal disease.
   2. Elevated creatinine.

   Several possible causes would include analgesic abuse syndrome as
   suggested by the pharmacist or an effect of high calcium on the kid-
   neys. The pharmacist also raises the question of milk alkali syndrome
   on the basis of Titralac and milk ingestion.

            Bone Marrow Report—Summary

Conclusion: Normal bone marrow.
```

tamide has been reported by Chapman et al.[4] A summary of the hemogram and bone marrow reports are shown in Figure 3.

Tolbutamide was discontinued and the patient was discharged after receiving a blood transfusion. Without the information obtained by this drug history, the patient probably would have been continued on tolbutamide. Subsequent follow-up indicated that the patient's hemogram had returned to normal.

*Case #3.* The drug histories obtained for hemograms may also be helpful in detecting other side effects of drugs besides blood dyscrasias, as demonstrated by this case. This 63-year-old-male was admitted with muscle twitching. A CBC showed a slight anemia, and an electrolyte panel showed an elevated serum calcium of 12.6 mg/100 ml (normal 8.5—10.5 mg/100 ml). His creatinine clearance was reported as 14 ml/min (normal 100—130 ml/min). The differential diagnosis included multiple myeloma and hyperparathyroidism. A bone marrow was ordered to determine if the patient had multiple myeloma. The drug history shown in Figure 4 was obtained by the pharmacist from the patient and from his charts from previous admissions. Two important considerations were revealed from the drug history. First, the patient had been taking numerous analgesics containing aspirin, phenacetin and caffeine for a number of years, which suggested the possibility of an "analgesic abuse syn-

drome." The association between analgesic abuse and renal impairment has been frequently discussed in the literature.[5,6] A review of the analgesic abuse syndrome has been presented by Gault et al.[7] This patient had the following symptoms which have been described in the analgesic abuse syndrome: renal impairment, musculoskeletal complaints, gastritis, hypertension, anemia and a psychiatric disorder. Second, the patient also stated that he was a "big milk drinker" (two or more quarts a day) and that he had been using Titralac tablets (calcium carbonate 420 mg/tablet) for over a year. This suggested a possibility of milk-alkali syndrome. The pertinent features of the milk-alkali syndrome are hypercalcemia, renal impairment and acid-base disturbances.[8]

A summary of the hematologist's report is shown in Figure 4. Based on the drug history report, the patient's physician instructed the patient to discontinue all intake of aspirin-, phenacetin- and caffeine-containing analgesics, all antacids containing calcium, and to restrict milk intake. The Demerol injections were gradually decreased and the patient was then discharged to be followed as an outpatient. Subsequent communication with the physician revealed a decreased serum calcium level and marked improvement in the patient.

## Comments

The preparation of drug history reports for all patients at Memorial Hospital Medical Center of Long Beach when hemograms and bone marrow studies are ordered is a clinical service provided by the pharmacy department to improve patient care. This pharmacist activity demonstrates specialization in the area of drug-induced blood dyscrasias. The pharmacists' time is directed toward a group of patients with a relatively high potential for this drug side effect. The pharmacist practicing in the clinical area is the most logical and qualified member of the health care team to provide this service. When a hemogram or bone marrow studies are ordered the physician receives not only a consult from the hematologist but also from the pharmacist.

A potential benefit of this service may be the detection of drug-induced blood dyscrasias previously unknown or unreported. This is particularly applicable to the many new drugs which appear on the market each year whose side effects may not be completely known. Of 94 drug histories obtained by pharmacists in this program, a significant association between the ingestion of drugs and blood dyscrasias was demonstrated in 14 patients. These included five patients with neutropenia, four with thrombocytopenia and five with anemia. Fifteen other patients in this group had other side effects associated with drug ingestion such as gastrointestinal bleeding, hepatotoxicity and lupus erythematosus.

In addition to drug-induced blood dyscrasias, the hematologist is also interested in ascertaining from the pharmacists' report which drugs the patient has ingested that may affect pharmacologically the hemogram, e.g., iron, folic acid, vitamin $B_{12}$ and steroids, although they may not be involved in the production of a blood dyscrasia.

In addition to improving patient care, this activity has enhanced the professional relationship and cooperation between the pharmacy department, the pathology department and the medical staff of the hospital.

## References

1. Weintraub, R. M., Pechet, L. and Alexander, B.: Rapid Diagnosis of Drug-Induced Thrombocytopenic Purpura, *J. Amer. Med. Ass. 180*:528–532 (May 19) 1962.
2. Bolton, F. G. and Dameshek, W.: Thrombocytopenic Purpura Due to Quinidine, *Blood 11*:527–546 (June) 1956.
3. Bolton F. G.: Thrombocytopenic Purpura Due to Quinidine, *Blood 11*:547–564 (June) 1956.
4. Chapman, I. and Cheung, W. H.: Pancytopenia Associated with Tolbutamide Therapy, *J. Amer. Med. Ass. 186*:595–596 (Nov. 9) 1963.
5. Murray, R. M., Lawson, D. H. and Linton, A. L.: Analgesic Nephropathy, *Brit. Med. J. 1*:479–482 (Feb. 27) 1971.
6. Gault, M. H. Blennerhassett, J. and Muehrcke, R. C.: Analgesic Nephropathy, *Amer. J. Med. 51*:740–756 (Dec.) 1971.
7. Gault, M. H., Rudwal, T. C., Engles, W. D. et al.: Syndrome Associated with the Abuse of Analgesics, *Ann. Intern. Med. 68*:906–925 (Apr.) 1968.
8. Wenger, J., Kirsner, J. B. and Palmer, W. L.: The Milk-Alkali Syndrome, *Gastroenterology 33*:745–769 (Nov.) 1957.

# 16 A Clinically Oriented Hospital Pharmacy Intern-resident Program

M. A. Riddiough, D. L. Sorby, and E. Owyang

A two-year training program designed to develop the skills necessary to implement, direct, and instruct clinical pharmacy programs is described.

Eligibility requirements for admission and selection of trainees are discussed. During the intern year, the trainee is a full-time senior student and has a service commitment of 250 hours. During the resident year, the trainee has a full-time service commitment. Participation of the trainees in seminars and supervision of the intern-residents are also described.

The University of California Hospital Pharmacy Intern-Resident Program is designed to provide an individual with two years of training in hospital pharmacy operations with special emphasis placed on developing the person's technical, administrative, and teaching skills necessary to implement, direct, and instruct clinical pharmacy programs. The basic intention is to develop leadership qualities in the trainee, which will enable him to effectively utilize his training, especially in the area of clinical pharmacy services. In order to do so, emphasis is placed on developing personal abilities in areas of effective communication, responsible service, and administrative finesse. In addition, we attempt to inform the trainee of professional obligations and trends of health care needs on a nationwide basis.

In an attempt to meet the professional demands being placed on our program graduates, the training goals of the program have changed quite significantly during the last few years. Until recently, major emphasis was placed on training in hospital pharmacy administration, with the intention of producing future chief pharmacists. A survey of the nature of practice of recent program graduates (since 1965) revealed that over 70% are currently developing and directing clinical pharmacy teaching and/or service programs. In an effort to meet this demand for pharmacists who are qualified to implement clinical pharmacy services, the Intern-Resident Program now provides broad based training in hospital pharmacy, with a heavy emphasis on the clinical practice of pharmacy.

Currently, there are eleven trainees in the program—five interns and six residents. Interns are fourth year students in the school of pharmacy who are enrolled in full-time course work in addition to having a minimum service commitment to the hospital of 1300 hours. Following successful completion of the intern year and receipt of the Doctor of Pharmacy degree, the trainee is appointed as a Resident in Hospital Pharmacy. Resident training consists of full-time practice, devoted mainly to serving in our clinical pharmacy programs, teaching pharmacy students, and performing administrative functions. Interns are salaried by the hospital and residents are salaried jointly by the hospital and the School of Pharmacy. These trainees serve as members of the hospital's clinical house staff.

Eligibility requirements for entering this training program at the intern level include admission to the University of California School of Pharmacy and completion of an academic course of study equivalent to the first three years of the professional curriculum at the University of California School of Pharmacy. Entrance at the resident level requires a Doctor of Pharmacy degree, in addition to academic and clerkship experience in clinical pharmacy equivalent to that offered in the intern year at the University of California. Trainees are selected by a committee comprised of members of the faculty and of the supervisory staff of the pharmaceutical services department.

Appointments are awarded on the basis of evidence of above average scholarship in professional studies, apparent interest in hospital pharmacy, leadership potential and individual personality.

## The Intern Year

The basic purpose of the intern year is to develop in the trainee an understanding of the overall scope of responsibilities of the pharmacy service in a hospital. Emphasis is placed on presenting the mechanisms employed in meeting these responsibilities. The intern is trained not only to practice in various pharmacy services, but also to analyze contributions of pharmacy service to patient care, to understand the administrative problems of operation, and to propose methods of improving existing services.

During this twelve month appointment, the intern provides a minimum of 250 hours of service in each of the following areas of pharmacy practice:

1. Outpatient Service
2. Pharmaceutical Services Administration
3. Inpatient Service: Distribution Systems
4. Parenteral Solutions Manufacturing Laboratory
5. Clinical Pharmacy Program.

*Outpatient Service.* When assigned to this area, the intern participates in three main activities:

1. Providing medications in a traditional outpatient dispensing system
2. Working with a clinical pharmacist in the pediatric outpatient clinic
3. Working with the department supervisor on various administrative tasks.

This scope of activities is designed to provide the intern with a working knowledge of existing methods of delivering outpatient pharmacy service, the need for expanded and more patient-oriented roles of the pharmacist in outpatient clinics, and the administrative problems encountered when implementing new services in an outpatient clinic.

*Pharmaceutical Services Administration.* During this assignment the intern encounters several of the responsibilities of the chief pharmacist, and gains insight as to the scope of pharmacy involvement at the administrative level. His experiences include working with interdepartmental operations, physical facilities planning, budgeting, personnel management, and interprofessional relationships. An attempt is made in this rotation, as well as throughout the program, to instill administrative tact in the trainee which will enable him to work effectively with people.

*Inpatient Service: Distribution Systems.* This assignment provides the intern with experience working with two drug distribution systems and the opportunity to analyze the advantages and disadvantages of each. At the University of California, San Francisco, we are in the process of converting our inpatient drug distribution from the individual prescription system to a centralized unit dose system, and the intern actively participates in both. In addition to learning the dispensing functions in both systems, he receives training in manufacturing-strip packaging procedures. He also monitors the unit dose system in the patient care areas, observing its utilization by patients, nurses and physicians. This range of activities allows the intern to view these distribution systems from several operational aspects. He is asked to evaluate our efforts in inpatient distribution, to determine which functions best allow the pharmacist to provide effective drug distribution, and to suggest methods of improving this service.

*Parenteral Solutions Manufacturing Laboratory.* While assigned to this service, the intern learns the responsibilities of the pharmacist in the formulation, manufacture, and control of parenteral solutions. He is taught to utilize aseptic technique, as well as the various methods of sterilization. We will soon be developing a centralized, hospital-wide intravenous additive program and the intern is now being brought into the administrative and technical aspects of its implementation.

*Clinical Pharmacy Program.* Intern participation in our clinical pharmacy services includes providing drug information, taking patient medication histories, monitoring patient drug therapy, and interacting with physicians and nurses on our surgical and medical floors. Since this clinical experience is essential to the trainee's ability to develop future pharmacy services, the intern serves approximately twice as much time in our clinical program as in other areas of service. Half of this time is spent on assignment to our drug information and analysis service.

As previously stated, in addition to fulfilling his service commitment, the intern is also a full-time senior student in our Doctor of Pharmacy curriculum. Since the academic content of this fourth professional year is comprised almost entirely of clinical pharmacy courses and clinical clerkship experience, the intern is able to incorporate this education into his training assignments.

At the end of the intern year, the trainee is considered to have a working understanding of all phases of our pharmacy services and is prepared to assume the responsibilities placed upon him as a pharmacy resident.

## The Resident Year

The resident year of training is designed to develop further the trainee's professional, administrative, and teaching skills, thus enabling him to gain the expertise necessary to coordinate future pharmacy service and/or teaching programs. The resident is a postdoctoral student in the school of pharmacy and provides full-time service to the hospital and the school. He receives eight months of training at the University of California, San Francisco, and four months at San Francisco Veterans Administration Hospital. Clinical pharmacy services are being developed at both institutions, thus the trainee is given exposure to a variety of implementation procedures and methods of program development. The resident assumes the responsibilities of a registered pharmacist in both hospitals, with the great majority of his activities involved with:

1. Practicing in clinical pharmacy services
2. Participating in clinical pharmacy teaching programs for senior students
3. Performing various administrative projects.

Approximately 60% of the resident's time (24 hr/week) is devoted to assigned practice in our clinical pharmacy services. He participates in surgical and medical work and teaching rounds; he interviews patients and determines their ability to receive medications; he consults with physicians and nurses concerning drug therapy; he monitors patients' drug regimens daily; and he participates as a member of the hospital's cardiac resuscitation team. The trainee also receives extensive training in our drug information service where he learns not only to retrieve and disseminate information, but also to employ his clinical knowledge and provide pertinent information which will lead to effective drug utilization. In addition, the resident staffs our central unit dose dispensing system, and contributes administratively to the improvement of the services operation. While practicing in these areas, the resident assumes full responsibility for his activities. He receives general supervision from the entire clinical pharmacy staff throughout the year.

A second major responsibility of our residents is that of providing teaching service. This includes supervising pharmacy students during their clinical clerkship assignments on the surgical and medical floors, as well as periodically leading conferences associated with the clinical teaching program. Residents also are teamed with an academic faculty member to serve as class advisors for freshmen pharmacy students. The intentions of this counseling assignment are to (1) provide the students with a person to whom they can relate clinical pharmacy practice, and (2) to introduce the approach of a recent graduate into the student counseling program. Occasionally, interns and residents provide lectures in pharmacology to nursing staff and students, dental hygiene students, and other paramedical personnel in the hospital.

At the San Francisco Veterans Administration Hospital, the residents provide several weekly in-service education seminars for the pharmacy staff concerning the clinical use of drugs. They also provide lectures in the basic sciences and pharmacology, and in addition, supervise on-the-job training in the pharmacy technician training program at the Veterans Administration Hospital. This latter teaching experience gives the resident an opportunity to gain better insight into the capabilities of pharmacy technicians and the level of training that is necessary in the development of nonprofessional pharmacy personnel.

These various teaching experiences, combined with working experience in clinical pharmacy services, provide the resident with the skills that are necessary to establish teaching programs related to the clinical use of drugs, whether it be aimed at professional students, pharmacists, physicians, nurses, or technical staff.

A third major area of resident training is that of performing various administrative services for the hospitals and the school of pharmacy. The phrase "administrative service" in this text does not carry the traditional connotation of budgeting, inventory control, etc. It refers to the planning and coordinating of activities that accompany implemtation and operation of new or improved pharmacy services. Each trainee is assigned an administrative research project or study area which he is to develop during his resident year. These projects are assigned on the basis of the trainee's interests and performance demonstrated during his intern year. Every attempt is made to appropriately match the individual's professional desire and ability to the designated administrative assignment. Examples of this year's resident projects include establishing plans and a proposal for a hospital-wide intravenous additive program; developing the groundwork for a local multihospital drug information service network; analyzing the clinical pharmacist's professional activities and defining his contributions to patient care; and assisting in the planning of physical facilities, service objectives, and methods of operation of decentralized outpatient clinical pharmacy services. As can be seen, these are not obscure assignments designed merely to keep the resident busy. They are areas of great concern to the development of our pharmacy services and require sincere effective effort. Whenever possible, it is intended for the resident to develop plans of operation, make proposals, and participate in implementation. Frequently, interns are asked to participate in these projects in order that they may continue these activities as residents. These assignments require extensive interaction with personnel at various levels of responsibility and provide the trainee with the opportunity of working with a multidisciplinary population. Various short term projects are also asked of the residents and interns throughout the program, i.e., drafting staff work schedules and performing drug utilization studies in the hospital.

## Seminars

Weekly seminars are held to provide additional administrative background. The majority of these seminars involve presentation and discussion of other hospital department operations; thus giving the trainee better insight of the hospital's total activities and responsibilities. In addition, these seminars provide training in various administrative managerial responsibilities, i.e., personnel management, communications techniques, and budgeting requirements. Visits to other hospitals and various types of health care treatment centers are offered in conjunction with these seminars.

## Supervision

The director of pharmaceutical services, who is also a member of the faculty of the school of pharmacy, is administratively responsible for the Intern-Resident Program. However, general supervision of the program is maintained by an Intern-Resident Program coordinator and the chief pharmacist. The program coordinator is a member of the clinical faculty of the school of pharmacy and devotes approximately 50% of his time to the Intern-Resident Program. His responsibilities in this respect include coordinating intern and resident work assignments to insure that they are consistent with program objectives; orienting of supervisory staff of the pharmacy service to the training objectives of interns and residents assigned to service functions; supervising and guiding administrative work projects of interns and residents; and making recommendations to the director and chief pharmacist concerning content and objectives of the Intern-Resident Program. The chief pharmacist instructs the interns and residents regarding the administrative aspects of hospital pharmacy service operations. He is also responsible for directing the staff of the pharmacy service to provide training to interns and residents.

## Conclusion

The University of California School of Pharmacy and University Hospitals are attempting to develop programs which will provide improved patient-oriented pharmacy services and will better train pharmacy students for their future roles in patient care. The Hospital Pharmacy Intern-Resident Program described here should provide the trainee with the framework of skills and knowledge needed for practice in innovative pharmacy programs whether his responsibilities involve professional practice, teaching or administration.

# 17 Clinical Pharmacy in the Small Hospital

Melvin Thomason

Clinical pharmacy practice in small hospitals is discussed.
Topics covered include implementation of clinical programs, patient chart review, drug histories, gaining clinical knowledge, and discharge interviews.

Can clinical pharmacy be practiced in the small hospital? Yes, it definitely can and should be practiced there, even more so than in large hospitals, which are usually teaching centers. If the physician in the large hospital feels that he needs advice, there are nearly always peers present whom he can ask; also, there may be a clinical pharmacologist no more than a telephone call away. In a small hospital, a clinical pharmacologist is usually not available. Someone must inform the physician about the recent developments concerning drugs and there are only two individuals available—the professional service representative and the pharmacist.

What is clinical pharmacy in the small hospital? It is the extrication of the pharmacist from the confines of the pharmacy and the contribution of his knowledge toward total patient care. What can the pharmacist in a small hospital do in order to accomplish this goal? The first thing is to stop performing the physical tasks of counting and pouring and obtain a competent technician to do these tasks under proper supervision. Also, what is so sacred about the pharmacist doing the purchasing? If adequate purchase records have been kept, a technician can be taught to keep inventories and initiate purchase orders under the supervision of a pharmacist. There are surely many other duties which could be adequately performed by a technician which would result in more time for the pharmacist to devote to other activities.

## How To Begin

Many things have been written and said about performing the professional tasks associated with clinical pharmacy, but how should a pharmacist in a small hospital begin? Does he simply present himself at the nursing station and start to monitor drug therapy? He might, if he never wanted cooperation from nursing again. The pharmacist should go to the director of nursing and discuss his plan with her and inform her of the possible benefits to the patients and her nursing staff. The pharmacist should inform physicians of his plans through the pharmacy and therapeutics committee. Even prior to talking to these people he must convince the hospital administrator of the need for a larger pharmacy budget. The pharmacist will need a very firm foundation for this request. After all, he is attempting to involve himself in an area that many people feel is out of the pharmacist's domain. The facts and figures should relate specifically to the hospital involved—data from another hospital may be used as a possible source of back-up material. In order to document a need for clinical pharmacy service in a small hospital, time must be spent searching medical records to determine:

1. How many patients received a drug potentially dangerous to them because of
   a. Allergy
   b. Drug interaction
   c. Idiosyncrasy
2. How many patients received a drug that interfered with a laboratory test
3. How many patients were discharged on drugs that may have been dangerous to them because of possible drug interaction
4. How many patients received warnings (as noted in the chart) concerning nonprescription and discharge medications

## The Patient Chart

The clinical pharmacist should become thoroughly familiar with the patient chart. The chart can be used for checking drug regimens and for bringing all aspects of the patient's medical treatment into perspective. The chart contains a patient's complete personal history, physical examination results, consultation reports by specialists, laboratory and other test reports. For example, if the patient is a diabetic, the chart should contain a complete record of blood sugar levels, urine sugar tests and insulin dosage, as well as the patient's diet. In addition, the nurses' notes are available which show the iv fluids, treatments, blood pressure, voidings and observations of the patient. The chart contains a progress record which gives a running picture of the patient's condition. Another record available in the chart is the treatment record where all drugs, radiotherapy and treatments are recorded. Graphic charts are also included which detail the blood pressure, temperature, weight, and fluid input-output information.

With the patient chart information, the pharmacist can make accurate judgements as to the effectiveness of the drug regimen. Under these circumstances the pharmacist can be of service to the patient by recommending to the physician, if necessary, that he might find a different drug or a different route of administration to be indicated. The pharmacist can help the nurse by bringing to light some of the side effects for which she should be alert. He can look for drug-drug, drug-food, and drug-laboratory test interactions or contraindications.

## Medical Rounds

I do not believe that the pharmacist can render a service on medical work rounds. The pharmacist is as much out of place here as the physician or nurse are when they compound an iv admixture. Some pharmacists go on medical work rounds, but they have not had the training of the physician to enable them to be of service at the bedside. How many pharmacists could consistently be accurate in their diagnosis of drug reaction? This is the function of the specialist — not the amateur — and the specialty of pharmacists is drugs.

To quote Palmer, "On clinical rounds, a drug is something that enters the discussion of a patients disorder at the very end as a mysterious but necessary intruder to an otherwise pristine discussion of differential diagnosis or surgical technique."[1] An editorial in *Medical Tribune* stated, "Without demeaning the importance of the hospital pharmacist . . . it is difficult

for us to visualize what could be offered by the pharmacist in hospital rounds at the patient's bedside."[2] However, there is a need for the pharmacist to check the patient's chart to determine if the drugs the patient is receiving are the best ones for his condition.

## Drug Histories

Some hospital pharmacists are presently taking drug histories upon admission of the patient to the hospital.[3] This history is placed in the chart as well as in the patient's medication profile. In a large metropolitan area where the patient may not have a family physician and in many cases is admitted via the emergency department, this interview could be very helpful. However, in the small hospital where most admissions are by a family physician, the patient interview may not be as important. However, if upon reading the patient's history, the pharmacist feels that there are some pertinent questions that should be asked about the patient's drug therapy, then he should determine the answers to his questions. After the pharmacist has interviewed a patient, he will necessarily evaluate the need and usefulness of the patient's drugs. There are many things which enter into his evaluation, e.g., sex, age, diagnosis and drug sensitivities. The pharmacist who wants to be a clinical pharmacist will have to have an increased knowedge of medical terminology, laboratory tests, and disease. If the pharmacist has this knowledge, he will be capable of making reasonable and well-founded decisions concerning a patient's health.

## Clinical Pharmacy Knowledge

How is the pharmacist going to gather this knowledge? Few pharmacists can stop working and go back to school for an extended period. Therefore, the pharmacist must move cautiously because he can do the patient, as well as himself and the profession, a great deal of damage if he sets himself up as a clinical pharmacist and is not prepared.

The pharmacist should talk to the physician of his choice and explain what is happening in the world of pharmacy and describe how he could be of help to the physician and his patients if he could get some exposure in the treatment areas. In the small hospital, the pharmacist can request to accompany the physician to the patients' bedsides for an explanation of the medical problems involved in each case. In this manner, he can learn what the physician must consider; this will aid the pharmacist later in his decision making.

Many people have stated that clinical pharmacy is the orientation of the pharmacist to the patient — this can be overdone. Knowledge of drug products is the greatest expertise of the pharmacist. This must not be allowed to deteriorate while the pharmacist learns about other aspects of patient care. What must be accomplished is a happy medium where the pharmacist maintains his basic pharmacy knowledge but applies it in a different manner.

## Other Functions

In the small hospital especially, there is an opportunity for the pharmacist to talk with patients upon their discharge. The pharmacist can ascertain that the patients know how to store and consume their home-going medications and that they are informed as to which preadmission drugs are not to be taken now or which nonprescription drugs are contraindicated.

Many times, the pharmacist in a small hospital knows the patient's community pharmacist. This enables the hospital pharmacist to call the community pharmacist and confer with him on matters concerning drug therapy for a specific patient. The community pharmacist should alert the hospital pharmacist of any potential problems if the patient is going into the hospital on an elective basis.

## Conclusion

The steps involved for a pharmacist in a small hospital to become a clinical pharmacist are as follows:

1. The pharmacist must remove himself from the confines of the pharmacy walls.
2. The pharmacist must document to the hospital administrator the need for his closer involvement in patient care.
3. The pharmacist must meet with nurses and physicians to explain the advantages of having a clinical pharmacist.
4. The pharmacist must learn medical terminology, laboratory and other tests, and more pharmacology in order to be prepared to answer questions and make decisions concerning drug therapy for a specific patient.
5. The pharmacist must interview patients upon admission when necessary.
6. The pharmacist must inform the discharged patient about his home-going medications.

## References

1. Palmer, R. F.: Drug Misuse and Physician Education, *Clin. Pharmacol. Therap. 10*:2 (Jan.-Feb.) 1969.

2. Anon.: Editorial, *Med. Trib.* (Oct. 7) 1968.

3. Wilson, R. S. and Kabat, H. F.: Pharmacist Initiated Patient Drug Histories, In *Clinical Pharmacy Sourcebook,* pp. 346-350.

# 18 The Role of a Pharmacist on the Pediatric Unit of a General Hospital

Paul Munzenberger, Sister Emmanuel, and Marilyn Heins

Seventy-five hospitalized pediatric patients and 40 pediatric patients discharged with prescriptions were studied to determine the role of a pharmacist on the pediatric unit of a general hospital.

During the 120-hour period the pharmacist was stationed on the pediatric patient care unit, 31 possible medication problems involving 14 patients were detected while monitoring patient charts, and 12 possible medication problems involving 12 patients were detected while taking admission drug histories.

Eight of the 31 (25.8%) possible medication problems involving six patients and detected while monitoring patient charts were considered by both the medical director of pediatrics and the pharmacist to be significant. Seven of the 12 possible medication problems detected while taking admission drug histories were allergies which had not been detected or recorded by medical or nursing personnel. The remaining five possible medication problems concerned medication the patients had been taking prior to admission which either should have been prescribed on admission or should have been removed from the patient's possession on arrival at the hospital.

While stationed on the pediatric unit, the pharmacist received and responded to a total of 55 drug information requests, 41 of which originated from the medical staff and 14 from the nursing staff. Forty-two percent of the requests concerned specific patients.

The pharmacist presented three formal lectures to the nursing staff and monitored medication storage conditions during which time three areas of potential hazards to the patients were discovered.

Six medication problems were detected in the homes of 20 patients who received a discharge consultation, while 11 medication problems were detected among 20 patients who did not receive a discharge consultation. A statistical test indicated that the patients who received a discharge consultation had significantly fewer medication problems in the home.

The results of this study suggest that a pharmacist's role on the pediatric unit of a general hospital may include the following: (1) monitoring patient charts, (2) providing admission drug histories, (3) providing discharge consultations, and (4) providing drug information to the medical and nursing personnel.

The care of the pediatric patient often presents unique problems. For example, the pediatrician is periodically confronted with congenital disorders such as phenylketonuria or cystic fibrosis which are present primarily during childhood. The nurse may be required to subdivide tablets or dilute injections in order to administer the correct dosage. The pharmacist, while monitoring pediatric dosages, must consider the degree to which certain organs have developed.

Certain pharmacists in the past have actively participated in the care of the pediatric patient. Ellis, for example, described a project conducted at the University of Texas Medical Branch Hospitals where a pharmacist was stationed on a pediatric unit.[1] At the Children's Memorial Hospital of Chicago, Illinois, Klotz has also participated in the care of the pediatric patient.[2] Other pharmacists have also shown an interest in becoming more directly involved in the care of the pediatric patient.[3,4]

The report of the Task Force on the Pharmacist's Clinical Role describes a number of areas where the pharmacist may function to the advantage of the patient.[5] Cited by the Task Force as clinical roles for pharmacists are the monitoring of drug therapy, obtaining drug histories, providing consultations to patients at the time of discharge from the hospital and others. Pediatric patients should be among those benefiting from the services mentioned in this report.

Whether or not pharmacists concerned with the pediatric patient assume these roles depends in part on whether they have the initiative, training and experience required to effectively function in these roles. It was the purpose of the study described in this chapter to provide additional data concerning the possible roles of a pharmacist on the pediatric ward of a general hospital.

## Methodology

The study was conducted in a 573-bed hospital located in the inner city area of Detroit, Michigan. This hospital provides medical care to many inner city residents and its facilities are utilized by Wayne State University in the education and training of medical, nursing, pharmacy and social work students.

In order to obtain the necessary data, the study was conducted in two settings: (1) in a pediatric patient care unit of the general hospital and (2) in the homes of patients discharged from this unit. The data gathered on the pediatric unit were collected over a six-week period from January 27 to March 14, 1971, and the data from home visits were accumulated over six and one-half weeks from July 7 to August 21, 1971. Additionally, from July 8 to July 28, 1971, the number and types of drug information requests directed to pharmacy personnel of the hospital by the medical and nursing personnel on the pediatric unit were monitored.

The pediatric unit had a capacity of approximately 30 beds; the children admitted to the unit ranged from six to fifteen years of age. All hospital physicians, representing a variety of services such as medical, surgical, etc., admitted patients to the unit. During the period of data collection, the pediatric unit had patients from a variety of medical services; hospital personnel assigned to the unit included nurses, a ward clerk, a psychologist, medical residents, a staff physician, a medical student and a number of volunteers. Prior to the study, a pharmacist had not been assigned to the pediatric unit.

The pharmacy department utilized a hall stock method of drug distribution whereby empty stock containers were replaced by the pharmacy at the request of nurses.

The pharmacist conducting the study was stationed on the pediatric patient care unit three hours a day, six days a week for six and one-half weeks (120 hours). During the period of data collection, all pediatric patients were included in the study as they were admitted to the unit. As a result, the patient sample consisted of patients with a variety of diagnoses who were being treated by pediatricians and specialists.

*Data Collected on the Unit.* The patient, on admission to the pediatric unit, or a member of his family, was interviewed by a physician, usually a resident or intern, who obtained a medical, social and, to a limited extent, a medication history. Following this, the pharmacist transcribed pertinent information from this history to his own admission history form.

Because of the nature of the physician's medication history, the pharmacist made an effort to obtain an admission drug history on all patients. Whenever possible, this additional drug history was obtained from the patient at the patient's bedside. In more than half the cases, however, the pediatric patients were either too young or lacked adequate knowledge concerning their medications to provide an accurate drug history. In these cases, the pharmacist interviewed the parent or guardian at the hospital or by telephoning them at home. The pharmacist-acquired drug history included known allergies and prescription and non-prescription medications taken by the patient prior to admission to the hospital. The drug history information obtained by the pharmacist was also recorded on his admission history form and later transcribed by the pharmacist to another form which was placed in the patient's chart and remained there until the patient was discharged.

The pharmacist reviewed each patient's chart daily and checked for possible drug-drug, drug-food, drug-diagnostic test interactions and other adverse drug reactions. When necessary, the pharmacist went to the patient's bedside to determine the sequelae of a possible drug-related problem. All possible drug problems were recorded. At the completion of this aspect of the study, these problems were reviewed with the medical director of pediatrics in regard to their clinical significance. The impressions of the medical director and of the pharmacist were recorded.

The pharmacist provided consultations for all patients receiving medication at the time of discharge either at the hospital or by telephoning the parent or guardian at home. Discharge medication consultations were provided directly to teenage patients where feasible. Instructions given included the proper administration and storage of the medication, possible side effects, the purpose of the medication and other pertinent information. The medications and the consultations given by the pharmacist were recorded.

The pharmacist responded to requests for drug information from the medical and nursing staff of the pediatric unit. Drug information requests and the pharmacist's response were recorded on a consultation form.

The pharmacist also presented lectures to the nursing staff, recorded possible adverse drug reactions and reviewed medication storage conditions. Possible adverse drug reactions were recorded on a special form while medication storage conditions were reported to the medical director of pediatrics and the nursing supervisor of the pediatric unit.

*Data Collected During Home Visits.* The pharmacist visited the homes of two groups of patients who had been discharged from the pediatric ward of the general hospital with prescriptions. The 20 patients in Group A were given a discharge consultation by the pharmacist; the 20 patients in Group B were not given a discharge consultation by the pharmacist. It should be noted that the patients in Group B were not among those who had been monitored by the pharmacist in the pediatric patient care unit. Prior to the home visit, the pharmacist contacted the parent or guardian by telephone to arrange for the visit. While in the homes of both groups of patients, the pharmacist questioned the parent, guardian or teenager in regard to: (1) the purpose of the medication, (2) frequency of administration, (3) times of the day medication administered, and (4) place of medication storage. Data collected during home visits were recorded by the pharmacist.

*Data Collected by Monitoring Drug Information Requests.* It was suspected that the availability of the pharmacist on the unit increased the number of requests for drug information. In order to test this hypothesis, the pharmacy department monitored the drug information requests from the pediatric unit directed to pharmacy personnel while the pharmacist was not available on the pediatric unit. Drug information requests were monitored over a 120-hour period, equivalent to the number of hours the pharmacist was on the pediatric unit during the first part of the study. During this time, data were collected concerning the source and type of drug information requested.

## Results

*Data Collected on the Unit.* During the 120-hour period the pharmacist was stationed on the pediatric patient care unit there was an average census of approximately 25 patients. A total of 75 patients were monitored requiring about one hour per day, and admission drug histories were completed on 74 patients requiring approximately 10 minutes for each history.

A total of 43 possible medication problems involving 25 patients were detected by the pharmacist during this period. Thirty-one of the possible medication problems involving 14 patients were detected while monitoring patient charts; possible medication problems involving 12 patients were detected while taking admission drug histories.

An analysis of the 31 medication problems detected during the chart review showed that: (1) 23 problems were drug-diagnostic test interferences, (2) one problem was a drug-drug interaction and (3) seven were miscellaneous problems including intravenous incompatibilities, medication administration, dosage and duration of therapy.

As shown in Table 1, eight of the 31 (25.8%) possible medication problems involving six patients and detected while monitoring patient charts were considered by both the medical director of pediatrics and the pharmacist to be significant. Seven of these involved miscellaneous problems and one involved a drug-drug interaction.

It is interesting to note that all drug-diagnostic test interferences encountered during this study were considered insignificant because the test results indicated that the predicated interference had not occurred, or a review of the pharmacology of the possible interference indicated that it was unlikely that an interference had actually occurred.

Penicillin G is reported to cause a decrease in the red blood cell count, but in all four possible instances of this interference the reaction did not occur. This is not surprising since the incidence of this reaction is low. Similarly, ampicillin is reported to increase the white blood cell count and in all three detected possible cases this reaction did not occur. The inactivation of oral penicillin G by gastric acid was considered significant in all three instances where it was suspected.

Out of the 74 drug histories completed, 12 possible medication problems involving 12 patients resulted. Seven of these possible problems were allergies to medication (such as aspirin, penicillin or ferrous gluconate) which had not been detected or recorded by medical or nursing personnel. The remaining five possible problems concerned medication (such as dephenhydramine, chlorpheniramine, phenylephrine, cyproheptadine, papaverine, ephedrine, diphenylhydantoin and phenobarbital) which the patients had been taking prior to admission; the patients did not have the medication ordered for them while in the hospital or were taking the medication unknown to the medical and nursing personnel.

The pharmacist received and responded to a total of 55 drug information requests, 41 of which originated from the medical staff and 14 from the nursing staff. Forty-two percent (23) of the requests concerned a specific patient while 58% (32) did not. Twenty-three of the requests concerned the pharmacology of specific medication. Eleven requests concerned side effects, 11 others involved dosage and 10 concerned the availability of certain medication from the pharmacy.

The pharmacist presented three formal lectures to the nursing staff of the pediatric unit on (1) the pharmacology, dosage, side effects and indications of

Table 1. Possible Medication Problems Detected During Daily Review of Patient Charts

| TYPE OF PROBLEM | MEDICATION | POSSIBLE MEDICATION PROBLEM | NO. OF TIMES MEDICATION PROBLEM DETECTED | PHYSICIAN-PHARMACIST IMPRESSION |
|---|---|---|---|---|
| Drug-drug | Codeine, meperidine and pentobarbital | CNS depression (excessive sedation) | 1 | Significant |
| Miscellaneous | Tetracycline | Impairment of teeth and bone development | 2 | Significant |
| | Oral penicillin G | Improper dosage schedule resulting in inactivation of penicillin from gastric acidity | 3 | Significant |
| | Gentamicin | Possible toxicity resulting from improper duration of therapy | 1 | Significant |
| | Intravenous Potassium penicillin G | Inactivation of penicillin resulting from ascorbic acid additive | 1 | Significant |
| Drug-diagnostic test | Penicillin G | False negative RBC count | 4 | Insignificant |
| | Acetaminophen | False negative RBC count | 1 | Insignificant |
| | Acetaminophen | False negative WBC count | 1 | Insignificant |
| | Corticosteroid | False negative serum potassium | 2 | Insignificant |
| | Corticosteroid | False positive serum sodium | 2 | Insignificant |
| | Potassium penicillin G | False positive serum potassium | 1 | Insignificant |
| | Ampicillin | False positive WBC count | 3 | Insignificant |
| | Aspirin | False negative serum potassium | 1 | Insignificant |
| | Corticosteroid | False positive or negative serum chloride | 1 | Insignificant |
| | Ferrous sulfate | False negative serum sodium | 1 | Insignificant |
| | Ferrous sulfate | False negative serum calcium | 1 | Insignificant |
| | Ferrous sulfate | False negative serum potassium | 1 | Insignificant |
| | Methicillin | False negative WBC count | 1 | Insignificant |
| | Sodium ampicillin | False positive serum sodium | 1 | Insignificant |
| | Isoniazid | False positive WBC count | 1 | Insignificant |
| | Cephalothin | False positive or negative WBC count | 1 | Insignificant |
| TOTAL | | | 31 | |

the penicillins, (2) the methods of detecting and reporting adverse drug reactions and (3) the methods used in calculating pediatric medication dosage.

The pharmacist examined medication storage conditions and discovered three areas creating potential hazards to patients: (1) unlabeled bottles from the diagnostic laboratory of the hospital were stored in the refrigerator, (2) physician samples of nonformulary medications were scattered throughout the regular medication supply and (3) reconstituted antibiotic suspensions were not labeled with either the date of reconstitution or the date of expiration. The pharmacist submitted a report to the medical director of pediatrics and to the nursing supervisor of pediatrics which resulted in immediate action to eliminate these potential hazards.

*Data Collected During Home Visits.* As shown in Table 2, six medication problems were detected with Group A patients while 11 problems were detected with Group B patients. A statistical test (z) indicated that significantly fewer patients (at the 0.95 confidence level) with a discharge consultation experienced medication problems at home.

Further analysis of the home visit data showed that eight of the 17 medication problems were a failure to follow the prescribed dosage schedule. The other nine included the following: (1) four problems involved incorrect storage, (2) four problems involved

## Table 2. Home Visit Medication Problems

| GROUP | MEDICATION | MEDICATION PROBLEM |
|---|---|---|
| A | Ampicillin | Dosage schedule not followed |
| | Penicillin G suspension | Incorrect storage |
| | Ampicillin suspension | Incorrect storage |
| | Atropine eye drops | Dosage schedule not followed |
| | Ampicillin suspension | Incorrect storage |
| | Penicillin G suspension | Medication not being taken |
| B | Aspirin | Dosage schedule not followed |
| | Ferrous sulfate | Medication not being taken |
| | Ferrous sulfate | Dosage schedule not being followed |
| | Penicillin G suspension | Medication discontinued prematurely |
| | Phenobarbital | Dosage schedule not followed |
| | Ampicillin suspension | Incorrect storage |
| | Theophylline | Dosage schedule not followed |
| | Phenobarbital and diphenylhydantoin | Dosage schedule not followed |
| | Multiple vitamins | Medication not being taken |
| | Atropine eye drops | Dosage schedule not followed |
| | Multiple vitamins | Medication not being taken |

medications not administered and (3) one medication was discontinued prematurely by the parent. Seven of the 17 medications involved were antiinfectives.

*Data Collected by Monitoring Drug Information Requests.* During the 120-hour period the pharmacy department monitored drug information requests, not one request originated from the personnel on the pediatric unit. At the time of this study, the pharmacy department of the hospital provided primarily a dispensing service.

## Discussion and Conclusions

The data resulting from this study support our contention that a pharmacist's role on the pediatric unit of a general hospital may include the following: (1) monitoring patient charts, (2) providing admission drug histories, (3) providing discharge consultations and (4) providing drug information to medical and nursing personnel.

During the study, eight significant medication problems involving six of 75 patients were detected by monitoring approximately 25 patient charts daily. While these appear to support the need for a pharmacist to monitor pediatric patient charts, the literature lacks support for this need. However, from experience gained on other patient units within the hospital, it appears

that the monitoring of patient charts by a pharmacist is relevant if done on a selective basis. A pharmacist can adequately screen 80 to 100 charts daily if the monitoring is restricted to those patients who present the greatest potential for drug problems. Closely monitored patients would include those with complex medical or surgical problems where multiple drug therapy is employed. Approximately 30 to 35 patient charts out of the 80 to 100 charts assigned to a pharmacist would actually require detailed monitoring which would require about two hours by a pharmacist possessing adequate clinical experience.

The medical director of pediatric services at the study hospital concurred that taking admission drug histories is a possible role for pharmacists. The data from this study support the conclusion that pharmacists can contribute to patient care by taking admission drug histories. Obviously, if pharmacist-acquired drug histories are to serve any useful purpose, they must be carried out at the time of admission. This presents a unique challenge to pharmacists who supply this service and to hospital administrators who finance such services. In the study hospital, patients are admitted around the clock and the usefulness of an admission drug history becomes questionable if completed several hours or more after admission. Consequently, pharmacists would have to be available on admission to take drug histories.

Data from this study also revealed that there appears to be a need for pharmacists to provide discharge prescription consultations. However, even when the pharmacist did provide a discharge consultation, six of 20 patients encountered a medication problem at home. Many of these problems resulted because patients forgot the detailed verbal instructions provided by the pharmacist. To circumvent this problem, the pharmacist should selectively supply patients with written instructions in addition to the usual verbal instructions. An example of a form which may be used for this purpose is shown in Figure 1. Additionally, in those cases where the patient is discharged with a number of drugs and in those instances where the proper administration or storage of the medication is vital to the health of the patient, a brief telephone follow-up may prove to be beneficial. A time for this follow-up could be suggested during the discharge consultation. If pharmacists assume the responsibility of providing discharge consultations, they will have to be available at the time of patient discharge.

It is of interest to note that not one request originated from the medical or nursing personnel on the pediatric unit during the study period when the pharmacist was not on the unit. Three conclusions may be drawn from the portion of the study dealing with drug information requests. First, the tendency of physicians and nurses to seek drug

*Figure 1. Pharmacy medication consultation form.*

Patient's Name   John Doe                                    Date  3-10-71
Chart No.        123456

DIRECTIONS FOR TAKING MEDICATION

| Name of your Medication and Color | Times for Taking Medications | | | | | Special Instructions |
|---|---|---|---|---|---|---|
| | morning a. m. | afternoon p. m. | evening p. m. | | | |
| Aspirin (white) | 2 at 8 | 2 at 1 | 2 at 6 | bedtime | before with meals after | This medication may also be taken with milk or antacids to reduce stomach pains. |
| | | | | bedtime | before with meals after | |
| | | | | bedtime | before with meals after | |
| | | | | bedtime | before with meals after | |
| | | | | bedtime | before with meals after | |
| | | | | bedtime | before with meals after | |
| | | | | bedtime | before with meals after | |
| | | | | bedtime | before with meals after | |

Additional Instructions:

Continue to take this medication until told otherwise by your physician.

Pharmacist  John Grant

information from a pharmacist is greatly enhanced when the pharmacist is available on the unit. Second, there appears to be a role for pharmacists as a source of drug information on the pediatric unit of a general hospital. Third, if pharmacists are to provide drug information on a pediatric unit, their unique form of knowledge must exceed that of the pediatrician.

Another factor influencing the utilization of a pharmacist as a source of drug information is the degree to which he is accepted on the unit by medical and nursing personnel. In this study, the pharmacist was initially introduced to the medical staff by the medical director of pediatrics who emphasized the pharmacist's role in drug information. The nursing supervisor of pediatrics followed the same procedure in introducing the pharmacist to nursing personnel. We believe it was the positive attitude on the part of the medical director of pediatrics and nursing supervisor which most influenced the readiness of medical and nursing personnel to accept and use the pharmacist.

Although this study was limited to 75 patients, we believe it shows that pharmacists may provide a valuable service to physicians, nurses and patients on the pediatric unit of a general hospital. However, if pharmacists are to provide the services explored in this study, they will have to be readily available on the patient care unit and the hospital administration will have to support these new roles for pharmacists.

### References

1. Ellis, M. D.: The Clinical Pharmacist on a Pediatric Unit, *Hosp. Topics 47*:60 (Nov.) 1969.
2. Klotz, R.: personal communication, May 3, 1971.
3. Gans, J. A.: personal communication, March 26, 1971.
4. Ward, C. O., Hanan, Z. I. and Durgin, Sister J. M.: The Practice of Clinical Pharmacy in Pediatrics, *Hosp. Pharm. 5*:15 (Aug.) 1970.
5. Anon.: Report of the Task Force on the Pharmacist's Clinical Role, *HSRD Briefs* (No. 4) Spring 1971.

# 19 Clinical Involvement for the Pharmacist in Chronic Care

Thomas J. Mattei

Pharmacist involvement in health care services for patients with chronic illnesses is discussed.

The pharmacist may become involved at four levels: (1) drug distribution, (2) patient education, (3) patient monitoring, and (4) primary health care. Specific functions associated with each of these levels are reviewed in relation to the concept of a pharmacy care plan.

The complexity of debilitation from chronic disease can best be described by the definition of chronic illness given by the Commission on Chronic Illness as:

> ... an impairment of health that requires an extended period of medical supervision. This may involve ambulatory, home, hospital or other institutional care, or various combinations of these. It may or may not be manifestly disabling. It may be progressive or stationary. The progression of the disorder and the degree of disability are not necessarily parallel. Disability results from an impairment of the biological, physiological or social efficiency of the individual and prevents him from pursuing normal or usual activities. Not unexpectedly chronic physical incapacitation often produces profound psychological effects on the patient and his family. Long-term illness changes the mode of living itself. It may tax to the utmost all of the patient's resources. Psychologically, his beliefs, his goals, interests, social contacts and daily pattern of living must be modified, while physically, his body is in the throes of continuing illness.[1]

The desired goal or endpoint in treating chronic disease is obvious. Physiological and psychosociological improvements of the patient are of paramount importance. This is the idealistic endpoint and often the target cannot be realized and we must settle for less. Then we must try to maintain the patient at his present point in the disease process.

A method must be designed to enhance the attainment of the goal. This method we can designate as the care plan or treatment. An important consideration for the care plan is that it be individualized; that is,

"ideal" treatment is not necessarily the most beneficial for a particular patient. Factors such as socioeconomics must be considered and incorporated into the care plan. For example, telling a patient he should be exposed only to a warm, dry, ecologically pure environment and eat only steaks to prolong life does little to help him if he lives in a damp attic in a Pittsburgh ghetto and has a monthly income of 80 dollars.

Perhaps the most frustrating aspect in the care of patients with chronic disease is the high rate of treatment failure. Temporary failure may be the result of external factors which can be controlled if the care plan is constantly reviewed and revised.

With this approach in mind, where do pharmacists fit in the care of patients with chronic illnesses? What are we prepared to do or what can we be prepared to do? What could we possibly accomplish if we freed ourselves from our frozen concept of pharmacy practice?

The common denominator for our involvement must be the chronically ill patients' need for medications and their need to know how to use these medications properly.

Four distinct levels of pharmacy practice can be isolated in sick-care services:

1. Distribution
2. Patient education
3. Patient monitoring
4. Primary health care.

## Distribution

There are two essential components to the distribution level of pharmacy practice. The pharmacist must assure an adequate supply of the drugs necessary for effective treatment. Many of the chronic illnesses necessitate the use of drugs to maintain the life of the patient, whereas other drugs are necessary only during periods of exacerbation. A patient with congestive heart failure may use a digitalis preparation daily for the rest of his life; whereas, a patient with allergies uses his drugs only on a seasonal basis. Pharmacists must define treatment schedules, using information derived from the patient, his physician, and the medical literature. Devices such as tickler files can be used as reminders to ourselves and patients. A patient with congestive heart failure could be reminded via postcard one week in advance that he is about to exhaust his supply of digitalis tablets and that if he would call us, we could prepare his prescription prior to his arrival. Tickler files are easy to develop and can be as simple as dividing a box by weeks of the year. While preparing the first prescription, the pharmacist can give the patient a postcard to fill out with his name, address, and telephone number. The pharmacist then records the number of the prescription or the name of the drugs to be compared to a patient profile and files the postcard into the tickler file. The card is then mailed at the appropriate time to the patient. Other, more complex devices for tickler files, such as the computer, make this task much more efficient and can be easily adapted.

Patients with allergies present a special problem. The patient profile should indicate the seasonal variation of the particular allergy and the patient can be notified of his need for medication in advance. True, this method does not lend itself well to all chronic diseases, but it is a service not available to many patients. Pharmacists should not only dispense the prescriptions but see to it that the patient takes his medications and gets more when he needs them.

Chronically ill patients may be their own worst enemies. Studies reveal that the course of the disease process, side effects, inability to adhere to schedules, the impact of outside sources of information, and economics are factors which make patients noncompliers with self-medication regimens. We are part of a society geared toward pleasure spending. People are willing to spend hundreds of dollars on color television and various automatic gadgets, and yet complain about medication which may cost, at the most 50 cents daily, while enhancing their life span by many years.

The pharmacist should call on every method possible to enhance patient adherence to treatment regimens. A number of techniques have been developed to identify noncompliers. Tagging methods, patient interviews, dosage unit counts, along with incorporating in the packaging sophisticated gadgetry, such as uranium imprinting and litmus paper, have been tried. The best solution is still in doubt. Perhaps, pretesting individuals, pharmacokinetics, and pricing prescriptions according to family income and number of dependents may help.

The importance of insuring an adequate supply of medicinals and the need for compliance are evident. The outcome of not taking prescribed medication is a self-perpetuating process which results in hospitalization, an extremely expensive alternative.

## Patient Education

To help eradicate noncompliance and thereby improve the treatment of chronic illness, pharmacists should direct their efforts toward patient education. This educational process should be designed to aid the patient in coping with his chronic illness while not increasing his despair about the future. It is important for pharmacists to recognize the psychology of chronic illness. Dr. Harry S. Abram, Professor of Psychiatry, Vanderbilt University School of Medicine, has discussed the psychological defenses of the chronically ill. He isolates the following defense mechanisms as common occurrences: regression, denial, intellectualization, projection, displacement, and introjection. The manner in which the patient uses the above defenses often determines his psychological responses to his illness. These responses take three forms: depression, overdependency and nonadherence to the therapeutic regimen. Dr. Abram continues by describing the "care giving" personnel attitudes which may significantly affect the patient's course, both positively and negatively. Negative attitudes come from overconcern and involvement, anger and rejection and lack of sensitivity. There are positive therapeutic and prophylactic measures which can be employed. They consist of:

1. Recognition that the patient does react to his illness with defenses that are unconscious and serve a purpose (to control anxiety) can reduce negativistic attitudes toward him. Thus regression, projection, etc., become comprehensible phenomena. If the reasons behind the patient's behavior are understandable, he is less likely to be labeled a "crock," "turkey," etc., and avoided by medical personnel.
2. A realistic approach to a patient's illness with an attempt to minimize the dependency and secondary gain allow the patient to lead a more fruitful and adaptive life. Overconcern and protectiveness to ease the physician's or family's anxiety may only increase the patient's inherent anxiety over his illness.
3. If a physician must "cure" his patients to prove his omnipotence, keep them dependent upon him to satisfy his own needs, or cause them overconcern because of his anxieties, his patients may suffer unnecessarily.[2]

The patient should be instructed about the disease, its relationship to the symptoms being manifested and how treatment can alleviate or curtail this process. Perhaps by using analogies with concepts patients understand, we might enhance this educational interaction (i.e., congestive heart failure compared to a malfunction of the carburetor of an automobile). How do we learn of these symptoms? Either by asking the patient or the physician, or by consulting the patient's medical record.

The patient should be counseled in regard to the treatment he is receiving. The drugs should be discussed in an attempt to correlate them with the disease. If the drug is digitalis, explain the overall effect it has on the heart and, in turn, how this will bring about positive changes in other systems. The patient should be made aware of methods to determine the effectiveness of the treatment (i e., symptoms, physical signs), so that ineffective regimens can be curtailed immediately.

At Mercy Health Center, we instruct patients to call us if a persistent increase in symptoms occurs. If the benefit of our program can be measured by the number of such calls we receive, we are having a significant impact on patient care.

The patient should be cognizant of common side effects and toxicities which may occur, when to expect them, what should be done about them, and to call the pharmacist if they persist. Patients started on methyldopa frequently incur dizziness on standing after three to four days of therapy. The body has auto-compensative processes which alleviate this problem in 24 to 72 hours. There are precautions which the patient should be familiar with in this compensation period (i.e., upon arising from sleep, he should sit on the bed for a few minutes; the change from a sitting to standing position should be slow and deliberate). Drug toxicities are usually manifested by certain symptoms which can act as signals to the patient. The patient could seek immediate attention if he were familiar with these signals.

The patient should be knowledgeable about when to take his medication and why a certain schedule may be crucial, how to store these items, and how to self-administer these agents, especially preparations such as eye and nose drops, injections, suppositories, and enemas.

Communications must be such that they can be accurately interpreted by the patient. Many institutions are employing audiovisual aids for this purpose. We must be careful not to become too far withdrawn from the patient. The personal touch is very important for patients with chronic diseases. Placing a patient in a room with a projector puts the pharmacist in no better circumstance than if a clerk hands the prescription to the patient.

Finally, the patient education process should also re-inforce preventive concepts of care. The pharmacist should reiterate aspects of diet, social habits, exercise, rest, methods of attaining comfort, other drugs or substances which should be avoided, and acute disease processes which can be harmful to a patient with chronic disease if not corrected immediately. An upper respiratory infection can be of serious consequence to a patient with chronic bronchitis. So can an antibiotic or antacid with a high sodium content to a patient with hypertension or congestive heart failure.

## Pharmacy Monitoring

It has been shown that patients use various resources for health care, including different physicians, different facilities, and different pharmacies for the same disease or many disease entities. It is possible for the patient to have the following occur:

1. A patient may receive a number of medications to treat one disease entity when one agent may be all that is necessary. The consequences of multiple therapy may be detrimental to the patient and/or his disease. The possibility of the same medication being prescribed and used simultaneously cannot be excluded and is compounded if two different pharmacies dispense two different brands of the same drug.
2. A patient's therapy for a primary disease may (a) aggravate a second pathological condition of the patient (i.e., diuretic and diabetes or gout); (b) be improperly absorbed, metabolized, detoxified, secreted, or excreted because of the existence of a second disease (i.e., digoxin and renal disease); or (c) be similar to medications to which he is allergic.

The pharmacist must act as the unifying force in this divergent system, sometimes without prior consents from the existing hierachy of health care. To do so, he must be competent in taking a medication history in order to identify allergies, current therapy, previous treatment for existing diseases, and the evaluation of the treatment's successes and failures. He must relate each drug to a specific disease process.

The integration of disease processes and drugs present a specific problem to pharmacists who do not have access to the medical record. At Mercy Hospital, we have found it useful to develop a series of questions about symptoms, physical examinations, and laboratory studies which are known to the patient. We also question the patient in regard to organ systems; for example, we ask if the patient has ever been told he has anything wrong with his eyes, heart, liver, kidneys, etc.

All of this information should be incorporated into the patient profile, and when possible, should be documented as a measurement (i.e., one or two plus edema) to be useful in therapeutic evaluation. I recommend that the patient record be structured according to the problem-oriented approach, with each block of space indicative of a disease, its treatment, its therapeutic failures and the toxicities of treatment incurred. Nonprescription drug products should be considered and treated similarly to prescription medications. Pharmacists must move away from a chronological listing of prescriptions as the concept of patient records.

The pharmacist at this level of practice should concern himself with the review and scrutiny of prescribed therapy. This activity differs from that in the fourth level of practice (primary health care practitioner) since the selection of therapy is still the responsibility of the physician and the pharmacist's role is limited to making recommendations. The pharmacist must concern himself with deciding if the drug of choice has been selected for a particular patient, if the drug is effective, and whether it interferes with any aspect of patient care.

Establishing models for these decisions should be our primary concern. Factors which may influence selection of therapy include the diseases present, laboratory tests to be performed, pharmacokinetics, the psychology and sociology of the patient, other drugs being used, their potential for adverse effects and toxicities, and documented allergies.

Patient symptoms, abnormalities present in the physical examination and laboratory studies should be used to measure the effectiveness of a treatment program. If these measurements indicate the existence of a disease, then the treatment can be evaluated by the effect it has on them. Let us not forget that drugs can interfere with these measurements. Perhaps another test can be performed or we can subtract the known amount of interference from the result to overcome this problem and, hence, not interfere with the care plan.

Medications have also been implicated in iatrogenic diseases, symptomatology, abnormal physical findings, and laboratory studies not related to the primary disease. Baseline studies should be performed with those which occur in high incidence and repeated at a predicted time to decrease the confusion caused by these abnormal results, and even more important, to negate the possible detrimental effects of a drug-induced disease.

## Pharmacists as Primary Health Care Practitioners

Universities and institutions are training individuals to perform a variety of primary health care functions under the direction of a physician. Anne R. Somers of Princeton University, a respected author in the field of health care, stated, "It's patently absurd that the whole medical field is agog over the need for training of new categories of health professionals while we stand by and watch the demoralization of two of our most respected members of the health care team." She was referring to pharmacists and nurses, and how right she was!

Drugs are used in the treatment of chronic diseases; most follow-up visits to the physician are aimed at evaluating the treatment. With the use of pharmacy care plans previously described, we should be able to perform this function and relieve valuable time for the physician. And isn't it possible for us, once a diagnosis is established, to develop into our pharmacy care plans, with the aid of participating physicians, methods of selecting and altering treatment based on our findings? Then instead of six to eight visits to the physician yearly, perhaps two to three will suffice. So level four, the pharmacist as the primary health care practitioner, could be the inclusion of the first three levels of pharmacy care, plus the selection and alteration of therapeutic plans. These roles must be carefully formulated based on tools available to the pharmacist and his ability to use these methods. Not all of us have renin values available to assess hypertension, but other methods can be used to evaluate therapy for hypertension. Physicians must always be the overseers of the entire system and agree upon all aspects of the pharmacy care plan.

The pharmacist practicing at level four is solely responsible for the functions we have described. He is expected to maintain the pharmacy care plan by those health professionals instrumental in its development. He must select and alter therapy, measure its effectiveness, and deter any untoward effects of therapy.

On each patient visit, the pharmacist interviews the patient, requests laboratory tests and does clinical measurements as specified in the pharmacy care plan, evaluates the data, and decides whether to continue the patient's medication, alter the dosage, or change the agent entirely.

The chart of each patient monitored by the pharmacist should be supplied with a flow sheet on which can be recorded specific parameters to aid the pharmacist in performing his delegated responsibilities. This flow sheet provides valuable information in summarizing and using the data of each patient.

## Why Should Pharmacists Become Involved?

George Allen, coach of the Washington Redskins, once remarked when asked why he was trading away all of his draft choices for veteran players. "The future is now." How true this is for the profession of pharmacy. There is much emphasis and money being placed on chronic diseases, as indicated by projects such as the National Hypertension Program and the possible development of a National Center for Health Education. The funding available for the hypertension program and for health education is for the creation of a more unified approach calling on all of the health disciplines to establish new methods of health care. Education for patients may become reimbursable under Medicare, Medicaid, and other health insurance programs. The manpower shortage, establishment of PSRO's, and the documented problems associated with the use of medications are but a few factors which should serve as positive reinforcements for our involvement.

The negative aspects, those forcing us in this direction, must be considered as even stronger catalysts. The news media continue to look at the practice of pharmacy, sometimes in a humorous fashion which tells a grim tale. Cartoons about pharmacy have appeared recently, reinforcing the unfavorable concept that some consumers, government officials, third party payers, and other professionals have about pharmacies and pharmacists.

The handwriting is on the wall; our profession has been weighed in the balance and found wanting. But there is already a group of creative, hard working pharmacists practicing at these higher levels in the care of patients with chronic illnesses. These are not responsibilities that are easily assumed. We could all profit if the American Society of Hospital Pharmacists would convene a group of pharmacists to develop pharmacy care plans. Such a group would be motivated by a certain idealism. There is nothing wrong with that, for idealism is often the stimulus for progress.

### References

1. Rapaport, H. G.: Chronic Illness, *Ann. Alergy 26*: 230-232 (May) 1968.
2. Abram, H. S.: The Psychology of Chronic Illness (Editorial), *J. Chronic Dis. 25*:659-664 (Mar. 6) 1972.

# 20 Hypertension: A Model for Pharmacy Involvement

Thomas J. Mattei, James A. Balmer, Lawrence A. Corbin, and
Sister M. Gonzales Duffy

Pharmacist involvement in a program for ambulatory hypertensive patients is described.
After physician diagnosis of essential hypertension, a pharmacist evaluates the severity of the hypertension, selects the drug therapy for the patient according to established guidelines, and continues to monitor the patient.

The data base used for making drug therapy decisions, classification of the severity of hypertension, treatment goals, method of therapy selection, and future evaluation of the program are discussed.

The National Health Survey of 1962 estimated that 26 million people in the United States had hypertension or hypertensive heart disease.[1] The disease is probably even more prevalent than this since it lacks overt symptomatology and therefore goes undetected in many people.

It has been shown that hypertension increases morbidity and mortality due to coronary heart disease, cerebrovascular accidents and renal failure. With the advent of antihypertensive agents, many investigators set out to study the effects of therapy on the morbidity and mortality of patients with hypertension. Hamilton reported in 1964 that of 22 hypertensive males followed from two to six years, 10 who received drug therapy did not incur the complications of hypertension.[2] Even before this study, investigators had concluded that survival in malignant hypertension could be extended with the use of antihypertensive therapy.[3]

A more recent prospective study on the effects of treating hypertension has been reported by the Veterans Administration Cooperative Study Group. This study has provided more conclusive evidence that lowering blood pressure is beneficial over a wide range of elevations.[4]

All available information, knowledge and studies stress the need for a more unified approach to the problem of hypertension. Former HEW Secretary Richardson called for this with the creation of the National Hypertension Program. Perhaps we as pharmacists should ask ourselves how we can become involved. Are there therapeutic responsibilities with chronic diseases such as hypertension that could be included in the practice of pharmacy?

Hypertension, like many other diseases, has measurable parameters which provide objective assessment in the choice of therapy and hence an excellent opportunity for pharmacy intervention. The following discussion represents pharmacy's involvement with hypertensive patients at Mercy Health Center, the ambulatory care facility of Mercy Hospital, Pittsburgh, Pennsylvania, and should be considered as one of many possible methods for pharmacy involvement.

## General Description of Program

Currently at Mercy Health Center there are two physicians involved in the program for ambulatory hypertensive patients. When a diagnosis of essential hypertension is confirmed by a physician, the patient is scheduled to be seen by a pharmacist at the Health Center. The pharmacist classifies the severity of the hypertension using the patient's data base. The parameters used to establish the data base determine the sequence of drugs used for treatment and are also useful in monitoring the course of disease and any untoward effects of therapy. The patient is seen by the pharmacist every two to three weeks until the desired response is attained, and then every one to three months, depending on the severity of the hypertension, the presence of other pathological entities and the antihypertensive agent being used.

The patient returns to the physician twice yearly unless other concurrent disease entities are being assessed and/or treated by the physician. The advent of new symptomatology secondary to hypertension may necessitate physician intervention at more frequent intervals.

## Data Base

The information essential for diagnosis, classification, assessment and treatment is derived from the patient's history, physical examination, laboratory and other tests, and is secured through a cooperative effort of the physician and pharmacist. These findings are included in the patient's medical record.

This data base is used by the pharmacist to classify the severity of the hypertension and select the appropriate drug regimen. Subsequent changes in data base parameters form the basis for measuring patient response to therapy, drug intolerance and side effects, and the progress of the disease. Changes in therapy, however, must ultimately be based on subjective evaluation of the patient's overall condition.

In compiling the data base, the physician or pharmacist questions the patient in regard to personal and social history since studies indicate that stress and emotion can play a role in hypertension.[5,6] The patient is also questioned as to the presence of symptoms such as chest pain, shortness of breath, orthopnea, nocturia or recurrent urinary tract infections to aid in determining the severity of the disease. An accurate and complete drug history is obtained with emphasis on prior treatment. The concomitant use of other agents (prescription or nonprescription) is determined so as to avoid any clinically significant therapeutic incompatabilities.

The physical examination includes initial height, weight, and both supine and upright blood pressure determinations. Treatment is indicated if the average systolic reading on three separate occasions is greater than 140 mm Hg and/or the average diastolic pressure is greater than 90 mm Hg and the patient is younger than 40 years of age, of if the average diastolic pressure is greater than 100 mm Hg and the patient is over 40 years of age.

Also included in the initial work-up are fundoscopy; apical heart rate; chest x-ray for cardiac size; electrocardiogram for ischemia, hypertrophy or arrhythmia; abdominal examination for the presence of bruits; and an intravenous pyelogram to assess the status of kidney function. These parameters are measured by the physician and, with the exception of an intravenous pyelogram, are repeated at yearly intervals. The initial findings are used in the classification of the severity of the disease. They also serve as base lines for comparison of subsequent findings and are utilized in assessing the overall status of the patient.

During subsequent sessions with the pharmacist, the patient's weight, pulse and blood pressure are again measured. Renal function is assessed at six-month intervals to monitor the progression of the disease and the effects of therapy, especially if the patient is receiving a drug which is known to alter blood flow to the kidney, e.g., reserpine or guanethidine. This parameter is assessed using blood urea nitrogen and serum creatinine determinations. Yearly urine cultures are obtained from women since the incidence of recurrent kidney infections is higher in this sex and such conditions can exacerbate the disease.

Other tests used by the pharmacist to establish baselines and assess the consequences of therapy are yearly complete blood count and differential (to detect allergic reactions, gastrointestinal ulceration and blood dyscrasias); and serum uric acid, glucose and electrolytes at six-month intervals. If the patient is receiving a potassium-depleting diuretic, such as one of the thiazides or furosemide, serum potassium is measured at monthly intervals until the patient is stabilized on the diuretic. Thereafter, the interval is increased to three months. All tests are performed at specified intervals unless symptomatology requires more immediate action.

Not included in the data base, unless the patient's symptoms or therapy warrant, are those complications of therapy which are rare occurrences (e.g., gynemastia with reserpine), the mental and emotional status of the patient, and questions in regard to postural hypotension or sexual abilities. Any abnormal findings are documented in the flow sheet section or under symptomatology in the progress notes section of the patient's medical record.

The pharmacist records the outcome of each visit in the patient's medical record using the problem-oriented approach. Abnormal findings are reviewed with the physician.

## Classification

The pharmacist uses the information from the data base to classify each individual patient according to the scheme of Melman and Morrelli.[7]

| | | |
|---|---|---|
| 1. Mild hypertension | | Blood pressure greater than 140/90 or 140/100 (age dependent) to 160/100—without complications. |
| 2. Moderate hypertension | | Blood pressure greater than 160/100 to 200/100 with or without left ventricular hypertrophy—and grade II retinopathy—without other complications. |
| 3. Severe hypertension | | Blood pressure greater than 200/100 or complications of cardiac or renal damage. |

## Treatment

The goals of treatment are (1) decrease the systolic and diastolic blood pressure as follows: (a) 40 years or younger, below 130 mm Hg systolic, 90 mm Hg diastolic, and (b) 41 years or older, below 140 mm Hg systolic and 100 diastolic; (2) to arrest the progression of hypertension using the data base items as indicators; and (3) to maintain the patient as comfortably as possible. An inadequate response is defined as not meeting any one of the above. These goals are achieved through the proper selection of an antihypertensive agent and patient education. The following agents have been approved by the participating physicians for selection and use by the pharmacists in treating hypertension:

1. Chlorothiazide
2. Reserpine
3. Methyldopa
4. Guanethidine
5. Hydralazine.

## Method of Therapy Selection

The choice of the agents by the pharmacist depends on the hypertensive classification (Figure 1), the abnormalities documented in the data base, the presence of other disease entities and the concurrent use of other medicinal agents. A description of each possible series of events that influences the pharmacist's choice of therapy is outside the scope of this chapter.

## Combinations of Agents

Those possible combinations of agents, other than the use of chlorothiazide plus one antihypertensive agent as described in Figure 1, is left to the discretion of the physician responsible for the patient's care. Other combinations are not used unless the sequence described in Figure 1 has failed to provide the desired response.

## Program Evaluation

There are currently 100 hypertensive patients being monitored in the manner described. A study to measure the effectiveness of this program is in progress. The study involves a group of examiners from the medical staff of the hospital as evaluators of quality of care. The study population consists of patients seen in Mercy Health Center and a number of private patients being seen by a physician in the community.

*Figure 1. Flow chart for the selection of antihypertensive therapy based only on classification and response*

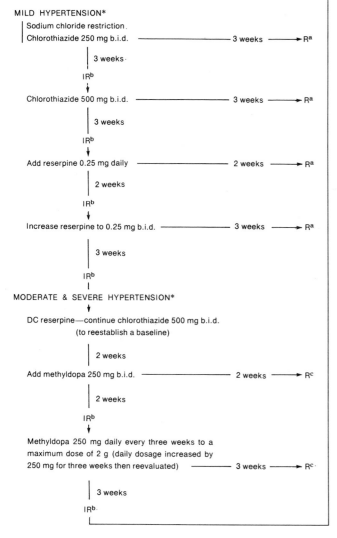

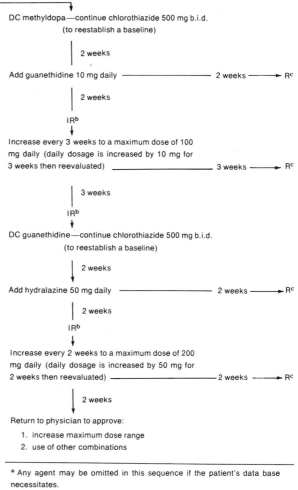

\* Any agent may be omitted in this sequence if the patient's data base necessitates.

$R^a$ = adequate response—patient returns every three months to pharmacist, every six months to physician.

$IR^b$ = inadequate response.

$R^c$ = adequate response—patient returns every 1½ months to pharmacist, every six months to physician.

## References

1. United States National Center for Health Studies: Vital & Health Statistics. Heart Disease in Adults: United States 1960–1962, PHS Publication No. 1000, Series 11, No 6, Government Printing Office, Washington, D. C., 1964.

2. Hamilton, M., Thompson, E. N., and Wisniewski, T. K. M.: The Role of Blood-Pressure Control in Preventing Complications of Hypertension, *Lancet 1:* 235–238 (Feb.) 1964.

3. McMichael, J. and Murphy, E. A.: Methonium Treatment of Severe and Malignant Hypertension, *J. Chronic Dis. 1:* 527–535 (May) 1955.

4. Freis, E. D.: Long-Term Treatment: Organization of a Long-Term Multiclinic Therapeutic Trial in Hypertension, Antihypertensive Therapy: Principles and Practice, edited by F. Gross, Springer-Verlag, New York, 1966, pp. 345–354.

5. Kunin, C. M. and McCormack, R. C.: An Epidemiologic Study of Bacteriuria and Blood Pressure Among Nuns and Working Women, *N. Engl. J. Med. 278:* 635–642 (Mar.) 1968.

6. Cruz-Coke, R., Etcheverry, R., and Nagel, R.: Influence of Migration on Blood Pressure of Easter Islanders, *Lancet 1:* 697–699 (Mar.) 1964.

7. Nies, A. S.: Cardiovascular Disorders in Clinical Pharmacology, Basic Principles in Therapeutics, edited by K. L. Melmon and H. F. Morrelli, Macmillan Company, New York, 1972, pp. 166–171.

# 21 Pharmacist Management of Ambulatory Patients Using Formalized Standards of Care

Philip O. Anderson and David A. Taryle

A report on the role of the pharmacist as a provider of maintenance care for ambulatory patients receiving chronic drug therapy at a 26-bed hospital is presented.

About 50 patients were managed utilizing protocols established by previous agreement between the pharmacist and physicians. In this system, the pharmacist interviews the patient, orders appropriate laboratory tests, evaluates the data, and makes the decision regarding refill of medications. It is concluded that the clinically-trained pharmacist can provide maintenance drug care; however, this role is limited by drug distribution responsibilities. It is suggested that in the future the drug distribution function and the direct patient care function may be served by two different types of pharmacy practitioners.

The Indian Health Service (IHS) of the U.S. Public Health Service has been likened to a system of prototype health maintenance organizations (HMO's) in which a number of innovative services have been implemented.[1] Several pharmacy services have been developed in the IHS which may have application in other organized health care settings.

It is the purpose of this chapter to discuss one of the direct patient care services provided to selected ambulatory patients by the pharmacist at the IHS hospital in Clinton, Oklahoma, from April 1972 to July 1973.

## The Maintenance Care Program

The Clinton Indian Hospital is a 26-bed inpatient facility offering general medical, obstetrical, and pediatric care to approximately 4,000 Cheyenne-Arapaho Indians in western Oklahoma.

During the period covered by this report, the Clinton medical staff of four physicians also maintained six smaller field clinics in addition to the inpatient and outpatient facilities at Clinton. Generally, only two physicians were at Clinton at any time during the four hours of each weekday that the outpatient clinic was open. The pharmacy was staffed by one pharmacist with part-time help provided by a pharmacy student intern. Over 10,000 patient visits per year were made to the hospital's outpatient department.

All outpatient prescriptions were dispensed directly from the patient's medical record which was organized in the problem-oriented format. The advantages of the problem-oriented record to the pharmacist and patient are many and are discussed elsewhere in this volume.[2]

To better serve patients with medical problems requiring the chronic use of medications, the pharmacist and physicians developed a program whereby the pharmacist may assume responsibility for the management of such patients. The medical problems included in the program are congestive heart failure, epilepsy, estrogen replacement, essential hypertension, isoniazid preventive therapy, oral contraception, and thyroid replacement.

## Methods of Pharmacy Involvement

There are two distinct methods by which to implement a program of maintenance care by the pharmacist. The first could be described as a "dependent" method in which the pharmacist interviews the patient, evaluates his health status, and then decides to either refill the patient's medication or refer the patient to a physician. The physician must countersign the pharmacist's chart entries for legal purposes and thereby assumes responsibility for the pharmacist's actions. This system, analogous to the functioning of a medical student or a physician's assistant under the preceptorship of a physician, was used at Clinton both prior to the development of the formalized program and to some extent afterwards. Other pharmacists have successfully functioned in this manner also.[3-5]

*Figure 1. Sample protocols which delineate the minimum standards applied to outpatients; time intervals for specific patients are determined by the physician and baseline data are collected by the physician at the designated* *intervals; monitoring data are collected on each patient visit unless otherwise stated; clinical data are obtained through the patient interview by either the physician or the pharmacist.*

### Definitions of Terms

*Baseline Data:* Information that will be collected by the physician before the patient is assigned to the protocol and as indicated on the particular protocol. The baseline data relates only to the monitoring of chronic drug therapy and does *not* attempt to define standards for any part of the patient's initial work-up.

*Monitoring Data:* Information that will be collected on each visit or at the specified interval by the pharmacist or physician.

*Clinical Data:* The pertinent clinical information which should be obtained on each visit by the physician or pharmacist through interview or observation of the patient.

### PHARMACY CHRONIC CARE MONITORING PROTOCOL
### ORAL CONTRACEPTION

Physician evaluation: Every 6 to 12 months.
Pharmacist evaluation: Every 3 months.

A. Drugs possible:
   norethindrone 1 mg and mestranol 80µg.
   norethindrone 1 mg and mestranol 50µg.
B. Baseline data:
   Breast exam, pelvic exam, and Pap smear:
      Women 35 years or under: every 12 months.
      Women over 35 years: every 6 months.
C. Monitoring data:
   1) Blood pressure.
   2) Weight.
D. Clinical data:
   1) Compliance with regimen.
   2) Breakthrough bleeding, vaginal discharges.
   3) Leg aches, calf pain, chest pain.
   4) Breast tenderness, lumps or discharge.

5) Fluid retention or swelling.
6) Headaches.
7) Mood changes.
8) Observe for jaundice.

### PHARMACY CHRONIC CARE MONITORING PROTOCOL
### CONGESTIVE HEART FAILURE

Physician evaluation: Every 3 to 6 months.
Pharmacist evaluation: Every 1 to 2 months.

A. Drugs possible:
   digoxin, digitoxin, hydrochlorothiazide, furosemide, spironolactone, potassium chloride solution.
B. Baseline data:
   1) EKG, chest X-ray every year.
   2) Serum creatinine every 6 months.
C. Monitoring data:
   1) Blood pressure.
   2) Weight.
   3) Pulse and regularity.
   4) BUN every 3 months.
   5) Urinalysis every 3 months.
   6) Serum potassium every 3 months unless unstable; then, every month.
   7) CBC every 6 months.
   8) FBS every 6 months if on hydrochlorothiazide.
D. Clinical data:
   1) Palpitations, arrhythmias.
   2) SOB, DOE, PND, orthopnea.
   3) Nocturia.
   4) Anorexia, nausea, vomiting, diarrhea.
   5) Visual abnormalities.
   6) Muscle weakness.

The logistics of this method can be cumbersome in a busy outpatient clinic, however. The pharmacist must repeatedly contact the physician throughout the day for approval and countersignature of his actions, and the routine of both practitioners may become disrupted.

The second method involves delegated responsibility to the pharmacist via a set of specified protocols previously agreed upon by both physician and pharmacist. This method is analogous to the use of "standing orders" under which a nurse is allowed to perform treatment in the absence of a physician. From April 1972 to July 1973, a similar method was employed at the Clinton Indian Hospital whereby the pharmacist followed selected patients with stabilized, chronic medical problems. The patients were selected by the medical staff and assigned to the program with the patient's consent. A total of about 50 stabilized patients were assigned to the maintenance program utilizing these protocols during the period covered by this report. Examples of two of the protocols are provided in Figure 1.

On each pharmacy visit, the pharmacist interviews the patient, requests laboratory and clinical measurements as specified in the protocols, evaluates the data and decides whether to refill the patient's medications.

Should the condition of the patient appear unstable, the pharmacist will consult a physician and a joint decision is made on the appropriate action to be taken.

The chart of each patient followed by the pharmacist is supplied with a flow sheet on which are recorded specific parameters and the patient's medications. The flow sheet, patterned after those described by Schulman and Wood,[6] is valuable in summarizing and correlating patient data, drug regimen, and patient response.

Conceptually, the protocols may be considered to be the minimum standards of care which are applied to patients with certain chronic medical problems. Once the standards have been agreed upon, it remains only to be decided which providers of care are best suited to carry out the indicated functions. At our facility, the authority for actions and decisions regarding the monitoring of a patient's condition between physician visits was delegated to the pharmacist. It should be emphasized that for any particular patient, the physician may decide that the pharmacist should acquire additional data to adequately monitor the patient's status.

Furthermore, the standards of care are necessarily limited by practical considerations such as laboratory capability and availability of specialized diagnostic equipment. For example, renal function is monitored via blood urea nitrogen (BUN) values with the realization that the serum creatinine level is a better index of renal function. However, in our laboratory it took the technologist about ten minutes to determine the BUN value versus about 40 minutes for the creatinine.

The protocols are quite like the minimum care criteria described by Kessner et al.,[7] except that ours are designed primarily for the application to maintenance care, whereas Kessner's are used in the initial work-up and stabilization of a patient. Our experience was similar to that described by the above authors in regard to the need for flexibility, periodic revision, and limitations dictated by practicality.

The use of formalized protocols by the pharmacist in the management of patients receiving long-term drug therapy was first developed in the IHS by Streit at the Cass Lake, Minnesota Indian Hospital in 1970.[8] Since then, this system has become widespread in the IHS and is described later in this book.[9] Pharmacists outside the IHS have also described similar programs utilizing formalized protocols.[10]

Although no review procedures were employed by us in conjunction with the maintenance care program at the Clinton Indian Hospital, the establishment of minimum care standards for both initial workup and maintenance care is appropriate for use with data obtained through a professional standards review organization (PSRO). Data collected by the PSRO serves as a feedback to aid in the refinement and periodic revision of the standards to insure that the standards are suited to the population being served.[7, 11] Cooperative physician-pharmacist ventures in professional standards review have been undertaken elsewhere with good results.[12-15]

## Success of the Program

Patients at the Clinton Indian Hospital readily accepted the pharmacist as a primary provider of health care and to our knowledge did not question his competency in this role. This acceptance was due in part to the explanation of the program to each patient when he was assigned to it. We believe that the further activities of the pharmacist are viewed by patients as a logical extension of the expanded role already played by the pharmacist in the Indian Health Service. The acceptance of a practitioner by a patient seems to be based more on the competency demonstrated by the practitioner than on the professional category into which he falls.

Acceptance of the program by physicians has been especially good. They feel that the protocols have been followed well and that the pharmacist is better utilizing his knowledge with the result that there is more

rational drug use. There has been no question of the pharmacist assuming responsibility beyond that agreed upon, nor do the physicians feel in any way threatened or that their "power" is being usurped. To the contrary, it is felt that more patients could be handled in this fashion. Indeed, the concept of the pharmacist managing chronic care patients has been given approval and support by the Senior Clinician of the Indian Health Service.[a] A three-year study is presently being performed at the Cass Lake Indian Hospital to attempt to determine the effectiveness of the pharmacist in the management of ambulatory patients using formalized protocols.

## General Applicability of the Role and Implications

The role that we have outlined for the pharmacist as a provider of maintenance care is but one of many roles which a clinically-trained pharmacist is capable of performing.[16] The role would be most suitably performed in a group medical practice, HMO, rural health care delivery system, or satellite facility such as a neighborhood health center. This view is consistent with the role of the pharmacist in the primary care setting of the emerging health care system as outlined by Dr. Edmund Pellegrino who sees the pharmacist as the person most responsible for proper drug therapy on a team of diverse health professionals.[17]

With the pharmacist assuming increasing responsibility for direct patient care, the question arises as to the type of practitioner that will assume the traditional drug distribution functions. In our experience at Clinton, the limiting factor in the utilization of the pharmacist in direct patient care was the pharmacist's involvement in drug distribution which was, by necessity, his top priority. We suspect that a conflict in priorities for the pharmacist's time will frequently exist when he must perform both drug distribution and direct patient care roles. Although subprofessionals can be used effectively to perform many tasks in the drug distribution process, the necessity of having a professional responsible for drug procurement, storage, and distribution is undeniable. In order to use pharmacy manpower most efficiently, one is led to the conclusion that two types of pharmacy practitioners must be formally recognized by the profession. Two recent dissertations have acknowledged this necessity and have related it to a perceived need for two distinct courses of study in pharmacy: a doctoral program emphasizing the clinical use of drugs and a baccalaureate program, perhaps of less than five years, emphasizing drug distribution.[16, 18]

---

[a] Maurice L. Sievers, M.D., in a memo to the Deputy Area Director of the Oklahoma City Area IHS, concerning the pharmacy chronic care monitoring protocols of the Clinton Indian Hospital, July 6, 1972.

## Conclusion

As the delivery of ambulatory care becomes more organized through the formation of HMO's and similar systems, the delivery of health care through a team approach draws closer to becoming a reality. The clinically-trained pharmacist promises to make a unique contribution to patient care as a drug therapy expert. A role for the pharmacist as a provider of maintenance care to ambulatory patients is presently being developed in several settings. By establishing and applying standards of care, not only can more uniform care be provided, but a medium is created through which the pharmacist can be integrated into the health care system and participate readily in peer review procedures.

From our experience at the Clinton Indian Hospital, we believe that a role for the pharmacist as a manager of chronic drug therapy is a viable one with considerable potential.

## References

1. Johnson, E. A.: Government's Role in Hospital-Based Health Care Delivery Systems, presented at the Seventh Annual ASHP Midyear Clinical Meeting, Las Vegas, Nevada, Dec. 3-7, 1972.

2. Borgsdorf, L. R. and Mosser, R. S.: The Problem-Oriented Medical Record: An Ideal System for Pharmacist Involvement in Comprehensive Patient Care, In *Clinical Pharmacy Sourcebook*, pp. 45-48.

3. Dunphy, T. W.: The Pharmacist in the Management of Chronic Disease, presented at the 119th Annual Meeting of the American Pharmaceutical Association, Houston, Texas, Apr. 22-28, 1972.

4. Miller, W. A. and Corcella, J.: New Member on the Team, *Ment. Hyg. 56*:57-61 (Spring) 1972.

5. Coleman, J. H., Evans, R. L., and Rosenbluth, S. A.: Extended Clinical Roles for the Pharmacist in Psychiatric Care, In *Clinical Pharmacy Sourcebook*, pp. 121-124.

6. Schulman, J., Jr. and Wood, C.: Flow Sheets for Charts of Ambulatory Patients. *J. Amer. Med. Ass. 217*: 933-937 (Aug. 16) 1971.

7. Kessner, D. M., Kalk, C. E., and Singer, J.: Assessing Health Quality—The Case for Tracers. *N. Engl. J. Med. 288*:189-194 (Jan. 25) 1973.

8. Streit, R. J.: Long-Term Drug Therapy—A Program Expanding the Pharmacist's Role, *J. Amer. Pharm. Ass. NS13*:434-443 (Aug.) 1973.

9. Ellinoy, B. J. et al.: A Pharmacy Outpatient Monitoring Program Providing Primary Medical Care to Selected Patients, In *Clinical Pharmacy Sourcebook*, pp. 115-120.

10. Mattei, T. J. et al.: Hypertension: A Model for Pharmacy Involvement, In *Clinical Pharmacy Sourcebook*, pp. 107-110.

11. Sanazaro, P. J., Goldstein, R. L., and Roberts, J. S.: Research and Development in Quality Assurance: The Experimental Medical Care Review Organization Program, *N. Engl. J. Med. 287*:1125-1131 (Nov. 30) 1972.

12. Ellinoy, B. J., Schuster, J. S. and Yatsco, J. C.: Pharmacy Audit of Patient Health Records—Feasibility and Usefulness of a Drug Surveillance System, *Amer. J. Hosp. Pharm. 29*:749-754 (Sept.) 1972.

13. Kunin, C. M. and Dierks, J. W.: A Physiciar-Pharmacist Voluntary Program to Improve Prescription Practices, *N. Engl. J. Med. 280*:1442-1446 (June 26) 1969.

14. Laventurier, M. F.: A Prototype Pharmacy Foundation Peer Review Program, *Calif. Pharm. 19*:36-38 (May) 1972.

15. Laventurier, M. F. and Talley, R. B.: The Incidence of Drug-Drug Interactions in a Medi-Cal Population, *Calif. Pharm. 20*:18-22 (Nov.) 1972.

16. Brodie, D. C., Knoben, J. E., and Wertheimer, A. I.: Expanded Roles for Pharmacists, *Amer. J. Pharm. Educ. 37*:591-600 (Nov.) 1973.

17. Pellegrino, E. D.: Relationship of Medical and Pharmacy Education, Proceedings, Conference on Challenge to Pharmacy in the 70's, University of Califonia School of Pharmacy, 1970, United States Department of Health Education and Welfare, National Center for Health Services Research and Development, Rockville, Maryland [DHEW Publication No. (HSM) 72-3000] pp. 83-91.

18. Goyan, J. E.: Pharmaceutical Education: A Ticket to Professional Survival or Extinction, The T. Edward Hicks Lecture, State University of New York at Buffalo, School of Pharmacy, Mar. 7, 1972.

# 22 A Pharmacy Outpatient Monitoring Program Providing Primary Medical Care to Selected Patients

Brian J. Ellinoy, John F. Mays, Paul V. McSherry, and
Lawrence C. Rosenthal

An operational program is described in which pharmacists provide primary outpatient medical care to patients with certain chronic illnesses.

Patients with stable, drug-controlled medical problems are referred to the pharmacist by a physician. General guidelines have been established by the medical and pharmacy staffs for each specific disease state covered. Using these guidelines and analyzing subjective and objective data, the pharmacist either continues the patient's drug regimen or refers the patient to the physician for further evaluation. In all cases a problem-oriented progress note is entered in the health record, reflecting the data obtained and the action taken on the problem. An appointment system has greatly facilitated surveillance of these patients, especially in the area of tuberculosis control.

The program has demonstrated that in a proper setting the pharmacist is capable not only of monitoring drug therapy but also of providing primary medical care.

An important component of the problem-oriented health record system[1-5] is the concept of standards of care. Under this system written minimal standards, reflecting the consensus of opinion of providers of care within a given environment, should exist for the management of each disease state. Specifically, such standards can be developed for stabilized patients with chronic diseases. The pharmacist, with his knowledge of drug therapy, is in an excellent position to utilize these guidelines to monitor such patients and expand his participation on the health team.

At the Shiprock Indian Hospital, the pharmacist has become involved in the management of drug-stable, chronic care patients through an outpatient monitoring program. The basic aim of the program is improved monitoring of drug therapy. In addition, the provision of primary medical care by the pharmacist is intended to allow more physician time for the treatment of acutely ill patients.

Serving the Northeastern Navajo reservation, the Shiprock Indian Hospital is a 75-bed facility with a medical staff of 15 physicians. The pharmacy staff consists of five pharmacists and one technician-interpreter. In fiscal year 1972, the average daily inpatient load was 57.4; there were 21,018 patient hospital days; outpatient visits numbered 59,306; and 95,662 outpatient

prescriptions were dispensed. In contrast to most institutions, all outpatient medications, including inpatient discharge medications, are dispensed directly from the patient's health record. Other pharmacy services include daily ward rounds, an i.v. admixture service, field health assignments, and cardiac arrest team membership. Hospital health records have been problem oriented since January 1970, and physicians and pharmacists are actively engaged in continuous peer review to improve the quality of patient care.[4, 6]

The monitoring program has developed in part from the pharmacist's past accomplishments in the problem-oriented system (the pharmacy audit[6]), his direct contact with the health record in his everyday activities, and physicians' attempts to lighten the workload in a very busy outpatient clinic. In addition, the pioneer work done at the Cass Lake Indian Hospital[7] definitely has served as an incentive.

## Program Design

Before any program of this type can begin, it is important to know what kind of patient is to be followed, how he is to be referred to the pharmacist, what questions are to be asked for followup, etc. The Appendix describes the design of the program and the screening questions asked by the pharmacist for each disease state, as determined for the Shiprock environment through the cooperative efforts of the medical and pharmacy staffs.

The concept of physician referral (Appendix, Item I.1) should be emphasized because it places the initial judgment responsibility about the patient in the proper hands. Patient choice of pharmacist or physician service (Appendix, Item I.3) is also very important and should be guaranteed. Obviously, program publicity and patient education are needed to make the service and its advantages (fewer physician visits, shorter waiting time, competent management) known. The program must be "sold" first to the medical staff so it in turn can help "sell" it to the patients. In view of the cultural and language barriers on the Navajo Reservation (a great number of the older people do not speak English), this is sometimes difficult to do. The Appendix applies to the Shiprock environment only and does not attempt to cover all situations or disease states. Every attempt has been made to keep all guidelines general in nature for easy tailoring to individual patients.

### Procedure

Once standards of operation have been established and the program initiated, the actual steps taken from the time the patient is entered into the system have to be documented. These steps for the Shiprock program are reviewed below.

The eligible patient, by his own choice, is entered into the program independently by the physician or at the suggestion of the pharmacist. The physician updates the problem list and indicates in a problem-oriented progress note the specific parameters he wishes to have followed (see Figure 1), e.g., time intervals between return visits to see the physician and to obtain refills, laboratory work to be done, acceptable limits of objective data, drug therapy, etc. If parameters which are felt to be needed are not mentioned, the pharmacist consults the physician for clarification.

The pharmacist reviews the health record after receiving it from the clinic, dispenses the patient's medication, counsels him on its proper use, reexplains the program and gives the patient an appointment to return to the pharmacy when it is time to obtain a prescription refill. An appointment slip is filled out showing the patient's name, chart number, the date and time of return, and the type of appointment. The patient's name, chart number, diagnosis and mailing address are entered in an appointment book under the date he is to return. Patients who are using *prn* medications, e.g., patients with some type of skin problem, arthritis, or aches and pains of old age, are not entered into the appointment book and therefore are not accounted for in the statistics. It is estimated that there are 30 to 40 of these patients.

When the patient returns for his appointment, his health record is sent directly to the pharmacy from the medical records department. The pharmacist reviews the problem list and pertinent information in the body of the health record. He then asks the patient the screening questions established for the problem(s) (see Appendix) and obtains any additional data base requested by the referring physician, e.g., weight, blood pressure (see Figure 1). Laboratory work is requested if indicated and medical advice may be sought as well if a problem exists. Collecting all the necessary data, evaluating it in light of the established standards, and using his professional judgment and experience, the pharmacist either refills the patient's medication or refers the patient back to the physician for evaluation. Hopefully in the future, using established standards, the pharmacist may also alter the drug therapy of these patients, e.g., change dosage regimens, add or delete drugs, etc.

A problem-oriented progress note (Figure 2) is entered in the health record by the pharmacist reflecting his contact with the patient—all subjective and objective data collected, any discussion, impression and a plan for each problem. This is done whether the pharmacist handles the patient completely or refers him to the physician.

Once the patient's medication is refilled and he is counseled about its use, another appointment to return to the pharmacy or to the physician is given, and the cycle is repeated when the patient returns to the hospital.

If the patient does not return to the pharmacy for his

*Figure 1. Physician progress note—entering a chronic care patient into the pharmacy program*

AMBULATORY CARE RECORD BRIEF
(CONTINUATION SHEET)

| 28. DATE And CLINIC | 29. DIAGNOSES AND CLINICAL NOTES |
|---|---|
| 6-1-72 | 9:50 AM |
| | #1 Diabetes |
| | Sx: Fractionals negative at home; feels fine; ō sxs of |
| Wt. 185 ¼ # | hypoglycemia |
| c̄ clothes + shoes | Obj. U/A ⟶ neg/neg |
| | Imp. Doing well off medication |
| | Plan ① Follow in pharmacy program q 2 months |
| | Weight ± 5# |
| | Fractionals no greater than 1+ |
| | ② Testape 1 roll |
| | ③ To MD in 6 months |
| | |
| | #2 Hypertension |
| | Sx: ō headaches or dizziness; taking meds |
| | Obj. BP 150/88 |
| | Cor: reg s̄ (m) |
| | Lungs: clear |
| | Eyes: Some arteriolar narrowing; ō H or E |
| | Ext.: ō edema |
| | Imp. Good control |
| | Plan ① Follow in Pharmacy Refill Program q 2 months |
| | BP not to be > 160 systolic or 95 diastolic |
| | ② Reserpine 0.25 mg Q AM #60 |
| | ③ Hydrodiuril 50 mg Q AM #60 |
| | ④ To MD in 6 months |
| | MD |

1. LAST NAME, FIRST, MIDDLE — 4. REGISTRATION NO.

HSM-45-3
REV. 7-72 (Continue on reverse)

*Figure 2. Pharmacy progress note—monitoring a chronic care patient*

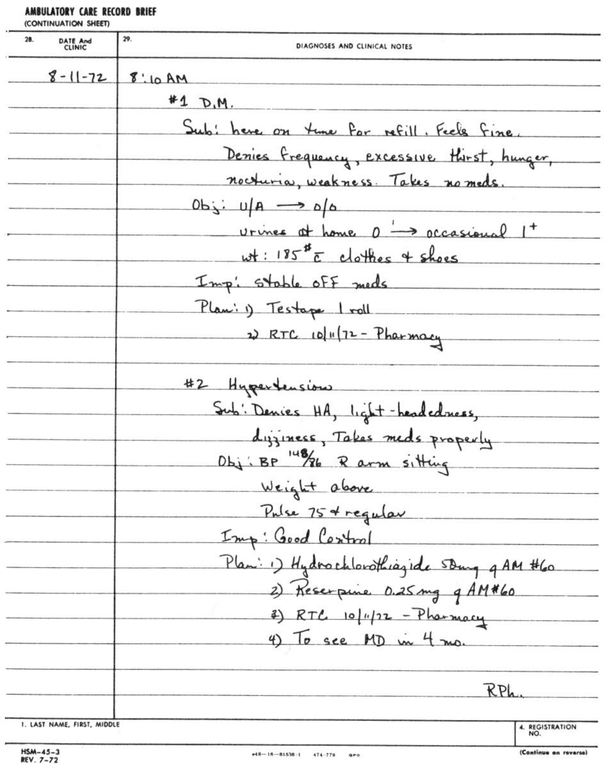

AMBULATORY CARE RECORD BRIEF
(CONTINUATION SHEET)

| 28. DATE And CLINIC | 29. DIAGNOSES AND CLINICAL NOTES |
|---|---|
| 8-11-72 | 8:10 AM |
| | #1 D.M. |
| | Sub: here on time for refill. Feels fine. |
| | Denies frequency, excessive thirst, hunger, |
| | nocturia, weakness. Takes no meds. |
| | Obj: U/A → o/o |
| | urines at home 0 → occasional 1+ |
| | wt: 185# c clothes + shoes |
| | Imp: stable off meds |
| | Plan: 1) Testape 1 roll |
| | 2) RTC 10/11/72 - Pharmacy |
| | #2 Hypertension |
| | Sub: Denies HA, light-headedness, |
| | dizziness, Takes meds properly |
| | Obj: BP 148/86 R arm sitting |
| | Weight above |
| | Pulse 75 + regular |
| | Imp: Good Control |
| | Plan: 1) Hydrochlorothiazide 50mg q AM #60 |
| | 2) Reserpine 0.25 mg q AM #60 |
| | 3) RTC 10/11/72 - Pharmacy |
| | 4) To see MD in 4 mo. |
| | RPh. |

1. LAST NAME, FIRST, MIDDLE | 4. REGISTRATION NO.

HSM-45-3
REV. 7-72   648—16—81538-1 474-779 GPO   (Continue on reverse)

scheduled appointment, his chart is pulled. A note indicating "no show" is entered and a reminder card (Figure 3) is mailed to him. A check is placed next to his name in the appointment book indicating that the card was sent. The followup of patients not responding to these cards is discussed in the results below.

## Results

Some interesting statistics have been generated by this program and are presented in Tables 1 and 2. It is encouraging to find a 49% return rate on appointments, especially at a hospital which does not have a general appointment system. Because of lack of transportation and long travel distances, patients usually arrive at the hospital when they are able and not necessarily when they are scheduled. Compliance with this program

*Figure 3. Reminder card sent by pharmacy to chronic care patients who fail to show for appointments*

*Dear Patient:*

*You recently missed a scheduled pharmacy appointment. Please return to the hospital as soon as possible and bring this card with you.*

*John F. Mays*
*Chief, Pharmacy Service*
*PHS Indian Hospital*
*Shiprock, New Mexico*

**Table 1. Some Results of the Pharmacy Program to Monitor Chronic Care Patients**

| | |
|---|---|
| Number of patients in program 10/1/71 to 5/1/72: | 477 |
| Total appointments made 10/1/71 to 5/1/72: | 712[a] |
| Number of appointments kept: | 352 (49%) |
| Number of appointments missed and cards sent: | 360 (51%) |
| Number of responses to cards: | 190 (53%) |
| Number of cards not receiving response | 170 (47%) |
| Ratio of cards not responded to total appointments made: 170/712 x 100% | (24%) |
| Number of patients on isoniazid who completed one year of therapy and received chest X-ray on program | 43 |
| Number of actual patient revisits to the pharmacy | 542 |

[a] During the next three months (5/1/72 to 8/1/72), 417 appointments were made, indicating that the program was expanding somewhat.

suggests that patients may be somewhat interested in keeping appointments; this might be an impetus to establishing a total appointment system. The 49% return rate on appointments does not imply that 51% of the people would not have returned for refills of their medications. Many patients responding to the cards were in fact not out of medicine. Although this indicates missed doses, the possibility exists that these patients would have returned when their medicine ran out. The 53% response to cards sent for missed appointments suggests that the time spent pulling charts, making notations and addressing cards has been useful. Because of time limitations, no repeat reminder cards have been sent to the remaining 170 patients who did not keep their appointments. These patients may be lost to the system, but because of time and staff limitations it was impossible to follow them more comprehensively. However, the fact that a note was made in the patient's chart stating that the appointment had been missed hopefully has enhanced future followup should the patient return to clinic. Anyone reviewing the chart can readily assess the patient's needs and take proper action.

**Table 2. Disease States Handled by the Pharmacy Monitoring Program[a]**

| DISEASE STATE | NO. PATIENTS |
|---|---|
| Tuberculosis prophylaxis (INH) | 431 (90%) |
| Diabetes insipidus | 1 |
| Diabetes mellitus | 10 |
| Epilepsy | 19 |
| Hypertension | 8 |
| Hypothyroidism | 1 |
| Oral contraception | 4 |
| Osteoarthritis | 1 |
| Rheumatic fever prophylaxis | 1 |

[a] Data collected from 10/1/71 to 5/1/72.

The majority (90%) of patients followed thus far are those taking isoniazid for tuberculosis prophylaxis (Table 2). The basic reasons for the lack of patients in other categories is discussed below. It should be noted here, however, that some of the conditions originally to be followed by the pharmacist (Appendix) were placed in the hands of other members of the health team in the interest of time and convenience. For example, patients on ethambutol and isoniazid dual therapy are followed in a weekly specialty chest clinic by a physician, and patients using oral contraceptives are monitored by the midwifery staff in charge of family planning.

### Analysis

The lack of adequate personnel in the face of an ever increasing outpatient workload has greatly limited the number and type of patients the pharmacist has been able to follow. This has also limited the amount of time he has been able to spend in chart review; in collecting and evaluating data; in writing proper, complete progress notes; and in serving the patient as he has been trained. Ancillary help would be beneficial in providing improved service and in eliminating the great amount of clerical work that is now being done by the pharmacist.

The lack of a separate consultation room has rendered privacy in the pharmacist-patient relationship almost impossible. All counseling is done at the pharmacy window which faces the waiting room. The setting is a rushed one and it is felt that the patient is put ill at ease by the asking of personal questions in front of others.

These deficiencies, well known at the program's outset, have limited the pharmacist's participation. Obviously it has been easier to take care of a patient on isoniazid because it takes less time to process his chart. His medical problem can be handled readily at the pharmacy window. Thus, priorities must be set as to what types of patients can be most readily taken care of under individualized circumstances.

In addition to the deficiencies, a few interesting discoveries have been made. At first there was some initial hesitance on the part of physicians to refer patients to the program. This can be attributed partially to a lack of knowledge of the program (a reflection of our failure to continuously advertise), forgetfulness, personal desires not to lose control of patients and perhaps a lack of confidence in the pharmacist's ability. As the program progressed and physicians reviewed charts of patients followed by the pharmacy, there was a considerable change of attitude. When they were subsequently asked by the pharmacist if a particular patient could be entered into the program, they agreed most of the time. We believe a bigger "sales pitch" would be a partial solution to this "problem," but it cannot be given because the pharmacy does not have the necessary resources to provide a complete service. The patients for the program are available, as daily chart reviews have revealed; and, faced with

such a busy outpatient clinic, the physicians are seeking help. The potential for greater pharmacy involvement in this program definitely exists.

Second, when physicians have referred patients to the program, many times they have understated the parameters to be followed and have had to be called by the pharmacy for clarification. By requiring proper planning in the care of patients, this action has promoted the problem-oriented system and has enabled the pharmacist to assume some responsibility for the maintenance of the system. As more experience has been acquired by the pharmacist, he has been asked by the physician to assist in the setting of acceptable standards for the individual patient. The pharmacist has also been asked to follow disease states not included in the original protocol, e.g., diabetes insipidus. Through this participation the pharmacist has been forced to increase his knowledge of disease states and clinical laboratory tests.

Third, there has been hesitance on the part of the patient to utilize the services of the pharmacist. This has resulted from a lack of general health education which should be continuously provided to the people by all members of the health team. Patients have been conditioned in the past to "come see the doctor" for any kind of problem. Some of them expect to see a physician, especially when driving to the hospital from as far as 60 miles away. Thus, even when the patient agrees to be seen by the pharmacist in the consultation program and seems to understand the advantages in doing so, occasionally he still returns to see the physician. Indeed, the patient must be made aware of the services available to him and must have the ability to select the level of service to suit his needs. This has not been easily accomplished on the Navajo Reservation because of language and cultural barriers, and a more organized effort is drastically needed.

Fourth, communication problems with patients have been identified. Patients have answered "yes" to questions when the answers really were "no," or vice versa, because the patients either did not understand the terminology used, wanted to avoid embarrassment, or wanted to be accepted by the questioner and answered to please him. It has also been found that the power of suggestion must be considered when asking or offering information. Telling patients what could happen to them by using a drug sometimes convinces them they have exactly that condition. When subsequently questioned about such side effects (e.g., poor appetite, lethargy) they will answer positively. Questions have to be formulated in such a manner that the patient explains his own problems and is not prodded with "helpful hints."

Fifth, thorough investigations have shown that patients whose chronic problems were controlled with drugs were not using the medications as instructed by the physician and/or pharmacist. Either the patient discovered by trial and error that he felt better when taking the medication a certain way or he had been taking the medicine one way so long that he would not change (even though a change was ordered). Breaking patients of this habit through consultation was often quite a chore. Often it was the physician who, based on the individual case, would allow the patient to use the medication "his own way" as long as his condition was controlled adequately.

Sixth, it is noteworthy to state that prior to the pharmacy department's monitoring of patients on isoniazid prophylaxis, no organized followup existed. The tuberculosis control office reviewed patient data from incomplete computer printouts provided by the State of Arizona on a time-available basis only. Public health nurses would check the health records of suspected delinquent patients and attempt to locate them for proper followup only as their busy schedules permitted. Further steps have been taken by the pharmacy to improve the program. Recently a tuberculosis clerk has been employed under the supervision of the pharmacy department and the field health department to update patient information for the computer so that all patients in the Shiprock Service Unit on isoniazid prophylaxis will receive up-to-date surveillance. It is felt that the use of the computer as a record-keeper and as an appointment book will help to minimize the clerical work now required and will facilitate the detection and management of delinquent patients. It will also facilitate the generation of statistical data and allow the pharmacist more time to spend with the patient. Even though only tuberculosis patients are followed by computer at present, other types of chronic care patients could be monitored similarly.

Finally, the pharmacist's participation in the monitoring of stable chronic care patients in a problem-oriented setting has rightfully made him a target of peer review by his colleagues and by the medical staff. The quality of care he provides is evaluated in light of established standards. He is expected to perform at certain levels of thoroughness, reliability, efficiency and competence. The educational feedback furnished by audits of his work assist him in improving the type of service for which he is responsible and in maintaining rapport with the rest of the health team.

## Conclusions

The future of the outpatient monitoring program and any effort toward expansion at Shiprock will depend upon the satisfaction of the needs discussed previously—staff additions and consultation space. Of course the continuous support of the medical staff will be needed. The continuing education of the pharmacist in clinical medicine and the problem-oriented system cannot be overlooked either in assuring his competence in such a program.

It has been shown that by using established guidelines the pharmacist has been able to provide primary medical care and monitor drug therapy for chronic disease patients in a problem-oriented environment. An ap-

pointment system has proved useful in following these patients and has lent itself easily to computerization of tuberculosis prophylaxis patients. It is hoped that the program can be expanded in the future to include a greater number of disease states.

### References

1. Weed, L. L.: Medical Records, Medical Education, and Patient Care: The Problem Oriented Record as a Basic Tool, The Press of Case Western Reserve University, Cleveland, Ohio, 1969.
2. Weed, L. L.: Medical Records That Guide and Teach, I, *N. Engl. J. Med.* 278:593–600 (Mar. 14) 1968.
3. Weed, L. L.: Medical Records That Guide and Teach, II, *N. Engl. J. Med.* 278:652–657 (Mar. 21) 1968.
4. Humphrey, J. B. and Schuster, J. S.: The Shiprock Experience in Introducing Problem Orientation, PHS Indian Hospital, Shiprock, New Mexico, June, 1971.
5. Bjorn, J. C. and Cross, H. D.: The Problem-Oriented Private Practice of Medicine: A System for Comprehensive Health Care, McGraw-Hill Book Company, Chicago, Illinois, 1970.
6. Ellinoy, B. J., Schuster, J. S., Yatsco, J. C. and Rosenthal, L. C.: Pharmacy Audit of Patient Health Records—Feasibility and Usefulness of a Drug Surveillance System, *Amer. J. Hosp. Pharm.* 29:749–754 (Sept.) 1972.
7. Streit, R. J. and Clark, T. C.: An Expanded Drug Refill Program: Building the Data Base to Aid in Patient Care, PHS Indian Hospital, Cass Lake, Minnesota, presented at the Sixth Joint Meeting of the Clinical Society and Commissioned Officers Association of the U.S.P.H.S., Galveston, Texas, April 1971.

### Appendix

#### Pharmacy Outpatient Monitoring Program

The following is a description of the pharmacy outpatient monitoring program which has been initiated at the Shiprock Indian Hospital for patients with stable, ongoing problems. An outline of the program design is followed by the screening questions asked by pharmacists for each disease included.

### I. DESIGN

1. Entrance to the program will be by physician referral only. Walk-in patients who refer themselves will be sent to the clinic where the physician may elect to enter them in the program if he feels they qualify.
2. Based on workload and staffing the pharmacy department will make the final determination as to whether or not the patient referred by the physician can be followed in the program.
3. The referring physician should make eligible patients aware of this pharmacy service and should give the patient the choice of accepting or rejecting this service.
4. At the time of referral the physician must certify that the problem list is complete and current based upon all the information recorded in the chart. It is suggested that where appropriate chronic disease flow sheets be established at the time of referral also.
5. The physician's referral will indicate the date of the patient's return to him (e.g., six months, one year) and the frequency of return to the pharmacy (e.g., every month, every two months). The pharmacy will keep an appointment book and remind all patients who fail to return by mailing out a postcard.
6. The physician should record in the chart at the time of referral

acceptable limits for any objective parameters that will be measured. If these limits are exceeded or if answers to screening questions indicate inadequate control of the disease state when the pharmacist monitors the patient, the patient will be referred to the physician before a refill is dispensed.

7. If the patient is taking medication incorrectly but reports no problems, the pharmacy will reinstruct him or consult the physician about the advisability of altering drug therapy. If on two consecutive visits the patient is taking medication incorrectly, he will be referred to the physician.

8. The pharmacist will enter a numbered, titled progress note in the chart detailing the subjective and objective data he obtained, his impression or assessment and his plan (e.g., medication dispensed). When flow sheets are present the necessary data will be recorded on them.

9. Program design and screening questions are subject to periodic review and revision by the medical and pharmacy staffs acting jointly.

## II. SCREENING QUESTIONS AND PARAMETERS MEASURED

1. Hypertension
   a. Have you developed headaches or dizziness?
   b. Do you feel light-headed after standing up?
   c. How do you take your medication?
   d. Are you taking medication from any other physician or pharmacy?
   e. (Weight)
   f. (Sitting blood pressure and pulse rate)
2. Diabetes Mellitus
   a. Are you having frequent urination? excessive thirst? to get up at night to urinate?
   b. Have you had spells of feeling weak, sweaty and hungry?
   c. Do you check your urine at home? What does it show?
   d. How do you take your medication?
   e. Are you taking medication from any other physician or pharmacy?
   f. (Weight)
   g. (Urine for glucose and acetone)
3. Epilepsy (Diphenylhydantoin and phenobarbital)
   a. Have you had any seizures since your last visit?
   b. Have you experienced headaches, bleeding gums or unsteadiness in walking?
   c. How do you take your medication?
   d. Are you taking medication from any other physician or pharmacy?
4. Arthritis (Salicylates)
   a. Does the medicine relieve your pain? Have you had any new pain?
   b. Does the medicine cause any stomach pain?
   c. How do you take the medicine?

d. Are you taking medication from any other physician or pharmacy?
5. Thyroid Replacement
   a. Have you developed nervousness, changes in appetite, diarrhea or constipation?
   b. How do you take the medicine?
   c. Are you taking medication from any other physician or pharmacy?
   d. (Weight)
   e. (Resting pulse)
6. Oral Contraceptives
   a. Are your periods regular? Have you had any bleeding between periods?
   b. Have you developed headaches, leg pain or swelling?
   c. How do you take the medicine?
   d. Are you taking medication from any other physician or pharmacy?
   e. (Blood pressure)
7. Antabuse Therapy
   a. Have you been drinking since your last prescription refill?
   b. How do you take the medicine?
   c. Are you taking medication from any other physician or pharmacy?
8. Eczema (Topicals)
   a. Does the medicine still control your rash?
   b. Have you had any new areas of rash or skin problems?
   c. How often and how much medicine do you apply?
   d. Are you taking medication from any other physician or pharmacy?
9. Antituberculosis Therapy
   Isoniazid Prophylaxis
   a. Have you developed abdominal pain, dark urine, or a rash?
   b. How is your appetite?
   c. How do you take the medication?
   d. Are you taking medication from any other physician or pharmacy?
   Ethambutol
   a. How do you take the medication?
   b. Are you taking medication from any other physician or pharmacy?
   c. (Color vision)
   d. (Visual acuity)
10. Anemia of Known Etiology
    a. Do you feel weak or tired all the time?
    b. How do you take the medication?
    c. Are you taking medication from any other physician or pharmacy?
    d. (Hematocrit—if requested by physician)
11. Paraplegics (Irrigation and Topical Medications Only)
    a. Are you having any problems?
    b. Are you taking medication from any other physician or pharmacy?

# 23 Extended Clinical Roles for the Pharmacist in Psychiatric Care

James H. Coleman, III, R. Lee Evans, and Sidney A. Rosenbluth

An interdisciplinary program which involves specially trained pharmacists in the care of ambulant psychiatric patients is described.

The pharmacist assesses stability of previously stabilized patients and may either refer a patient to the psychiatrist or work with the patient personally. If judged stable, the patient may be continued on the previous drug regimen. However, if the patient is mildly unstable or experiencing drug side effects, the pharmacist may alter dosage(s) or schedule(s), discontinue drug(s), and/or add drug(s). The pharmacist occasionally administers intramuscular injections of a long-acting phenothiazine and performs venipunctures to collect blood for lithium determinations. These activities make use of the pharmacist's special knowledge of drugs but also depend on additional training, including didactic material and field experiences. Training of this type is offered under supervision of pharmacists, psychiatrists, and psychologists in an elective 11-week rotation for doctor of pharmacy candidates.

The program shows great promise for improving access to care and reducing costs, and it makes better use of available mental health manpower.

Many of the problems in mental health care involve drugs in one way or another,[1-5] a fact which itself suggests the possibility for contributions by the pharmacist. Poland has focused attention on mental illness[6] and mental hospitals[7] and has called for deeper involvement by pharmacists in mental health.[8] In addition, he has indicated that pharmacy schools have not prepared their students for such involvement.[8] Some pharmacy schools have sponsored continuing education seminars in mental health and published proceedings,[9,10] and the National Institute of Mental Health is currently supporting two training projects to develop and evaluate behavioral science training for pharmacists.[11,12] There has been a recent surge of activity in specialized extended roles for pharmacists in psychiatric care. For example, Kohan and associates described a number of clinical roles for pharmacists in the care of institutionalized psychiatric patients.[13] In recent years approaches to mental health care have included a dramatic shift in emphasis from institutional and custodial care toward convenient, accessible ambulatory care in the community. In this regard, Miller and Corcella have made innovative strides in bringing the pharmacist into a team effort in the care of patients in a community mental health center.[14] Similarly, Kaufman and associates have developed a program in which the pharmacist actively participates in reducing tranquilizer abuse in a large American Indian clinic population.[15]

The purpose of this chapter is threefold: (1) to describe experiences with extended model roles developed specifically to help resolve existing problems in treatment of psychiatric patients in the community, (2) to review the training of pharmacists for such roles, and (3) to present a limited evaluation of this program through subjective observations and questionnaire surveys of participating medical and nursing personnel and pharmacists who received the training and participated in the program.

## Model Roles

Through service contracts, the University of Tennessee College of Pharmacy is now responsible for pharmacy services in several mental health facilities: Tennessee Psychiatric Hospital and Institute, Oates Manor Community Mental Health Clinic, and the Memphis and Shelby County Mental Health Center. In each location, pharmacists are responsible for all dispensing functions and are also deeply involved with medication maintenance of previously stabilized patients.

The hospital and clinics have gained full service pharmaceutical departments, the College has obtained specialized teaching programs and the patient has acquired a new member of his health care team.

All of the patients seen by pharmacists have been previously diagnosed and stabilized by psychiatrists. Many of the patients are indigent. The purpose of the maintenance clinics is to keep patients stabilized on medications, out of the hospital and functional in the community. Patient populations include those with alcohol and drug abuse problems. Pharmacists are involved in alcohol and drug detoxification programs and the subsequent medication maintenance of these patients.

Additional assistance to medical and nursing practitioners has been instituted in all the clinics in the form of inservice education programs. The participating staff has access to the University of Tennessee Drug and Toxicology Information Center, and many are utilizing this information service through the pharmacy department.

Although the pharmacist can become proficient in interviewing psychiatric patients and performing medication maintenance functions, he does not function independently. Rather, he is an integral part of a system closely coordinated with the psychiatrist and based on common patient records. Functions of the pharmacist in the medication maintenance of the mentally ill are outlined in Figure 1.

The pharmacist reviews the patient's chart prior to initiating the interview. A drug history is taken during the initial interview and is updated during subsequent visits. Patients are seen at times by different pharmacist interviewers, a fact which requires very rigorous record keeping to insure desired continuity. A key function is the assessment of patient stability using the techniques learned during formal training programs and reinforced by subsequent experiences. If judged stable, the patient may be continued on the previous drug regimen. The stable patient represents at least temporarily successful therapy which in this program is primarily chemotherapy. Efforts are immediately made to assure continued compliance and patient confidence in this course of treatment. Such reinforcement attempts involve displays by the pharmacist of concern and confidence in the treatment regimen. In addition, the patient is complimented for his cooperation and good progress. However, if the patient appears unstable, the pharmacist must

take a different approach. First, he attempts to determine what has precipitated the instability. The most common problems involve patient noncompliance, drug side effects or interference by medications other than those prescribed in the mental health program. Other possible factors include alterations in the patient's mental status and/or diagnosis. Frequently, the pharmacist's uncovering of precipitating factors leads to correction through patient education rather than alterations in therapy.

If the patient is mildly unstable or experiencing drug side effects, the pharmacist may decide to alter the dosage(s) or schedule(s), discontinue drug(s) and/or add drug(s). In this case the pharmacist decides whether or not a psychiatric consult is necessary. If the patient has become uncontrolled, the pharmacist immediately consults the psychiatrist who may elect to assume the entire responsibility for the patient's subsequent therapy, continue to involve the pharmacist to whatever degree appropriate or even hospitalize the patient.

In all cases, whether the patient is stable or experiencing any degree of instability, the pharmacist discusses with the patient critical aspects of his medication regimen such as: purposes of the drugs, possible consequences of noncompliance, dosage and administration questions, side effects which might be experienced and major contraindications. A medication profile is maintained on all patients, originating from the medication history taken on the initial visit to the clinic.

At the end of the interview, the pharmacist enters his impressions and any new information about the patient into the chart. The pharmacist then writes the prescription(s) for the patient's medication(s) just as he entered them in the chart. Prescription blanks are presigned by the sponsoring psychiatrist and cosigned by the pharmacist when he issues the prescription. In the clinics, the pharmacist routinely performs any treatment procedures necessary to complete the patient's care. For example, he administers intramuscular injections of psychotherapeutic drugs and performs venipunctures to collect blood specimens primarily for serum lithium determinations. In cases where the patient appears to be noncompliant or his drugs have been therapeutically ineffective, the pharmacist occasionally performs simple urinalyses to determine if the drugs have been taken by the patient.

Drug side effects and adverse reactions are not difficult to detect and correct. Often only minor adjustments of the patient's medication program are necessary. Patients may experience less obvious medical complications such as changes in blood pressure which sometimes occur with some antidepressant drugs. The pharmacist takes blood pressure readings of patients taking such medications. Other examples include hyperirritability when withdrawing from various sedative-hypnotic drugs, diminished thyroid function with lithium therapy and other endocrine imbalances attributable to some psychotherapeutic agents. If the patient is experiencing any of these problems or complications, the pharmacist notes them in the chart and notifies the physician. The physi-

*Figure 1. Functions of the pharmacist in medication maintenance*

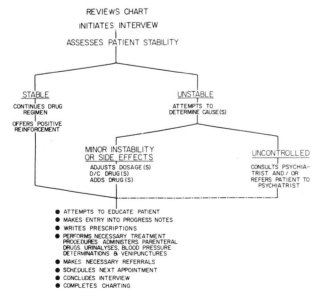

REVIEWS CHART

INITIATES INTERVIEW

ASSESSES PATIENT STABILITY

STABLE
CONTINUES DRUG
REGIMEN

OFFERS POSITIVE
REINFORCEMENT

UNSTABLE
ATTEMPTS TO
DETERMINE CAUSE(S)

MINOR INSTABILITY
OR SIDE EFFECTS
ADJUSTS DOSAGE(S)
D/C DRUG(S)
ADDS DRUG(S)

UNCONTROLLED
CONSULTS PSYCHIA-
TRIST AND/OR
REFERS PATIENT TO
PSYCHIATRIST

- ATTEMPTS TO EDUCATE PATIENT
- MAKES ENTRY INTO PROGRESS NOTES
- WRITES PRESCRIPTIONS
- PERFORMS NECESSARY TREATMENT
  PROCEDURES: ADMINISTERS PARENTERAL
  DRUGS, URINALYSES, BLOOD PRESSURE
  DETERMINATIONS & VENIPUNCTURES
- MAKES NECESSARY REFERRALS
- SCHEDULES NEXT APPOINTMENT
- CONCLUDES INTERVIEW
- COMPLETES CHARTING

cian may treat the complication himself or instruct the pharmacist to do so under his close supervision. Occasionally, it is necessary to refer a patient to another medical specialist if he is experiencing complications which are not associated with his psychiatric therapy but which are adversely affecting the course of this therapy. In no case is any treatment instituted for a nonpsychiatric condition without full supervision by the physician. Such activities make use of the pharmacist's special knowledge of drugs but also depend heavily upon the additional training which he has received. If the patient requires the services of a social worker, the pharmacist will refer the patient. The pharmacist frequently will continue to work with the patient and social worker over an extended period of time. After setting the date for the patient's return visit, the pharmacist concludes the interview and completes the progress notes. Actual dispensing of prescribed medication is handled in a more traditional manner, and the dispensing pharmacist is not necessarily the interviewing pharmacist. The limited number of drugs, the routine scheduling of patient visits and the highly predictable patterns of prescribing lead to extensive use of prepackaging. Supportive personnel assist with label typing, and together with the prepackaging program, tend to minimize dispensing procedures in the clinics. The pharmacist controls the dispensing program but also has additional time freed for the clinical functions previously described. The overall effect is a highly efficient dispensing system, very short waiting periods for patients and much improved utilization of manpower.

## Training Program

The training program is encompassed in an 11-week (220 clock hour) elective rotation in the doctor of pharmacy curriculum. It is primarily conducted at Tennessee Psychiatric Hospital and Institute and the Memphis and Shelby County Mental Health Center. The clinical background of the participating pharmacists includes advanced courses in therapeutics, disease processes and clinical pharmacy as well as experience in such rotations as internal medicine, pediatrics, chest diseases, critical care, drug information and others.

The psychiatric training is presented by the staffs (primarily the psychiatrists) of these institutions. Two students are assigned to each psychiatrist for the clinical aspects of training while the didactic portion is presented simultaneously as a block of material to all students. While the psychiatrist presents the majority of both the clinical and didactic training, pharmacists, staff psychologists, social workers and special therapists present lectures in their areas of specialization in the care of the mentally ill. The pharmacists instruct the students in psychopharmacology and pharmacotherapy and serve as role models.

The training involves two phases: first, orientation to the care of the psychiatric patient by all members of the mental health team, current concepts in mental illness and principles of psychopharmacology; and second, involvement in the Alcohol and Drug Unit of the hospital which prepares the student to participate in the detoxification and subsequent management of the alcoholic patient and drug user. The students are also given technical training in the administration of parenteral dosage forms and the performance of venipuncture techniques for the collection of blood specimens. There is also some experience in a methadone maintenance program. Additional material presented by the Tennessee Psychiatric Hospital and Institute staff includes:

1. A general introduction to the principles of psychiatry, techniques and methods of interviewing the psychiatric patient, and psychotherapy appropriate to the type and degree of mental illness.
2. The development and some current philosophies of psychiatry.
3. Discussion of electroconvulsive therapy.
4. Lectures defining mental illness and describing associated symptomatology.
5. Principles of psychological testing and its significance to psychiatric diagnosis.

The students are acquainted with the functions of the paramedical staff and the roles which they play in the rehabilitation of the mentally ill patient. The students are introduced to the roles of psychiatric social workers, adjunctive therapists and group therapists in those phases of patient rehabilitation which do not involve pharmacotherapy.

The majority of the didactic material is presented in the first three to five weeks of the rotation. During this time the student is also actively participating in patient interviews and pharmacotherapy sessions with the psychiatrist and pharmacist. As the students gain experience, the instructors gradually shift more and more of the interview and therapy session to the students so that after completion of the formal training period, the students themselves conduct patient interviews independently, under the supervision of the psychiatrist.

## Evaluation

In the first two years of the rotation, 27 pharmacists received the training, including two clinical faculty members who participated for the purpose of personal development. It is interesting that this relatively short but intensive block of training and experience has helped influence five graduates to select positions primarily concerned with the care of mentally ill patients and with additional responsibilities to serve as role models and faculty members in four pharmacy schools. Another graduate is chief pharmacist in a small community hospital and serves as a clinical pharmacy consultant to a mental health center in a neighboring community. Several additional graduates have participated in interviews at mental health facilities which appear intent on incorporating pharmacy services similar to those described in this chapter. Similarly, several additional pharmacy schools have interviewed graduates with this training for faculty positions with teaching responsibilities in psychiatric care.

Because of interest and opportunities in this specialized field, plans are being developed to offer a one-year clinical pharmacy residency program in psychiatry. Several individuals have already applied for such a training program even prior to its formal approval.

Questionnaire surveys of psychiatrists and nurses revealed a very high level of acceptance of the program by participating individuals. They unanimously felt that this program resulted in patient care of a quality at least equal to that produced by more traditional methods. About one-third of the respondents felt the level of care to be superior to that resulting from traditional methods. Medical and nursing team members also envisioned a number of program benefits which included more economical treatment, improved accessibility, better manpower utilization and a vast improvement in education of students and health team members. The doctor of pharmacy students in a similar survey also expressed enthusiasm and acceptance of the psychiatric rotation and cited this training as a very sound basis on which to build competence.

## Conclusion

The opinions of psychiatrists, nurses and doctor of pharmacy students involved with this service and education program indicate a degree of success in developing a team approach which shows great promise in improving access to care and reducing costs, and which makes better use of available mental health manpower. These opinions also suggest the possibility of a level of care above that provided by more traditional systems. A rigorous scientific approach to evaluation of these factors is necessary before any valid conclusions are possible. There are two major barriers which would tend to limit the movement of pharmacists into such types of practice: reimbursement mechanisms and legal questions. However, as model programs withstand scientific scrutiny and display real value, the experimental data will become a major force in overcoming such barriers.

### References

1. Dolly, P.: Chemotherapy of Psychiatric Disorders, Plenum Press, New York, New York, 1967, p. 4.
2. Klein, D. F. and Davis, J. M.: Diagnosis and Drug Treatment of Psychiatric Disorders, The Williams & Wilkins Company, Baltimore, Maryland, 1969, pp. 18-23.
3. Lennard, H. L., Epstein, L. J., Bernstein, A. and Ransom, D. C.: Hazards Implicit in Prescribing Psychoactive Drugs, Science 169:438–441 (July 31) 1970.
4. Hollister, L. E.: Mental Disorders—Antipsychotic and Antimanic Drugs, N. Engl. J. Med. 286:984–987 (May 4) 1972.
5. Hollister, L. E.: Mental Disorders—Antianxiety and Antidepressant Drugs, N. Engl. J. Med. 286:1195–1198 (June 1) 1972.
6. Poland, D. M.: Schizophrenia and Related Drug Therapy, Hosp. Pharm. 6:20–22 (Dec.) 1971.
7. Poland, D. M.: The Psychiatric Hospital Evolution, Hosp. Pharm., 7:128–130 (Apr.) 1972.
8. Poland, D. M.: Psychiatric Fundamentals Are a Must for Pharmacists, Hosp. Pharm. 7:55–58 (Feb.) 1972.
9. Seminar on the Pharmacist's Role in Mental Health, University of North Carolina School of Pharmacy, Chapel Hill, North Carolina, 1968.
10. Seminar on the Pharmacist and Community Mental Health, St. Louis College of Pharmacy, St. Louis, Missouri, 1968.
11. Grant MH-12301, Human Behavior for Students of Pharmacy, University of Southern California School of Pharmacy, Los Angeles, 1970–74.
12. Grant MH-12306, A Multidisciplinary Role for a Health Professional, University of Tennessee College of Pharmacy, Memphis, 1971–74.
13. Kohan, S., Chung, S. Y. and Stone, J.: Expanding the Pharmacist's Role in a Psychiatric Hospital, Hosp. Comm. Psych. 24:164–166 (Mar.) 1973.
14. Miller, W. A. and Corcella, J.: Professional Pharmacy Functions in Community Mental Health Centers, J. Amer. Pharm. Ass. 12:68–73 (Feb.) 1972.
15. Kaufman, A., Brickner, P. W., Varner, R. and Mashburn, W.: Tranquilizer Control, J. Amer. Med. Ass. 221:1504–1506 (Sept. 25) 1972.

# 24 The Pharmacist in the Care of Ambulatory Mental Health Patients

Marianne F. Ivey

Pharmacy services in a community mental health center are described.

Services include traditional dispensing functions and clinical activities which involve medication group sessions conducted by a nurse and a pharmacist and patient drug profiles. After initial physician diagnosis and prescription of a drug regimen, the pharmacist evaluates patient drug therapy using a psychiatric rating scale. Based on this evaluation, the pharmacist and nurse decide whether to continue present drug therapy or initiate altered drug therapy. The patient education function of the pharmacist, evaluation of the program, and long-range plans for the program are discussed.

It is estimated by various studies that from 9 to 24%[1-5] of our population is sufficiently ill to require psychiatric attention. Kline estimates 50 million psychiatric patients are being seen by the country's 25,000 psychiatrists, thus making a case load of 2,000 patients per psychiatrist.[6] Applying this information to the 110,000 people residing in the Harborview catchment area in Seattle, Washington, nine percent, or 9,900 people, are at risk. If these patients should seek care at the rate of one physician visit per month, there would be 118,800 patient visits per year to the psychiatric facilities of the catchment area.[7] Having this indication for the need of psychiatric services, the Harborview Community Mental Health Center was developed out of funding from the Seattle Model Cities Program, the National Institute of Mental Health, the Mental Health and Retardation Board and the University of Washington. The services include emergency room, inpatient, outpatient, and partial hospitalization or day treatment facilities.

In the ambulatory care area (outpatient, partial care and day treatment) there are 15,000 patient visits per year. The equivalent of three-and-a-half full-time psychiatrists, two psychiatric nurses, several social workers, and numerous community volunteers shoulder a major part of the patient care responsibility. In December 1971, the University of Washington School of Pharmacy and the Harborview Medical Center Department of Pharmacy were contacted by the Physician-Director of the Mental Health Center. It was his desire that pharmacy be included in solving some of the problems relating to drug therapy, drug distribution, and drug education within the center.

The objectives in developing the pharmacist's role were to provide the patient with the convenience of a pharmacy within the center, to provide the center with a pharmacist whose training in psychotherapeutics would increase rational drug therapy, and to provide a pharmacist who could educate the professional staff, the volunteer staff and the patients on the uses and abuses of drugs. At the same time this pharmacist would serve as a model in both the clinical role and in the unique dispensing function for pharmacy students rotating through the center.

In July 1972, a pharmacist who was concerned with psychotherapy in general and who was committed to pursuing the objectives outlined above was assigned to the center. He was located in the satellite pharmacy which contains the psychotherapeutic drugs on the center's formulary, appropriate reference texts, copies of pertinent articles from the current psychiatric literature, a medication profile system, and other routine equipment necessary for the dispensing of prescriptions.

## Use of Profiles During Medication Groups

One of the few assumptions in psychiatry that arouses little or no controversy is that the major tranquilizers are extremely useful in the treatment and control of schizophrenia. Schizophrenia in its variable forms is one of the most frequent diagnoses in a psychiatric patient population. One of the greatest burdens on the country's psychiatrists is the post-discharge schizophrenic who fails to take his medication and then relapses. Thus, medication and patient compliance are important for the ambulatory mental health patient.

In the center, the patients' medications are regulated mainly through medication groups. These groups are a modification of a commonly used form of treatment in the psychiatric field. The purpose of group therapy is to get patients together who have common problems and to allow them to support, empathize with, or challenge each other concerning these problems. The medication group therapy session is a refinement of the above in that patients are further selected for a specific concern they share, i.e., medication control. Patients in the day treatment program have a medication group every week and the outpatients meet about once a month. "Med groups" meet six to seven times per week with from five to ten patients in each group. The day treatment groups are conducted by the psychiatric nurse and the pharmacist. Since the medication group patients are all on return visits or are in day treatment, the pharmacist has a medication profile on each patient.

The profile information is acquired by direct interview and is augmented by the patient chart. The profile has the usual demographic information, the patient's diagnosis, his concurrent medications, including both prescription and nonprescription drugs, allergies, current psychotherapeutic drugs and refill information. On the back of the profile is a psychiatric rating scale (Figure 1). Symptoms which are rated include depressive mood, unusual thought content, suspiciousness, and so on. These symptoms are rated from zero to six with zero representing symptoms not present and six representing a symptom which is extremely severe. Adjacent to the scale, the pharmacist notes what medication or medications the patient is taking. Over several visits he can detect from the rating scale and from subjective patient information a presence or lack of improvement. On the basis of this information, the

pharmacist and the nurse decide whether to continue the present medication or to initiate different therapy. The patient is also observed for and questioned about specific symptoms which would indicate side effects of therapy. Such effects are the motor restlessness, dystonias, and parkinsonian syndromes of phenothiazine therapy. If they are present, an anticholinergic drug is added to the regimen or the phenothiazine dosage is decreased. After the medication groups are over, the prescriptions are reviewed by a physician and then given to the pharmacist for dispensing. Patients who are having unusual problems with their medications meet in a special medication group, and in this group, a physician joins the nurse and pharmacist.

The pharmacist asks the patients to go to the waiting room while he dispenses the prescriptions. The dispensing procedure is facilitated by the use of prepackaged medications. When the prescription is dispensed the patient either returns to the pharmacy or the pharmacist goes to the waiting room to give the patient instructions and cautionary warnings. Auxiliary labels such as "Do not drink alcohol while taking this medication," or "This medication may cause drowsiness—care should be exercised in driving a vehicle or operating machinery," are placed directly on the prescription bottle and reinforced verbally. Warnings about sunburn, postural hypotension, or other appropriate remarks are also made to the patient, and he is encouraged to discuss with the pharmacist any questions he might have. The pharmacist reminds the patient about his next scheduled medication group, which usually coincides with the patient's refill date. If the patient misses two consecutive, regularly scheduled refill dates, the pharmacist contacts a social worker who then contacts the patient.

### Rational Therapy

The pharmacist's role in educating the professional staff further benefits the patient. With the aid of a visiting psychiatrist, the mental health center's pharmacist has cooperated with the center physicians and encouraged them to modify several of their prescribing habits:

1. The pharmacist has encouraged the prescribing physicians to change from multiple daily dosing of long-acting antipsychotics to a once per day or twice per day schedule with the largest dose being given at bedtime. This recommendation is based on both biopharmaceutic and patient considerations. First, the half-life of many antipsychotic drugs, including the phenothiazines and butyrophenones, is about 24 hours, thus dosing every half-life yields a once-a-day schedule. Second, if the patient takes his whole dose or major portion of the dose at bedtime, he will be sleeping at the time of the occurrence of the most intense side-effects—sedation, dryness of mouth, blurred vision and postural hypotension. Third, it is felt that patient compliance will be increased when he is required to take the medication less often. Fourth, the cost of a single large dosage is usually less expensive than an equal dosage consisting of several smaller doses.

*Figure 1. Back side of patient profile contains psychiatric rating scale*

| | NOT PRESENT = 0 | MODERATE = 3 |
| | VERY MILD = 1 | MODERATELY SEVERE = 4 |
| | MILD = 2 | SEVERE = 5 |
| | | EXTREMELY SEVERE = 6 |

2. The pharmacist has encouraged prescribing physicians to evaluate a patient more carefully before he is automatically placed on an anticholinergic drug to prevent extrapyramidal side effects. If the physician finds it necessary for the patient to be placed on an anticholinergic medication, it is recommended that the physician discontinue the anticholinergic drug after three months. These recommendations are again based on several factors. First, the antipsychotics vary greatly in their potential for producing extrapyramidal effects with the high-dose type of antipsychotics having a lesser potential than the low-dose types. Second, individual patient variation is great. Third, anticholinergic drugs are not innocuous in that they potentiate the anticholinergic effects of the antipsychotics and can at toxic levels cause a psychosis themselves. Fourth, the anticholinergic drugs place an economic burden on either the patient or a third party. The last part of the recommendation, that is, discontinuation of anticholinergic therapy after three months, is based on the fact that many patients, although initially manifesting extrapyramidal side effects, apparently become tolerant. After three months of therapy, withdrawal of the anticholinergic causes only about 10% of the patients to experience a relapse of the side effects.[8]

3. The pharmacist has recommended that the physicians consider drug-free weekends for their patients on anti-psychotic drugs. This is in an attempt to prevent some of the cumulative levels of the drugs and their attendant effects and is based on the work of DiMascio[9] and Hollister.[10]

The pharmacist is also cooperating with physicians in an attempt to curb minor tranquilizer abuse among the center's patients. Prescriptions for drugs such as chlordiazepoxide and diazepam are written for only a week's supply with no refills permitted. The patient must appear in person for reevaluation before a new prescription is considered. The physicians are conducting gradual withdrawal programs for some of the chronic users. These patients need psychological support and the pharmacist contributes in this area by listening to the patient and reinforcing the reasons for the prescribing policy.

The pharmacist also provides information to the staff on an *ad lib* basis and has access to the University of Washington Health Sciences Library and the Drug Information Center of the School of Pharmacy for researching questions and reviewing the current literature. The pharmacist has personal subscriptions to some of the specialty journals such as *Diseases of the Nervous System*.

Regular lectures are given to the volunteer staff on the topic of drug use. The pharmacist has lectured University of Washington School of Nursing students on psychopharmacology.

## Patient Education

The mental health center's pharmacist provides patient education in the discourse that occurs during the medication groups and during the dispensing function. He also encourages the patients to visit the center's pharmacy or telephone if they have any questions between appointments. The pharmacist also provides information on drug use and abuse to the day treatment patients. The sessions, held once a week for an hour, cover street drugs, prescription drugs and social drugs such as coffee, alcohol and cigarettes. The sessions are sometimes a formal lecture but more often are informal discussions with the patients encouraged to do most of the talking. The pharmacist tries to guide the patients in discussing the psychological needs that drugs answer and alternative methods for satisfying those needs. The patients are informed of agencies that provide treatment and rehabilitation programs that they might utilize. The discussions also involve talking about long-term complications of drug abuse such as the possibility of developing staphylococcal endocarditis after heroin use. Some principles of pharmacology and physiology are also discussed with the patients such as the patterns of alcohol addiction, the phenomenon of tolerance and the long-term physiologic changes involving organ toxicities. The lectures are repeated every six weeks with subjects modified as the pharmacist deems appropriate for the different patients entering day treatment.

## Relationship to the Main Pharmacy

The mental health center's limited inventory of psychotherapeutic agents is purchased through the Harborview Medical Center's pharmacy. An addendum to the main pharmacy's policy and procedure manual is concerned with the activities at the center. The pricing schedules are that of the main pharmacy. No money is exchanged at the center for services. If the patient is able to pay he or she is billed through the main hospital's central accounting office. This circumvents a security problem as the center is an old, converted apartment building in the central city.

In case of illness or a greatly increased workload, the center pharmacist can call on the main pharmacy or the clinical faculty at the School of Pharmacy for support.

## Evaluation

An evaluation of the center pharmacist's contribution to improve patient care is needed to justify continued support of his position and to convince directors of other ambulatory mental health clinics of the economic feasibility of the inclusion of such a professional. The evaluation is difficult because of many variables inherent in such a program. Recognizing this, the evaluation of the Harborview Community Health Center pharmacist will measure patient compliance, patient understanding and hospital readmission rates. Several other mental health clinics in the area are without the services of a pharmacist, and recognizing the variables introduced here, these centers will be used as a control. To this point in time the evaluations have come informally from the professional staff. The psychiatric nurses who did much of the medication management until the pharmacist came are much more confident with the pharmacist's presence in the medication groups. They also feel that there is increased patient understanding concerning medications.

The community volunteers who have requested and are receiving information concerning drug therapy and drug abuse have indicated that this education has increased their usefulness in the center by increasing their understanding of the patients' problems.

The center physicians continue to utilize the pharmacist's formal training and encourage the pharmacist to be more aggressive in offering his skills and information that concern the care of individual patients.

### Long-Range Plans

In addition to the formal evaluative studies which are planned, the pharmacist and his colleagues at the School of Pharmacy are planning an audit program. Essentially this is a system of peer review and will require further development of standards of care similar to those indicated above under rational therapy. It is planned that the audit be jointly conducted by the psychiatric nurses, physicians and pharmacist because of the responsibility of this team in the therapeutic management of the patient.

### Summary

The pharmacist in the Harborview Community Mental Health Center ambulatory clinic serves the patient by participating actively in medication management, dispensing the medication to the patient, offering formal sessions in patient education concerning drugs, contributing to policies whose goals are rational drug therapy and providing drug education for the clinic's professional and volunteer staffs. Evaluation procedures of the importance of these contributions are being developed.

### References

1. Lemkau, P., Tietze, C. and Cooper, M.: Mental-Hygiene Problems in an Urban District, Part 1, *Ment. Hygiene 25*:624–646 (Oct.) 1941.
2. Lemkau, P., Tietze, C. and Cooper, M.: Mental-Hygiene Problems in an Urban District, Part 2, *Ment. Hygiene 26*:100–119 (Jan.) 1942.
3. Lemkau, P., Tietze, C. and Cooper, M.: Mental-Hygiene Problems in an Urban District, Part 3, *Ment. Hygiene 26*:275–288 (Apr.) 1942.
4. Lemkau, P., Tietze, C. and Cooper, M.: Mental-Hygiene Problems in an Urban District, Part 4, *Ment. Hygiene 27*:279–295 (Apr.) 1943.
5. Srole, L. et al.: Mental Health in the Metropolis: The Midtown Manhattan Study, Volume 1, McGraw-Hill, New York, New York, 1962.
6. Peck, R. L.: What Every Doctor Should Know About Drug Therapy for Psychotics, *Hosp. Phys. 8*:32 (Apr.) 1972.
7. Sata, L. S.: A Mental Health Center's Partnerships with the Community, *Hosp. Commun. Psychiat. 23*:242–245 (Aug.) 1972.
8. Orlov, P. et al.: Withdrawal of Antiparkinson Drugs, *Arch. Gen. Psychiat. 25*:410–412 (Nov.) 1971.
9. DiMascio, A. and Shader, R. I.: Clinical Handbook of Psychopharmacology, Science House, New York, New York, 1970.
10. Hollister, L. E.: Clinical Use of Psychotherapeutic Drugs: Current Status, *Clin. Pharmacol. Ther. 10*:170–198, 1969.

# 25 Clinical Pharmacy in a Methadone Program

Willard L. Harrison and Susan P. Flinkow

Pharmacist involvement in a methadone treatment and detoxification program is discussed.

The use of methadone to treat heroin addiction is briefly reviewed. Clinical and traditional functions of pharmacists involved in a methadone program are described. These functions include service on the screening committee which admits addicts to the program, methadone dosage calibration, patient counseling, and establishment of detoxification schedules. To succeed in these duties, the pharmacist must supplement his scientific knowledge with patient sociological and psychological factors.

The overall success of the methadone program is briefly discussed.

"Drug abuse is a human problem. However, its range, extent, and growth are calculated; numbers alone cannot measure its real costs to society and to the individual victims. The human price is paid in lives wasted and talents lost, and in the social by-products of crime, disintegration of communities and despair."[1]

Society has attempted for years to develop a "cure" for drug addiction. Trials have included such things as incarceration, self-evaluation, groups for addicts patterned after Alcoholics Anonymous, religion, psychotherapeutic drugs, carbon dioxide treatment and live-in addict "families." Success in these trials has been minimal. Federal hospitals such as the facility at Lexington, Kentucky report a 3–5% success rate; jails, almost zero; and live-in therapeutic communities, 10–20%. Although satisfaction accrues when any addict reaches the point of being able to live without drugs, such elation must be tempered by an honest appraisal of how to best help the greatest number of people with the minimum of funds available.

There is no treatment modality which is a "cure" for drug addiction and no specific treatment which is best for all addicts. Millions of dollars are being spent annually, however, to produce a small handful of ex-addicts.

Are the words "cure" and "success" synonymous in the treatment of drug addiction? What determines a successful patient: if he stops using heroin or opiates, if he stops his criminal behavior, if he begins to work or goes to school, if he returns to a normal home life, or if he begins therapy to eventually learn to live with himself and without drugs? It seems foolish to call a man anything other than successful if he is making progress in any of these areas even though he may not fit the clinical picture of being "cured."

## Methadone as a Tool

The Drug Treatment Program of the Department of Pharmacy Services, Medical College of Virginia Hospitals, has been involved in treating heroin addiction for more than three years. The staff of 32 professionals and paraprofessionals has adapted an old three-story building separated from the hospital setting in a commercial-residential area of central Richmond.

Of the 295 active client load, approximately 170 are on methadone. Along with the spectrum of problems facing any treatment program, a very basic problem is faced by any treatment program which uses methadone. The use of a "narcotic drug" as a treatment approach antagonizes many people in the medical community who consider this technique as "substituting one addiction for another." Insulin, antidepressants, tranquilizers, hormone preparations, etc., are used routinely and are widely accepted as excellent therapeutic tools on either a short-term treatment regimen or as maintenance drugs. However, since methadone is a synthetic opiate, it causes much greater alarm among health professionals as well as the lay public. The alarm among health professionals perhaps relates to a regimented educational background which has assigned an extreme and, in fact, illegal connotation to narcotic drugs. In the problem of the disease state termed addiction—a problem still without a clearly defined treatment answer—much panic

129

ensues when an attempt at treatment involves the use of methadone.

There have traditionally been both criticism about the validity of methadone usage and concern about its proper handling. Having observed both sides of these questions, we can understand these attitudes. In any program, a real possibility of diversion of methadone exists. Any time medication is allowed to leave the premises, it is no longer under strict control. For this reason, both federal and state regulations have severely restricted the ability of a patient to obtain take-home privileges. Only after an extended and cooperative period of active participation may a person be considered for such rights. Each case must then be reviewed individually; the patient must present evidence of rehabilitation; all doses must be in a liquid form, as noninjectable as possible; and the program must conscientiously monitor the patient's progress and attitudes.

Although lifelong high-dose maintenance was once an accepted mode of methadone therapy, we rarely allow a patient to follow such a line. Each person is encouraged to reach a drug-free state and a graduated detoxification must be part of any sound rehabilitative effort. Rather than using methadone as an end-point in therapy, it is used as a temporary restructuring tool.

A further change in the use of methadone has been the alteration in dosage levels. To encourage people to detoxify and to ease this process, low-dose therapy has been encouraged. Research has shown that high doses do not produce a corresponding effectiveness, and thus average clinic doses of 40 - 50 mg are much more common.

With decreasing emphasis on high-dosage maintenance has come a correlated emphasis on the psychology of addiction. More and more therapists are beginning to treat addiction as a behavioral disorder, and clinics are reflecting these changes. Staffing patterns have expanded from medical personnel to incorporate psychologists, social workers, counselors and former addicts. The belief held by many in the field is that drug-seeking behavior is only partially the result of threatened withdrawal discomforts. Much more important is the effect—"the feeling," if you will—produced by the drug. It is that high, that relaxation, that escape which makes the drug so enticing. Frequently, a close examination of the patient reveals a person with a poor family relationship, difficulty in social adjustment and a weakened self-image. For such a person, a chemical with an euphoric erasing ability can easily become a panacea. The emphasis of treatment, therefore, is on training the patient to face daily anxieties and to cope with them using learned mechanisms rather than blocking them with an opiate.

This reasoning has resulted in such treatment techniques as one-on-one counseling, group therapy, transcendental meditation, yoga and behavior modification. Efforts are frequently made to bring the family into counseling with the patient since support will be needed when the impact of treatment is finished. Ancillary services incorporated into more rehabilitation schedules include legal assistance, vocational rehabilitation, job placement and financial training. The thrust of such a comprehensive program is toward a better-adjusted person, both physically and mentally.

## Pharmacist Involvement

Our drug treatment program is unique because of the tremendous involvement of pharmacists in the total system (see Figure 1). The project director and program coordinator are both pharmacists. Two additional pharmacists are responsible for the methadone distribution and control functions as well as carrying out other program responsibilities.

Psychiatric rehabilitation is carried out by a full-time counseling staff with guidance and training provided by the chairman of the Department of Psychiatry and two psychiatrists from the School of Medicine of the Medical College of Virginia. This staff includes people with degrees in such areas as social work, psychology, guidance counseling, rehabilitative counseling and vocational counseling.

Medical support, including the prescribing of methadone, ongoing medical follow-up and the general treatment of medical problems related to drug abuse is carried out by an affiliate agency of three physicians who each spend 16 hours per week at the program.

The community services supervisor is involved in job development, job placement, and most important, working to develop an understanding within the general community to promote acceptance of the individual who carries the reputation of former addiction.

## Clinical Pharmacy Applications

Clinical pharmacy has been defined to encompass varying roles, functions and responsibilities. The common denominator in most definitions is patient-oriented practice. There is no better opportunity for a close pa-

*Figure 1. Organizational chart of the Drug Treatment Program*

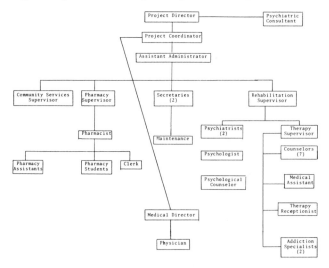

tient-pharmacist-physician relationship and a true health care team approach than that available to a pharmacist actively practicing in a drug abuse treatment program.

The best way to realize the opportunities for clinical involvement of pharmacists in a program such as the MCV program is to follow a hypothetical patient who has voluntarily requested help for his heroin addiction. The entire intake procedure or induction period spans approximately 48 hours. The patient's first contact is with the pharmacy where a monitored urine specimen is obtained which will be tested within 24 hours for the presence of opiates. This test aids in the required medical determination of physiologic addiction. The patient is then directed to the therapy receptionist who, after verification of name and age, arranges for an intake interview. This first interview is accomplished by an addiction specialist who is a former addict now drug-free and trained by the staff. In the intake interview, the addiction specialist obtains all basic demographic information and tries to determine the addict's purpose, motivation and potential for rehabilitation. This first interview also includes a basic, yet complete, orientation to the program, explaining all the services that are offered, program goals and the applicant's obligations. In addition to an explanation of his obligations and requirements, the applicant is advised of possible disciplinary action resulting from infraction of program regulations.

After the intake interview is completed, the therapy receptionist schedules the applicant's appointment with the medical assistant. This should also occur within the first 24 hours. The medical assistant obtains a medical history and appointments are made for the second day.

The applicant is seen twice during the second day, first for an appearance before the screening committee and second for a visit with the physician to receive a medical examination and a prescription for methadone, if indicated. It is the function of the screening committee to determine if the patient is an acceptable candidate for admission to the program. The screening committee consists of two members of the counseling staff, a psychiatrist, a pharmacist, an addiction specialist and a patient who is currently doing well in the program. This committee attempts to evaluate the patient's basic motivation, attitude and general responsiveness to the treatment approach offered. As a key member of this committee, the pharmacist has a specific responsibility to counsel the patient regarding the probable physiological effects of methadone and possible untoward effects he might encounter, and to generally inform him as to what he should and should not expect to happen when taking methadone.

If the screening committee decides favorably upon the patient's request for admission, he is then assigned an individual counselor and a therapy program. He signs a consent form, receives an identification card and a copy of the program's rules (Figure 2). At this point, a medical chart is developed for his file. Later during the second day the patient visits the physician for a complete

Figure 2. Drug Treatment Program rules

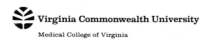
Virginia Commonwealth University
Medical College of Virginia

DRUG TREATMENT PROGRAM
of
THE DEPARTMENT OF PHARMACY SERVICES

PROGRAM RULES

Because of the serious nature of the following rules, a violation of any of them constitutes grounds for termination.

1. Absolutely no selling or giving your methadone to another person whether that person is on the program or not, nor will you be allowed to pick up for other persons on the program.

2. Absolutely no violence or threat of violence, which includes carrying concealed weapons of any kind.

3. No illegal actions may be permitted while on the premises, such as, vandalism, stealing, gambling, loitering, and so on.

4. Methadone must be consumed within the immediate confines of the dispensing area, and must be completely consumed in clear view of, and to the complete satisfaction of, the dispensing staff member.

To insure consistency in our Program's operation, and also to ensure fairness and equality, each patient must abide by the following regulations.

1. You must appear daily for your methadone. Three consecutive days missed result in termination.

2. Broken, lost, or stolen bottles will not be replaced.

3. You must give a monitored urine sample on the day requested or it will be counted as a dirty urine.

4. You must keep and be on time for all appointments. You must also pick up methadone during your assigned time slot.

5. You must always have with you and present upon request, your patient ID card.

6. Non-cooperation with the program rules and regulations, or hasseling the staff will not be tolerated.

SIGNED_____

Health Sciences Center • Richmond, Virginia 23219

physical examination and the obtaining of various specimens for the required laboratory tests. Only after all these procedures have been carried out does the patient actually have an order written for methadone and receive an initial dose. The physician has at his disposal all of the intake records on the patient during this visit, including any comments from the counselor, the pharmacist or the screening committee. In addition, a positive opiate test result must have been received from the urine specimen obtained during the intake process.

If all professionals are in agreement, the patient is now ready to begin receiving methadone on a daily basis. The initial dose prescribed is normally rather low and is based upon value judgments of the counselor, pharmacist and physician who attempt to evaluate the size and duration of the heroin habit, the quality of heroin on the street at the time (which fluctuates greatly) and the general distress the patient will be experiencing if withdrawal symptoms are present. The pharmacist plays a key role in dosage calibration during the first few days of treatment and conveys any recommendations for a change in the patient's dosage to the physician.

The patient is normally assigned to individual counseling sessions with his specific counselor and may also be assigned to one of the several therapy groups which exist in the program.

Because of the counseling workload which does not permit individual sessions with the counselor on a daily basis, the pharmacist becomes the primary contact individual for the patient on a daily basis during the first six months of enrollment. The pharmacist rapidly learns much about the patient, such as his medical and psychological condition, and acts as an intermediary to essentially become a triage officer to screen the patients who really need to visit a physician. It is well established that drug addicts have a high incidence of medically-related problems, but it is equally well understood that they exhibit an extraordinary high incidence of imagined or distorted medical problems. The pharmacist serves a valuable role in sorting out these complaints at the time the patient reports for his daily administration of methadone. He likewise has an opportunity to observe any side effects or adverse reactions which may develop from methadone administration.

As previously stated, the basic philosophy of the MCV Drug Treatment Program is that the drug-free state is the optimal goal toward which all treatment techniques are directed. This means that many patients are on decreasing dosage schedules. Detoxification may be accomplished in a few days or may take several weeks. The patient and counselor work together to determine when this schedule should begin. This information is relayed to the physician, who, after seeing the patient and evaluating his progress, either accepts or denies the counselor's recommendation. If detoxification is agreed upon, it becomes the responsibility of the pharmacist to work out the detoxification schedule and insure that the schedule is carried out.

### Team Approach

The team approach to patient care is exemplified by the daily interaction of all members of the staff. One and one-half hours per day are devoted to interdisciplinary communication to insure that each member of the team is aware of the progress as well as problems of individual patients. The interaction may take the form of general staff meetings, continuing education programs, staff groups or meetings of the medical and paramedical groups. The pharmacist is a key input person in all these sessions since the daily contact he has with the patient may well indicate necessary changes in the treatment approach to adapt to changing attitudes which are manifested at the pharmacy window.

In addition to the previously-mentioned responsibilities, the pharmacist is involved extensively in a review board. This board acts as an "appeals court" for those patients who have committed rules infractions such as missed counseling appointments, "dirty" urines, etc. More importantly, however, this board reviews a certain number of patient case records each week to evaluate progress or lack of progress in the program. Such evaluations allow the staff to encourage those who are doing well and to give additional needed support to those showing negative behavioral characteristics before they fail.

The pharmacist's overall impact and success in functioning in the many clinical roles mentioned depends largely upon his ability to adapt a purely scientific base of knowledge to one which considers the sociological and psychological factors which affect the patient's well being. The pharmacist must learn to consider and evaluate the emotions and attitudes of patients as well as physical effects which indicate medical progress.

### Traditional Pharmacy Roles

Some traditional roles of the pharmacist have proven very valuable in the evolution of the MCV program. Pediatric overdosages of methadone often occur when patients who are parents of small children have take-home privileges. A dosage formulation developed at the program has overcome this problem and there have been no pediatric toxicity problems over the past 20 months. Although each dose is given in a thick orange syrup base, a mixture of powdered dextrose and psyllium is added to each bottle of syrup containing methadone which leaves the clinic. This mixture forms a gel which must be diluted with approximately five ounces of water to reach a normal drinking consistency. Since it must be scraped out of the original container and does not pour, it greatly reduces the chance of pediatric toxicity.

Another traditional role of the pharmacist which is extremely important in any drug treatment program using methadone is inventory control. A commercial posting machine has been adapted to use for this purpose. Each client has a ledger card which becomes his daily record of medication administered or dispensed (Figure 3). The daily totals on the machine tape give the pharmacist an opportunity to check the day-end physical inventory with the theoretical balance. The ledger card also serves as the message center for patients. If a counselor or physician wishes to see a patient for any reason, a message is attached to the ledger card and given to him when he appears for his daily methadone administration.

### Program Results

The management of and active participation in a drug abuse treatment program is a role foreign to most pharmacists. Are the results worth the frustrations, the periods of depression when a "favorite" patient backslides, and the difficulty in defining "success" for this type of treatment? All of the pharmacists involved in the program feel that the results justify the intense efforts necessary to maintain the program.

An addict on the street costs his community a minimum of approximately $10,000 per year. Therefore, a patient load of approximately 300 patients will save the city from 2.5 to 3 million dollars per year. The crime rate in Richmond, Viriginia has decreased regularly for the past 18 months. This decrease cannot be definitively attributed to the Drug Treatment Program but indications are that it has been an important factor.

Additional results of the program which are even more important to the staff members and patients include:

*Figure 3. Example of patient ledger card which is a daily record of medications administered or dispensed*

PATIENT'S LEDGER

Name: EXAMPLE, HARRY    Dr.: Bright    Acct. #: 1204

Address: 3708 Forest Hill Ave. Telephone: 233-6554    Age: 23

| Memo | Date | Account Number | Number of Units | Dosage | Charges | Credits | Balance |
|------|------|---------|---------|--------|---------|---------|---------|
| | | Payment Source | | Dosage Forward | | | Balance Forward |
| | VOCATIONAL REHABILITATION | | | | | | |
| Atarax 2 X/day | 3/12/72 | 1204 | 2 | 50 | 1.00 | | 1.00 |

1. Over 150 people who are working, attending school or receiving vocational training who formerly exhibited strong antisocial and/or criminal behavior patterns.
2. A large majority of patients are on decreasing dosage schedules and progressing toward the drug-free state which over 100 patients have already attained.
3. Program costs per patient per year per treatment slot is $1,350. Cost per year per patient seen is $710.
4. Of patients contacted, approximately 55% remain in treatment to a point of detoxification.
5. The program has recently added an outreach and follow-up staff to provide ongoing aftercare and more extensive contact within the community. Inherent in this effort will be the ability to evaluate the status of those patients who have left the program.
6. A multidisciplinary team of professional workers from both the social and physical sciences who are uniformly oriented toward finding better approaches to the treatment of the drug abuser.
7. A training program for pharmacy, medical and social work students to better orient and train these individuals to deal with the common problems of the drug abuser.

Pharmacy and medicine have long been involved in discussions of the problem of drug abuse. The time for discussing the problem is past. Pharmacists and physicians must now become aggressive in fulfilling their professional responsibilities in the area of drug abuse treatment and rehabilitation.

### Reference

1. Special Action Office for Drug Abuse Prevention. Brochure distributed by Executive Office of the President, Washington, D.C., October 1972, p. 6.

# 26 Use of Medication Profiles to Detect Potential Therapeutic Problems in Ambulatory Patients

David K. Solomon, R. Paul Baumgartner, Lyle M. Glascock, Shirley A. Glascock, May E. Briscoe, and Norman F. Billups

The effect of using a patient medication profile on the pharmacist's ability to detect potential therapeutic problems in ambulatory patients was studied.

Phase I of the study consisted of obtaining and recording patient information on medication profile cards. Data were collected on 23,657 prescriptions representing 14,069 patients. During Phase I, the pharmacist did not utilize the medication profile cards to detect potential therapeutic problems. Phase II consisted of the detection (using the medication profile cards) and recording of potential therapeutic problems for 25,197 prescriptions representing 14,975 patients. Phase I data were compared with Phase II results.

In Phase II, 1,497 potential therapeutic problems were identified, compared to only 13 potential therapeutic problems in Phase I. The incidence of detection of potential problems was 5.8% in Phase II and 0.1% in Phase I (a statistically significant difference). Over 65% of the total therapeutic problems in Phase II resulted from potential patient over-utilization of medications while 22% resulted from potential patient under-utilization. Data are presented to show the relationship between (1) potential therapeutic problems detected in new and refill prescriptions, (2) the method of financing prescription payment and patient utilization of drugs, (3) therapeutic drug classification and patient utilization of drugs, and (4) potential therapeutic problems and various patient age groupings.

Patient medication profiles, when properly utilized by the pharmacist, demonstrated their effectiveness in aiding in the detection of potential therapeutic problems.

The literature abounds with articles which promote the use of patient medication profile systems by the pharmacist.[1-10] In addition, the Report of the Task Force on the Pharmacist's Clinical Role[11] suggests that one function for a pharmacist in a clinical role would be documenting professional activities. Such activities entail pharmacist preparation of adequate records to assure a documented source of expanding clinical experiences which enhance his services as a drug specialist and consultant. However, most of these articles[1-10] are concerned primarily with inpatient hospital pharmacy systems. Furthermore, few articles quantitate how the pharmacist can effectively utilize the profile to detect and/or avert potential therapeutic problems either in an inpatient or outpatient environment.

In recent years there has been an increase in the percentage of total prescriptions dispensed by hospital outpatient pharmacies in the United States: 10.9% of all prescriptions dispensed in 1968 originated in hospital outpatient pharmacies; 11.8% in 1969.[12] With this increase in prescription volume comes the proportional increased responsibility of the pharmacist for assuring safe and proper utilization of the medication by the patient. In fact, the patient in modern medical care deserves, and should demand, the pharmacist's professional judgment resulting from the use of patient medication profiles.[13]

It has been our experience,[14] and that of others,[15] that ambulatory patients frequently misuse medications and have therapeutic or drug-related problems concerning their medication regimen. To further measure the value of the patient medication profile as a tool for use by the pharmacist in the detection of potential therapeutic problems, a study was outlined by the Appalachian Regional Hospitals pharmacy staff to be conducted at the Wise, Virginia Appalachian Regional Hospital (ARH).

## Wise Appalachian Regional Hospital

The Wise ARH is located in rural Southwest Virginia and serves the 40,000 residents of Wise County plus much of the population in the surrounding counties (Lee, Dickenson and Russell) as well as some patients from the nearby areas of Kentucky. This 68-bed, non-profit, community health care center—in addition to rendering the traditional services of a community hospital—has an intensive care unit, cardiac care unit, a home health care agency, and supportive services (e.g., social services).

The community is served by a physician group practice clinic which at the time of this study was located within the hospital. The clinic is comprised of 16 physicians with disciplines ranging from general practice to specialties including obstetrics and gynecology, pediatrics, surgery and internal medicine. Additionally, one of the few mental health clinics serving the Appalachian area is located nearby.

The hospital pharmacy staff consists of two pharmacists, two pharmacy helpers and two clerk typists. The pharmacy provides inpatient and outpatient services.

## Purpose of the Study

The major goal of this study was to determine the pharmacist's ability to detect potential therapeutic problems by utilizing a patient medication profile. The following hypotheses were considered in this study:

1. Far more potential therapeutic problems will be detected by the pharmacist when utilizing a patient medication profile as compared to the pharmacist not using a profile.
2. The incidence of potential therapeutic problems will be higher with new prescriptions than for refill prescriptions.
3. The over-utilization[a] of medications as measured by the patient medication profile will present the greatest number of potential therapeutic problems.
4. The over-utilization of medications for prescriptions financed by a third-party payor will be more common than the under-utilization of prescriptions which are financed by the same method.
5. The under-utilization[b] of medications by patients paying directly for prescriptions will be more common than the over-utilization of prescriptions which are financed by the same method.
6. The over-utilization of psychotherapeutic drugs will occur more often than for any other drug classification.
7. The potential misuse of medications (that is over-utilization and under-utilization) is considered to be more prevalent among patients age 65 years and over than among patients in any other age grouping.

---

[a] Potential over-utilization of medication occurred when a patient returned twice in succession for a refill or with a new prescription for a drug seven days or more *before* his supply should have been exhausted.
[b] Potential under-utilization of medication occurred when a patient returned twice in succession for a refill or with a new prescription for a drug seven days *after* his supply should have been exhausted.

## Methodology

*Experimental Design and Scope of Study.* In June 1971, a two-part study was initiated to determine the effect that a patient medication profile would have on the pharmacist's ability to detect potential therapeutic problems with ambulatory patients presenting prescriptions at the Wise ARH outpatient pharmacy. To accomplish this objective the study was divided into two phases.

Phase I consisted of the pharmacist's:

1. Obtaining and recording the patient information on medication profile cards in order to establish baseline data for comparison with Phase II.
2. Dispensing medications in the usual manner without the aid of the patient medication profile card.
3. Detecting potential therapeutic problems *without* the aid of the patient medication profile card.

Over a period of 150 working days (approximately 5½ months) patient information data were collected for every medication dispensed—this amounted to 23,657 prescriptions (20,843 new and 2,814 refill) for 14,069 patients during Phase I.

Phase II consisted of the pharmacist's:

1. Continuing data collection on the patient medication profile card.
2. Dispensing medications utilizing the patient medication profile card.
3. Detecting potential therapeutic problems *with* the aid of the patient medication profile card.

Phase II involved 14,975 patients and also lasted 150 days, during which time 25,197 prescriptions (21,237 new and 3,960 refill) were analyzed for potential therapeutic problems.

In both phases of the study, the two pharmacists involved each dispensed approximately one-half of all medications. However, in Phase II, both pharmacists employed the record system to detect potential therapeutic problems, and these problems were noted prior to dispensing the medication. Finally, one pharmacist reviewed all prescriptions and profiles in Phase II in order to provide uniformity and to reduce possible pharmacist-to-pharmacist variation in the ability to detect potential therapeutic problems.

Each patient having a prescription filled or refilled was included in this study during the 300 working days of Phases I and II. Regarding the patient population, it is our subjective opinion that the patient samples in Phases I and II were similar, since a majority of patients included in the baseline Phase I study were also included in Phase II.

It should be noted that professional bias may have improved the pharmacists' performance in Phase II since they were aware of the study. The pharmacists intervened only in cases where they thought the potential therapeutic problem could be harmful to the patient.

(However, the current practice, which was implemented after the study, calls for pharmacists to continually monitor for potential therapeutic problems using the patient medication profile and when problems occur, to take appropriate action to solve these problems.)

For purposes of this study, prescription drugs and the problems associated with them, rather than patients, constituted the unit of analysis.

*Definition of Potential Therapeutic Problems.* A potential therapeutic problem was defined as an undesirable situation which, in the judgment of the pharmacist, could potentially hinder the proper and safe utilization of medications by the ambulatory patient. In order to clarify these potential therapeutic problems, the following categories, definitions and examples are given:

1. *Physician duplicates active prescription on file with the same drug.* If the patient should still have an adequate supply of the drug on hand from a previous prescription, this was considered a potential therapeutic problem.

   Example (A): On May 1, 1971, a patient has a prescription filled with 60 digitoxin 0.1 mg tablets with directions–take one tablet daily; and on May 15, 1971, a prescription is written for 30 digitoxin 0.1 mg tablets with directions–take one tablet daily.

2. *Physician duplicates active prescription on file with similar therapeutic entity.* This was considered a potential therapeutic problem when the use of both drugs simultaneously could be potentially detrimental to the patient if he or she were to continue taking the first medication in addition to the second similar medication.

   Example (B): A patient on May 1, 1971, has a prescription filled with 60 digitoxin 0.1 mg tablets with directions–take one tablet daily; and on May 5, 1971, he has a prescription filled with 60 digoxin 0.25 mg tablets with directions–take one tablet daily. (This example was considered a problem.)

   Example (C): A patient on May 1, 1971, has a prescription filled for 90 meprobamate 400 mg tablets with directions–take one tablet three times a day; and on May 15, 1971, the patient has a prescription filled for 90 chlordiazepoxide 10 mg capsules with directions–take one capsule three times a day. (Due to the frequent practice of prescribing more than one minor tranquilizer, this example was not considered a problem.)

3. *Patient over-utilizes drug.* When a patient returned twice in succession for a refill or with a new prescription for a drug seven days or more before his supply should have been exhausted, this was considered a potential problem.

   Example (D): A patient has a prescription for 90 diazepam 10 mg tablets, with directions–take one tablet three times a day, filled on May 7, 1971. The patient returns with the same prescription on May 25, 1971 and again on June 18th.

4. *Patient under-utilizes drug.* This was considered a potential problem with chronic illness medications such as digitalis or tolbutamide when the patient received a refill or when a new prescription was dispensed more than seven days after his supply should have been exhausted. For this situation to count as a problem, it had to occur twice in succession.

   Example (E): A patient has a prescription for 30 digoxin 0.25 mg tablets, with directions–take one tablet daily, filled on May 1, 1971; he returns June 8 and again July 15th, which was considered a problem.

5. *Potential drug-drug interaction.* This was considered a problem when the potential interaction could be verified by Hartshorn's *Handbook of Drug Interactions* and in the pharmacist's judgment was considered to be potentially detrimental to the patient's well being.

   Example (F): A patient has been self-administering warfarin 10 mg tablets, one daily for five months, and then propoxyphene compound, one capsule every six hours, is prescribed for pain.

6. *Potential disease-drug contraindication.* When a drug was prescribed, the action of which the pharmacist considered to be potentially detrimental to the patient's well being, this was considered a potential therapeutic problem.

   Example (G): A patient with severe hypertension on a low salt diet is given a prescription for sodium salicylate 300 mg, one tablet four times a day.

7. *Prescription discrepancies.* This was considered a potential therapeutic problem when the drug strength or dosage was not indicated on the prescription, or the strength or dosage was different than previously prescribed. This was important in cases of chronic disease states in which dosages and strengths of medications usually remain constant over a period of time.

   Example (H): A patient has been self-administering digitoxin 0.1 mg, one tablet daily for three months, then the patient obtains a prescription for digitoxin 0.2 mg with directions of one tablet daily.

*Patient Medication Profile Card.* The patient medication profile card utilized for ambulatory patients at the Wise ARH has proven to be very adequate—both from the standpoint of completeness of data and ease of recording. The form and specific procedures for its use may be obtained from the authors upon request.

### Results and Discussion

The study data were subjected to statistical analysis to test the seven hypotheses. All statistical methods used are described in Siegel[16] and McNemar.[17]

The number of potential therapeutic problems detected in new and refill prescriptions according to medications dispensed in Phases I and II is shown in Table 1. In Phase II, 1,497 potential therapeutic problems were identified with 1,459 prescriptions from a total of 25,197 prescriptions dispensed. Some prescriptions exhibited more than one potential therapeutic problem. Only 13 problems were detected for 23,657 prescriptions dispensed in Phase I. The average incidence of potential therapeutic problems was 5.8% in Phase II as compared to only 0.1% for the control (Phase I).

The detection of potential therapeutic problems by the pharmacist was hypothesized to be far greater when utilizing a patient medication profile, as compared to the pharmacist not using the profile. To test this hypothesis, a chi-square test was performed on the data in Table 1. Results of the test strongly support the hypothesis ($\chi^2 = 1373.3$, df = 1, $p < 0.001$).

These data illustrate the effectiveness and value of the patient medication profile—when properly utilized by the pharmacist—to aid in the detection of potential therapeutic problems.

*Incidence of Potential Therapeutic Problems.* The incidence of potential therapeutic problems was expected to

**Table 1. Potential Therapeutic Problems Detected in New and Refill Prescriptions in Both Phases of Study**

| PRESCRIPTION TYPE | PHASE I | | | PHASE II | | | PHASES I & II | | |
|---|---|---|---|---|---|---|---|---|---|
| | NO. RX'S DISPENSED | PROBLEMS | | NO. RX's DISPENSED | PROBLEMS | | NO. RX'S DISPENSED | PROBLEMS | |
| | | NO. | % | | NO. | % | | NO. | % |
| New | 20,843 | 7 | 0.03 | 21,237 | 1,111 | 5.2 | 42,080 | 1,118 | 2.7 |
| Refill | 2,814 | 6 | 0.2 | 3,960 | 348 | 8.8 | 6,774 | 354 | 5.2 |
| New & refill | 23,657 | 13 | 0.1 | 25,197 | 1,459[a] | 5.8 | 48,854 | 1,472 | 3.0 |

[a] A total of 1,497 potential therapeutic problems were detected in Phase II for 1,459 prescriptions. Prescriptions for which problems were detected—rather than the number of problems per se—constituted the dependent variables for statistical analyses based on these data.

be higher for new prescriptions than for refill prescriptions. To test this hypothesis, a chi-square test was performed on the combined Phase I—Phase II data in Table 1. The chi-square test was highly significant ($\chi^2 = 131.8$, df = 1, $p$ <0.001), indicating that—contrary to expectations—a significantly greater proportion of potential therapeutic problems was detected for the refill prescriptions dispensed in Phases I and II than for the new prescriptions dispensed. Although refill prescriptions comprised only 13.9% of the total prescriptions dispensed, they accounted for almost one-fourth (24.0%) of the total prescriptions for which therapeutic problems were detected. In this regard, it has been our experience that the bulk of refill prescriptions are prescribed for chronic diseases whereas a substantial proportion of new prescriptions are prescribed for acute conditions. Thus, the opportunity for detection of potential therapeutic problems under the conditions of this study is possibly greater for chronic disease therapy than for acute conditions.

*Distribution of Potential Therapeutic Problems by Categories.* It was predicted that the "over-utilization of medications" category would present the greatest number of potential therapeutic problems. The distribution of potential therapeutic problems in the seven predefined categories is shown in Table 2. When the data were

combined for Phases I and II, over-utilization accounted for 65.2% of the total potential therapeutic problems detected, while under-utilization accounted for another 22.1% of the total problems.

Both the overall chi-square test and the chi-square test for the comparison between over-utilization and under-utilization problems were highly significant ($\chi^2 = 3561.9$, df = 6, $p$ <0.001; and $\chi^2 = 320.6$, df = 1, $p$ <0.001, respectively) and provided strong support for the third hypothesis. These results parallel findings of another study[18] which demonstrated patient over-utilization of medication.

*Misuse of Drugs by Financing Method.* The data concerning the relationship between method of financing prescription payment and the detected incidence of potential misuse of drugs in Phase II is presented in Table 3. For this study, the potential misuse of drugs consisted only of the over-utilization and under-utilization categories.

A one-sample chi-square test was performed on the data in Table 3 for third party financed prescriptions to assess the validity of the fourth hypothesis. This analysis was based on Phase II data only, since only 13 potential therapeutic problems were noted in Phase I. Results of the test strongly support the hypothesis ($\chi^2 = 390.9$, df = 1, $p$ <0.001) that the over-utilization of medications for prescriptions financed by third-party payors (United Mine Workers of America Welfare and Retirement Fund and the state welfare program) will be more common than the under-utilization of prescriptions financed by the same method. This pattern of patient drug over-utilization frequently has been observed in patients who are not directly responsible for paying for their prescription medications. However, it should be pointed out that, in this study, the under-utilization of prescriptions by third-party beneficiaries is also a matter of concern.

**Table 2. Potential Therapeutic Problems According to Category and Phase of Study**

| CATEGORY | PHASE I | | PHASE II | | PHASES I & II | |
|---|---|---|---|---|---|---|
| | NO. | % | NO. | % | NO. | % |
| 1. M.D. duplicates active Rx with same drug | 4 | 30.8 | 101 | 6.8 | 105 | 6.9 |
| 2. M.D. duplicates active Rx with similar drug | 3 | 23.0 | 19 | 1.3 | 22 | 1.4 |
| 3. Patient over-utilizes drugs | 3 | 23.0 | 981 | 65.5 | 984 | 65.2 |
| 4. Patient under-utilizes drugs | 2 | 15.4 | 332 | 22.2 | 334 | 22.1 |
| 5. Potential drug-drug interaction | 0 | 0 | 4 | 0.3 | 4 | 0.3 |
| 6. Potential drug-disease contraindication | 1 | 7.8 | 9 | 0.6 | 10 | 0.7 |
| 7. Prescription discrepancies | 0 | 0 | 51 | 3.4 | 51 | 3.4 |
| Total[a] | 13 | 100 | 1497 | 100 | 1510 | 100 |

[a] The number of potential therapeutic problems detected—rather than the number of prescriptions involving problems—constituted the dependent variables for the statistical analyses based on these data.

**Table 3. Incidence of Potential Over-Utilization and Under-Utilization of Medications According to Method of Prescription Payment in Phase II of Study**

| CATEGORY | THIRD PARTY PAYMENT | | SELF-PAYMENT | |
|---|---|---|---|---|
| | NO. | % | NO. | % |
| Over-utilization | 885 | 79.7 | 96 | 47.5 |
| Under-utilization | 226 | 20.3 | 106 | 52.5 |
| Total | 1,111 | 100 | 202 | 100 |

**Table 4. Incidence of Potential Over-Utilization and Under-Utilization of Medications According to Drug Class in Phase II of Study**

| DRUG CLASSIFICATION | PRE-SCRIPTIONS DISPENSED | | OVER UTILI-ZATION | | UNDER-UTILI-ZATION | |
|---|---|---|---|---|---|---|
| | NO. | % | NO. | %[a] | NO. | %[a] |
| Psychotherapeutic | 3,202 | 12.7 | 300 | 9.4 | 0 | 0 |
| Antihypertensive | 2,705 | 10.7 | 251 | 9.3 | 142 | 5.2 |
| Cardiovascular | 1,861 | 7.4 | 120 | 6.4 | 95 | 5.1 |
| Analgesic | 3,016 | 12.0 | 100 | 3.3 | 0 | 0 |
| Antispasmotic | 1,130 | 4.5 | 69 | 6.1 | 10 | 0.9 |
| Antidiabetic | 799 | 3.2 | 54 | 6.8 | 44 | 5.5 |
| Antiasthmadic | 931 | 3.7 | 29 | 3.1 | 5 | 0.5 |
| Hormones | 892 | 3.5 | 19 | 2.1 | 14 | 1.6 |
| Antiinflammatory | 351 | 1.4 | 11 | 3.1 | 0 | 0 |
| Others | 10,310 | 40.9 | 28 | 0.3 | 22 | 0.2 |
| Total | 25,197 | 100 | 981 | 3.9 | 332 | 1.3 |

[a] Percent based on total number of drugs dispensed in the corresponding drug category.

Table 3 also presents the data relevant to the fifth hypothesis which predicted a greater incidence of under-utilization than over-utilization for prescriptions payed for directly by patients. Although under-utilization was detected slightly more often than over-utilization, the difference was not statistically significant ($\chi^2 = 0.50$, df $= 1$, $p > 0.50$).

*Misuse of Drugs by Drug Category.* The relationship between drug classification and the incidence of potential misuse of drugs in Phase II is presented in Table 4. To assess the prediction that potential over-utilization of psychotherapeutic drugs would be detected more often than for any other drug category, the data in Table 4 were first subjected to an overall chi-square analysis. The results were significantly beyond the 0.001 level ($\chi^2 = 904.1$, df $= 9$). Next, separate comparisons were made between the incidence of over-utilization detected for psychotherapeutic drugs and the incidence of over-utilization of drugs in each of the nine remaining drug categories. Results indicated no significant difference in the incidence of over-utilization between psychotherapeutic and antihypertensive classes ($Z = 0.1$, $p > 0.50$). However, all other comparisons yielded statistically significant results with $Z$ values ranging from 2.4 ($p < 0.02$) for the comparison between psychotherapeutic and antidia-

betic classes to 29.2 ($p < 0.0001$) for the comparison between the psychotherapeutic and the "others" category.

It is of interest to note that the psychotherapeutic and antihypertensive drug categories demonstrated a significantly greater potential for over-utilization than any of the other drug classes studied. Inspection of Table 4 further indicates that the antidiabetic, cardiovascular and antispasmodic classes were associated with a greater potential for over-utilization than either the antiinflammatory, antiasthmatic, analgesic or hormone categories.

The "others" category accounted for 40.9% of the total prescriptions dispensed and yet comprised only 2.9% of the detected potential drug over-utilization. Possible explanations for this small tendency for over-utilization are (1) the majority of drugs used to treat *acute conditions* fall into the "others" category, and (2) the patient is less likely to "stockpile" medication for acute conditions.

There may be some tendency for patients on chronic medications to "stockpile" drugs which they know will be needed at a later date. Due to the distance, rugged terrain and lack of transportation facilities[19] in the area served by the Wise ARH pharmacy, it is common for the patient to request prescription medication in advance. According to the definition of over-utilization established for this study, patients requesting medication seven days or more before their supply should have been exhausted were counted as potential over-utilizers. Perhaps, in some cases, they could have more accurately been termed "stockpilers."

Although no specific predictions were made concerning under-utilization of drugs in each of the ten classes, a chi-square analysis was used to compare the frequency of under-utilization associated with the three drug classes cardiovascular, antidiabetic and antihypertensive against the remaining seven classes. Results indicated that under-utilization problems were detected significantly more often for cardiovascular, antidiabetic and antihypertensive drugs than for the seven remaining categories ($\chi^2 = 749.3$, df $= 1$, $p < 0.001$).

*Misuse of Drugs by Age.* The relationship between the potential misuse of medication and the age of the patient in Phase II is presented in Table 5. To test the hypothesis that misuse of medication is more prevalent among patients 65 years and older, the data in Table 5

**Table 5. Incidence of Potential Over-Utilization and Under-Utilization of Medications According to Age Group in Phase II of Study**

| AGE RANGE | TOTAL RX'S DISPENSED | | OVER-UTILIZATION | | UNDER-UTILIZATION | | COMBINED | |
|---|---|---|---|---|---|---|---|---|
| | NO. | % | NO. | %[a] | NO. | %[a] | NO. | %[b] |
| 0–12 | 2,122 | 8.4 | 17 | 77.3 | 5 | 22.7 | 22 | 1.0 |
| 13–20 | 573 | 2.3 | 17 | 77.3 | 5 | 22.7 | 22 | 3.8 |
| 21–40 | 3,187 | 12.6 | 57 | 72.2 | 22 | 27.8 | 79 | 2.5 |
| 41–64 | 15,495 | 61.5 | 656 | 84.3 | 122 | 15.7 | 778 | 5.0 |
| 65 and over | 3,820 | 15.2 | 234 | 56.8 | 178 | 43.2 | 412 | 10.8 |
| Total | 25,197 | 100 | 981 | 74.7 | 332 | 25.3 | 1313 | 5.2 |

[a] Percent based on total misuse for the corresponding age category.
[b] Percent based on total number of prescriptions dispensed for the corresponding age category.

were first subjected to an overall chi-square analysis. Results of this analysis were highly significant ($\chi^2 = 367$, df = 4, $p < 0.001$). Next, individual comparisons were made between the incidence of over-utilization detected for the 65-and-over age category and for each of the four remaining groups. For the individual comparisons, $Z$ values ranged from 5.2 ($p < 0.001$) for the $13 - 20$ vs. 65-and-over groups to 14.0 ($p < 0.001$) for the difference between the 65-and-over vs. the $0 - 12$ groups. From these findings it was concluded that over-utilization was detected significantly more often for patients 65 years and older than for patients in any of the younger age categories. Inspection of the data in Table 5 indicates that under-utilization is also a problem for patients 65 years and older.

Potential over-utilization and under-utilization of drugs by the age group 65 and older was more common than for any other group. This finding may be due to the relatively greater transportation problems experienced by the elderly which could either result in stockpiling or an undersupply of medications.

## Summary and Conclusion

The goal of this study was to determine the pharmacist's ability to detect potential therapeutic problems in ambulatory patients by utilizing a medication profile.

When the medication profile card was used by the pharmacist, 14,975 patients presented 25,197 prescriptions which resulted in the identification of 1,497 potential therapeutic problems. When dispensing medications in the traditional manner without the assistance of the profile, 14,069 patients presented 23,657 prescriptions which resulted in the identification of only 13 potential therapeutic problems. The numbers of patients and prescriptions in both phases of the study were comparable in size.

The study results support the effectiveness and value of the patient medication profile—when properly utilized by the pharmacist—to aid in the detection of potential therapeutic problems.

A significantly greater proportion of potential therapeutic problems was detected for refill prescriptions than for new prescriptions. In fact, refill prescriptions comprised only 13.9% of the total prescriptions dispensed but accounted for 24.0% of the total prescriptions for which potential therapeutic problems were detected.

Possible improper utilization of medications accounted for approximately 88% of the total potential therapeutic problems. Potential over-utilization occurred more frequently (65.2%) than did potential under-utilization (22.1%).

Over-utilization of prescriptions financed by a third-party payor was found to occur significantly more frequently than under-utilization of prescriptions financed by the same method.

Under-utilization was detected slightly more often than over-utilization for prescriptions financed by the self payment method. However, this difference was not statistically significant.

Psychotherapeutic and antihypertensive drugs demonstrated a significantly greater potential for over-utilization than any other drug class studied.

Over-utilization was detected significantly more often for patients 65 years and older than for patients in any other age category. Under-utilization was also found to be more common for the 65 and over group.

*Implications of Study.* Stewart and Cluff[15] reviewed published reports dating back as far as 1955 pertaining to medication errors and noncompliance in ambulant patients. Their review indicates the percentage of patients making errors in the self-administration of prescribed medications, with few exceptions, ranged between 25 and 59%. In addition, 4 to 35% of the patients were misusing their medications in such a manner as to pose serious threats to health. Thus, it is an obvious conclusion that serious problems related to ambulant drug therapy do exist in a variety of health care settings.

Following the studies by Barker et al.,[20] which quantitated the problem of medication errors in hospitals, pharmacists were shocked into action and took substantial steps to correct the problems by instituting improved systems of drug distribution. These improved systems are now commonly referred to as unit dose and intravenous admixture services. Thus, hospital pharmacy practice met a challenge for patients served at institutional levels of care. However, despite a clear need on the part of ambulant patients, no far-reaching campaign has been launched to correct deficiencies in ambulatory drug distribution systems. To some extent this is understandable insofar as ambulatory care tends to be given at the behest of the patient, and communications between the various health care providers, especially physicians and pharmacists, are less than efficient.

This study covers only one of several factors which should be considered before conclusively stating that pharmacist maintenance and utilization of patient medication profiles are necessary. Additional studies are recommended to (1) further quantitate the extent to which pharmacists can detect and avert actual problems, (2) determine costs, (3) evaluate benefits and (4) determine patient acceptance and cooperation. Also, a validation study is suggested to assess the extent to which medication over- and under-utilization, as measured by the patient medication profile, corresponds to actual over- and under-utilization of medications by ambulatory patients.

Although this study is not conclusive in all respects, the results indicate that more pharmacists and health care administrators should strongly consider utilizing patient medication profiles when providing care for ambulatory patients. While this study does not purport that patient medication profiles result in the elimination of potential therapeutic problems, it nonetheless clearly indicates that such a system will place the pharmacist in a position of being able to detect such problems. It follows that many pharmacists, if given the opportunity to understand the scope and magnitude of ambulatory drug-related problems, will feel a legal if not moral responsibility to take positive action in the best interests of their patients.

### References

1. Almquist, D. D.: Manual Patient Drug Profiles as a Part of a Drug Distribution System, *Amer. J. Hosp. Pharm.* 27:988–993 (Dec.) 1970.

2. Davis, N. M.: Patient Profile Draws the Whole Picture, *Hospitals* 45:110–115 (Sept. 1) 1971.

3. Minor, M. F.: Patient Drug Profile, *Hosp. Pharm.* 5:10–13 (Dec.) 1970.

4. Klotz, R. O.: Pediatric Patient Drug Profiles, *Hosp. Pharm.* 7:27–28 (Jan.) 1972.

5. Stevens, R. and Wolfert, R.: Three Years Experience with a Patient Medication Record and Charge Ticket, *Amer. J. Hosp. Pharm.* 25:569 (Oct.) 1968.

6. Stevens, R. and Wolfert, R.: A Ramdom Filing System for Inpatient Medication Records, *Amer. J. Hosp. Pharm.* 26:290–293 (May) 1969.

7. Slining, J., Cole, P. and Sister Emmanuel: Development of a Drug Incompatability File and Its Use in Patient Medication Profile Reviews, *Amer. J. Hosp. Pharm.* 27:459–467 (June) 1970.

8. Hernandez, L. and Boutet, J. C.,: Outpatients Get Better Service, *Hospitals* 46:81–85 (Jan. 1) 1972.

9. Cain, R. M. and Kahn, J. S.: The Pharmacist as a Member of the Health Team, *Amer. J. Pub. Health* 61:2223–2228 (Nov.) 1971.

10. Tice, L. F.: Outpatient Pharmacy Services, *J. Amer. Pharm. Ass. NS7*:622–623 (Dec.) 1967.

11. Report of the Task Force on the Pharmacist's Clinical Role, HSRD Briefs, No. 4 (Spring) 1971. (A publication of the National Center for Health Services Research and Development, Health Services for Mental Health Administration, Department of Health, Education, and Welfare, Rockville, Maryland.)

12. Anon.: Hospital Prescriptions at Record Level; More Pharmacists are Employed, *Amer. Drug.* 162:25–26 (Aug. 10) 1970.

13. Smith, W. E.: Using the Patient Drug Profile, *Drug Intel. Clin. Pharm.* 4:73–76 (Mar.) 1970.

14. Solomon, D. K. and Muha, K. M.: Patient Medication Profiles: Pharmacist Contribution in Monitoring and Improving Drug Therapy, *Appal. Med.* 4:50–53 (Sept.) 1972.

15. Stewart, R. B. and Cluff, L. E.: A Review of Medication Errors and Compliance in Ambulant Patients, *Clin. Pharmacol. Ther.* 13:463–468 (July–Aug.) 1972.

16. Siegel, S.: Nonparametric Statistics For the Behavioral Sciences, McGraw-Hill, New York, 1956.

17. McNemar, Quinn: Psychological Statistics, 2nd Ed., Wiley, New York, 1959.

18. Latiolais, C. J. and Berry, C. C.: Misuse of Prescription Medications by Outpatients, *Drug Intel. Clin. Pharm.* 3:270–277 (Oct.) 1969.

19. U.S. Census of Housing, U.S. Dept. of Commerce, Bureau of the Census, 1970.

20. Barker, K. N., Kimbrough, W. and Heller, W. M.: A Study of Medication Errors in a Hospital, University of Arkansas, November 1966.

# 27 A Patient Profile System for Monitoring Long-term Anticoagulant Therapy

Diane Bernstein, Earl C. Harrison, and Margaret M. McCarron

A patient profile system for monitoring anticoagulant therapy of patients with prosthetic heart valves is discussed.

The patients are seen by a pharmacist every two weeks for anticoagulant dosage adjustment, and by a physician every two months for a physical examination. The profile system provides (1) rapid access to information useful in determining the anticoagulation sensitivity and stability of a patient, (2) a means of analyzing and categorizing symptoms suggestive of an embolus, and (3) a method of monitoring for specific changes in patient parameters such as blood pressure, pulse, weight, electrolytes, etc.

It is suggested that the profile system could serve as a prototype for programs monitoring other types of long-term drug therapy.

An anticoagulation clinic was established to assist the cardiologists in caring for a large number of anticoagulated patients and to provide for an organized and consistent approach to patient management. The clinic is managed by a pharmacist and consists of 65 patients selected from a cardiology clinic of approximately 130 prosthetic valve patients.

Problems anticipated in anticoagulation management were outlined by the cardiologist. He taught the pharmacist how to recognize anticoagulant complications, symptoms suggesting deterioration of the primary disease and the clinical significance of such symptoms. The patients in this clinic are essentially managed by a physician-pharmacist team. The pharmacist has been given the responsibility for careful patient monitoring, while the physicians continue to see the patients on a routine basis for cardiac evaluation. The pharmacist sees the patients every two weeks for adjustment of their anticoagulant dosage, detection of adverse drug effects and drug interactions, and early recognition of symptoms suggesting deterioration of the patient's medical status. The physician sees the patients every two months for routine evaluation unless the pharmacist refers a patient sooner.

This chapter explains the monitoring system that was developed by the patient care team. It also describes in detail the pharmacist's use of the forms which were developed for this clinic. This system is presented as a prototype that could be utilized by a clinical pharmacist participating in the management of medically stabilized patients on long-term drug therapy.

## Need for a Monitoring System

Since the patients were to be seen so frequently by the pharmacist, it was obvious that a large volume of data was going to accumulate. In addition, it was vital to keep track of all the data collected for effective monitoring of the patients as well as for later research purposes. It was evident that an outpatient profile system had to be developed to aid the pharmacist in handling the data.

## Materials Used

The reusable Plannit[a] folder with its 20 5 × 8-inch cards provided a means for developing a highly organized and compact monitoring system for regularly obtaining patient data. All the necessary information is printed on both sides of the cards. The cards are notched to fit into the precut slots provided on the folder. One folder is used for each patient in the clinic (Figure 1). When the cards are completely filled they can be removed and placed alphabetically in a file box. New cards can then be inserted.

The entire profile system consists of only four different printed cards. Two of these cards provide basic information on the patient. Card 1 is concerned with patient identification and card 2 with drug and allergic histories. The other two cards are repeated consecutively through

---

[a] Oxford Supply Company, Inc., Clinton Rd., Garden City, NY 11530.

Figure 1. The patient folder

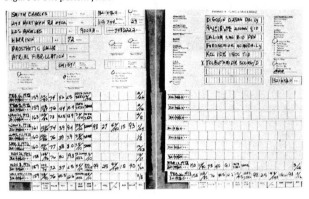

the folder and accommodate information collected at each of 18 patient interviews. Card 3 is concerned with the symptoms of the patient, while card 4 allows for notes of interest, referrals and specific laboratory data. Cards 3 and 4 are used together as a set at the time of each interview (Figure 2).

## Utilization of the System

Card 1 is completed by the pharmacist at his initial visit with the patient (Figure 3). Background information such as name, address, telephone number, patient file number, sex, age, birthdate, referring physician, height, race and the referring clinic is collected here. Information such as cardiac rhythm, the date of the heart valve replacement and the type of valve replaced is obtained from the patient's original hospital record. With the clinic presently restricted to patients with prosthetic heart valves, certain information required on the cards is specific for this. With eventual expansion of the clinic, however, such specific details could be exchanged for other information.

Figure 2. Cards 3 and 4 which are used as an interview set.

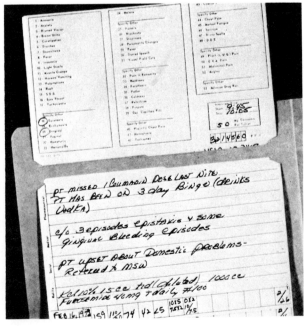

Figure 3. Card 1, for basic patient data, is completed by the pharmacist at his initial visit with the patient

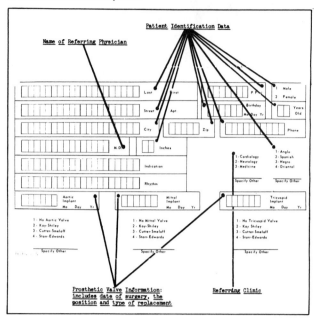

Card 2 is used when a complete drug history is taken from the patient by the pharmacist (Figure 4). The pharmacist asks the patient to tell or show him what medications he is currently taking. This list of drugs is then compared with the categories on the "cue" list printed on this card. When the patient does not report therapy in a category, he is specifically asked if he is taking any drugs for a particular purpose, such as convulsions, anxiety, indigestion, etc. Medicines that are being taken by the patient which were originally prescribed by a physician in a specialty clinic such as diabetes are indicated on the card by an "X."

Once the therapy is determined and entered on the

Figure 4. Card 2 is used in taking the drug history

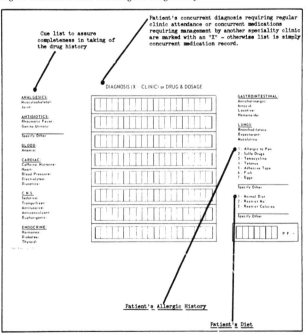

card, it is checked for therapeutic incompatibilities or potential drug interactions with warfarin. If such incompatibilities are noted, the problem is discussed with the patient's physician and a change in the therapy is initiated. Should potential interactions exist, the pharmacist either standardizes the dosing of the interacting drug or recommends the substitution of a noninteracting drug whenever possible. If a patient's concurrent medical diagnosis requires special clinic attendance, this is indicated on the card by an "X." An allergic history and any special dietary restrictions are also noted and serve as guides in making future recommendations.

On subsequent visits this drug history is updated by reviewing the hospital chart and also by asking the patient if there has been any change in his medicines since his last visit to the anticoagulation clinic. Any changes are noted, and again, the potential for incompatibility or warfarin interaction is assessed.

On card 3, data regarding weight, blood pressure, pulse, packed cell volume and thrombotest, are recorded at each clinic visit (Figure 5). The weight, blood pressure and pulse are obtained by clinic attendants before the patient is seen by the pharmacist. The packed cell volume and thrombotest are obtained in the laboratory, and the patient usually hand carries these results to the pharmacist. Additional spaces are available to record electrolyte values which are ordered monthly by the pharmacist, primarily to monitor serum potassium values in digitalized patients. From data previously entered in this fashion, the pharmacist is able to monitor the stability of these parameters and to make the appropriate recommendations and referrals to the physician.

*Figure 5. Card 3 is used for recording patient parameters at each clinic visit*

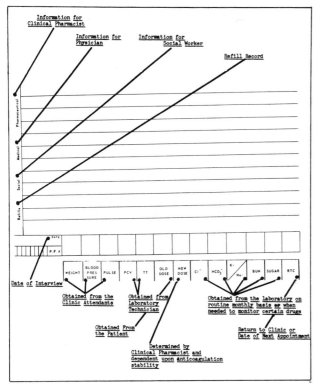

For example, if the pharmacist notes a sudden weight loss, he questions the patient about anorexia, malaise, blurred vision, diarrhea and headache, symptoms suggestive (although not diagnostic) of digitalis intoxication. He would then refer the patient to a physician with a note stating the reasons for referral. Similarly, by observing changes in blood pressure and pulse rate, the pharmacist can pursue questions which may indicate a need for a change in antihypertensive or antiarrhythmic therapy. By referring the patient to a physician when such observations are made, the pharmacist assists in early diagnosis and prompt treatment. Detecting a fall in the packed cell volume value helps detect internal hemorrhage and suggests its severity. A modified prothrombin test, known as the thrombotest, is used exclusively in the anticoagulation clinic to monitor warfarin therapy. By observing previously entered values, the pharmacist can assess at a glance the patient's sensitivity to warfarin. He can decide whether to continue or alter the dose of the anticoagulant. He can correlate the administration of a new medication or the altered dose of an old medication with sudden changes in the coagulation of the blood-changes which could result in an embolic episode or hemorrhage if not detected early. The space marked "RTC" indicates the return to clinic date or the date of the patient's next thrombotest appointment.

Card 4 is used after the above data have been entered and the patient has been asked how he is feeling or how he has been feeling since his last visit (Figure 6). He is specifically asked if he has noted any signs of bleeding. If the patient offers any significant symptoms corresponding to those on card 4, the number printed by the symptom is circled. The symptoms printed on the card are grouped to help detect commonly overlooked problems found in these anticoagulated patients. For example, symptoms numbered 18 through 24 represent indi-

*Figure 6. Card 4 is used for recording patient symptoms*

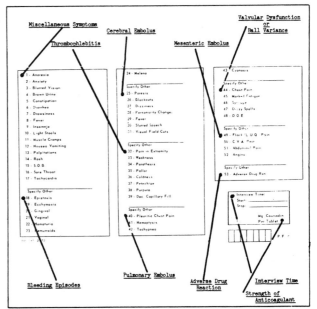

vidual bleeding episodes; those numbered 32–39, 40–43 and 49–51 may indicate a thrombophlebitis, a pulmonary embolus or a mesenteric embolus, respectively. The variety of symptoms grouped into numbers 1–17 and classified simply as miscellaneous include such problems as digitalis intoxication, electrolyte depletion, serum hepatitis, etc. The signs and symptoms grouped into numbers 44–48 are related to valvular dysfunction or to ball variance, indicating the deterioration of the prosthetic valve. Item 52 is for angina, and item 53 is used to indicate when an adverse drug reaction has been noted. By offering a means to analyze and categorize medical symptoms suggestive of an embolus, card 4 serves as a guide for the interviewer to pursue other questions. This often leads to important symptoms which suggest the need for immediate referral of the patient to a physician or to the hospital emergency room. A record of the interview time is also kept on the card; an average visit takes 12 minutes. The patient is also routinely asked the strength of his warfarin tablets to insure the proper terminology in explaining new dosage regimens, as well as to help reinforce the importance of knowing which strength he is taking.

Once the initial inquiries are completed, the necessary warfarin adjustments are made. The patient is then asked about anything which may have influenced the stability of his anticoagulation such as improper dosage, concurrent illnesses or the concurrent use of other medication. This information is then entered under the pharmaceutical note section on card 3. The patient is routinely asked how he had been taking his warfarin since his last visit. This dosage is then compared with that dosage listed on the form under "old dose," which is the dose the patient should be taking. If the patient has taken the warfarin incorrectly because of noncompliance with instructions, a misunderstanding or self-adjustment of dosage, the problem is discussed with the patient and noted in the record. Readjustment is then recommended on the basis of the actual dose which had been taken. Similarly, any symptoms of a medical or psychiatric nature which may have become evident during the interview are recorded on the card and the appropriate referrals are made. A record of all prescription refills is also kept to assess the patient's drug utilization.

## Conclusion

The pharmacy monitoring system and the forms used to record necessary patient information in a specialized cardiology clinic have been presented. These forms constitute a system useful for monitoring a specific kind of drug therapy. The detailed content of each form was presented to explain how the system functions. With adaptations, this format could be used to assist a physician-pharmacist team in establishing a similar program for monitoring other types of long-term chronic drug therapy.

# 28 Problems Encountered by Pharmacy Students Conducting Patient Interviews

V. A. Lomonte, Jr., Jon J. Tanja, Charles N. Bell, and
Ronald A. Young

The experiences encountered by students conducting patient interviews in an outpatient clinic are documented relative to the deficiencies in a clinical course within a traditional pharmacy curriculum.

Student experiences indicated communication problems with allied health personnel in the clinic, difficulty in reviewing patient charts and in conducting patient interviews, and communication problems with patients. The difficulties experienced by students in the clinical program revealed deficiencies related to four principal areas: (1) preclinical education, (2) knowledge of the clinical environment, (3) practical experience, and (4) student motivation.

As clinical pharmacy education and practice develops, educators must realize the importance of the student in the program, the impact of traditional pharmacy practice on the profession, the attitudes of other health professionals toward pharmacy and the limitations of the present curriculum relative to a clinical pharmacy course.

The consensus of the ASHP-AACP Invitational Workshop on Clinical Pharmaceutical Practice and Education[1] suggested essential requirements for clinical pharmacy programs. Particularly, the workshop noted: (1) patient orientation should begin early in the curriculum, (2) the pharmacy curriculum should culminate in an intensive clinical experience, and (3) clinical practitioners should be in charge of clinical instruction. The importance of these three points cannot be overemphasized. However, another factor relative to clinical pharmacy education which was not presented must be considered. Derzon[2] raised the question, "Is this program of sufficient attractiveness to increase the quality of the student body entering schools of pharmacy?" Maybe of more importance is the question, "How does the present pharmacy student fit into a clinical pharmacy program?"

The proceedings of the workshop will serve as a useful guide to schools of pharmacy as clinical pharmacy is implemented into the curriculum. In the interim, problems which may be common to clinical pharmacy programs throughout the country must be recognized. Therefore, the objective of this paper is to support the consensus of the ASHP-AACP Workshop and to document the problems encountered by students conducting patient interviews in a clinical pharmacy program.

## Background: The Patient Interview

One of the objectives of clinical pharmacy education is, "To develop in the student a facility for effective interaction with the patient and practitioners of other health professions."[3] The patient interview provides one mechanism for accomplishing this objective, and a brief description of it is presented to further illustrate the appropriateness of this technique in clinical pharmacy education.

The patient interview for hospitalized patients is composed of four parts: (1) the initial interview, (2) communicating the information obtained to the physician, (3) the interim visit and (4) the discharge interview.[4] In contrast, the initial interview in an outpatient facility requires a review of the patient's chart just prior to the interview. The pharmacist determines the patient's medication regimen and patterns of drug usage and passes the information to the physician, either orally or by use of a patient medication profile. If the profile is used, the pharmacist should be available for consultation with the physician. Next, the physician sees the patient, and depending on the patient's condition, the physician may decide to continue all drugs, to discontinue one or more of the drugs, to increase or decrease the dosage or to prescribe additional drugs. Pursuant to the actions of the physician, the pharmacist advises the patient on his drug therapy. When the patient returns to the facility, the pharmacist conducts the follow-up interview. This visit gives the pharmacist an opportunity for assessing the patient's response to the prescribed drugs.

## The Clinical Course

The School of Pharmacy at Northeast Louisiana University incorporated one semester of clinical practice into its curriculum in the fall of 1969 on an elective basis. The following year the clinical course became a requirement for graduation. As in other schools of pharmacy, the course was taught for 14 weeks in the third professional year of the curriculum. With the exception of this addition, only minimal modifications were made in the curriculum. Other course contents were not appreciably altered to reflect clinical philosophy and application.

The clinical course consisted of two three-hour laboratory sessions in various clinical environments supplemented by a weekly, one-hour conference dealing with disease states. Throughout the course, students were rotated through clinical environments to provide experiences in the hospital, outpatient clinic and community pharmacy.

The outpatient clinic is operated as part of a 160-bed, general acute care state hospital. The medical staff of the hospital is composed of staff physicians and residents. The residents are available through an agreement with medical schools in the state which lends somewhat of a "teaching hospital" atmosphere to the facility. As for pharmacy coverage, inpatient service is limited to a traditional floor stock system and outpatient prescription service is not provided.

Student experiences with patient interviews were limited to this outpatient clinic. The School's agreement with the clinic provided access to the patients, patient charts and interview rooms, but it did not provide for incorporating the pharmacy program into the clinic routine. Thus, students functioned independently of the clinic operation. The initial objectives established for the student included:

1. Securing patient medication histories:
   a. Prescription medications
   b. Nonprescription medications
   c. Drug sensitivities
2. Reviewing patient charts
3. Observing physician examination and diagnostic techniques
4. Observing functions and interview techniques of social workers
5. Consulting with allied health personnel
6. Advising patients on their drug regimens and pertinent drug information
7. Participating in follow-up visits to patients' homes with social workers and public health nurses.

## Patient Interviews

Over the past two years, two basic forms have been utilized by students in conducting interviews with patients seen primarily by the medical service in the outpatient clinic. The forms used and the experiences of the program are not unique. In fact, they probably parallel those of other schools of pharmacy.

As stated earlier, students functioned in the clinic independent of its operation. They were not familiar with the operating procedures of the clinic and were not able to establish rapport with the clinic personnel. As a consequence, the feeling pervaded that students were "in the way," and meaningful interaction with physicians and other allied health personnel was practically nonexistent.

Initially, only the patient profile form was used by students in reviewing patient charts and conducting interviews. On this form students noted: (1) general patient information, (2) admitting diagnosis, (3) doctor and clinic specialty, (4) medication history, (5) drugs taken with water, foods, etc., (6) surgery history, (7) laboratory and other tests, (8) nurses' notes and (9) comments on drug advice given and conclusions. During the first semester, students had difficulty in reviewing patient charts due to their inexperience with abbreviations used and the physicians' handwriting. Difficulty was also encountered by students in trying to conduct the patient interview. Particularly, they were uncertain as to what questions they should ask of the patient. Recognizing the problem, the clinical instructor modified a patient questionnaire[5] which dealt with the misuse of medications by the patient and patient opinions and attitudes relative to the physician, the pharmacist and the patient himself. This form was called the clinical questionnaire and was used in conjunction with the patient profile form. Thus, students were reviewing patient charts and then conducting interviews using the questionnaire format. Although this process did not produce a patient medication history in the truest sense, it did give students a sense of direction when interviewing patients.

Another interview-related problem was the communications gap between students and patients due to the students' unfamiliarity with communication techniques.[6] Concurrently, the interviews, in most cases, were not only the students' first contact with patients but also brought students in contact with individuals from different socioeconomic strata. In addition to communicating with patients, students must be able to interpret and assess the validity of the patients' responses. This is of particular importance if the information obtained in the interview is to be used by the physician. Due to their inexperience, it is doubtful if the students were able to adequately assess the interviews during the semester.

## Discussion

The difficulties experienced by students conducting patient interviews in an outpatient clinic revealed deficiencies in the clinical program which are related to four principal areas: (1) preclinical education, (2) knowledge of the clinical environment, (3) practical experience and (4) student motivation.

*Preclinical Education.* It has been said that "present pharmacy graduates are not prepared to work in a health-care system."[7] Similarly, the present preclinical training of the pharmacy student does not suitably prepare him for a training period in the clinical environment. Unfortunately, the clinical course in most curricula is merely an add-on program in which students are supposed to acquire a patient awareness. Yet, the remainder of the curriculum is not amended or integrated to reflect clinical aspects of pharmaceutical practice. In many cases, the acquired knowledge is still basically product-oriented and leaves the student without an appreciation for disease states and therapeutics. This is also manifested by the student's lack of exposure to the medical literature and his inability to interpret or evaluate it. This is evidenced by the fact that many students still consider the *Physicians' Desk Reference* as a reliable source of drug information. As a result, the student placed in a patient care area with his present educational background is ill-prepared to function in this new environment.

*Knowledge of the Clinical Environment.* Hand-in-hand with the inadequacy of the student's preclinical training is his lack of knowledge of the clinical environment. Generally, the student does not know the scope, facilities, departments or operations of the hospital or clinic. In particular, he is unfamiliar with the patient chart and its composition. Also, the student is inept in dealing with patients, physicians, nurses and other allied health personnel. To function effectively in the clinical environment requires communicative skills which pharmacy students lack.[8] Hence, valuable time must be spent to orient the student in the clinical environment in the add-on course.

Students still face the traditional attitudes of medical personnel toward the pharmacist who is stereotyped as a drug supplier.[9] In the facility where pharmacy services are minimal, traditional attitudes are perpetuated. Outpatient pharmacy services such as patient interviews and patient medication profiles in addition to prescription services offer the pharmacist the opportunity to participate with physicians and other allied health personnel in providing patient care. Only until the pharmacist has demonstrated his ability to function in this environment will he be accepted by other health professionals. These barriers must be scaled by both student and clinical faculty alike in implementing clinical pharmacy programs.

Any pertinent information obtained during the interview by the student in our initial program was not communicated to the physician. Thus, needed student-physician interaction was not present and patient benefit was not realized. The student was disadvantaged because he functioned in the clinic under an agreement dictating observation which did not provide a mechanism for effective interaction. Meaningful experiences are only possible when the activities of the student contribute a service to the patient and the facility.

*Practical Experience.* Pharmacy students may be deprived of valuable experience when they choose to forego summer employment in pharmacies because of the relatively low pay. Summer employment may also be discouraged in states where the experience gained does not shorten the mandatory internship time. Thus, it is not uncommon for many fifth-year students to lack experience in all areas of pharmacy practice. In many instances even those students who have participated in the traditional areas of pharmacy practice have had very little patient contact.

*Student Motivation.* The literature is replete with articles describing clinical pharmacy educational programs. However, it is somewhat ironic that in the process, educators have seemingly overlooked the student. The success or failure of clinical pharmacy practice is not only dependent on the quality of the graduates in the program but also the quality of students entering the program. Therefore, it is fitting that some basic statements be made as to the quality, attitudes and motivations of pharmacy students. It must be realized that it is difficult to separate these three interrelated aspects of students.

Primarily, the quality of the student who enters pharmacy is influenced by his views of pharmacy. His exposure to pharmacy is usually confined to community practice, namely the drugstore, which has been characterized as a "commercialized jungle."[10] As a result, the professional role of the pharmacist may not be discernible to the student and may only instill in him thoughts of business and personal economic gain. Another factor which affects the quality of students is the admission procedures of pharmacy schools. It is not that the requirements are not stringent enough, even though this may sometimes be the case, but in many schools there is a lack of competitiveness in entrance requirements.

Also, for whatever the reason, students, like some pharmacists, are just not interested in the clinical role of the pharmacist.[11] In conjunction with this, there has been an apparent failure of pharmacy educators to stimulate students professionally. Pharmaceutical education is composed of educators who are research-oriented rather than practitioners.[12] Overall, one cannot help but feel that the profession lacks a philosophy, pride and *esprit de corps* which transcends pharmacy.

### Program Improvement

Changes in pharmaceutical education necessary for the development of clinical pharmacy programs will take time to evolve. This is of little solace to programs presently in existence. However, improvements can be made in a clinical course to aid the student during this transition period.

Probably the biggest problem of the contemporary student is his inability to correlate the knowledge he has acquired with patient care. However, he can, with effort, bridge the gap. To help the student in this task, changes are being made in the clinical course at Northeast Louisiana University.

Prior to being assigned to the clinic, students will receive a more intense orientation directed toward reviewing patient charts, interview techniques and disease states. Improvements can be summarized as follows:

1. *Revising Student Objectives.* The objectives have been revised in terms more realistic to the student's actual clinic involvement. A clinic procedure has been developed which clearly defines what is expected of the student.
2. *Disease States Orientation.* Emphasis will be placed on student efforts in dealing with diabetic and hypertensive patients. These two disease states will be discussed in the conferences prior to the students' involvement in the clinic.
3. *Chart Familiarization.* Students will be exposed to outpatient charts in case studies. This will increase their familiarity with handling and interpreting the charts.
4. *Interview Techniques.* Patient interview techniques will be stressed. An attempt is being made to develop videotaped interviews for instructional purposes.
5. *Patient Profile Worksheet.* Students will use a revised patient profile worksheet for the chart review and patient interview. A predetermined format will be followed to aid the student in conducting the interview.
6. *Drug Therapy Plan and Information Assignments.* After interviewing patients, students will be required to prepare a drug therapy plan.[13] Each student will also have a drug information assignment on a subject pertaining to one of the patients he has interviewed. In preparing this report the format of "the DIAS rounds"[14] will be followed. Hopefully, these types of assignments will help the student integrate his knowledge and teach him the proper use of medical literature.

The above improvements should provide the student with more meaningful experiences in the outpatient clinic. However, he will still be limited by a lack of time and a minimal interaction with allied health personnel.

### Conclusions

The ASHP-AACP Workshop will have a tremendous impact on the development of clinical pharmacy education and practice.[15] During this period educators must also realize the importance of the student, the impact of traditional pharmacy practice on the profession, the attitudes of other health professions toward pharmacy and the limitations of the present curriculum relative to clinical pharmacy practice.

Concurrent with this, community pharmacy practitioners must demonstrate a more patient-oriented attitude which will improve the image of pharmacy. In this atmosphere, properly structured externships could provide an invaluable source of needed student experiences. Likewise, all segments of pharmacy must develop and foster a philosophy of service, pride and *esprit de corps* which is essential in any profession.

Admission to pharmacy schools must become competitive to ensure that properly motivated students enter the profession. Similarly, pharmacy educators must assume a more responsible role in educating students. As part of this, curriculum reforms must be instituted to provide the preclinical education necessary for a training period in the clinical environment.

In the clinical facility, student activities should provide a service which contributes to the patient's well-being. Also, effective interaction with physicians and other health personnel should be an integral part of the program. Effective interaction will demonstrate the need for the pharmacist in the clinical environment and hasten his acceptance as part of the health care team.

Finally, the patient interview can be used by clinical educators as a test of the adequacy of the student's preclinical training because it integrates all aspects of knowledge and skills which are required of the pharmacist to function in the clinical environment.

### References

1. Anon.: ASHP-AACP Program Adds Insight Into Patient-Oriented Pharmacy, *ASHP Newsletter 4*:2 (Sept.) 1971.
2. Derzon, R. A.: Should the Role of the Pharmacist Be Redefined?, *In* Proceedings of an Invitational Workshop on Pharmacy Manpower, DHEW Publication No. (HSM) 72-3000 (Sept.) 1970, p. 12.
3. Lemberger, A. P.: Standing Committee Reports: Committee on Curriculum, *Amer. J. Pharm. Ed. 32*:435 (Aug.) 1968.

4. Gonzales, Sister M.: An Added Dimension. . . , *Amer. J. Hosp. Pharm. 28*:496 (July) 1971.

5. Groth, P. E.: Outpatients' Use of Medications: Survey of Attitudes and Behavior of Selected Iowans, Thesis for the Master of Science Degree, University of Iowa (Aug.) 1970.

6. Covington, T. R. and Whitney, H. A. K., Jr.: Patient-Pharmacist Communication Techniques, *Drug Intel. Clin. Pharm. 5*:370 (Nov.) 1971.

7. Ulan, M. S.: The Future of the Health Care System, *Amer. J. Pharm. Ed. 32*:724 (Dec.) 1968.

8. Miller, R. A.: Experiences at a School of Pharmacy Within a Health Center, *Amer. J. Pharm. Ed. 32*:772 (Dec.) 1968.

9. Thompson, C. O. et al.: Pharmaceutical Communications in the Clinical Environment, *Amer. J. Hosp. Pharm. 27*:277 (Apr.) 1970.

10. Francke, D. E.: Medicines, Medical Care, Manpower and Mankind, *Amer. J. Hosp. Pharm. 28*:410 (June) 1971.

11. Durant, W. J. and Zilz, D.A.: Some Deficiencies of the Pharmacist in the Clinical Environment, *Amer. J. Hosp. Pharm. 25*:172 (June) 1968.

12. Francke, D. E.: Let's Separate Pharmacies and Drugstores, *Amer. J. Pharm. 141*:161 (Sept.-Oct.) 1969.

13. Herfindal, E. T. and Levin, R. H.: Clinical Pharmacy Training in an Outpatient Clinic, *Amer. J. Pharm. Ed. 36*:72 (Feb.) 1972.

14. Hirschman, J. L. and Maudlin, R. K.: Drug Information Analysis Service—The DIAS Rounds, *Drug Intel. Clin. Pharm. 4*:10 (Jan.) 1970.

15. Anon.: Foreword to the Proceedings, *Amer. J. Hosp. Pharm. 28*:843 (Nov.) 1971.

# 29 Drug Defaulting Part I: Determinants of Compliance

James R. Boyd, Tim R. Covington, Walter F. Stanaszek, and R. Timothy Coussons

Literature reports on drug defaulting—failure of a patient to comply with the physician's directions for taking prescribed medication—are reviewed.

The reports are categorized according to method of determining compliance: (1) urine testing, (2) dosage unit counting, and (3) patient interviews. Reports on measurement of comprehension and efforts to improve compliance are also reviewed.

Comprehension and recall of prescription directions, as determinants of compliance, are discussed. Pharmacists can have an impact on comprehension through patient education efforts and attempts to inform physicians of the need for complete directions on written prescriptions.

Drug defaulting by ambulatory patients, a public health problem of great significance, is becoming an increasing concern of pharmacists as their logical role in promoting patient compliance to a prescribed drug regimen continues to develop. The drug defaulting dilemma, although well documented, has not been sufficiently analyzed and understood as evidenced by the paucity of activity directed toward the solution of the problem. A contribution to therapeutic compliance by ambulatory patients can be made by pharmacists as they better appreciate and understand this complex problem, including the social and behavioral aspects of medication consumption.

In order to provide better appreciation and understanding of this complex problem, this chapter will present a review of previous studies and present a model of many of the determinants of compliance in a manner which will illustrate the interrelationship between these factors. For the purpose of identifying the problem, the following definition is offered:

> *Drug defaulting* is the failure to comply (intentional or accidental) with the physician's directions (expressed or implied) in the self-administration of any medication.

This definition is not to be confused with medication errors committed by health professionals in prescribing, dispensing or administering medication to institutionalized patients or with problems of self-medication with nonprescription drugs by ambulatory patients.

The problem of drug defaulting has undoubtedly existed since the first crude extracts were prescribed by ancient physicians. The significance of this problem, however, was probably not realized until the twentieth century with the beginning of chemotherapy. One of the first reports on drug defaulting was published in 1954 by Jenkins.[1] Although quite limited in scope, this study revealed that the "average patient" takes only about one-half of the doses prescribed. This finding remains consistent with most subsequent investigations.

## Methods of Investigation

Three basic mechanisms have been utilized to study drug defaulting patterns: (1) urine testing, (2) dosage unit counting and (3) patient interviews. Each method has inherent advantages and disadvantages and varies as to the nature of the results obtained. Theoretically, a combination of all three methods would prove most valuable; however, the magnitude of this methodology is generally prohibitive.

*(1) Urine Testing.* In studies of a group of patients taking the same drug for which a suitable analytical procedure is available, compliance can be measured by the presence of the drug or its metabolite(s) in the urine. This method has been applied to several studies of patients taking the antitubercular drugs isoniazid and/or aminosalicylic acid.[2-16] Similarly, urine testing has been used in studies of patients taking penicillin,[17-21] phenylbutazone,[22] and chlorpromazine and imipramine.[23]

Although urine testing provides an objective measurement of consumption, a quantitative measurement is usually lacking. The presence of the drug in the urine fails to differentiate between underdosing and overdosing, and gives little insight into the overall rate of consumption.

(2) *Dosage Unit Counts.* The technique of providing an exact quantity of medication to the patient and counting the number of remaining doses at a later time has been used in many compliance studies.[1,6,7,15,17,21,24-32] This method provides an advantage over the urine test method in that presumed total consumption may be determined. The basic assumption of this method is that the medication that is removed from the container is consumed by the patient, hopefully in the manner prescribed. Wide variation has been reported in the range of error allowed in determining compliance. When comparing the results of urine tests and dosage unit counts in the same patient, a significant difference is frequently noted.[6,10,17,30] This discrepancy may be explained by overdosage or underdosage on a continuous basis which is not evident in the urine tests.

The dosage unit count method will fail to identify problems of noncompliance when the contents of the bottle are consumed in an erratic manner, disposed of, shared with others or otherwise not properly consumed by the patient.

When dealing with liquid medications, a large error of dosage measured by the patient may be attributed to the variation in measuring devices. One study investigating the liquid capacity of teaspoons used to administer medications found a range of 2.8 ml to 4.2 ml.[21] This physical error must be evaluated in a different manner than other types of noncompliance.

(3) *Patient Interview.* Although urine testing and dosage unit counts are more objective means of directly measuring compliance, the personal interview has been used either alone or in combination with other methods.[17,21,24-27,30,32-36] The major advantage of the interview is that it permits a more in-depth study of subtle types of errors.

The inherent disadvantage of the patient interview is reliance upon the patient to respond truthfully. Mechanisms for checking the reliability of responses (i.e., dosage count) have been built into several studies.[17,21,24-27,30] In comparing verbal reports to dosage unit counts a discrepancy often exists, but it has been found that accuracy is not seriously in error when noncompliance is large.[30] Another mechanism to improve accuracy of interviews includes phrasing questions and conducting interviews in a manner that does not impose guilt upon the patient. The investigator must be familiar with interviewing techniques for proper interpretation of responses.[37] The pharmacist's ability to detect previously ignored factors in the patient's medication history is documented elsewhere in this book.[38]

**Drug Defaulting—Previous Findings**

The wide variation of defaulting rates as previously mentioned is summarized in Tables 1, 2 and 3. Table 1 summarizes the results of 18 studies of noncompliance in tuberculosis patients as evidenced by negative urine tests. Over 50% of the studies reported a noncompliance rate between 21% and 40% of the population studied.

Although these studies cannot be directly compared due to variations in methodologies and definitions of noncompliance, a weighted mean based on the number of noncompliant patients in each study is approximately 36%.

Table 2 summarizes the results of 12 studies utilizing the dosage unit count method to determine noncompliance. The range of defaulting reported is from 11% for a group of 162 patients to 87% for a group of 30. Over half of the studies reported defaulting rates between 25% and 51%. The weighted mean of all studies cited reveals approximately 47% noncompliance.

Table 3 summarizes the results of eight studies based on patient reporting in interviews. The defaulting rates reported range from 17% for a sample of 59 patients to 90% for a sample of 40 patients. Over half of the studies reveal a defaulting rate between 27% and 59%. The weighted mean of all studies cited indicates approximately a 38% noncompliance rate. Although a wide variation of results has been reported, the total evidence serves well to document the problem of drug defaulting.

**Association of Demographic Variables with Compliance**

Most drug defaulting studies have attempted to detect relationships between noncompliance and demographic variables. The literature fails, in most cases, to offer any consistent conclusions.

The majority of studies fail to find a significant difference in defaulting patterns between age groups. The exceptions to this general finding indicate increasing noncompliance with increasing age.[26,33,35] One study suggested a decrease in error rate through the 71–80 year age group, followed by a substantial increase in the 81–90 year group. The lower error rate in the 71–80 year age group was attributed to "fewer daily distractions in their lives."[24] The effects of aging on compliance could easily be multiple in nature and require more detailed research.

Several studies have indicated that females are more likely to discontinue taking their medications than males.[5,9,11,16] Most investigators, however, could not find a significant difference between the sexes in drug defaulting.[10,18,23,26,41]

Increased education was found to have no effect on compliance in four studies,[10,19,26,34] however, a positive effect has also been reported.[11] In general, defaulting has been found to increase with increases in duration of treatment,[7,9,17,24] number of concurrent medications,[10,24,26,34] and total number of daily doses.[1,24]

The effects of socioeconomic status on defaulting rates have also been investigated. The conclusions, however, remain obscure. Most studies have failed to show a significant difference in defaulting rates between socioeconomic groups.[7,10,11,33] There is, however, some evidence that a higher incidence of defaulting is found in lower socioeconomic groups.[33] A major problem in studying socioeconomic influences is the lack of a balanced socioeconomic distribution in any given study population.

**Table 1. Drug Defaulting Rates in Various Studies of Tuberculosis Patients Taking Isoniazid and/or Aminosalicylic Acid as Determined by Negative Urine Tests for the Drugs**

| INVESTIGATOR | DRUG | NO. OF PATIENTS | % DE-FAULT-ING[a] |
|---|---|---|---|
| Berry[2] | INH | 26 | 6 |
| | PAS | 26 | 8 |
| Breite[3] | PAS | 76 | 65 |
| Chaves[4] | PAS | 2622 | 40 |
| Dixon[5] | PAS | 151 | 50 |
| Fox[6] | PAS | 79 | 4 |
| Ireland[7] | PAS | 87 | 18 |
| Leggat[8] | PAS | 50 | 22 |
| Luntz[9] | PAS | 705 | 34 |
| Maddock[10] | INH | 50 | 19 |
| | PAS | 33 | 33 |
| Marrow[11] | INH | 350 | 32 |
| Pitman[12] | PAS | 61 | 41 |
| Preston[13] | PAS/INH | 25 | 28 |
| Simpson[14] | PAS | 100 | 23 |
| Velu[15] | INH | 27 | 23 |
| | INH | 35 | 21 |
| Wynn-Williams[16] | PAS | 153 | 21 |

[a] Criteria for determining defaulting rates vary.

**Table 2. Drug Defaulting Rates in Various Studies as Determined by Dosage Unit Count Methods**

| INVESTIGATOR | DRUG | NO. OF PATIENTS | % DE-FAULTING[a] |
|---|---|---|---|
| Arnhold[32] | Penicillin | 104 | 19 |
| Bergman[17] | Penicillin | 59 | 82 |
| Clinite[24] | Mixed | 30 | 87[b] |
| Feinstein[25] | Penicillin | 109 | 45 |
| | Sulfadiazine | 120 | 56 |
| Jenkins[1] | Mixed | 22 | 50 |
| Leistyna[21] | Penicillin | 162 | 11[b] |
| Libow[39] | Placebo | 20 | 25 |
| Lipman[27] | Meprobamate | 125 | 42 |
| | Placebo | 129 | 49 |
| Nugent[28] | Prednisolone | 20 | 25 |
| Park[40] | Imipramine | 36 | 51 |
| Porter[29] | Mixed | 301 | 77 |
| Velu[15] | Calcium | 58 | 19 |
| | INH | 62 | 20 |

[a] Criteria for determining defaulting rates vary.
[b] Data obtained from dosage unit count and interview.

**Table 3. Drug Defaulting Rates of Various Studies as Determined by Patient Report**

| INVESTIGATOR | DRUG | NO. OF PATIENTS | % DE-FAULTING[a] |
|---|---|---|---|
| Bergman[17] | Penicillin | 59 | 17 |
| Clinite[24] | Mixed | 30 | 87[b] |
| Feinstein[25] | Penicillin | 113 | 27 |
| | Sulfadiazine | 126 | 33 |
| Latiolais[26] | Mixed | 180 | 43[b] |
| Malahy[34] | Mixed | 40 | 90 |
| Mohler[33] | Penicillin | 245 | 34 |
| Porter[29] | Mixed | 301 | 25 |
| Schwartz[35] | Mixed | 178 | 59 |

[a] Criteria for determining defaulting rates vary.
[b] Data obtained by interview and dosage unit count.

Comparisons among studies with similar parameters for determining compliance indicate a lower defaulting rate in a private practice setting as compared to a clinic setting.[17,21] Assuming a socioeconomic difference between the populations, the data suggest increasing compliance in the higher socioeconomic group. It is, however, quite possible that the differences found are more appropriately attributed to the practice setting and the influence of the providers of health care. In one study in private practice by Leistyna et al.,[21] each patient was given a detailed information sheet explaining the importance of continuing the medication as prescribed. It is not surprising, therefore, that the defaulting rate was found to be a low 11%.

**Measurements of Comprehension**

In order to obtain a more thorough understanding of the problem of drug defaulting, it would seem logical to measure the patient's comprehension of directions for use of the medication. Only seven of the studies reviewed, however, made any reference to the patient's comprehension.[10,17,18,21,26,27,36]

Maddock found that 90% of the patients studied "understood perfectly the directions" for use of the medication.[10] Bergman states that "95% were familiar with the proper directions."[17] Stewart defined comprehension as knowing the name and purpose of the drug. Only 37.5% correctly identified the medication, while 86.2% knew the general purpose of the medication.[36] Charney found that all 96 of his patients knew the correct dosage.[18] Leistyna states that "those parents who failed to give the medication (to the child) seemed to comprehend the original instructions."[21]

Only one drug defaulting study directly addressed itself to a formal inquiry into comprehension. Although the mechanism and parameters used were not disclosed, Arnhold et al. found only four of 104 patients who "seemed to have misunderstood the instructions."[32] Latiolais and Berry attributed 33.3% of the patient errors structions.[26] Obviously, lacking any formal parameters to measure comprehension, it is difficult to draw valid conclusions from the above data.

A study by Hermann, which appears later in this volume, suggests that ambulatory patients are generally incapable of establishing an appropriate schedule for medication administration given b.i.d., t.i.d. or q.i.d. directions. As contrasted with directions specifying a given hourly interval, these directives rely on the patient to establish the timing of administration. Findings indicated that for 15.5% of the directions given, patients were completely unable to interpret the implied schedule, and interpretations of 33.3% of the directions varied greatly among patients.[42]

**Mechanisms of Improving Compliance**

Pratt et al. found that physicians overestimate the level of medical knowledge in a patient population and that patients generally make no aggressive demand for more information.[43] It is, therefore, necessary for the physician to develop a better understanding of the patient's level of medical knowledge and to provide additional information, as patients given more thorough explanations were found to be more compliant.[43]

A later chapter in this section documents that through therapeutic counseling by a pharmacist prior to hospital discharge, patients make fewer self-administration errors.[44] It should be noted, however, that counseling is "not simply a matter of giving clear instructions or labeling medications."[32] Validation of patient understanding by questioning must be included in the discussion.

In studying public attitudes toward physicians and pharmacists in the dissemination of health information, Knapp found the physician to be more readily accepted. In further study, however, it was found that after presentation of the pharmacist's capabilities, he became equal to the physician in knowledgability, in the eyes of the lay person.[45]

> Thus, it would appear that efforts aimed at informing the public about the educational background of pharmacists could improve their credibility, perceived expertise, and overall effectiveness in areas involving drugs . . .[45]

The use of fear arousal or threatening techniques has been studied as to its effectiveness in counseling patients:

> Fear-producing messages generated the desired effects among lower socioeconomic status groups, and more reassuring messages had better results among higher socioeconomic status groups.[46]

Based on the findings previously noted in the literature, it appears that one primary aspect of the drug defaulting problem has been neglected. Does the patient have adequate comprehension of the directions for use of the medication? If noncompliance is related to insufficient information, the cause of the drug defaulting lies in the inadequacies of the health care delivery system and not solely in the patient. To further examine the roles of the physician, the pharmacist and the patient in achieving compliance, the following model was developed to serve as a basis for determining which links in this complex chain of events are weak.

### Determinants of Compliance

The fundamental prerequisite to compliance in the use of prescription medications is a thorough understanding of the directions for use. Initial comprehension must then be maintained throughout the duration of therapy. Both comprehension and recall of directions are prerequisites to compliance. Successful achievement of the goal of compliance involves a complex interaction among the patient, the physician, and the pharmacist,

each having duties and responsibilities to the other (see Figure 1).

*Comprehension.* To examine the determinants of comprehension, one must identify the contributions of each party to establishing a given level of comprehension in the patient. The responsibility for establishing the dosing schedule generally belongs to the prescribing physician. Undoubtedly, most physicians provide directions; the written description of the dosing schedule and related information is not always adequate, however. Elements of the directions are frequently implied but not expressed to the patient. The physician and other health professionals, being quite familiar with the proper use of medication, may fail to appreciate the patient's level of understanding. For example, consider a mother receiving a prescription for ampicillin suspension for a child's earache. It is not beyond possibility for the medication to be instilled into the child's ear rather than being administered by the desired oral route. In order to avoid such problems, we suggest six essential elements of complete directions for proper self-administration: (1) amount of drug to be taken in a single dose, (2) total number of doses to be taken daily, (3) the timing or sequence of administration of the medication, (4) the route of administration (5) the purpose of the medication and (6) the name of the medication. Although there is frequently additional information which should be given to the patient, these six elements are common to all prescriptions.

The pharmacist, being an intermediate party to this relationship, is often placed in a rather difficult position. Being the provider of the medication, he has the responsibility to insure that the patient understands the direc-

Figure 1. Determinants of compliance

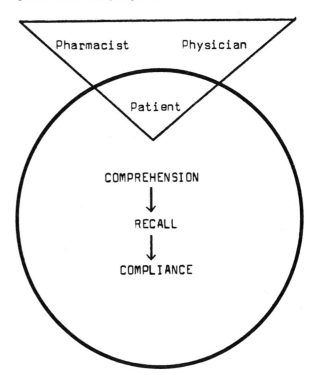

tions for proper usage. If complete directions are provided by the physician, the pharmacist must provide this information on the prescription label in a manner easily interpreted by the patient. Ideally, the pharmacist should reinforce the written directions with verbal instructions. A second, and probably more common, situation often faces the pharmacist. When presented a prescription with incomplete directions, the pharmacist has the alternatives of perpetuating the negligence of the physician or expanding the directions based upon his professional judgment. A common example of the alternatives to this dilemma is illustrated by the following labels prepared for a prescription written for ampicillin capsules, with the directions "1 q.i.d."

A. 1 capsule 4× daily.
B. Take ONE capsule FOUR times daily, every six hours, on an empty stomach. Take all capsules until gone for infection. Ampicillin 250mg

Obviously, label B would be much more informative to the patient.

A problem, however, arises when the physician previously has verbally instructed the patient to take the medication with meals and at bedtime. This conflict should ultimately be resolved through increased dialogue between physicians and pharmacists. The principle to be investigated in this dialogue is the need for the patient to be informed of such information, and the need for it to appear on the prescription label.

The third but most vital party to this interaction is the patient. It is necessary that the patient possess the ability to understand the directives given him. Thus, in most patients comprehension is basically an educational parameter. A patient with limited or impaired mental acuity must be given directions on a level more easily understood. One cannot assume any basic knowledge on the part of the patient. When dealing with a non-English speaking or illiterate patient, appropriate labeling and counseling techniques must be utilized. Pathological conditions such as chronic brain syndrome or cerebral vascular accident must also be considered and appropriate measures instituted.

*Recall.* With respect to recall, the physician can be a strong motivating force by placing emphasis on the importance of proper self-medication in achieving a successful outcome. Positive thinking can also potentiate the placebo effect which may dominate many therapeutic regimens.

Dosage schedules, as prescribed by the physician, may also affect recall. The basis of this assumption is that a patient is more likely to recall a "once daily" medication time than three or four separate times. In a previous chapter in this section, it was advocated that longer acting drugs be used when available to minimize such problems.[47] The effect of multiple prescriptions may also contribute to the patient's difficulty in recalling which drug to take at a given time.

The pharmacist also has an opportunity to affect recall. By reinforcing the importance of proper medication usage, the impression may be more firmly set in the patient's mind. The prescription container label, however, is likely to provide the greatest influence on recall. The label, serving as a permanent record of the complete directions for use, will prevent the patient from relying completely on memory. The memory itself is strongly influenced by the label as a visual educational aid. In studies conducted to compare the effects of various educational media, subjects were found to retain only 10% of information provided solely by verbal communications, whereas 20% of visual information was retained. When information was presented by both visual and verbal means, the three-day recall level was 65%.[48] Thus, a complete prescription label in addition to appropriate verbal counseling should be an important factor in improving recall.

The patient-related factor in recall is basically the patient's perceived importance of the proper use of the medication. Educationally, this is dependent upon the information provided by the physician and the pharmacist. There are, however, behavioral factors involved in the patient's belief in, reliance upon and retention of such information. The type and severity of pathology may also affect the patient's capability to recall information.

*Compliance.* As previously stated, compliance should be directly dependent on comprehension and recall of instructions, the above factors being influenced largely by the providers of health care. The actual act of compliance is, nevertheless, ultimately dependent upon the individual patient. The behavioral characteristics which dictate the overt act of compliance or noncompliance are factors which are often beyond outside influence. Another patient-related factor influencing compliance is financial status which may dictate the patient's fiscal inability to comply.

## Summary

The problem of drug defaulting has been explored through review of numerous studies in the medical and pharmaceutical literature. Examination of the factors which influence compliance indicate those areas in which the pharmacist has the greatest opportunity to contribute to patient education. Although lack of comprehension is only one of many factors which contribute to noncompliance, it is an easily remedied problem. Pharmacists have a dual opportunity to affect this problem by (1) aggressive efforts to fill the gaps in patient education and (2) efforts to educate physicians of the need for more complete directions on written prescriptions.

## References

1. Jenkins, B. W.: Are Patients True to TID and QID Doses?, *GP 9*:66–69 (June) 1954.
2. Berry, D. et al.: Self-Medication Behavior as Measured by Urine Chemical Tests in Domiciliary Tuberculous Patients, *Amer. Rev. Resp. Dis. 86*:1–7 (July) 1962.

3. Breite, M. J.: Urine Test for the Detection of PAS in Ambulatory Tuberculous Patients, *Amer. Rev. Resp. Dis. 79*:672 (May) 1959.

4. Chaves, A. D.: Results of the PAS Urine Test (Phenistix) Study Done in May and June, 1959, *Amer. Rev. Resp. Dis. 81*:111-112 (Jan.) 1960.

5. Dixon, W. M., Stradling, P. and Wootton, I. D. P.: Outpatient PAS Therapy, *Lancet 2*:871-872 (Nov. 2) 1957.

6. Fox, W.: The Problem of Self-Administration of Drugs with Particular Reference to Pulmonary Tuberculosis, *Tubercle 39*:269-274 (Oct.) 1958.

7. Ireland, H. S.: Outpatient Chemotherapy for Tuberculosis, *Amer. Rev. Resp. Dis. 82*:378-383 (Sept.) 1960.

8. Leggat, P. O.: PAS and the Patient, *Lancet 2*:1283 (Dec. 21) 1957.

9. Luntz, G. R. W. N., and Austin, R.: New Stick Test for PAS in Urine, *Brit. Med. J. 1*:1679-1684 (June 4) 1960.

10. Maddock, R. K.: Patient Cooperation in Taking Medicines, *J. Amer. Med. Ass. 199*:137-140 (Jan. 16) 1967.

11. Marrow, R. and Rabin, D. L.: Reliability in Self-Medication with Isoniazid, *Clin. Res. 14*:362 (Apr.) 1966.

12. Pitman, E. R. et al.: Clinic Experience with a Urine PAS Test, *Dis. Chest 36*:1-2 (July) 1959.

13. Preston, D. F. and Miller, F. L.: The Tuberculosis Outpatient's Defection from Therapy, *Amer. J. Med. Sci. 247*:21-25 (Jan.) 1964.

14. Simpson, J. M.: Simple Test for the Detection of Urinary PAS, *Tubercle 37*:333-340 (Oct.) 1956.

15. Velu, S. et al.: Progress in the Second Year of Patients with Quiescent Pulmonary Tuberculosis after a Year of Chemotherapy at Home or in Sanatorium, and Influence of Further Chemotherapy on Relapse Rate, *Bull. WHO 23*:511-533, 1960.

16. Wynn-Williams, N. and Arris, M.: On Omitting PAS, *Tubercle 39*:138-142 (June) 1968.

17. Bergman, A. B. and Werner, R. J.: Failure of Children to Receive Penicillin by Mouth, *N. Engl. J. Med. 268*:1334-1338 (June 13) 1963.

18. Charney, E. et al.: How Well Do Patients Take Oral Penicillin? A Collaborative Study in Private Practice, *Pediatrics 40*:188-195 (Aug.) 1967.

19. Gordis, L. et al.: Studies in the Epidemiology and Preventability of Rheumatic Fever. Part 4. A Quantitative Determination of Compliance in Children on Oral Penicillin Prophylaxis, *Pediatrics 43*:173-182 (Feb.) 1969.

20. Gordis, L. et al.: The Inaccuracy in Using Interviews to Estimate Patient Reliability in Taking Medications at Home, *Med. Care 7*:49-54 (Jan.-Feb.) 1969.

21. Leistyna, J. A. and Macaulay, J. C.: Therapy of Streptococcal Infections. Do Pediatric Patients Receive Prescribed Oral Medications?, *Amer. J. Dis. Child. 111*:22-26 (Jan.) 1966.

22. Joyce, C. R. B.: Patient Cooperation and the Sensitivity of Clinical Trials, *J. Chron. Dis. 15*:1025-1036 (Nov.) 1962.

23. Willcox, D. R. C. et al.: Do Psychiatric Outpatients Take Their Drugs?, *Brit. Med. J. 2*:790-792 (Oct. 2) 1965.

24. Clinite, J. C. and Kabat, H. F.: Errors During Self-Administration, *J. Amer. Phar. Ass. NS9*:450-452 (Sept.) 1969.

25. Feinstein, A. R. et al.: Controlled Study of Three Methods of Prophylaxis Against Streptococcal Infection in a Population of Rheumatic Children, *N. Engl. J. Med. 260*:697-702 (Apr. 2) 1959.

26. Latiolais, C. J. and Berry, C. C.: Misuse of Prescription Medications by Outpatients, *Drug Intel. Clin. Pharm. 3*:270-277 (Oct.) 1969.

27. Lipman, R. S. et al.: Neurotics Who Fail to Take Their Drugs, *Brit. J. Psychiat. 111*:1043-1049 (Nov.) 1965.

28. Nugent, C. A. et al.: Glucocorticoid Toxicity; Single Contrasted with Divided Daily Doses of Prednisolone, *J. Chron. Dis. 18*:323-332 (Apr.) 1965.

29. Porter, A. M. W.: Drug Defaulting in a General Practice, *Brit. Med. J. 1*:218-222 (Jan. 25) 1969.

30. Rickels, K. and Briscoe, E.: Assessment of Dosage Deviation In Outpatient Drug Research, *J. Clin. Pharmacol. 11*:153-160 (May-June) 1970.

31. Roth, H. P. and Berger, D. G.: Studies on Patient Cooperation in Ulcer Treatment, *Gastroenterology 38*:630-633 (Apr. 4) 1960.

32. Arnhold, R. G. et al.: Patients and Prescriptions: Comprehension and Compliance with Medical Instructions in a Suburban Pediatric Practice, *Clin. Ped. 9*:648-651 (Nov.) 1970.

33. Mohler, D. N. et al.: Studies in the Home Treatment of Streptococcal Disease, *N. Engl. J. Med. 252*:1116-1118 (June 30) 1955.

34. Malahy, B.: The Effect of Instruction and Labeling on the Number of Medication Errors Made by Patients at Home, *Amer. J. Hosp. Pharm. 23*:283-292 (June) 1966.

35. Schwartz, D. et al.: Medication Errors Made by Elderly, Chronically Ill Patients, *Amer. J. Pub. Health, 52*:2018-2029 (Dec.) 1962.

36. Stewart, R. B. and Cluff, L. E.: A Review of Medication Errors and Compliance in Ambulant Patients, *Clin. Pharmacol. Ther. 13*:463-468 (July-Aug.) 1972.

37. Francke, D. E. and Whitney, H. A. K.: Perspectives in Clinical Pharmacy, Drug Intelligence Publications, Hamilton, Illinois, 1972, pp. 226-227.

38. Covington, T. R. and Pfeiffer, F. G.: The Pharmacist-Acquired Medication History, In *Clinical Pharmacy Sourcebook*, pp. 351-354.

39. Libow, L. S. and Mehl, B.: Self-Administration of Medications by Patients in Hospitals or Extended Care Facilities, *J. Amer. Geriat. Soc. 18*:81-85 (Jan.) 1970.

40. Park, L. C. and Lipman, R. S.: A Comparison of Patient Dosage Deviation Reports with Pill Counts, *Psychopharmacologia 6*:299-302 (May) 1964.

41. Davis, M. S.: Physiologic, Psychological and Demographic Factors in Patient Compliance with Doctors' Orders, *Med. Care 6*:115-122 (Mar.-Apr.) 1968.

42. Hermann, F.: The Outpatient Prescription Label as a Source of Medication Errors, In *Clinical Pharmacy Sourcebook*, pp. 175-179.

43. Pratt, L. et al.: Physicians Views on the Level of Medical Information Among Patients, *Amer. J. Public Health 47*:1277-1283 (Oct.) 1957.

44. Cole, P. and Sister Emmanuel: Drug Consultation: Its Significance to the Discharged Hospital Patient and Its Relevance as a Role for the Pharmacist, In *Clinical Pharmacy Sourcebook*, pp. 168-174.

45. Knapp, D. E. and Knapp, D. A.: Perceived Credibility, Expertise and Effectiveness: Pharmacist vs. Physician, *Soc. Sci. Med. 4*:253-256 (Aug.) 1970.

46. Holder, L.: Effects of Source, Message, Audience Characteristics on Health Behavior Compliance, *Health Serv. Rep. 87*:343-350 (Apr.) 1972.

47. Ivey, M.: The Pharmacist in the Care of the Ambulatory Mental Health Patient, In *Clinical Pharmacy Sourcebook*, pp. 125-128.

48. Meyer, J., 3-M Corporation, personal correspondence, October 7, 1972.

# 30 Drug Defaulting Part II: Analysis of Noncompliance Patterns

James R. Boyd, Tim R. Covington, Walter F. Stanaszek, and
R. Timothy Coussons

A study was conducted among outpatients of a teaching hospital to determine (1) the extent of drug defaulting, (2) the clinical significance of specific errors, and (3) the interrelationship among several variables.

The study included 134 patients who received 380 prescriptions. The study instrument was an in-depth personal interview of the patient at home seven to ten days after his clinic visit.

Only 22% of the prescriptions studied were being consumed properly and 31% were being misutilized in a manner that posed a serious threat to the patients' health. The most frequent errors concerned improper dosing intervals and premature discontinuance of medication. A positive relationship was found between prescription label information provided and patient comprehension of directions, and between comprehension and compliance. It was concluded that a major contributing factor to the drug defaulting problem was lack of complete and comprehensible directions from either the pharmacist or the physician. It is suggested that pharmacists can play a dual role in minimizing the drug defaulting problem by providing complete label information to the patient and by influencing physicians to include on prescriptions more complete directions for proper self-administration of medications.

This chapter will present the findings of a study conducted to investigate the relationships between a group of variables and compliance.

The objectives of this study were to:

1. Determine the incidence of noncompliance by specific type of error in the study population.
2. Determine the clinical significance of various errors of noncompliance.
3. Measure comprehension of directions for self administration.
4. Determine the relationship between these variables: a. label information and comprehension, b. comprehension and compliance, and c. demographic variables and compliance.

## Methodology

This research was conducted between July 1 and September 30, 1972, in cooperation with the Outpatient Clinics, Department of Medicine, University of Oklahoma Health Sciences Center. Although patients treated in this department come from throughout the state, subjects were limited to those living within the greater Oklahoma City area (within approximately a 20-mile radius of the University of Oklahoma Health Services Center). This restriction was imposed to enable the investigator to visit each patient at home. Socioeconomically, the majority of the population studied were medically indigent patients unable to obtain health care services from the private sector. Although the economic status of the patients was not determined directly, the Hollingshead Two-Factor Index of Social Position was utilized.[1] This tool is used to define five socioeconomic classes based on the subject's education and occupation.

Selection of subjects from the clinic patients each day was based upon: (1) receipt of one or more written prescription(s) at a clinic visit, (2) living in the defined geographical area and (3) being available for interview when contacted by the investigator. Physicians were provided duplicate prescription blanks for all prescriptions written during the study. The carbon copy of each prescription was placed in the patient's chart by the physician. The investigator collected the prescription copies each evening and submitted a request for the charts of those patients living within the geographical limitations of the study.

The age, sex, race, clinic visited and diagnosis were recorded from the chart. It was further determined what medications, other than those for which a new prescription had been written, the patient should be taking. In each case all medications in the patient's current regimen, as indicated by the chart, were studied. Patients were classified by pathology into one of 17 major groups based on the International Classification of Diseases.[2]

The patient was visited in his home within seven to ten days after his clinic visit, all interviews being conducted by the principal investigator. This time interval was selected so as to include short-term therapy while allowing enough time for the patient to establish his pattern of medication utilization.

The interview was conducted in an informal manner. The patient was first asked to bring all of his prescribed medication(s) into the room and was told that we would like to discuss his drug therapy. The interview proceeded considering one medication at a time, first measuring comprehension, then compliance and finally the miscellaneous information.

Great effort was made to ask questions at a level easily understood by the patient. When possible, open-ended questions were asked in an attempt to elicit a more spontaneous, complete and truthful response. Proper phrasing of questions was necessary so as not to impose a feeling of guilt upon the patient, thus prompting a false response. For example, asking a patient, "Do you ever skip a dose?" will often elicit a negative response. However, by asking, "How often do you skip a dose?" the patient is more inclined to respond truthfully.

In spite of the inadequacies of the interview procedure, it remains the only mechanism available for both qualitative and quantitative assessment of the drug defaulting problem. Undoubtedly, relying on patient reports will tend to underestimate the degree of the problem of drug defaulting. It is felt, however, that this inadequacy is overcome by the depth of inquiry obtainable through the interview. We also believe that the inadequacies of the interview procedure are minimized by our considerable clinical experience in interviewing the type of population studied.

An objective check evaluating the validity of patient responses was available to the investigator at the time of the interview. The number of tablets or capsules remaining in the container could be counted as a check on total consumption. This was not possible in all cases, as many prescriptions were refills or samples. It should be noted that because no outpatient pharmacy services were available at the clinic, all patients were patrons of various community pharmacies. In some cases, patients were provided unknown quantities of samples by the prescribing physicians. The bottle contents were counted in all cases, however, to indicate to the patient that his accuracy in reporting was being checked. This check served as the basis for further probing when the investigator determined that false responses were being given. The interview was concluded with a discussion of the patient's therapy with positive reinforcement of the necessity for proper technique of self-medication.

Appendix A shows the interview form used to measure comprehension and compliance. Comprehension was indicated as either correct, incorrect or no knowledge. Appendix B indicates the criteria for determining noncompliance. The clinical significance of the error was indicated for the specific error committed. The criteria for defining the clinical significance of an error is listed in Appendix C.

In addition to the interview data, the prescription label information and the written prescription directions were recorded (Appendix D). The copy of the original prescription order and the prescription container label were examined for the inclusion of the six elements of the directions previously mentioned (Appendix B).

## Results and Discussion

Data were collected on 380 prescriptions from 134 patients. The individual prescription, rather than the patient, is the study unit for purposes of data presentation. Patient characteristics are therefore duplicated for patients taking more than one prescription drug.

*The Patient Population.* Table 1 compares the absolute and relative distribution of demographic variables of the prescription and patient populations. Approximately two-thirds of the patient population was female, over three-fourths was over 45 years of age, and slightly over one-half was white. Approximately three-fourths of the population studied was classified as Hollingshead Social Class V. Comparison of the patient population with the prescription population reveals very close correlation. Patients with circulatory diseases, primarily hypertension and congestive heart failure, appear to take slightly more medications per patient than the other disease groups; however, statistical analysis of this discrepancy indicates no significance at $p = 0.05$.

During the study period, 6,570 patients from the Oklahoma City area were seen in the clinics utilized in this study. Preliminary information from the prescription copy and the patient chart was collected on 194 patients. Six patients were eliminated from the study because of a history of acute psychiatric disturbance. Of the remaining 188 patients, interviews were conducted with 134. Several patients could not be located due to an incorrect address, several others had moved, and the remainder could not be found at home or contacted by phone on at least two consecutive days. Due to the fact that attempts to contact patients occurred during the day, the population studied may be under-represented by working patients and over-represented by the elderly, the unemployed and housewives. The 134 patients selected represented 8.53% of the patients eligible for inclusion in the study by geographic limitations. Assuming that patients were seen that did not receive any prescriptions at a clinic visit, the 134 patients studied almost certainly represent over 10% of the patients receiving prescriptions during the study period.

*Significance of Drug Defaulting.* Table 2 indicates the incidence and significance classification of specific self-administration errors. Significance group 1 represents no errors and groups 2, 3 and 4 represent increasing degrees

**Table 1. Distribution of Demographic Variables in Patient and Prescription Populations**

| VARIABLE | PATIENTS (N = 134) | | PRESCRIP-TIONS (N = 380) | |
|---|---|---|---|---|
| | N | % | N | % |
| *Sex* | | | | |
| Male | 45 | 33.6 | 118 | 31.1 |
| Female | 89 | 66.4 | 262 | 68.9 |
| | 134 | 100 | 380 | 100 |
| *Age* | | | | |
| Under 24 | 3 | 2.24 | 4 | 1.05 |
| 25–44 | 26 | 19.4 | 85 | 22.4 |
| 45–64 | 63 | 47.0 | 184 | 48.4 |
| 65 and over | 42 | 31.3 | 107 | 28.2 |
| | 134 | 100 | 380 | 100 |
| *Race* | | | | |
| White | 73 | 54.5 | 213 | 56.0 |
| Black | 55 | 41.0 | 145 | 38.2 |
| Native American | 5 | 3.73 | 19 | 5.00 |
| Other | 1 | 0.75 | 3 | 0.79 |
| | 134 | 100 | 380 | 100 |
| *Social class* | | | | |
| I or II | 1 | 0.75 | 1 | 0.26 |
| III | 7 | 5.22 | 21 | 5.53 |
| IV | 27 | 20.2 | 82 | 21.6 |
| V | 99 | 73.9 | 276 | 72.6 |
| | 134 | 100 | 380 | 100 |
| *Clinic* | | | | |
| General medicine | 100 | 74.6 | 264 | 69.5 |
| New medicine | 6 | 4.48 | 15 | 3.95 |
| Cardiology | 7 | 5.22 | 29 | 7.63 |
| Renal-metabolic | 1 | 0.75 | 3 | 0.79 |
| Hypertension | 9 | 6.72 | 30 | 7.89 |
| Oncology | 4 | 2.98 | 10 | 2.63 |
| Pulmonary | 6 | 4.48 | 23 | 6.05 |
| Gastrointestinal | 1 | 0.75 | 6 | 1.58 |
| | 134 | 100 | 380 | 100 |
| *Disease* | | | | |
| Neoplastic | 1 | 0.75 | 2 | 0.53 |
| Endocrine | 14 | 10.4 | 27 | 7.11 |
| Blood | 1 | 0.75 | 1 | 0.26 |
| Mental | 9 | 6.72 | 14 | 3.68 |
| Nervous system | 7 | 5.22 | 19 | 5.0 |
| Circulatory | 70 | 52.2 | 233 | 61.3 |
| Respiratory | 15 | 11.2 | 46 | 12.1 |
| Digestive | 6 | 4.48 | 9 | 2.37 |
| Genitourinary | 9 | 2.98 | 7 | 1.84 |
| Musculoskeletal | 5 | 3.73 | 18 | 4.74 |
| Ill-defined symptoms | 2 | 1.49 | 4 | 1.05 |
| | 134 | 100 | 380 | 100 |

of significance (see Appendix C). The 0 response column indicates the 24 prescriptions not filled, thus posing no potential for errors numbered 1–10, 13 and 15. Additionally, 30 prescriptions contained p.r.n. directions and were therefore considered separately from those specifying a given frequency of administration.

Table 2 also shows the distribution of errors in the top three significance groups. The most frequently occurring error was that of improper dosing intervals which occurred on 143 of 256 prescriptions. Prematurely discontinuing the medication occurred on 116 prescriptions, doses were forgotten on 90 prescriptions and doses were knowingly skipped on 89 prescriptions. With respect to significance group, improper dosing interval, although being the most frequently occurring error, was of minor clinical significance. Of the 143 errors committed on dosing interval, 87.4% were determined to be clinically insignificant and the remaining 12.6% were of intermediate significance. The most clinically significant error was that of not having the prescription filled, being of major significance in all 24 cases. The most frequently occurring errors of major significance were associated with the 67 prescriptions which patients discontinued taking.

The significance of defaulting on each prescription was determined by the highest significance rating assigned to any specific error committed on the prescription. Table 3, therefore, indicates the distribution of prescriptions with respect to significance of errors. Errors of major clinical significance were committed on 118 prescriptions or 31% of those studied. Only 145 or 38% of the prescriptions were either taken correctly or with insignificant errors.

Table 4 indicates that the written prescription, and subsequently the prescription label, was deficient in providing information concerning timing of administration and purpose of the medication on the majority of the prescriptions studied. The greatest discrepancy between the written prescription and the label was with respect to including the name of the medication on the label. This finding clearly indicates negligence on the part of the pharmacists dispensing these prescriptions, since the prescriptions contained printed instructions for the pharmacist to label the name of the medication.

Comparing patient comprehension to the prescription label information indicates close correlation with respect to amount of single dose, number of daily doses and route of administration. With respect to timing and purpose, the patient's comprehension is found to be greater than the label information. Although many patients were able to establish an acceptable timing schedule without receiving specific label directions, the approximately 25% of the population which could not do so emphasizes the necessity to include this information. When summarizing comprehension, the patient was aware of all six elements of the directions on only 31% of the prescriptions.

Compliance was below comprehension in all cases with the exception of purpose of the medication. For 20% of the prescriptions, patients did not know the purpose of the medication, but only 3% of the prescriptions were taken for an inappropriate use. Errors of compliance relating to the number of daily doses and of timing of administration show the greatest discrepancy with comprehension. This finding suggests that inconvenience in administering a dose at a given time during a patient's daily routine is likely to lead to intentional noncompliance.

The association between label directions provided and comprehension, and between comprehension and compliance, on each of the six elements of the directions evaluated, was tested statistically using chi-square analysis. The association between label directions and com-

**Table 2. Incidence and Significance of Compliance Errors**

| | NO. ERRORS/SIGNIFICANCE GROUP | | | | | ERRORS IN TOP 3 SIGNIFICANCE GROUPS | | | |
| --- | --- | --- | --- | --- | --- | --- | --- | --- | --- |
| ERROR | 0 | 1 | 2 | 3 | 4 | TOTAL NO. | 2 | 3 | 4 |
| 1. Reduced amount of single dose | 24 | 340 | 2 | 8 | 6 | 16 | 12.5% | 50.0% | 37.5% |
| 2. Increased amount of single dose | 24 | 333 | 5 | 12 | 6 | 23 | 21.7 | 52.2 | 26.1 |
| 3. Decreased number of daily doses | 54 | 237 | 21 | 53 | 15 | 89 | 23.6 | 59.6 | 16.8 |
| 4. Increased number of daily doses | 54 | 295 | 7 | 15 | 9 | 31 | 22.6 | 48.4 | 29.0 |
| 5. Took p.r.n. dose when not needed | 350 | 28 | 0 | 1 | 1 | 2 | 0 | 50.0 | 50.0 |
| 6. Omitted p.r.n. dose when needed | 350 | 14 | 5 | 5 | 6 | 16 | 31.25 | 31.25 | 37.5 |
| 7. Improper dosing intervals | 24 | 213 | 125 | 18 | 0 | 143 | 87.4 | 12.6 | 0 |
| 8. Improper timing with meals | 24 | 354 | 0 | 2 | 0 | 2 | 0 | 100 | 0 |
| 9. Improper technique of administration | 24 | 352 | 0 | 4 | 0 | 4 | 0 | 100 | 0 |
| 10. Use of medication for wrong purpose | 24 | 346 | 8 | 1 | 1 | 10 | 80.0 | 10.0 | 10.0 |
| 11. Prescription never filled | 0 | 356 | 0 | 0 | 24 | 24 | 0 | 0 | 100 |
| 12. Taking outdated medication | 0 | 379 | 0 | 0 | 1 | 1 | 0 | 0 | 100 |
| 13. Forgot to take medication | 24 | 266 | 30 | 55 | 5 | 90 | 33.3 | 61.1 | 5.6 |
| 14. Taking discontinued medication | 0 | 276 | 0 | 2 | 2 | 4 | 0 | 50.0 | 50.0 |
| 15. Discontinued taking medication | 24 | 240 | 10 | 39 | 67 | 116 | 8.6 | 33.6 | 57.8 |

**Table 3. Significance of Drug Defaulting on 380 Prescriptions[a]**

| ERROR SIGNIFICANCE GROUP | PRESCRIPTIONS | |
| --- | --- | --- |
| | NO. | % |
| 1 | 82 | 21.6 |
| 2 | 63 | 16.6 |
| 3 | 117 | 30.8 |
| 4 | 118 | 31.0 |
| | 380 | 100 |

[a] Determined by the highest significance rating assigned to any error associated with a specific prescription.

prehension was found to be statistically significant with respect to number of daily doses ($p = 0.05$) and name of the medication ($p = 0.001$). The elements of timing and purpose of medication were found to have no significant association. The elements of amount of dose and administration appear to have an association, but statistical testing by chi-square was not possible due to small cell size.

The association between comprehension and compliance was statistically significant ($p = 0.05$) in all cases, with the exception of administration. Again the association is apparent but could not be tested due to small cell size. Although a cause and effect relationship cannot be unequivocally proven, the results of this study indicate a positive relationship between increased information provided via the prescription label and increased comprehension and compliance, with few exceptions. The occurrence of intentional error, or noncompliance associated with correct comprehension, was only large with respect to errors of timing and number of daily doses. This finding again suggests the desirability of prescribing a convenient dosing schedule, which is compatible with rational therapeutics.

*Effects of Demographic Variables.* The effects of the demographic variables—sex, age, race, education, occupation and social class—on comprehension and compliance were tested. The following discussion represents

**Table 4. Presence and Positive Responses to Elements of Directions on Written Prescription, Prescription Label, Comprehension and Compliance on 380 Prescriptions**

| | PRESENCE | | CORRECT RESPONSE | |
| --- | --- | --- | --- | --- |
| ELEMENT | WRITTEN PRESCRIPTION | PRESCRIPTION LABEL | COMPREHENSION | COMPLIANCE[a] |
| Amount of dose | 99.1% | 98.8% | 91.3% | 89.3% |
| Number of doses | 94.0 | 92.7 | 85.8 | 63.8 |
| Timing | 12.6 | 12.8 | 70.5 | 60.1 |
| Administration | 97.0 | 98.2 | 94.5 | 98.9 |
| Purpose | 15.1 | 15.3 | 80.5 | 97.2 |
| Name of medication | 98.9 | 59.6 | 40.3 | — |

[a] Based on the 356 prescriptions actually dispensed.

only those variables found to have statistically significant relationship.

*(1) Sex.* Females were found to have a higher comprehension level than males ($p = 0.05$). No significant difference, however, was found with respect to compliance or the number of errors committed. It was also noted that women received verbal instructions more frequently from both the pharmacist and the physician. Male patients received verbal instructions from the physician on only 66.1% of the prescriptions, whereas female patients received instructions on 83.6% of the prescriptions studied. The pharmacist was found to give verbal instructions to male patients on only 8.5% of the prescriptions and to female patients on 17.9%. While it is interesting that both physicians and pharmacists took more time to educate the female patients, it is most alarming to note the overall low incidence of pharmacists providing verbal instructions.

*(2) Age.* The 45–64 age group was found to have the highest level of comprehension. The 65 and over group had the lowest comprehension level. This difference was found to be significant at $p = 0.05$.

The 45–65 age group had the least number of errors per prescription ($p = 0.001$). A possible explanation for this finding might be that patients in the 25–44 age group are preoccupied with the working world and are not acutely health conscious. The 45–65 group is becoming more aware of their health while concurrently decreasing their other activities. The increase in errors in the 65 and over group is then attributed to more complex health problems combined with decreasing ability to care for oneself.[3]

*(3) Race.* A significant relationship was found between race and comprehension level ($p = 0.001$), the white population having a higher comprehension level than the nonwhite population. No difference was noted between the races with respect to the number of errors committed per prescription. There was, however, a significant relationship between race and the significance of the errors committed. The nonwhite population was found to make more clinically significant errors ($p = 0.05$).

*(4) Education.* No relationship was found between education and the number of errors committed; however, a significant relationship exists between education and comprehension level ($p = 0.01$). Patients in education classification 7 (least number of years of education) had a significantly lower comprehension level than patients with more education.

*(5) Social Class.* A significant relationship was found between social class and comprehension level ($p = 0.01$). The 276 patients in social class V had a lower comprehension level than patients in the other groups.

## Summary

As has been documented previously, this research revealed a substantial degree of drug defaulting by ambu-latory patients. Over 60% of the population studied was found to be making self-administration errors that precluded optimal response to their drug therapy. Additionally, comprehension of the directions for proper utilization of the medication was measured and found to be directly related to compliance. Thus, it is concluded that a major step towards improving compliance would be increased patient education. This stresses the importance of the pharmacist including complete directions on the prescription label. The pharmacist was found to be negligent in providing verbal instructions to the patient; patients received such counseling less than 15% of the time.

Two errors, that of never having the prescription filled and of prematurely discontinuing the medication, contributed to the majority of the highly significant "errors." Of the 380 prescriptions studied, 24 were never filled and 116 were prematurely discontinued; thus, approximately 35% of the prescriptions studied were not taken continuously as prescribed.

## Recommendations for Further Study

Further study of the problems of drug defaulting should be directed at measuring the effects of mechanisms aimed at improving compliance. Therapeutic counseling by pharmacists and improved labeling practices are the most promising mechanisms which need further study. The use of calendar packaging has proven successful with oral contraceptives and should be expanded to include other medications. This study might be expanded to provide multiple drug packages personalized to the patient. Subjects with a wider variation of educational and socioeconomic backgrounds are needed to verify the relationships suggested by this research.

## Conclusions

The association between the written prescription and the prescription label, and consequently the effect on comprehension and compliance, should be a mandate to physicians to improve prescription writing habits. Likewise, pharmacists should attempt to improve labeling procedures and encourage improved prescription writing by physicians. The solution to the problems of drug defaulting should be through a coordinated effort by both physicians and pharmacists.

The great strides in the development of new medications for the successful treatment of disease are of little value if the patient does not obtain and consume the medication as prescribed.

## References

1. Hollingshead, A. B.: Two-Factor Index of Social Position, August B. Hollingshead, New Haven, Connecticut, 1957.

2. Anon.: International Classification of Diseases and Accidents, PHS Pub. No. 1693, U.S. Department of H.E.W., Eighth Revision, December 1968.

3. Clinite, J. C. and Kabat, H. F.: Errors During Self-Administration, *J. Amer. Pharm. Ass. NS9*:450–452 (Sept.) 1969.

## Appendix A

### Patient Interview Form

| | | | |
|---|---|---|---|
| Level of comprehension | 6  5  4  3  2  1  0 | | |
| How much do you take as a single dose? | 1. Correct | 2. Incorrect | 3. No. Knowledge |
| How often do you take the medication? | 1. | 2. | 3. |
| When do you take each dose? | 1. | 2. | 3. |
| How do you administer the medication? | 1. | 2. | 3. |
| What are you taking this medication for? | 1. | 2. | 3. |
| What is the name of the drug? | 1. | 2. | 3. |

*Compliance*

| Error Classification | Specific Error | Significance of Error |
|---|---|---|
| Amount of single dose | 1. None | 2. Error |
|   Decreased single dose | | 0  1  2  3  4 |
|   Increased single dose | | 0  1  2  3  4 |
| Frequency of dosage | 1. None | 2. Error |
|   Omitted scheduled dose | | 0  1  2  3  4 |
|   Extra dose | | 0  1  2  3  4 |
|   Ommitted p.r.n. dose | | 0  1  2  3  4 |
|   Extra p.r.n. dose | | 0  1  2  3  4 |
| Timing/sequence | 1. None | 2. Error |
|   Improper interval (± 30 min.) | | 0  1  2  3  4 |
|   Improper timing with meals | | 0  1  2  3  4 |
| Administration | 1. None | 2. Error |
|   Improper route | | 0  1  2  3  4 |
|   Improper technique | | 0  1  2  3  4 |
| Purpose | 1. None | 2. Error |
|   Use for wrong purpose | | 0  1  2  3  4 |
| Miscellaneous | 1. None | 2. Error |
|   Prescription never filled | | 0  1  2  3  4 |
|   Taking outdated medication | | 0  1  2  3  4 |
|   Forgot to take medication | | 0  1  2  3  4 |
|   Taking duplicate medications | | 0  1  2  3  4 |
|   Taking discontinued medication | | 0  1  2  3  4 |
|   Discontinued taking medication | | 0  1  2  3  4 |
| Number of error types committed | 0  1  2  3  4  5  6 | |

## Appendix B

### Criteria for Determining Errors of Drug Defaulting

*Single Dose.* The amount of single dose was considered an error if any single dose was increased or decreased by more than 20% of the dose prescribed.

*Frequency of Dosing.* The frequency of dosing was considered in error if the total number of doses consumed in any 24-hour period exceeded or was less than the number of doses prescribed. In the case of prescriptions written "as needed" (p.r.n.) an error was considered as taking a dose when not needed or omitting a dose when it was needed.

*Timing Sequence.* An error of timing or sequence was counted if the medication was not consumed within 30 minutes of the time prescribed. (Considerable latitude was allowed on prescriptions written as b.i.d., t.i.d. or q.i.d. The important consideration was establishing a fixed dosing time with uniform intervals.)

*Administration.* An error of administration was considered the use of a medication by the wrong route or improper technique of administration.

*Purpose.* Use of a medication for a purpose other than that for which it was prescribed was considered an error of purpose. Taking a medication properly without knowledge of purpose was not considered an error of noncompliance.

*Miscellaneous.* The following cases were also considered errors:

  a. Failure to have the prescription filled.
  b. Taking a prescription medication previously prescribed, but not in the current therapeutic regimen.
  c. Forgetting to take a dose of the medication.
  d. Taking the same medication from two or more duplicate bottles.
  e. Taking an out-dated medication.
  f. Discontinuing the medication without the consent or notification of the physician.

## Appendix C

### Classification of the Clinical Significance of Errors of Drug Defaulting

0. Does not apply, no opportunity to commit error.
1. *No Error.* Absolutely no errors committed.
2. *Insignificant Error.* A minor or infrequent error which has no potential of increasing morbidity.
3. *Intermediate Error.* An error that, if continued, has the possibility of increasing morbidity or causing mortality, but not posing any immediate threat to the health of the patient.
4. *Significant Error.* An error that is currently, or has the probability of increasing morbidity or causing mortality, thus posing an immediate threat to the health of the patient.

*Miscellaneous Questions*

When did you have your prescription filled?
                Day 0  1  2  3  4  5  6
Did the doctor tell you how to take this medication?
                1. Yes 2. No
Did the pharmacist tell you how to take this medication?
                1. Yes 2. No

## Appendix D

### Prescription and Label Information

Elements appearing on written prescription

|  |  | 6 | 5 | 4 | 3 | 2 | 1 | 0 |
|---|---|---|---|---|---|---|---|---|
| Dose | 1. Yes | | | | | 2. No | | |
| Frequency | 1. Yes | | | | | 2. No | | |
| Timing | 1. Yes | | | | | 2. No | | |
| Administration | 1. Yes | | | | | 2. No | | |
| Use | 1. Yes | | | | | 2. No | | |
| LABEL | 1. Yes | | | | | 2. No | | |

Elements appearing on prescription label

|  |  | 6 | 5 | 4 | 3 | 2 | 1 | 0 |
|---|---|---|---|---|---|---|---|---|
| Dose | 1. Yes | | | | | 2. No | | |
| Frequency | 1. Yes | | | | | 2. No | | |
| Timing | 1. Yes | | | | | 2. No | | |
| Administration | 1. Yes | | | | | 2. No | | |
| Use | 1. Yes | | | | | 2. No | | |
| Name of drug | 1. Yes | | | | | 2. No | | |

Prescription filled on day     0   1   2   3   4   5   6

Net days deviation (from H below)

1. +4
2. +3
3. +2
4. +1
5.  0
6. −1
7. −2
8. −3
9. −4

A. Days since Rx was filled   ————

B. Number of doses per day   ×————

C. Theoretical doses used   =————

D. Number of doses prescribed   ————

E. Number of doses remaining   −————

F. Actual doses used   =————−C———— =G————

G———— ÷ B———— =H——

# 31 The Pharmacist's Role in Patient Discharge Planning

Gary E. Greiner

A pilot study to explore the pharmacist's role in discharge planning revealed a significant need for pharmacy involvement. This relates to several areas of concern, including the patient's understanding of medications to be taken and their contraindications and precautions; continuation of therapy after discharge; and overall relationship of the pharmacist, nurse, and physician in the clinical setting.

During the study, the pharmacist met three times a week in discharge planning conferences with the physician, nurse, and social worker. The needs of each patient were evaluated from the standpoint of the patient's post hospital care. Following the conferences, the physician wrote discharge orders. From this point, the pharmacist filled the orders after reviewing the medications and the patient's chart and consulting the physician when indicated. In a final interview with the patient, the pharmacist instructed the patient regarding the correct use of the medications and plans for continuation, if indicated.

Evaluation of the pharmacist's contribution was made after counseling 156 patients who received discharge medications during this two-month study. Several of the more interesting case studies are presented from among the complete record of patients interviewed.

Follow-up of the patient group over a six-month period showed a slight, but statistically insignificant, decrease in readmission rate.

As the role of the pharmacist continues to change and progress, it becomes clear that exploration into all possible areas of involvement is essential if he is to realize his full potential. My residency program at the Veterans Administration Hospital, Cincinnati, Ohio, was designed to explore these possible roles and prepare a practitioner who is capable of functioning in a setting more compatible with his professional training. The purpose of this chapter is to share some of my experiences in an area in which the hospital pharmacist can make a unique contribution to improved patient care. However, this contribution can be made only if the pharmacist is willing to leave the confines of his pharmacy and is eager to interact with his fellow professionals and with patients.

## Stimulus for the Program

A patient may receive the best of medical, pharmaceutical and nursing care while hospitalized. However, we are increasingly aware that if provisions are not made for his needs after discharge from the hospital, he may soon return, suffering from the same problems for which he was previously treated. A survey at the Veterans Administration Hospital in Cincinnati revealed that 24% of patients treated on acute medical wards were readmitted to the hospital within six months of discharge.

As a result of this high readmission rate, and because of the frequency with which the outpatient nursing supervisor was being called about needs at home by patients after discharge, an in-depth study of the hospital's discharge procedure was felt to be in order. The study revealed that the procedure employed for patient discharge was a possible contributing cause to this high readmission rate. Under this system, it was the discharged patient's responsibility to (1) report to the clinic office to make an appointment for his next visit, (2) go to the pharmacy to have his discharge prescriptions dispensed, and (3) reclaim any belongings left at the clothing and valuables storage area during his stay. In some cases, this procedure was found to require six hours because the discharged patient had to compete for attention with the large numbers of outpatients seen daily in the clinics and at the pharmacy. After an ordeal like this there is little likelihood that a patient would remember any special instructions or directions given to him regarding care at home. When one considers that this was likely to be the patient's first full day of activity since entering the hospital, the magnitude of the task becomes clear to the observer.

Pharmacy service was invited to participate in the assessment of the problem for the following reasons: (1) the outpatient pharmacy was one area where the discharged patient was forced to spend considerable time trying to complete his discharge procedures, (2) a large number of calls received by the outpatient nursing supervisor were related to the medications the patient was taking at home, and (3) pharmacy service had shown the interest and ability to become more involved with patient care through the development of patient oriented services, such as the iv additive program, and through its work with the pharmacy-nursing committee.

Therefore, in an effort to improve patient care and decrease the high readmission rate, a pilot program of coordinated discharge planning was initiated on the acute medical wards. The program was designed to minimize the active involvement of the patient in the physical tasks of preparing for discharge so that he would be free to concentrate on any special instructions about his needs for care at home. During the two months of the pilot study, 156 patients were discharged under the plan about to be described. The program involved three to four hours per day of the pharmacy resident's time in servicing the 80 beds on the two wards.

## Conferences

Three times a week the head nurses, medical nursing supervisor, outpatient nursing supervisor, pharmacist and social worker met with physicians to discuss the progress and needs of each patient. The physician discussed the patient's disease problems, drug and physical therapy and prognosis. The nurse then described the patient's condition at that time, adding additional information about the patient pertinent to his care in the hospital and at home. The social worker discussed the patient's home life and future plans, emphasizing those aspects which were pertinent to problems of returning to a normal way of life after discharge. At this time the pharmacist could raise any questions he felt were relevant. These would be directed to the physician and nurse regarding drug therapy and any condition of the patient which might alter his response to a drug or require some alteration of the dosage form routinely available from the pharmacy. Specific attention was then given to discussing the ability of the patient or his family to provide care, if needed, in the home. The social worker and nurses were able to provide much useful information regarding the patient's attitude, reliability, etc., and information about the patient's background and home life important in determining the individual's needs and adequately preparing for his discharge.

More detailed discussion was held in the case of patients to be discharged within a day or two of the conference. Each member of the conference discussed a particular aspect of the patient's discharge and how he would relate to it. The physician discussed the drugs and treatments the patient would require at home; the nurse discussed any tests, dressing changes, dietary teaching, etc., about which she had instructed the patient; and the social worker described plans which had been made in the home for the patient's return. The pharmacist would then recommend instructions for the patient taking his medications at home and any special steps required to instruct the patient on the correct use of his drugs.

The day before the patient was to be discharged, the physician wrote discharge orders and a discharge summary of the patient's stay in the hospital. The discharge orders included medications, period of time before the next clinic visit and special needs of the patient such as equipment for use in the home. The ward secretary then telephoned the clinic to make the patient's clinic appointment, ordered the necessary equipment, helped the patient arrange transportation home and informed the pharmacy that the patient was to be discharged the next day. The pharmacist went to the floor to compile additional information regarding the patient's discharge medications.

## Functions of the Pharmacist

The pharmacist first reviewed the patient's chart, paying particular attention to the discharge summary, medications to be taken at home and the patient's most recent laboratory test results. Next, he reviewed the nursing notes, noting the medications the patient received during his stay in the hospital and any other pertinent information. The pharmacist then compared the prescriptions orders the physician had written for the patient with the discharge summary and nursing notes.

The pharmacist consulted the physician and nurse regarding any questions which may have arisen during examination of the patient's chart. Examples of questions included such areas as possible drug interactions, therapy regimens and electrolyte requirements. In two instances the pharmacist noted that a patient had been receiving warfarin and chloral hydrate while hospitalized but was being discharged on warfarin alone. The pharmacist alerted the physician to the possibility of an altered response by the patient to the warfarin, and the physician decided to gradually reduce the dose of chloral hydrate and concurrently adjust the warfarin dose rather than abruptly discontinue the chloral hydrate.

In another case, a physician had written orders for

warfarin and phenobarbital to be taken concomitantly. The directions were such that the patient was given the option of continuing the phenobarbital or discontinuing it, depending on how he felt. Since the patient's next clinic appointment was scheduled for a month later, the pharmacist felt there was a possibility that the patient might stop taking the phenobarbital and encounter bleeding problems due to decreased warfarin metabolism. After consultation with the physician it was decided to give the patient specific directions for gradually tapering off the dose of phenobarbital and arrange to adjust the warfarin dose with the aid of a physician in his home town. On eight different occasions the pharmacist found laboratory values which prompted him to consult with the physician; in all cases the patients were suffering from congestive heart failure and were being treated with digitalis preparations and diuretics. The laboratory results showed low normal or below normal serum potassium levels. Because of the relatively high incidence of digitalis toxicity and its relation to serum potassium levels, the pharmacist felt obligated to check with the physician regarding the possibility of toxicity developing at home while the patient continued the use of the digitalis preparation and the diuretic. In all eight cases the physician concurred with the pharmacist and either ordered supplementary potassium for the patient or instructed the patient to increase his dietary intake of potassium by including bananas or other foods high in potassium in his daily diet.

With questions such as these answered, the pharmacist consulted the ward secretary to learn the date of the patient's next clinic appointment and, when indicated, made appropriate adjustments in the quantities of medication prescribed. Since the pharmacy supplied diabetic patients with insulin, needles, syringes, cotton, alcohol and testing kits for home use, the pharmacist checked with the nurse and patient to be sure that the patient had been adequately trained in the use and care of the insulin administration equipment and had a sufficient supply of the necessary equipment and supplies for use until his next clinic visit. In four cases it was discovered that the patient did not have sufficient supplies to meet his needs until the clinic visit. In the case of individuals returning to treatment by a private physician, a ten-day supply of medication was dispensed to enable the patients to make the transition from the V.A. system to private health care.

After reviewing the prescription orders as described, the pharmacist proceeded to the pharmacy where the medications were dispensed. At the same time a set of instructions for the patient was initiated. The initial step consisted of preparation of a record with the patient's name and prescription numbers on it. The following morning—the morning the patient was to be discharged—the pharmacist was ready to take the medications to the ward to discuss each of them with the patient or a member of the patient's family. His first stop was at the nursing station where he briefly discussed the patients to be discharged with the head nurse. After gathering any last bits of information he felt pertinent, the pharmacist then proceeded to visit the individual patient and discuss each medication with him.

Through discussions held at the planning conferences it had become evident that, because the Veterans Administration treats individuals from all cultural and sociological backgrounds, instructions for taking medications would have to be highly individualized. These discussions had also led to decisions as to exactly what information should be relayed to the patient concerning his medications and condition. The amount of information relayed to the patient was based on the patient's ability to comprehend, the possible effects of the information on the patient's psychological response to treatment and the relevance of such information to the patient's ability to care for himself at home.

Armed with this background and information, the pharmacist spent a short time acquainting himself with the patient before actually beginning to discuss medications with him. The pharmacist then discussed each medication with the patient, explaining, as previously decided, the medication's intended use, how it was to be taken and what precautions should be observed in use of the drug. The work of previous investigators had shown that verbal directions had little effect on the frequency with which patients made errors in taking medications at home.[1] For this reason, it was felt that written instructions should be supplied. In an attempt to aid the patient further, it was decided that the written instructions should be put in the words of the patient to ensure understanding of the directions at home. The pharmacist first discussed the medications with the patient and then let the patient repeat, in his own words, the directions and information about each. When the pharmacist was sure the patient understood the information presented to him, he then completed the form which had been started when the prescriptions were dispensed. Using the patient's words, the pharmacist wrote a brief description of the appearance of the drug, its intended use and how the patient should take it. In the case of diabetic patients, the pharmacist had the patient perform a urine sugar test and a simulated needle and syringe sterilization procedure. In two cases it was discovered that patients had not been taught the sterilization procedure and the nurse was called upon to instruct the patient in the correct technique. This situation arose because of the somewhat paradoxical situation at our hospital whereby patients are taught on the ward to give their own insulin injections using disposable needles and syringes. At discharge, however, the pharmacy supplies the patients with glass syringes and needles which must be reused.* In the two cases mentioned, a new nurse not completely familiar with all hospital procedures had been caring for the patients and had assumed they would receive disposable equipment when discharged. When the pharmacist completed his instructions to the patient, he explained the procedure to be followed in acquiring refills for prescriptions, when indicated, or the steps to take if the patient was returning to treatment by a private physician. In all cases the pharmacist emphasized that the patient should bring his medications with him to the clinic or when he visited his private physician so that the physician would have some basis for determining if the medications had been taken correctly and whether or not an additional supply might be needed, as in the case of patients on long term therapy for such conditions as congestive heart failure, diabetes, etc. The pharmacist then asked the patient if he had any questions or comments regarding his medications, the entire discharge procedure or anything concerning his stay in the hospital. It was during this time that the pharmacist became aware of factors that can influence a patient's progress at home. Two cases will serve as examples to illustrate this point.

Case 1: Patient E. G., a 43-year-old male, had been admitted to the hospital suffering from congestive heart failure. His stay had been uneventful and he had been maintained on a regimen of digoxin, 0.25 mg/day and hydrochlorothiazide, 50 mg/day. He was to return to his private physician for treatment after discharge. During the discussion the patient casually mentioned that he had a large supply of digoxin and furosemide at home that had been prescribed for him by a different physician. He felt that he might just as well take these after he finished the medications with which he was being sent home. He felt in that way he would not have to bother seeing his physician at home and would be spared the expense of purchasing additional medications. It took quite a bit of explanation by the physician and the pharmacist to convince the patient that he would have to see his physician at home and follow directions if he expected to stay well and out of the hospital.

Case 2: Patient T. W., a 64-year-old male, was admitted to the hospital with severe congestive heart failure approximately three months after having undergone open heart surgery. After a lengthy stay in the hospital he was ready to go home. In addition to his drug therapy he was placed on a severely restricted sodium diet about which he and his family had been carefully instructed by the dietary department. The patient appeared to understand his medications well, knew his dietary restrictions and was quite eager to go home to his family. Two weeks after his discharge, he was readmitted to the hospital suffering from severe congestive heart failure which did not respond to treatment; the patient died a week later. On talking with the patient's family, the physician discovered that the patient had been home alone during the day, had not felt up to preparing his diet as directed and began heating a "can or two" of canned soup for lunch each day. These soups supply approximately two to three grams of sodium per can.[2] When one considers that a patient may seem to grasp everything explained to him in the hospital and yet go home and do the exact opposite, it becomes obvious that much work is still to be done in learning how to communicate effectively with the patient and in assessing the effect of this communication accurately. The literature is replete with similar examples.[3-6]

## Evaluation

Follow-up of the patient group over a six-month period showed a slight decrease in the readmission rate which was not statistically significant.

Because of the potential contributions of the program to improved patient care, however, plans have been made to repeat it in an altered form. Rosenberg has reported that patient education, if begun early in the course of hospitalization, can have a significant effect on the patient's performance in self-management of disease problems.[7] We plan to alter our procedure by increasing the contact between the pharmacist and the patient, including follow-up consultation during the patient's clinic visits. The repeat study will employ some aspects of Rosenberg's methodology, and it is hoped that it will show more favorable results.

The short term effects of the program were most gratifying. All health care professionals involved felt that the team concept was most helpful, both in improving patient care and in making all the members of the team more aware of the problems and the capabilities of each other. This was especially gratifying to the pharmacist, who, as the neophyte member of the direct patient care team, was somewhat unsure of the response by both health care practitioners and patients to his presence in the patient care area. Acceptance by physicians and nurses was excellent because in the words of one physician, the pharmacist was able to make a significant contribution to improved patient care by making himself available and readily accessible.

As time progressed, the physicians began consulting the pharmacist about other problems as well.

---

*This procedure has since been changed and all patients are to be supplied with disposable equipment.

The pharmacist was, for instance, able to provide significant information about biopharmaceutical aspects of drug therapy on several occasions, enabling the physician to obtain a therapeutic response he had not been able to attain previously. The pharmacist also profited from this experience by observing and learning firsthand that many factors are involved in the course of a patient's stay in the hospital. It became quite evident that all aspects of a patient's condition must be considered when arriving at a sound decision regarding what should or should not be done for a patient. Without clinical exposure pharmacists risk being too narrow in their view of factors influencing a patient's condition. We may attribute too much to drugs and drug therapy if we are not aware of all factors involved.

Patient reaction to the program also appeared to be excellent. With four or five exceptions, patients discharged under the program were most appreciative, especially with regard to medication instructions. One can imagine the surprise and pleasure the day a patient stopped the pharmacist in the hall and wanted to know when the program would start on his ward.

## Conclusion

The pharmacist has a definite place in discharge planning which can lead to improved patient care. As professionals, our responsibility is clear: if a problem exists for which we can offer any portion of a solution, we must become actively involved.

### References

1. Malahy, B.: The Effect of Instruction and Labeling on the Number of Medication Errors Made by Patients at Home, *Am. J. Hosp. Pharm.* 23:283-292 (June) 1966.

2. Bowes, A. and Church, C. F.: Food Values of Portions Commonly Used, 11th ed., J. B. Lippincott Company, Philadelphia, Pennsylvania, 1970, pp. 66-67.

3. Latiolais, C. J., and Berry, C. C.: Misuse of Prescription Medications by Outpatients, *Drug Intel. Clin. Pharm.* 3:270-277 (Oct.) 1969.

4. Clinite, J. C., and Kabat, H. F.: Errors During Self-Administration, *J. Amer. Pharm. Ass.* NS9:450-452 (Sept.) 1969.

5. Maddock, R. K.: Patient Cooperation in Taking Medicines, *JAMA 199*: 169-172 (Jan. 16) 1967.

6. Neely, E., and Patrick, M. L.: Problems of Aged Persons Taking Medications at Home, *Nursing Res. 17*:52-55 (Jan.) 1968.

7. Rosenberg, S. G.: A Case for Patient Education, *Hosp. Formulary Management 6*:14-17 (June) 1971.

# 32 Drug Consultation: Its Significance to the Discharged Hospital Patient and Its Relevance as a Role for the Pharmacist

Philip Cole and Sister Emmanuel

A study of 75 hospitalized patients was undertaken to determine whether patients discharged from the hospital with prescriptions self-administer these medications at home as prescribed.

The patients were divided into three groups of 25 patients each. To the first group of patients, pharmacist medication consultation was provided at the time of their discharge from the hospital. The second group received no pharmacist medication consultation prior to discharge. The third group received pharmacist medication consultation and were taught how to self-administer medications prior to discharge from the hospital.

Seventy-six percent of the 25 patients who received no consultation prior to discharge deviated significantly from their prescribed drug regimen at home. Of the two groups of patients who received consultation, only 8% of the patients who received only pharmacist discharge consultation deviated from their prescribed drug regimens; only 12% of the patients who were also taught to self-administer their medications while in the hospital deviated from their regimen after discharge.

Overall, 90% of the patients who had received pharmacist discharge drug consultation showed no deviation from prescribed drug regimens at home; these patients had fewer medication problems than those who were not provided consultation service prior to discharge. Only 24% of the patients who did not receive consultation showed no signs of deviation from their prescribed drug regimens.

The study appears to indicate that the most common reason for not following prescribed regimens was forgetfulness; the next most common reason was the appearance of undesirable side effects. Most instances of deviation were found among medical patients, particularly among patients for whom antibiotics and tranquilizers had been prescribed.

Contemporary health care concerns itself with a vast number of long term chronic illnesses which necessitate therapeutic use of new and highly potent medications. To illustrate the incidence of chronic disease, in 1967 the incidence of circulatory diseases was 29,944, and the number of patients under treatment for diabetes mellitus in the same year was 35,049.[1]

Many chronic illnesses are treated by long term oral medications and many patients with chronic disorders who are poorly educated about their prescribed medications do not follow their therapeutic regimens properly at home.[2] If a drug therapy regimen for the discharged hospital patient, especially patients with long term chronic disorders, is to be effective, patients should be well educated about their medications and the importance of following drug regimens in detail should be impressed upon them.

From personal conversation with discharged hospital patients, it appears that some are uncertain about self-administration of drugs prescribed for them. For example, one patient in the hospital under study, who was discharged with a prescription for an antibiotic vaginal cream, admitted having received no instructions as to how the cream should be applied, nor did she understand the reasons for which the cream had been prescribed. Still another patient stated that no explanation had been given for removing the foil wrapping from rectal suppositories prior to use. Doubts such as these in the mind of the patient result in apprehension as to the rationale of the physician in prescribing certain forms of treatment. According to Latiolais and Berry, if the patient is not cognizant of what his illness is or why he is taking medication, he may resort to superstitious-like behavior and have misapprehensions about his disease and the drugs prescribed.[3]

Further, according to Kane, it appears that explanations are often lacking as to the importance of administering all medications in a drug regimen regularly and at appropriate intervals.[4] Prior to our study, one patient on a daily maintenance dose of digitalis admitted that when he occasionally forgot to take his daily dose, he made up the missed dose by doubling the dose the following day. It has been pointed out by Jenkins that the average patient takes only about half the doses of medication which are prescribed.[5]

Without proper knowledge or communication with either the physician or the pharmacist at the time of discharge, self-evaluation of apparently improved physical progress may lead the patient to terminate his prescribed drug regimen. If the patient sees no apparent effectiveness resulting from the prescribed medications, this may also lead him to discontinue them. If the importance of continuing dosage regularly at home is properly stressed, such problems as the above might well be greatly reduced. This belief is based on the premise that problems of this nature result from a failure to provide adequate information to the patient, a failure to communicate effectively, and a false assumption that the patient is knowledgeable concerning his drugs and that he will automatically follow a drug therapy regimen.

Failure to discuss side effects or possible adverse drug reactions also leads the patient to misunderstand the primary purpose for which the medications are prescribed. For example, awareness of possible urine discoloration with the use of certain medications, or of side effects such as vertigo or gastrointestinal upset, will help to prevent the development of fear in the patient at the onset of these symptoms. Likewise, knowledge of this type could possibly prevent discontinuation of the medication by the patient and reduce the possibility of further complicating the disease state by disrupting a much needed course of drug therapy.

Additionally, if a patient does not know what side effects he may experience from a drug, he might fail to identify unusual reactions as side effects and conclude that the reaction is part of the normal mechanism of the medication action. In a discussion with one patient, the authors learned that she was being maintained on a tranquilizer administered three times a day. The patient admitted she had not been informed of side effects which might be expected and stated that she lacked her usual ambition and spent most of her day sleeping. She related that "her vacuum cleaner and iron were too heavy to lift and use."

Although this worried the patient to some extent, she was under the impression that loss of ambition and strength was to be accepted as part of the "cure" of her nervous disorder. Since the physician and pharmacist failed to describe the side effects to the patient, it could not be expected that she would necessarily complain about the side effects at a future office visit.

### Assistance of a Pharmacist — A Remedy?

It seems apparent that there should be effective patient-physician discussion at the time of prescribing. To accomplish this there must be adequate time available to the physician to provide a complete discussion of medications prescribed, or perhaps a pharmacist could assist the physician in providing total patient drug education. Present high patient-to-physician ratios arising from the existing physician shortage combined with the rapid development of new drugs seems to indicate a need for pharmacist involvement in a clinical role on the health care team, both in the community setting as well as in the hospital. Current education of the patient in the use of drugs is, in most instances, accomplished haphazardly. The typical busy physician claims he lacks the time to inform himself of all data concerning side effects and reported adverse reactions of drugs, and to discuss information he does possess with his patient.

It would appear beneficial, therefore, to examine some of the underlying factors which contribute to the uninformed nature of the patient in regard to drug therapy. First, we must not make the assumption that failure of the patient to maintain an acceptable dosage regimen is due solely to his own irresponsibility. Considering the "pampering" which the patient receives and most often graciously accepts while hospitalized, it is not difficult to understand why patients make poor judgments as to their medication regimen after discharge from the hospital. Several earlier studies, especially that of Clinite and Kabat, indicate that patients are somewhat unreliable when charged with the responsibility for self-administration of prescribed drugs upon discharge from the hospital.[6] It has also been suggested by Latiolais and Berry that unreliability of patients in this regard may be due in part to the fact that a patient's drug therapy while in the hospital is entirely controlled for him.[3] The physician prescribes, the pharmacist dispenses and the nurse, in most institutions, administers.

Another factor contributing to the failure of patients to maintain acceptable dosage regimens is related directly to the physician. In a study by Jaco of a group of physicians who claimed they were providing adequate discharge medication consultation, it was shown that relatively few physicians actually had the time to provide this type of consultation.[7] In Jaco's study involving 50 physician-patient consultations, information on reasons for diagnostic laboratory tests, results of these tests, etiology of the patient's illness, outcome from the prescribed treatment and prognosis or possible future complications was presented to the patient only through a series of isolated facts.[7]

Because of the physician's apparent lack of time for consulting with patients and because of the authors' interest in the problem, a study was undertaken to determine whether patients actually encounter problems with medications prescribed upon discharge from a hospital, and whether discharge drug consultations with a hospital pharmacist would be helpful in imparting to patients a proper understanding of their prescribed drug regimens.

## The Research Setting

This study was conducted at Providence Hospital, a 400-bed, short-term, general hospital, during the period January 1971 through March 1971. The average daily census for the hospital under study was 349 patients with an average daily discharge rate of 41 patients.

For the purpose of this study, it was necessary to evaluate two methods of teaching the patient how, when and why to self-administer drugs prescribed at the time of discharge. Patients to be studied were divided into three groups:

> Group I —Pharmacist consultation provided to patients at time of discharge
>
> Group II —Patients who neither received pharmacist consultation nor were permitted to self-administer medications prior to discharge
>
> Group III—Pharmacist consultation provided to patients at time of discharge in addition to consultation prior to self-administration of medications for two days while in the hospital.

In order to determine the impact of pharmacist consultation on patient self-administration of medications at home, Groups I and III were compared to Group II patients who had no interaction with a hospital-based pharmacist prior to discharge.

The objectives of this study were to:

1. Establish whether medication administration patterns at home are improved when patients have been counseled by a pharmacist prior to discharge from the hospital as compared to administration patterns which patients establish at home when discharged without pharmacist consultation
2. Establish whether patients discharged from the hospital have problems at home with prescribed medications and, if so, the nature of the problems
3. Investigate the possible advantages which result when patients are taught how to self-administer medications while still in the hospital.

The latter objective offered the opportunity to teach each patient how to self-administer medications based on a somewhat individualized schedule while still maintaining the physician's intent.

## Methodology of the Study

The study sample consisted of 75 randomly selected hospitalized patients between the ages of 18 and 80. These patients were divided into three groups, as previously described; the first 25 patients were assigned to Group 1, the next 25 patients to Group 2 and the remaining 25 to Group 3.

The medical records of the 75 patients were reviewed by the interviewing pharmacist and appropriate identifying information was abstracted from the charts and transcribed to the upper portion of an Initial Interview Data Form (Figure 1). To reduce the possibility of introducing bias, two pharmacists were involved in the study. One pharmacist, a graduate student at Wayne State University and a candidate for the Doctor of Pharmacy degree, served as the interviewing pharmacist and conducted the initial consultation with patients in Group 1 and Group 3. A second pharmacist, the senior author and a candidate for the Master of Science degree in Hospital Pharmacy, was responsible for the patients in Group 2 and performed the follow-up consultation of all patients in their homes. The inter-

*Figure 1. Initial interview data form*

```
                   INITIAL INTERVIEW DATA FORM

GROUP   1                                   January 23, 1971
                                            Date of Discharge
PATIENT NAME___JOHN SMITH_____AGE_52____  SEX  (M) F

TELEPHONE_____222-0000_____

PRIMARY DIAGNOSIS_____

              PRESCRIPTIONS WRITTEN UPON DISCHARGE
     MEDICATION        SIGNATURE      QUANTITY   RENEWAL
  Combid Spansules      i bid           50         0

  Lomotil 2.5 mg        i qid prn       50         1

  Lasix  40 mg          i qd            30         1

                   CONSULTATION NOTES
     Patient has colostomy.  Patient also takes Bufferin for arthritis.
Patient does not use ASA because it upsets his stomach.  Informed
patient of Tylenol in the event Bufferin upset his stomach.  Patient
is also on a digoxin preparation at home.  Recommended to the physician
that the patient have a potassium supplement.  Potassium chloride
20mEq per day was prescribed.

DOSAGE SCHEDULE REVIEWED /X/  Combid is long-acting, take q 12 h
DRUG SIDE EFFECTS DISCUSSED /X/  Dryness of mouth
ANTICIPATED PROBLEMS WITH OTC PREPARATIONS /X/   Psychological
                                                  (Bufferin)
RENEWAL DISCUSSION /X/  Lomotil and Lasix may be renewed once

                   ADDITIONAL COMMENTS
     Upon talking further with the patient, it was discovered that he
was already taking Combid.  It was explained to him that he should
complete taking the first prescription for Combid at home before
beginning the new prescription.
INTERVIEWING PHARMACIST_____Thomas Jones, R.Ph._____
```

viewing pharmacist is so designated throughout this paper and the senior author is referred to as the primary investigator.

The Initial Interview Data Form, completed for each patient in the study, provided sections for listing personal patient data, medications prescribed at the time of discharge from the hospital, quantities of each medication prescribed and renewal instructions, if any. The data sheet also included space for special consultation notes, such as comments the patient made to the pharmacist, as well as any special advice provided by the pharmacist. The form provided, in check-off style, items which were to be discussed with each patient.

To assess the effectiveness of this study, it was necessary to follow up patients after discharge. All patients in Groups 1, 2 and 3 were telephoned at home by the primary investigator, who in no case conducted the discharge consultation. The follow-up interview by telephone was carried out approximately two weeks after each patient's discharge from the hospital. A standard form (Figure 2) was used for collecting data and was designed to include questions on prescribed medications and their quantities and renewal instructions; prescription numbers, the name and telephone number of the dispensing pharmacy and the date of dispensing; the original quantity dispensed and the quantity remaining at the time of the follow-up call. The latter quantity was obtained by requesting the patient to count the dosage units remaining in the prescription container. This method of determining dosage deviation, although not accurate in some instances, has been proven satisfactory in a study by Rickels and Briscoe.[8] The count supplied by the patient was recorded on the Follow-Up Interview Form (Figure 2) and was compared to the theoretical balance for each medication as determined by the primary investigator. The theoretical balance was determined by calculating the number of days from the date the medications were dispensed (obtained from the pharmacy from which the medication was dispensed) to the date and time of the follow-up telephone call. Variations between the theoretical balance and the actual balance, as reported by the patient, were interpreted as errors in self-administration. When the count disclosed the actual balance to be in excess of the theoretical balance, this was considered to represent an error of omission. Counts disclosing balances less than the theoretical balance were considered to be errors of overdosage; patients were questioned as to the number of doses taken each day when this occurred. If errors were cited, an attempt was made to correct the error through additional consultation with the patient at the time of the follow-up telephone call.

The patient was also questioned as to dosage times. For example, if a patient was to take a medication three times a day, the primary investigator conducting the follow-up interview determined what time the patient actually took his medications and made recommendations to the patient regarding his drug regimen if necessary. The primary investigator further questioned the patient about the occurrence of side effects and noted those which had occurred. Finally, the primary investigator made a total evaluation of the patient based upon information received and placed his comments and recommendations at the bottom of the Follow-Up Interview Form.

Upon completion of the follow-up interviews of the 75 patients, it was shown that patients in Group 1, who had received pharmacist consultation at the time of discharge, were least negligent in all phases of self-administering medications at home. Of the 25 patients in this group, 23 (92%) correctly self-administered their medications at home (Table 1). The primary investigator is of the opinion, based upon information received at the time of the patient follow-up interview, that the two patients in Group 1 who did not take their medications as prescribed were opposed to the concept of self-administration after leaving the hospital, regardless of any benefits which could be cited from such a practice.

The data obtained from follow-up interviews of patients in Group 3 indicates that patients who had been taught to properly self-administer medications in the hospital, and who had received consultation at

***Figure 2. Follow-up interview form***

FOLLOW-UP INTERVIEW FORM

GROUP 1
PATIENT NAME John Smith
DATE February 5, 1971

MEDICATIONS PRESCRIBED AT TIME OF HOSPITAL DISCHARGE

| MEDICATION | Rx No. | PHCY& TELEPHONE | DISPENSING DATE | ORIGINAL QTY | BALANCE[a] | DIFF |
|---|---|---|---|---|---|---|
| Combid Sp. | 236001 | Community 333-0000 | 1-23 | 5C | 21 | 29 |
| Lomotil 2.5 | 236002 | Same | 1-23 | 50 | 18 | 32 |
| Lasix 40 mg[b] | 236003 | Same | 1-23 | 30 | 16 | 14 |
| KCl 20 mEq | 236004 | Same | 1-23 | 16oz. | 2oz. | 14oz. |

PATIENT CLAIMS TO BE ADMINISTERING MEDICATIONS AS PRESCRIBED:
/X/ YES
/ / NO
COMMENT patient is familiar with dosage schedule of all medications

DISCUSSION OF DOSAGE TIMES

| MEDICATION | SIGNATURE | PATIENT ADMINISTERS AT: | COMMENT |
|---|---|---|---|
| Combid Spansule | i bid | 10 AM & 10 PM | Has good pattern |
| Lomotil 2.5 mg | i qid prn | 10 AM & 10 PM | Uses prn as prescribed |
| Lasix 40 mg. | i daily | 11 AM | Taking as prescribed |
| KCl 20mEq/15cc | i tblsp bid | 11 AM & 6 PM | Takes with food |

OCCURENCF OF SIDE EFFECTS...../X/ YES
/ / NO
COMMENT patient has experienced some xerostomia

| MEDICATION | ACUTAL BALANCE | THEORETICAL BALANCE | COMMENT |
|---|---|---|---|
| Combid Spansules | 21 | 21 | Taking |
| Lomotil 2.5 mg. | 18 | none established | prn use |
| Lasix 40 mg. | 14 | 14 | Taking |
| Potassium Chloride | 2oz. | 2oz. | Taking |

EVALUATION: Patient is following directions as well as can be determined from interview. Patient was also quite pleased with the concern and follow up afforded her.

[a] obtained by having patient count remaining tablets
[b] note inclusion of KCl supplement per pharmacist recommendation to physician

## Table 1. Survey of Discharged Patients' Medication Administration Habits

| CRITERIA | GROUP 1[a] | GROUP 2[b] | GROUP 3[c] |
|---|---|---|---|
| Patients self-administering medications at home as prescribed at the time of hospital discharge | 23 (92%) | 6 (24%) | 22 (88%) |
| Patients not self-administering medications at home as prescribed at the time of hospital discharge | 2 (8%) | 19 (76%) | 3 (12%) |
| Total Patients | 25 | 25 | 25 |

[a]Patients who received pharmacist discharge medication consultation
[b]Patients who did not receive pharmacist discharge medication consultation
[c]Patients who were taught to self-administer medications at their bedside and received discharge medication consultation

the time of discharge, did not perform significantly better than patients in Group 1 who had received pharmacist medication consultation only. The follow-up interviews disclosed that 88% of the patients in Group 3 were self-administering prescribed medications at home as directed by the interviewing pharmacist at the time of discharge (Table 1).

A review of the data from the follow-up interviews of patients in Group 2 of the study (Table 1) disclosed that 76% of these patients, who had neither received medication administration instruction while in the hospital nor pharmacist consultation upon discharge, deviated significantly from directions for self-administration of medications at home.

Table 2 categorizes the major problems documented from the data collected on patients who did not self-administer medications as prescribed. Seventy-six percent of the patients in Group 2 accounted for 84% of the total problems documented on follow-up. The most common error of the Group 2 patients was underdosage relating to a failure to remember to self-administer specific doses. The most common error among this group was administration at improper times. One patient was to take an antiarrythmic cardiac drug four times a day. Upon follow-up, the primary investigator learned that this patient, on the basis of personal convenience and lack of understanding of the rationale for the use of the medication, had established a regimen of two tablets in the morning (one at 8:00 AM and the other at 9:00 AM); the remaining two tablets were administered at 9:00 and 10:00 PM respectively. Such a schedule was a considerable deviation from the physician's original intent.

Premature discontinuation of medication by patients in Group 2 was the next most common error noted. Patients claiming to have discontinued their medications gave as their reason the fact that they could no longer detect symptoms of the disease for which they

## Table 2. Reasons Medications Were Not Taken as Prescribed Following Discharge From Hospital

| | GROUP 1[a] | GROUP 2[b] | GROUP 3[c] | |
|---|---|---|---|---|
| Total Patients Not Self-administering Medications at Home as Prescribed at Time of Hospital Discharge | 2 (8%) | 19 (76%) | 3 (12%) | Total Incidence of Problem |
| **PROBLEMS NOTED:** | | | | |
| Underdosage due to Forgetfulness | 1 | 10 | 1 | 12 |
| Underdosage due to Misunderstanding of Directions | 1 | | | 1 |
| Premature Discontinuation of Drug Regimen due to Self-Evaluated Physical Improvement | | 4 | 1 | 5 |
| Administration of Doses at Wrong Times | | 5 | 1 | 6 |
| Overdosage due to Duplication of Prescriptions | | 1 | | 1 |
| Overdosage due to Exceeding Prescribed Dosage at any one Administration Time | | 3 | | 3 |
| Premature Discontinuation of Drug Regimen due to Side Effects of Drugs as Observed by the Patient | | 2 | | 2 |
| Patient Claimed to be Taking all Drugs but Tablet Count did not Balance | | 1 | | 1 |
| **TOTAL PROBLEMS NOTED** | 2 | 26 | 3 | |
| **TOTAL PROBLEM INCIDENCE** | | | | 31[d] |

[a]Patients who received pharmacist discharge medication consultation
[b]Patients who did not receive pharmacist discharge medication consultation
[c]Patients who were taught to self-administer medications at their bedside and received discharge medication consultation
[d]Based on 75 patients

thought they were being treated. Several patients included in this category were on antibiotics which proved to be the class of medication most frequently discontinued by this group. These same patients also failed to follow their entire drug regimen and they did not have their prescriptions renewed because, in their opinion, the medication was too expensive and their physical condition had improved.

There were two incidents in which Group 2 patients discontinued their drug regimen because of distressing side effects. In both instances, the two drugs involved were irritating to the gastrointestinal tract; this complaint was relayed to the primary investigator on follow-up of these patients. It is interesting to note that four patients in Groups 1 and 3 (those who had received pharmacist discharge consultation) also experienced some gastrointestinal upset. All these patients, however, had been counseled on how to manage an upset stomach and they did not discontinue their drug regimens.

The relationship of patient deviations from prescribed drug regimens at home to patient diagnosis and drug classes was also studied. Deviation, for the purpose of this study, was defined as any instance in which the medication regimen, as prescribed by the physician at the time of patient discharge from the hospital, was not followed, and it includes all the reasons listed in Table 2. A large number of cardiac patients deviated from their drug regimens. The largest number of patient deviations occurred with tranquilizers and the second most frequent deviation occurred with antiarrythmic agents. Of the 13 cardiac patients on tranquilizers, nine patients from Groups 1 and 3 showed no deviations, while all four patients in Group 2 who were on tranquilizers deviated from their regimen.

Patients diagnosed with gastrointestinal disorders, particularly those with acute cholecystitis, showed the next highest incidence of failure to follow their drug regimen. Of four patients with a diagnosis of acute cholecystitis, who were taking antibiotics, the only deviations were shown by the two patients in Group 2 who had not received pharmacist discharge consultation.

## Conclusion

Data collected from patients in the three groups of this study yielded interesting and revealing facts. By examining data collected from follow-up telephone calls to the patients involved, it was determined that patients in Groups 1 and 3, who had been provided pharmacist consultation, showed less deviation from prescribed drug regimens and had fewer medication problems at home than did patients in Group 2 who received no consultation. Ninety percent of the patients in Groups 1 and 3 showed no deviation from their prescribed regimens. Patients in Group 2 represent "average" hospitalized discharge patients who, upon discharge from a hospital, do not receive a pharmacist consultation. This study indicates that most patients have problems with discharge medications. These patients, apparently not realizing the importance of their medications, deviate significantly from their prescribed regimens.

Patient acceptance of the pharmacist consultation service was unanimous. Many patients expressed appreciation that someone was interested enough to provide information which they desired but for which they had been reluctant to ask.

In several instances, physicians responded positively when facts which they had not known about their patients' drug histories were presented to them. A patient who continued to administer digitalis received from a physician while concurrently administering an identical digitalis product prescribed on discharge from the hospital, is one example which was of interest to physicians.

From the authors' experience, providing discharge consultation service is not a check-list procedure nor a matter of routine. It is necessary for the interviewing pharmacist to be warm, sincere, and understanding of the patient. He must be able to relate to the patient and win the patient's confidence. Only then will the pharmacist have some assurance that his patient will be fully receptive to instructions regarding the medications prescribed for him. Such an approach develops a sense of trust in the patient and encourages the patient to freely discuss all aspects of his drug therapy with the pharmacist.

In discussing drug therapy with the patient, the following points are recommended for discussion:

1. Determination of medication already being taken which may duplicate or interfere with newly prescribed medications
2. The optimum dosage administration schedule to be followed
3. Measures to be taken in the management of side effects of the prescribed medications
4. The importance of administering all doses of the medications as prescribed.

Although there are many other points which could be discussed, these are perhaps the most significant.

In the present study, which took place in a hospital setting, the interviewing pharmacist required approximately 15 minutes per patient to carry out uncomplicated discharge consultations—those which required neither further discussion with the attending physician nor identification of existing medications at home. For more complicated consultations, 30-45 minutes per patient could be anticipated. The latter cases, however, rarely occurred. These time determinations were obtained from records kept at the time of the discharge interview and the follow-up telephone call.

Based on the telephone follow-up procedure of the discharged hospital patients in this study, an average of 5 minutes per patient should be anticipated. An additional 5 minutes per patient will be required to complete follow-up forms and to contact the pharmacy from which the medications were dispensed. For complicated cases (those requiring consultation with the attending physician, or drug identification), an average of 10 to 15 minutes per patient will be required in addition to the time required to complete the follow-up forms and to contact the dispensing pharmacy.

From these time determinations, and considering that the 400-bed hospital under study discharged an average of 41 patients per day, it is projected that one full-time pharmacist would be required to provide drug consultation to the patients discharged with prescriptions. It must be kept in mind that of the 41 patients who were discharged daily from this hospital, not all had prescription orders for their continued care at home.

The most suitable time for providing discharge consultation service in the hospital under study was in the morning while physicians were available, and just prior to the patient's discharge. Conceivably, a pharmacist could spend the morning hours of an eight-hour shift obtaining the necessary information about the patients to be discharged. This information would be obtained from the patient charts just prior to the discharge interview with the patient. The afternoon hours could be utilized in carrying out telephone follow-ups on discharged patients who had received pharmacist consultation. Although the original purpose of the follow-up telephone calls was to collect data for the study, the pharmacist frequently was able to give further advice to patients regarding their medication habits. For this reason, the follow-up telephone call is recommended as a regular service. The afternoon hours could be further utilized in obtaining preadmission drug histories by telephone from patients scheduled for admission to the hospital within a few days. This could be of value to the attending physician in prescribing hospital medications and might also help the anesthesiologist in determining preoperative medications.

### References

1. U.S. Bureau of the Census, *Statistical Abstract of United States*: 1969 (90th edition) Washington, D.C., 1969.
2. Galluzzi, N.: Automedication at the Hospitalized Patient's Bedside—Advantages and Disadvantages, *Hosp. Formulary Management 3*:25 (June) 1968.
3. Latiolais, C. and Berry, C.: Misuse of Prescription Medication by Outpatients, *Drug Intel. Clin. Pharm. 3*:270 (Oct.) 1969.
4. Kane, R.: What Happens When Your Patient Goes Home? *Resident and Staff Physician 16*:124 (Feb.) 1970.
5. Jenkins, W.: Are Patients True to T.I.D. and Q.I.D. Doses?, *GP 9*:68 (June) 1954.
6. Clinite, J. and Kabat, H.: Errors During Self-Administration, *J. Amer. Pharm. Ass. NS9*:450 (Sept.) 1969.
7. Jaco, E.: Patients, Physicians and Illness, 8th printing, Collier-MacMillan Limited, London, 1968, p. 255.
8. Rickels, K. and Briscoe, E.: Assessment of Dosage Deviation In Outpatient Drug Research, *J. Clin. Pharmacol. New Drugs 10*:160 (May-June) 1970.

# 33 The Outpatient Prescription Label as a Source of Medication Errors

Freya Hermann

Patient interpretation of outpatient prescription label directions was studied by asking patients to state the times they planned to take their medications.

A total of 451 medication schedules were recorded. The results showed that (1) directions on 48.8% of the prescriptions did not necessitate scheduling, (2) for 15.5% of the directions, patients were unable to state an interpretation of the dosage schedule, and (3) interpretations of 33.3% of the directions varied greatly among patients.

It is suggested that pharmacists take the responsibility for scheduling doses for outpatients whenever necessary, rather than leaving it up to the patient to interpret directions that may be ambiguous to him.

Outpatients schedule their own medications. If a physician writes for a *t.i.d.* dose, the pharmacist will type on the label *three times daily,* and at some time between picking up his medication at the outpatient window and taking the first dose, the patient will decide when to take the three daily doses.

Nurses or pharmacists schedule doses for inpatients. They follow guidelines which may have been developed by physicians, pharmacists and nurses together. Adjustments can be made on the basis of patient criteria, therapeutic category of the medication, possible side effects, dosage form and concurrent therapy. Deciding the time of day at which a dose is to be taken does require judgment. Pharmacists may use judgment for inpatients, but for an outpatient, the pharmacist usually translates the *t.i.d.* of the direction to *three times daily* on the label and leaves the scheduling of doses to the patient. Yet most patients have no knowledge of the factors involved in deciding on an optimal schedule.

Much has been written about medication errors committed by patients. Concern has been voiced over the extent to which incorrect drug administration may affect the outcome of therapy. Verbal reports by patients, "pill counts," and monitoring of urine samples have served to assess deviation from the medication schedule which the patient had been expected to follow.[1] Reasons for patient noncooperation in scheduling medications have been proposed ranging from forgetfulness to excessive independence.[2] Measures have been suggested which would improve patient cooperation.[3,4] However, looking for the reasons behind noncooperation by the patient presumes that the patient was aware of the schedule.

Could not the vagueness of a direction lead the patient into underestimating the importance of adhering to a schedule, or to the adoption of a less than optimal schedule, resulting perhaps in therapeutic failure or in unnecessarily pronounced side effects which in turn might cause the patient to abandon therapy altogether? Perhaps before measures can be designed which will lead to better patient cooperation with dosage regimen, it must be established whether the prescription label directs a patient clearly and positively to adopt an optimal drug administration schedule.

This study was undertaken to examine the scheduling of doses by outpatients. The objective was to determine how outpatients interpret their prescription label directions.

## Experimental

The subjects of this study were patients of The Ohio State University Hospitals' Outpatient Department. Data were collected on all patients during one shift over a one-week period. Patients were handed their medication in the usual manner and were asked to read the directions on the label while the pharmacist recorded the name of the drug and the directions. Then patients were asked to specify at which hour(s) of the day they planned to take their medication. This was recorded.

Almost all patients were willing and able to give this information; some seemed pleased to receive extra attention and were eager to show their ability to handle their medications. Since outpatients in a large metropolitan teaching hospital were the subjects of the study, the re-

175

sults apply only to a similar population. However, with respect to medications, many of these patients appeared, if anything, more knowledgeable than patients in general. Many of the outpatients showed a surprising familiarity with hospital dosage schedules, possibly because some were former hospital patients who were now being treated in a clinic and who had been alert patients while they were in the hospital.

## Results

A total of 451 medication schedules were recorded. The prescription rather than the patient was considered the sampling unit. Out of the 451 patient responses, 57 could not be used for evaluating intended dose intervals because patients gave insufficient information, such as "morning and evening," instead of an exact hour of the day. Another 13 observations were excluded from the evaluation because the patients insisted that they did not know how to decide on a time for taking their medication. When they were asked what they planned to do about this, most of them stated that they would ask someone, a relative perhaps, or phone the doctor. Some patients appeared to be under stress and apparently wanted to defer their decision, perhaps regarding this problem as one of minor priority.

Medication schedules tabulated for evaluation numbered 381. Table 1 shows the directions occurring in the study. Fifty-eight prescriptions were for *prn* medication, most of them analgesics, some anticoagulants, tranquilizers and antacids. As these were unscheduled doses, problems of scheduling should not arise.

Thirteen prescriptions directed the patient to take medication by stating specific intervals, such as *every two hours* (for antacids), *every four hours* (for analgesics), *every six hours* (for antibiotics), *every twelve hours* (for long-acting dosage forms). In all of these instances patients were well aware of when to take their medication.

The largest number of medications in one category of directions was 149 medications prescribed for a *once daily* schedule. They were diuretics, cardiac glycosides, vitamins, oral contraceptives, oral hypoglycemics, hormones, antihypertensives, hypnotics, laxatives, topical creams, anticoagulants and potassium supplements. The responses showed that patients were able to plan a daily dose. Generally, patients scheduled doses in the morning, but patients taking oral contraceptives scheduled nighttime doses. Hypnotics and laxatives were scheduled at bedtime, and all except one carried the addition *at bedtime* in the direction. Without exception, patients expressed the intention to take their one daily dose at the same hour each day.

All other medications were prescribed on a *b.i.d.*, *t.i.d.* or *q.i.d.* schedule. There were 47 *b.i.d.* medications, 52 *t.i.d.* medications and 62 *q.i.d.* medications. Each patient's dose schedule was translated into medication intervals to gain a basis for comparison by eliminating differences that were based only on differences in daily living patterns of patients. For example, a schedule of 10 a.m., 2 p.m., 6 p.m. and 10 p.m. was considered not to be different from a 9 a.m., 1 p.m., 5 p.m. and 9 p.m. schedule.

Results of comparisons are shown in Figures 1 to 9 which illustrate the frequency distribution of intervals as they occurred in patients' dose schedules. For the first interval of *b.i.d.* medication the patients' times ranged from 3 to 16 hours, and the second interval showed a range of 8 to 21 hours. The first interval of the *t.i.d.* medications ranged from 0 to 12 hours. For the second interval, the range was also 0 to 12 hours, and the third interval ranged from 7 to 24 hours. For *q.i.d.* medications, patients scheduled the first, second, and third interval with ranges of 0 to 7 hours, 1 to 12 hours, and 0 to 8 hours. The fourth interval showed a range of 6 to 21 hours on the patients' schedules.

Standard deviations for each of the intervals are shown in Table 2. Standard deviation is a measure of variation within a set of observations. Variation of intervals was highest on a *b.i.d.* schedule. There was less variation, on the average, among intervals on a *q.i.d.* schedule than among intervals on a *t.i.d.* schedule. The first interval in each case was the one following the first dose of the day, and there was the least variation in this interval.

### Table 1. Occurrence of Prescription Label Directions in the Study

| DIRECTIONS | FREQUENCY |
|---|---|
| q. 2 h. (or other specific interval) | 13 |
| prn | 58 |
| q.d. | 149 |
| b.i.d. | 47 |
| t.i.d. | 52 |
| q.i.d. | 62 |

### Table 2. Mean Length and Standard Deviation of Dosage Intervals

| DOSE INTERVAL | MEAN LENGTH (hr) | STANDARD DEVIATION |
|---|---|---|
| b.i.d., first interval | 10.40 | 3.65 |
| second interval | 13.60 | 3.65 |
| t.i.d., first interval | 4.48 | 1.85 |
| second interval | 6.23 | 2.82 |
| third interval | 13.30 | 3.49 |
| q.i.d., first interval | 4.17 | 1.48 |
| second interval | 4.74 | 2.31 |
| third interval | 4.09 | 2.04 |
| fourth interval | 10.93 | 3.51 |

Figure 1. *Frequency distribution of the first interval of* b.i.d. *medications*

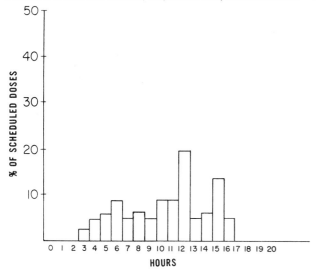

Figure 4. *Frequency distribution of the second interval of* t.i.d. *medications*

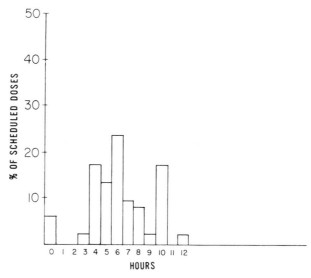

Figure 2. *Frequency distribution of the second interval of* b.i.d. *medications*

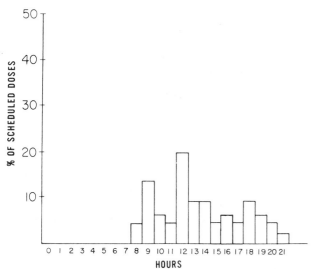

Figure 5. *Frequency distribution of the third interval of* t.i.d. *medications*

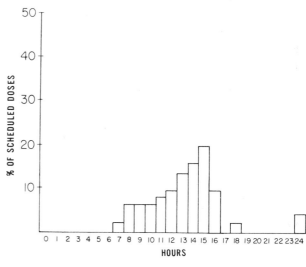

Figure 3. *Frequency distribution of the first interval of* t.i.d. *medications*

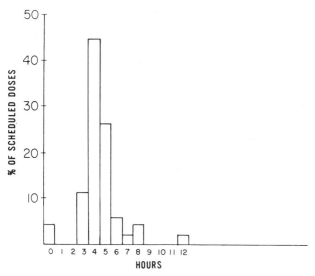

Figure 6. *Frequency distribution of the first interval of* q.i.d. *medications*

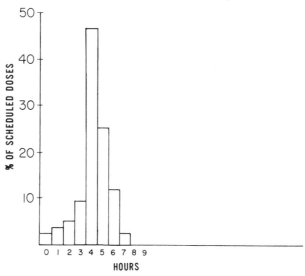

*Figure 7. Frequency distribution of the second interval of q.i.d. medications*

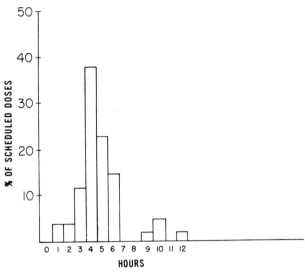

*Figure 8. Frequency distribution of the third interval of q.i.d. medications*

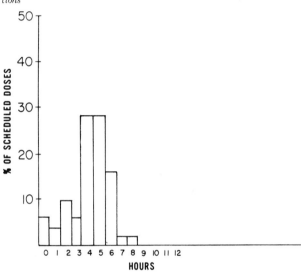

*Figure 9. Frequency distribution of the fourth interval of q.i.d. medications*

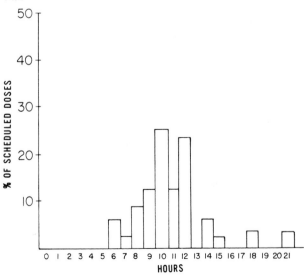

## Discussion

Does the prescription label provide a definitive instruction to the patient? From this study one must conclude that it depends on the type of directions. Some directions, about half of the ones encountered in this study, were definitive, the others apparently were not.

On the positive side were 149 medications prescribed for one daily dose, 58 *prn* medications and 13 directions which stated exact intervals, for a total of 220 medications, or 48.8% of the sample. They were either medications which did not need to be scheduled or the directions were clear to the patient.

On the negative side, there were 70 medication schedules, or 15.5% of the sample, which could not even be included in the tabulation because patients either did not know at all how to schedule the medication, or knew only vaguely so that they could not specify exact times. While their responses cannot be used for comparison of scheduling, the directions did not have a clear meaning to the patients.

Also on the negative side were the 161 medications for *b.i.d., t.i.d.* or *q.i.d.* administration. Patients' interpretations of directions varied greatly, apparently these directions did not carry a precise meaning for all patients.

The objective of the study was to determine how patients interpret prescription label directions. It appears that whenever scheduling was called for, the resulting schedules showed great variation.

What conclusions can be drawn from this study? Are some patients planning to take their medications at the wrong time, thereby creating the chance for a medication error? Administration of a medication more than 30 minutes before or after a set time has been defined as a medication error.[5] But this "set" time is not always the same for a given direction. *Three times daily* can be correctly interpreted to mean either *every eight hours,* as in the case of an antiinfective, or *with meals,* as in the case of iron salts. Traditionally, timing of medication is done within a 12-hour period of time, and *three times daily* generally is associated with mealtime. *Four times daily* adds another dose at bedtime. But the timing of doses has become more demanding. For example, antibiotics are most rationally scheduled in divided doses over 24 hours, and some are most effective if taken away from meals, whereas other medications are poorly tolerated unless taken with food. Dosage schedules may be recommended on the basis of the biological half-life of the drug and should be followed accordingly. Not all *t.i.d.* schedules would be the same even if they were scheduled by pharmacists, because a schedule is set according to medication criteria and patient criteria. Pharmacists can take all factors into account and arrive at an optimal schedule.

Admittedly then, variation per se among schedules planned by patients does not mean that doses were scheduled at the wrong time. On the other hand, it seems unlikely that patients were able to consider both medication and patient criteria and schedule medication in a rational manner; therefore, it seems unlikely that variation among schedules would mean variation among optimal schedules.

This study was not designed to evaluate dose schedules of individual drugs, but several examples of scheduling indicated that patients' dose schedules violated scheduling principles. Frequently, patients did not schedule antiinfectives in divided doses over 24 hours. For example, two sulfamethoxazole doses per day were scheduled within four hours of each other; four tetracycline doses per day would have been taken at two-hour intervals; and four methenamine mandelate doses would have been taken at 9 a.m., 10 a.m., 11 a.m. and 12 noon. Several examples suggested that multiple medications for one patient complicated the problem of scheduling. The patient who planned to take his methenamine mandelate at one-hour intervals, planned to take his other medications—ascorbic acid, *q.i.d.*, stilbestrol, *q.d.*, and digoxin, *q.d.*—one after another, at one-hour intervals.

Can we conclude that because some patients did not take their medications at optimal times, their clinical progress was seriously jeopardized? Clinical significance of deviation from an optimal schedule has been shown in a study of diuretics[6] and in the case of quinidine when it is used for the prevention of arrhythmias.[7] But it has not been established for most drugs. This study points out a need to investigate the clinical significance of an optimal schedule.

Should the pharmacist even before he has proof of clinical significance make a change in his traditional labeling practice and assume the additional function of consulting with the patient to obtain patient criteria and then actually schedule doses for the outpatient? Among the prescriptions in this study, 13 directed the patient to the exact interval at which the medication should be taken. It has been suggested that physicians prescribe the frequency of administration in this manner, thereby decreasing their contribution to hospital medication errors.[8] One would think that physicians could not possibly object if pharamacists translated inexact times into exact hours. Certainly, physicians would prefer the pharamacist to do this rather than the patient.

Perhaps such clinical service cannot yet be justified economically unless the medical significance of adhering to an optimal schedule can be proven. Or should pharmacists assume this responsibility on the mere chance that they could decrease the incidence of less than optimal therapy? Opportunities for pharmacists to contribute their knowledge toward better patient care are not so numerous that they can afford to waste one.

### References

1. Rickels, K. and Briscoe, E.: Assessment of Dosage Deviation in Outpatient Drug Research, *J. Clin. Pharmacol. 10*:153–160 (May–June) 1970.
2. Leistyna, J. A. and Macauley, J. D.: Do Pediatric Patients Receive Prescribed Oral Medication? *Amer. J. Dis. Child. 111*:22–26 (Jan.) 1966.
3. Arnhold, R. G.: Do Your Patients Take Their Drug? *Clin. Pediat. 6*:139 (Mar.) 1967.
4. Malahy, B.: The Effect of Instruction and Labeling on the Number of Medication Errors Made by Patients at Home, *Amer. J. Hosp. Pharm. 23*:283–292 (June) 1966.
5. Barker, K. N. and McConnell, W. E.: The Problem of Detecting Medication Errors in Hospitals, *Amer. J. Hosp. Pharm. 19*:360–369 (Aug.) 1962.
6. Murphy, J., Casey, W. and Lasagna, L: The Effect of Dosage Regimen on the Efficacy of Chlorothiazide in Human Subjects, *J. Pharmacol. Exp. Ther. 134*:286–290 (Dec.) 1961.
7. Bloomfield, S. S.: Conducting the Clinical Drug Study, *In* Proceedings of the Institute on Drug Literature Evaluation, American Society of Hospital Pharmacists, Washington D. C. 1968, pp. 141–154.
8. Anderson, R. D.: The Physician's Contribution to Hospital Medication Errors, *Amer. J. Hosp. Pharm. 28*:18–25 (Jan.) 1971.

# 34 Prescription Dispensing to the Problem Patient

Philip Liberman and Allan J. Swartz

This chapter reviews some of the reasons outpatients make mistakes in taking their medications and suggests actions that pharmacists may take to remedy this problem.

A case study of an illiterate patient who failed to take her medications properly is presented. Pharmacists designed a special patient medication sheet to assist the patient.

The aspects of self-medication errors discussed include the inability to comprehend directions, patient attitude toward taking drugs, and unclear directions. Included among the solutions to these problems are supplemental directions, pharmacist-patient consultations, better packaging, and patient follow-up. The pharmacist must consider it his responsbility to assure the correct self-administration of drugs by outpatients.

Studies indicate that a staggering percentage of outpatients take their prescription medication incorrectly.[1-3] Yet it is a rare hospital pharmacist who feels personally responsible if the medications he dispenses are not taken properly.

## Case Study

The case study of an illiterate patient treated at City of Hope will illustrate a number of points to be discussed. This patient was taught how to take her discharge medication correctly, although she had failed to do so following her previous discharge.

Mrs. K. had been hospitalized at City of Hope for three months. She was discharged, but returned two weeks later in acute distress. It was discovered that Mrs. K. had not been taking any medication while at home. Since she could not read, the labeled directions on her prescription containers were meaningless to her; she did not know what to do with her drugs, so she did nothing. She was ashamed of her inability to read and did not ask for help.

Due to her inability to read, a somewhat complicated dosage schedule, and her previous failure, it seemed unlikely that the patient would be able to take her medications correctly after discharge. Verbal reinforcement of her prescription directions was important, but probably not sufficient. It was clear that unless something was done to assure that the patient would take her medications properly, she soon would experience another relapse and readmission.

Her discharge medications were digoxin 0.25 mg, one tablet daily; furosemide 40 mg, two tablets every other day; and prednisolone 5 mg, ten tablets every other day (to alternate with furosemide). A special patient medication sheet utilizing visual and mechanical aids was designed for Mrs. K. so that she was able to take her medications without having to read any written instructions (Figure 1). Each medication sheet contained a one-week supply of drugs. The dose to be taken each day was placed in mini-Brewer boxes opposite the date. The mini-sleeves were permanently attached to the sheet; the mini-trays were removable. We took advantage of the fact that Mrs. K. was able to recognize the numerical representation of the date. All she had to do was to slide out the mini-tray opposite the appropriate date and take the drugs inside. She was given fresh medication sheets

Figure 1. Patient medication sheet

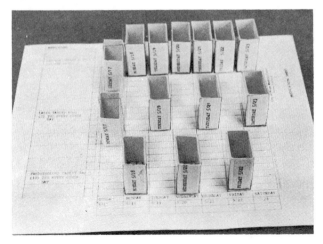

by a pharmacist following her weekly outpatient clinic visits. After four weeks, Mrs. K. was sufficiently used to taking her drugs so that she no longer needed the patient medication sheet. Through continuing follow-up on this patient, at home and in the clinic, we were able to determine that she was taking her medication exactly as ordered.

## Inability to Comprehend Directions

To a semiliterate or illiterate patient, such as the one discussed above, the typewritten directions on a prescription container are useless. The problems of the foreign-language patient who may have difficulty speaking and reading English are essentially the same. There is, however, a solution for patients who cannot read English, but do read another language: Dispense his prescriptions with directions in his native language. This may seem obvious, but the vast majority of pharmacies in this country probably have no provision for writing directions in any language but English. There are language guides available which translate common prescription directions into many foreign languages.[4,6] Such guides would be useful additions to any prescription department.

Even though a patient may speak a language other than English, we cannot assume that he also can read that language. In the case of certain American Indian tribes, no written language exists. In order to overcome this handicap, the United States Public Health Service Indian Hospital at Fort Defiance, Arizona originated an excellent pictorial label. It consists of four boxes showing a rising sun, a noon-day sun, a setting sun and a night scene. A picture of a tablet or tablets, teaspoon or drops is placed in the appropriate box by means of a rubber stamp (Figure 2).

Many other individuals face severe obstacles to the proper use of their medication. These include mentally or emotionally disturbed individuals, patients with physical handicaps and elderly patients. If the pharmacist feels that any of these patients are unable to safely medicate themselves, he has a duty to see to it that someone will medicate them. There should be one responsible individual—usually a relative or a neighbor—who knows exactly what to do for the patient.

## Patient Attitudes

Many patients have a generally lax attitude toward taking drugs. They simply cannot be bothered with the nuisance of maintaining a dosage schedule. Some patients have a subconscious desire to be sick or to die. Others feel fine and see no reason to continue

*Figure 2. Pictorial prescription label for illiterate patients*

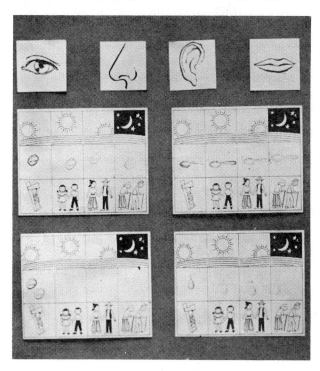

taking their medication. A prime example is the tuberculosis patient who must take medication steadily for prolonged periods of time with no apparent effects and while feeling healthy. Then there is the individual who stops taking his antibiotic as soon as the symptoms of his infection subside.

Many patients decide on their own that the dosage the physician prescribed is not right for them.[7] They may take substantially less medication than prescribed. This is not necessarily undesirable, however, these patients rarely inform their doctor of what they are doing. There also are some who take substantially more medication than they should. Some patients are quite forgetful. Alcoholics, in particular, are notoriously absentminded when it comes to taking medication.

These poorly motivated patients are the most difficult to assist; many of them cannot be helped. However, it is imperative that pharmacists become aware that such problems exist.

## Unclear Directions

A high incidence of errors can be expected when certain labeling practices are used. A majority of all prescriptions dispensed do not state what the drug is to be used for. Yet, it is likely that many patients will forget what a drug is for unless its use is stated on the label. This is especially true when a patient is receiving a drug for the first time, when he has many medications to take, when a drug is to be taken "when needed" or when a significant amount of time has elapsed between the time the prescription was dispensed and the medication is taken. Pharmacists have been extremely timid when confronted with the need to expand upon the prescriber's directions. Yet, the pharmacist knows that propoxyphene is for pain, kaolin-pectin for diarrhea and digoxin for the heart. Why not label drugs with their routine use, even if the prescriber neglects to state that use?

What can be done in cases where drugs have multiple uses? Ask the patient what he was told to use the medication for. If he knows the use, type it on the label so he cannot forget. If the patient does not know or states a use that is not indicated for that drug, check with the prescriber. In either case, note the use on the prescription blank and on the prescription label.

The worst results occur when prescription medications are labeled "take as directed." The patient frequently forgets part or all of any verbal directions by the time he arrives home. His problems are compounded if he has many medications labeled "as directed." When such a prescription order is received, ask the patient what directions the doctor gave him. If the patient has forgotten or states unusual directions, check with the prescriber.

The importance of taking certain drugs regularly is often not stressed. A patient may receive prescriptions for digoxin and for multivitamins. Both are labeled: "Take one daily." While it is critically important for him to take the digoxin every day exactly as directed, the vitamins are of less importance.

Many prescribers write prescriptions using technical language which is beyond the comprehension of the average layman. It is the duty of the pharmacist to "translate" medical jargon into easily understandable English. For example, a pharmacist should routinely substitute "under the tongue" for "sublingually," "to the skin" for "topically," "arm pit" for "axilla," "under the skin" for "subcutaneously," and "labored breathing" for "dyspnea."

Vague terms are frequently used in prescription writing. Many patients, for example, are unclear as to the proper definition of taking a drug "on an empty stomach." It may be necessary to question the patient about his eating habits and suggest specific times when it would be best to take his medication.

Prescription directions can be expanded and modified in many other ways to make them clearer to the patient. For example, instead of labeling a nitroglycerin prescription "one sublingually when needed," it may be labeled "allow one tablet to dissolve under the tongue when needed for chest pain. Nitroglycerin."

A great deal of caution, judgment and tact must be exercised so that the label represents only what the prescriber originally intended. Of course, it would be better if all prescribers would write complete directions in the first place. But until someone can devise a technique to convince or compel them to do so, alternative methods must be used.

## Supplemental Directions

It is often desirable to give the patient supplemental written directions in addition to the typewritten directions on the prescription label. Small gummed labels with short warning phrases such as "avoid alcoholic beverages," "may cause drowsiness" and "may discolor urine" can be attached directly to the prescription container where applicable.[8,9]

Often there is literature available that can be given to the patient with his prescriptions. For example, Eaton Laboratories has a booklet for patients taking levodopa.[10] "Understanding Tuberculosis Today, a Handbook for Patients" is a valuable booklet for anyone on tuberculosis drug therapy.[11] Griffith's *Instructions for Patients* is an excellent collection of instruction sheets giving valuable information about a wide range of drugs and many common illnesses.[12] This type of literature can be a valuable aid to the patient. More of such aids are needed; unfortunately, available aids are not finding their way into the hands of patients. The pharmacist can help correct this situation by taking the initiative in distributing literature of this type (Figure 3).

A word of caution: Supplemental directions may be received by the patient from the physician, the nurse and the pharmacist. All of these directions must be compatible to avoid confusing the patient. The pharmacist must take care not to give contradictory information.

There is also the risk that the patient will be bombarded with so much information that he cannot assimilate all of it. For example, a patient may be told to take tetracycline suspension four times a day, one hour before meals or two hours after meals and

*Figure 3. Patient guides for self-administration of medications*

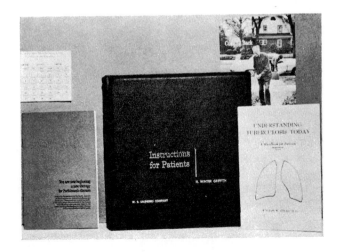

at bedtime; take until gone; may take with fruit juice, but not with milk or other dairy products, ferrous sulfate, or antacids; shake well; discard after March 1974. All of this information, although useful, may be too much for a patient to quickly assimilate, especially if recited rapidly across a crowded, noisy prescription counter.

## Pharmacist-Patient Consultations

Brands[13,14] has advocated that pharmacists utilize a private office where the patient can be told about the medicine he is taking. This is an excellent idea which would go far toward helping a patient fully understand his medications. But even without a private office the pharmacist can render a valuable service by spending a few minutes with each patient to see if he really knows what to do with his medications. We do not mean simply reading the labeled directions—a true dialogue between patient and pharmacist is needed.

## Better Packaging

Better prescription directions, both oral and written, can go far toward solving the problem of patient error. However, a redesigned prescription package also must be considered a key factor when attacking this problem.

Ideally, the drug manufacturing and packaging industry should offer a "mistake-proof" container which would virtually guarantee the correct self-administration of medications. This ideal has been closely approached by manufacturers of oral contraceptives. The success of "the pill" is in no small part due to the fact that it is dispensed in a form that helps assure its proper use.

The "Calendar-pak" and "Dialpak" concept could easily be applied to any drug that must be taken regularly. There are, however, very few instances (other than oral contraceptives) where manufacturers provide their drugs in special packages.

We should not sit idly by and wait for the pharmaceutical industry to hand us a better package. Individual pharmacists and pharmacies must take the initiative. The patient medication sheet utilized in the case study discussed earlier is but one example of the type of action that can be taken. Once we free our thinking from the limitations of the traditional prescription container, the possibilities are unlimited.

## The Follow-Up

There is one critical element that is still missing: the follow-up. A tuberculosis patient is usually checked

upon at regular intervals by the local public health department. But who checks on cardiac or diabetic patients to see if they are still taking their drugs properly a week, a month, or a year after the initial prescription? A pharmacist can help monitor a patient's drug therapy by checking the time intervals between refills for maintenance drugs. The patient to really be concerned about, however, is the one who does not come in for scheduled refills.

There are a growing number of health maintenance organizations concerned with continuity of care. Pharmacists should become actively involved in such organizations which are designed to facilitate patient follow-up.

## Conclusion

It is a rather new and revolutionary idea that a pharmacist should take interest in a patient once he leaves the pharmacy. However, it is about time that pharmacists take a good look across the prescription counter and redefine their responsibilities to include the correct self-administration of drugs by outpatients instead of strictly mechanical tasks involved with plastic vials and multicolored "pills."

## References

1. Bergman and Werner: Failure of Children to Receive Penicillin by Mouth, *New Engl. J. Med.* 268:1334-1338 (June 13) 1963.
2. Friend, D. G.: Everyone Should be Concerned with Drug Safety, *J. Amer. Pharm. Ass. NS4*:528-529 (Nov.) 1964. 1964.
3. Malahy, B.: The Effect of Instructions and Labeling on the Number of Medication Errors Made by Patients at Home, *Amer. J. Hosp. Pharm.* 23:282-292 (June) 1966.
4. Bartilucci, A. J. and Durgin, J. M.: Language Guide for the Clinical Pharmacist, St. John's University Press, New York, New York, 1971.
5. Strauss, S. and Blumberg, M.: A Multi-Lingual Guide for Pharmacists, *Pharm. Times* 36:50-52 (Aug.) 1970.
6. Strauss, S. and Blumberg, M.: A Multi-Lingual Guide for Pharmacists, *Pharm. Times* 36:54-63 (Sept.) 1970.
7. McClellan, T. A. and Cowan, G.: Use of Antipsychotic and Antidepressant Drugs by Chronically Ill Patients, *Am. J. Psychiat.* 126:1271-1273 (June) 1970.
8. Fox, L. A.: Written Reinforcement of Auxiliary Directions for Prescription Medications, *Am. J. Hosp. Pharm.* 26:334-341 (June) 1969.
9. Silnutzer, A.: Are We Ready to Face New Challenges in Rx Labeling?, *Pharm. Times* 36:44-50 (Dec.) 1970.
10. Anon.: You Are Now Beginning a New Therapy for Parkinson's Disease, Eaton Laboratories, Norwich, New York.
11. Stead, W. H.: Understanding Tuberculosis Today: A Handbook for Patients, 2nd Ed., Marquette University Press, Milwaukee, Wisconsin, 1970.
12. Griffith, H. W.: Instructions for Patients, W. B. Saunders Company, Philadelphia, Pennsylvania, 1968.
13. Brands, A. J.: Quality Comprehensive Pharmacy Services, presented at Annual Meeting of the District of Columbia Pharmaceutical Association, Lancaster, Pennsylvania, (June 26) 1969.
14. Brands, A. J.: Complete Directions for Prescription Medication, *J. Amer. Pharm. Ass. NS7*:634-635 (Dec.) 1967. 1967.

# 35 Therapeutic Judgments

Charles C. Pulliam

Participation by pharmacists in the therapeutic decision making process is discussed. Six prerequisites to rational therapy are reviewed, and the steps involved in making therapeutic decisions are explored. The need for a systematic approach in making therapeutic judgments is emphasized.

Contemporary pharmacy practice has its philosophical base in a responsibility for optimal safety and efficacy in the distribution and use of medication.[1] Accountability, however, provides the credence which must accompany responsibility; moreover, it is the recognition of an accountability, both within and beyond the profession, which strengthens respect for that responsibility.

In recent years pharmacists have moved steadily toward a greater participation in the therapeutic decision process. Clearly, an accountability for the safe and efficacious use of medications requires this participation. Perhaps less clearly, but just as surely, the participants in this decision process must be intellectually worthy of their responsibility. That is to say, they must be both knowledgeable about the use and effects of medication, and possess the ability to apply their knowledge in a meaningful way.

Individually, many pharmacists have earned the respect of the medical profession for their sound, well-based judgments in contributing to the decisions of therapy. The clinical success enjoyed by these individuals reflects their own strides in developing and continually improving their pattern of practice. Through this effort they have become increasingly sophisticated and accomplished in applying the principles of rational therapeutics.

For these pharmacists, their participation is the product of their pharmaceutical knowledge and their respected clinical judgments. They contribute somewhat in the fashion of partners in participative management. The physician is the participative manager who seeks the knowledge, judgments and unique perspective of each team member and incorporates their contributions in formulating a treatment plan. Their intellectual acceptance and effective participation in this role reflects favorably on the integrity of their therapeutic judgments.

## Prerequisites to Rational Therapy

Effective participation in the therapeutic decision process is gained through methodical and disciplined attention to detail and a strong respect for its implications. One objective of such participation should be safety and efficacy in drug use. Unfortunately, rational therapeutic practices are neither the result nor an assurance of safe and efficacious drug use. On the other hand, attention to the prerequisites of rational therapy will provide the foundation for progress toward that goal. Smith and Melmon have listed six prerequisites to rational therapy in the text, *Clinical Pharmacology: Basic Principles in Therapeutics.*[2] They pertain to the contributions of each participant in the decisions of drug therapy.

The rational choice of therapeutic agents involves these prerequisites:
1. An accurate diagnosis
2. A thorough knowledge of the data related to the pathophysiology of the disease
3. A knowledge of the basic pharmacology and biochemistry of the drug and its metabolites, and the kinetics of the compound in normal and diseased man
4. The ability to transfer such knowledge to effective bedside action
5. Reasonable expectations of the relation of pathophysiology and pharmacology so that the drug's effect can be anticipated

6. A plan to make specific measurements that will reveal efficacy and toxicity and will set the course for continued therapy.

These quite purposeful prerequisites dramatize the challenge of rational drug use. Therapeutic success is at risk if each of these prerequisites is not assured. For this reason, participants in decisions of therapy must give attention to each point listed. The pharmacist's contribution will be greater in some instances (e.g., pharmacology and kinetics) than in others (e.g., pathophysiology), but in working to assure safe and efficacious drug use he must contribute to achieving each prerequisite

Meeting that challenge demands acquiring (or refurbishing) the skills, abilities and knowledge base to which each prerequisite alluded. It is diagnostic skills which are most remote from pharmacy's education and training; nevertheless, this capability is essential to the exercise of therapeutic judgment in the decision process.

Diagnosis is the recognition of a derangement or disease from its signs and symptoms. The objectives of diagnosis are to characterize the derangement and evaluate its consequences to the patient. According to Judge, diagnosis provides a frame of reference suggesting what to do and what to expect.[3] Of course, diagnosis in its most strict tradition is within the realm of medical practice. It relates to those complaints which cause a person to seek the physician's services; it relates to the dysfunction and abnormality associated with those complaints.

But in a broader view, as the team concept of health care becomes more widely implemented, other health professionals are acquiring and utilizing diagnostic skills in their practice. Nursing personnel have long used diagnostic skills in their contribution to patient care. And as pharmacists begin to seek greater participation in patient care they will renew the heritage of their profession's potential for diagnostic contribution.[a] Recognition and evaluation of intended therapeutic response, adverse drug reactions and side effects are contributions to patient management which require diagnostic skill.

Certainly, the need to distinguish between iatrogenic processes and disease processes is obvious. Incomplete knowledge of either the pathophysiology involved or the pharmacologic and kinetic characteristics of the drugs in use create a potential for misinterpretation of observed changes in the patient's status. Participative evaluation of therapy allows for the pharmacist to make judgments on the strength of his pharmaceutical knowledge which can compliment the physician's knowledge of the natural course of the disease process.

The ability and willingness to make judgments, and the confidence to stand accountable for those judgments, are hallmarks of full stature among professionals. Making judgments is the process of evaluation by comparison; making therapeutic judgments is the process of selecting from among several reasonable alternatives a logical or appropriate fact which will contribute to a therapeutic decision. Judgments are necessary at each step in the therapeutic decision process. Typically, the judgment at one step in the process will dictate the alternatives to be considered at the next step. Thus, judgments are related and only as sound as those which were reached earlier in the process. This should become more evident as the decision process is reviewed.

### Making Therapeutic Decisions

Therapeutic decisions are reached through a series of considerations, observations, evaluations and reevaluations. The series is actually a cycle which recurs throughout a course of treatment; it is a cycle because with each reevaluation a new decision is reached. The decision may be active (alter therapy) or inactive (change nothing), but the consequences of that decision must be evaluated. Several organized approaches to therapeutic decisions are possible. For purposes of discussion, however, the problem-solving approach seems to be most thorough and logical in its sequence. Briefly, it involves six steps: (1) recognition, (2) investigation, (3) analysis, (4) assessment, (5) plan and (6) follow-up. A review of what each step contributes to the decision and the judgments made at each step follows.

*Recognition.* Recognition of real therapeutic problems (and anticipation of potential therapeutic problems) is an essential first step in evaluating drug therapy. It is the initial challenge of participation in the decision process. It requires that the observer anticipate changes in patient status and be alert to their occurrence as well as their failure to occur. Judgment at this point involves a distinction between drug effects and disease effects. One example is recognition of the fact that symptoms of congestive heart failure are similar to symptoms of digitalis toxicity. It is indeed a challenging therapeutic dilemma when a patient has received "usual daily doses" of digoxin and presents with nausea, vomiting and other overt symptoms of heart failure.

*Investigation.* This essentially involves a collection of pertinent clinical evidence in consideration of the problem. It organizes both the subjective and objective findings of importance. A complete investigation requires a knowledge of the data relevant to the disease pathology and the drug's kinetic and pharmacologic characteristics. Judgment here involves selection of evidence. For example, recognition that dose, route, frequency of administration, serum potassium values, time course of the symptom development, concurrent therapy, and so forth are pertinent facts in the evaluation shows good judgment; however, failure to select data which will reflect renal function shows poor judgment.

---

[a] From the Policy and Procedure Manual of an Italian hospital (1762): "The pharmacist is not only compelled to follow the physician during the visit to the patient, but also he will make other visits every day to examine the seriously ill patients, for needs which might suddenly arise."[4]

186

*Analysis.* This involves an interpretation of the data collected. It draws upon knowledge and experience in that relationships between and among certain elements of evidence must be appreciated. Judgment is exercised in sorting the possibilities according to the probability of their causing or influencing the problem. In the situation presented above, a serum potassium value which has changed from 4.9 to 3.6 mEq/liter over 72 hours might lead one to suggest increased cardiac sensitivity, but a serum creatinine value which has changed from 1.9 to 1.2 mg/100 ml over that same period would make therapeutic failure (secondary to an increased rate of drug elimination) a more probable cause of the observed symptoms.

*Assessment.* An assessment of the clinical implications of a problem should precede any decision to alter therapy. If the implications of a changing patient status are deemed severe enough, immediate action may be indicated; on the other hand, if they are considered to be insignificant or self-limiting, no therapeutic action may be called for. Judgment is employed here in deciding what to expect; what to anticipate; and what treatment objectives, if any, should be outlined. It is possible that the diuresis accompanying improved renal function will bring a resolution of the failure; it is also possible that the patient will be unable to tolerate even this transient cardiac failure because of other clinical complications. These judgments must be made in order that recommendations for resolving the problem may be formulated.

*Plan.* A plan of action is developed through consideration of those therapeutic alternatives with potential to resolve the problem. In formulating a recommendation for resolution of the problem, potential complicating difficulties associated with each alternative must be considered. As each alternative is considered, the treatment objectives outlined in the assessment process provide a basis for judgment in selecting a plan of action. A plan for our patient might include an adjustment in dose based on pharmacokinetic calculations, two days of moderate potassium supplements, and a recommendation to follow electrolytes and parameters of renal function.

*Follow-up.* This completes the decision process by beginning the cycle again. Follow-up is an evaluation of the course of action taken. Among the judgments which might be considered are how often and how frequently should reevaluations be made. Follow-up can avert serious problems before they occur. It is a very important step in the decision process.

### Need for a Systematic Approach

Therapeutic judgments can be lost among the many steps and the many patients being evaluated. So that no stone is left unturned, these judgments must be made within an orderly, systematic approach to the evaluation process. Valid, rational decisions depend on a meticulous collection of evidence and an orderly means of reviewing therapy; these can only be accomplished using a pattern, a logical and systematic approach.

Several approaches to managing therapeutic data for its review and evaluation have been developed, but few have been published (the most recent, by Bennett et al, appears elsewhere in this volume.[5]) furthermore, there is no evidence of attempts to achieve consistency of function among pharmacists directly involved with patient care; there are only indications that each program is pursuing its own course in relative isolation of others. While such activities have identified certain neglected or poorly met needs of the health team, they have also been viewed as an effort to be all things to all people. It is reasonable to say that, beyond activities improving distribution of drugs, the pharmacist's efforts in the patient care area have been fragmented in the broad view. As a result, the physician remains the practitioner accountable and, therefore, responsible for safe and efficacious use of medication. My only knowledge of a probable exception to this is the situation which exists on Docent Teams at the University of Missouri-Kansas City Medical Center.

Utilizing the participative management analogy once more, pharmacists might do well to express their wish for accountability and encourage their own active use of the patient's medical record. Consistency in approach could be served simultaneously if active pressure to incorporate the problem-oriented medical record (POMR) accompanied efforts to use the medical record. Those outside of pharmacy who would encourage and welcome pharmacy's participation in the therapeutic decision process would then realize their expectations of consistency among pharmacists in their contributions.

### References

1. Brodie, D. C.: Drug-Use Control: Keystone to Pharmaceutical Service, *Drug Intel.* 1:63–65 (Feb.) 1967.
2. Melmon, K. L. and Morrelli, H. F. (eds.): Clinical Pharmacology: Basic Principles in Therapeutics, The MacMillan Co., New York, New York, 1972, p. 3.
3. Judge, R. D. and Zuidema, G. D. (eds): Physical Diagnosis: A Physiological Approach to the Clinical Examination, Little, Brown and Co., Boston, Massachusetts, 1963, p. 8.
4. Koup, J. R.: Déjà Vu: We Have All Been Here Before (Letter), *Drug Intel. Clin. Pharm.* 7:191–192 (Apr.) 1973.
5. Bennett, R. W. et al.: Development of a Pharmacy Care Plan, In *Clinical Pharmacy Sourcebook*, pp. 49-52.

# 36 A Systematic Approach to Drug Therapy for the Pharmacist

Donald T. Kishi and Arthur S. Watanabe

A systematic and orderly thought process which can be used by the pharmacist in approaching rational therapeutics is presented.

The approach is based in part on the concepts of the problem-oriented medical record. Six steps of the approach are discussed: (1) defining the problem, (2) defining the therapeutic goal or end-point, (3) defining the therapeutic alternatives, (4) establishing the final therapeutic plan, (5) monitoring parameters to evaluate the therapy, and (6) determining nonresolution or treatment failure. A patient case study is presented to illustrate the steps.

Traditionally, the pharmacist's role in the health care delivery system has been one of procurement, storage, preparation, and distribution or dispensing of medications. Although this traditional role is a valid and necessary function, it is incomplete since the emphasis on medications which results has led traditional pharmacy toward a product orientation and away from a patient orientation. In such a product-oriented environment, little concern is directed toward the rationale and propriety of the prescribed medication for a given patient. Similarly, little concern is given to the patient-medication interaction once the medication has been dispensed.

The trends in pharmacy and pharmaceutical education reflect an awareness of the limited nature of the traditional practice of pharmacy. This awareness is reflected by the increasing emphasis on the medication as a therapeutic agent which elicits both beneficial and adverse effects, as well as the concern for the patient as a recipient of such agents. Patient-oriented pharmacy practice is known as clinical pharmacy.

The evolutionary process which these trends reflect will require the reorientation and reeducation of the existent pharmacist. Similarly, graduates of schools of pharmacy which do not provide an experience in the application of clinical didactic materials may require an orientation to clinical practice. To use an analogy, a pharmacist with a good background in didactics without clinical experience is not unlike the new diabetic patient who is given a syringe, needle and bottle of insulin without any instruction in their use; he has the tools but does not know how to apply them. This chapter will attempt to facilitate the requisite reeducation and reorientation by describing a systematic and orderly thought process which can be used as an approach to rational therapeutics.

The concepts described are, in part, an application of Weed's problem-oriented medical record (POMR) approach to medical practice. The basic criterion of the practicing clinician, according to Weed, is "how well he can identify the patient's problems and organize them for solution." Similarly, the multiplicity of problems related to medications—therapeutic, pharmacologic, pharmacokinetic, and toxicologic—rely on their identification and organization before a rational solution can be reached.

The data base is central to the POMR and the concepts of this chapter (Figure 1). The data base consists of the patient's (1) age, sex, race, (2) chief complaint, (3) history of present illness, (4) past medical history, (5) family medical history, (6) review of systems, (7) physical examination, (8) medication history,[a] (9) social history and (10) laboratory data and other diagnostic studies. It should be emphasized that the data base, by its intrinsic nature, is not a static source of information. Rather, the data base of a patient begins as the initial work-up. The dynamic state of the human body and the influence of medications and disease states constantly result in new parameters of the data base, or alterations of those previously noted.

The pharmacist's approach to rational therapeutics is in essence a thought process followed by the appropriate

---

[a] Includes present and significant past medications, allergies and adverse medication reactions, and exposure to chemicals or other toxins, including alcohol.

Figure 1. *Flow diagram of the thought processes involved in establishing a systematic approach to drug therapy*

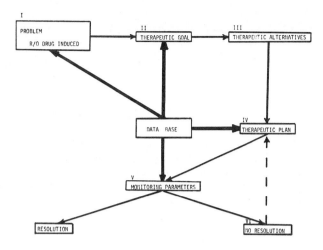

action or behavior. With reference to the flow diagram (Figure 1), it can be seen that these thought processes occur in a defined and orderly sequence. Each step is presented for consideration and results in a specific action or behavior before proceeding to the next step. The consideration of each of these steps, sequentially and in context of the data base, lends itself to the prevention of oversights and random, inefficient approaches. Thus, a complete data base is essential for accurate diagnosis and rational therapeutics.

For purposes of simplification, the following scheme is intended for single problem application. However, it is important to understand that although a given patient may present simultaneously with multiple problems, the concepts of this chapter are easily applied keeping in mind that the interaction between medications and all physiologic systems is on-going.

### Step I: The Problem

The problem is defined as: (1) a proven diagnosis, e.g., diabetes mellitus; (2) a physiologic entity or syndrome, e.g., hemolytic anemia; (3) a symptom, e.g., arthralgia; (4) a physical sign or finding, e.g., elevated blood pressure; or (5) an abnormal laboratory value or other diagnostic study, e.g., hypokalemia. In the approach advocated by this chapter, the problem represents the portal of entry for the pharmacist. The pharmacist must screen and separate the multiple problems with which a given patient may present into those amenable to drug therapy or potentially induced by drug effect or toxicity. He should never lose sight, however, of the entire picture with which the patient presents.

Once a problem is identified, the pharmacist must exclude the possibility of a drug induced etiology. This is accomplished by referring to the medication portion of the patient's data base and either applying pharmacologic knowledge or researching the literature to exclude the relationship between the problem and medication(s) received by the patient. Assuming that a relationship

may exist, feasibility of designating that the problem is the result of the medication must be evaluated. The dose, duration of therapy, mechanism and incidence relationship must be established.

For example, in a patient with extrapyramidal Parkinsonian-type movements, the medication history should be examined for drugs known to cause extrapyramidal side effects, most prominently, the phenothiazines. If the patient has recently received or is currently receiving a phenothiazine, a correlation of the dose, time and duration of therapy with the known facts concerning phenothiazine-induced extrapyramidal side effects should be made. If the correlation is positive, the appropriate counteracting measures should be evaluated and instituted, e.g., discontinuance, decreasing dose or counteracting therapy. For phenothiazine-induced extrapyramidal effects in a patient with psychiatric problems, the patient should be evaluated for possible contraindications to anticholinergic therapy. If none exist, an appropriate agent is instituted.

If the problem cannot be related to the patient's medications, the pharmacist must conclude that the problem is not drug-related. The pharmacist must then progress to Step II: The Therapeutic Goal or Endpoint.

### Step II: The Therapeutic Goal or Endpoint

The therapeutic goal or endpoint is defined as the criteria or results toward which therapy is directed. This goal or endpoint is dependent on the pathophysiology, severity and/or stage of the problem as denoted by the patient's data base. For example, the goal or endpoint of therapy of an iron deficiency anemia due to a chronic inflammatory disease differs from that for an iron deficiency anemia due to malabsorption of iron. Similarly, the goal of therapy for a 65-year-old Caucasian patient with a blood pressure of 150/100 differs from that of a 32-year-old black patient with the same blood pressure.

In all cases where feasible, the therapy should be directed toward the goal or endpoint of correction of the problem and not simply the correction of symptoms, signs, abnormal studies or laboratory test manifestations of the underlying problem. In such instances where curative therapy is not available, the goal of therapy may be symptomatic, palliative or simply supportive. The approach may be related to the different types of therapy available for the problem, the patient's data base and the desired therapeutic results.

### Step III: The Therapeutic Alternatives

The therapeutic alternatives are defined as those currently accepted and approved regimens for accomplishing the desired endpoint or goal. Once established, the alternatives for achieving the endpoint or goal by the desired approach must be evaluated. The basic alternative is the decision to treat (medicinal or nonmedicinal) or not to treat. Nonmedicinal intervention is exemplified by the obese maturity onset diabetic who is placed on a restricted calorie diet. If the decision is to intervene with medication, the various agents which will achieve the goal or endpoint by the designated approach must be considered. Additionally, the advantages and disadvantages, the dosages, idiosyncracies, toxicities, the degree of anticipated response and the possible routes of administration must be noted.

## Step IV: The Final Therapeutic Plan

The final therapeutic plan is defined as the most appropriate therapeutic alternative which is consistent with the desired goal or endpoint and approach to the problem in the individual patient under consideration. The selection of an alternative to be the basis of the final therapeutic plan involves a correlative thought process. This correlation involves the integration of the known facts about each agent and the known facts—the data base—of the patient. Such a thought process must include the following considerations: possible patient predisposition to the toxicity of agent(s) being considered—age, sex, race, concurrent pathophysiologic processes, reactivation of old disease, drug-drug interactions, drug-drug physicochemical incompatibility, allergic history, the rapidity of response desired and the duration of response desired. This correlative process is exemplified by the patient with a history of angina who is now hypertensive. Hydralazine is one agent which may be considered. Since hydralazine causes tachycardia, there would be a relative contraindication to its use in this patient. Another example is the patient with rheumatoid arthritis who has congestive heart failure. If glucocorticoids were indicated, prednisone or other glucocorticoid with low mineralocorticoid properties would be preferred to hydrocortisone.

Once the basic agents of the final therapy plan have been selected, the time course of expected response, modification of dosing regimen, prophylactic therapy for the prevention of avoidable side effects and adjunctive therapy must be considered. Examples of this process would include: dietary sodium restriction in the patient with congestive failure; modification of the dose and/or regimen of digoxin in a patient with anuria; and advising the patient on guanethidine to sleep with the head of his bed elevated and to arise slowly in the morning to minimize orthostatic hypotension.

## Step V: Monitoring Parameters

Monitoring parameters are defined as those subjective and objective criteria which are utilized to evaluate the patient's response to therapy, both therapeutic and toxic. Subjective criteria are those which are not quantitatively measurable and require a value judgment, including, general appearance, complaints, state of mind, strength or weakness. Objective criteria are those which are measurable, for example, vital signs, laboratory values.

Once the final therapy plan is developed, monitoring parameters based on therapeutic response and drug pharmacology must be established. The parameters which are to be used for therapeutic response should be consistent with and/or appropriate for the established therapeutic endpoint or goal. These parameters should include both objective and subjective evaluations. For example, a patient with hypertension may notice a decrease in headache as a subjective finding and his blood pressure will be lower as an objective finding as a reflection of therapeutic response.

The parameters which are to be used for monitoring for toxic effects of therapy are based on the pharmacologic properties of the drug(s) and were considered in the final therapeutic plan. Both subjective and objective parameters can be used to monitor for toxicity. A patient taking digoxin may complain of gastrointestinal distress as a subjective parameter of toxicity, while a digoxin plasma level may provide objective evidence of toxicity.

In addition to the parameters directly associated with the therapeutic and toxic effects of the drug(s), the parameters which will influence the drug's excretion should be noted. If a patient is taking digoxin, for example, the plasma potassium and calcium level, as well as renal function, should be checked periodically.

An awareness of potential drug-induced laboratory interferences which might alter the evaluation of therapy should also be included in the monitoring of drug therapy. The most common examples are the drugs which may cause false positives on the urine test (Clinitest) for glucose.

## Step VI: Nonresolution or Treatment Failure

With appropriate management, the therapeutic goal or endpoint would be achieved with subsequent resolution of the patient's problem. However, in many cases nonresolution or treatment failure occurs. Nonresolution or treatment failure can be defined as failure to attain the designated therapeutic goal or endpoint. This unfortunate set of circumstances is heralded by one or more of the following occurrences: (1) drug inappropriateness as documented by poor therapeutic response, (2) manifestations of drug toxicity, or (3) changing data base requiring alteration of therapy. A situation of this nature requires the pharmacist to determine the etiology of the treatment failure. This may require reevaluation of the therapy plan and consideration of any recent changes in the data base. Based on this reevaluation, appropriate changes or corrections in the current plan, or assignment of new therapeutic goals, alternatives, plan, and monitoring base must be established.

## Example of a Case

The following simplified case can be used as a model to demonstrate the thought processes involved in applying the concepts of this chapter.

> C.C.: The patient is a 32-year-old Caucasian female with fever and with frequency and urgency of urination for 24 hours.
> H.P.I.: One day prior to admission the patient developed an increased frequency and urgency of urination. This was associated with dysuria. Temperature at that time was 101 F. The symptoms have persisted since that time.
> PM Hx: Noncontributory, no previous history of U.T.I.
> Soc. Hx: Married, school teacher.
> R.O.S.: Noncontributory.
> P.E.: T 102 F, P 100, R 20, B.P. 125/84. No C.V.A. tenderness noted, otherwise noncontributory.
> Medication History: As per pharmacist history.
> Admitting Labs:
> CBC: Hct 40, WBC 14,000, Diff: P 80%, M 5%, E 2%, L 15%, Cr/BUN: 1.0/10
> U/A: sp. gr. 1.020, pH 6.0, many WBC's, many bacteria, otherwise noncontributory. Gram stain: many gram-negative rods.
> IMP: UTI secondary to gram-negative rods.

The case is referred to the pharmacist for consultation and evaluation, which initiates his involvement and the application of the systematic approach to drug therapy. (Refer to Figure 2 in conjunction with each step below.)

*Step I.* The pharmacist, noting the diagnosis of an acute urinary tract infection along with its clinical implications, proceeds to obtain a drug history from the patient and ascertains the following information:

1. Current medications: none, with the exception of birth control pills.
2. Nonprescription medications: aspirin occasionally for headaches.
3. Allergies: penicillin, oral, two years prior characterized by rash, hives. Denies any other allergies or adverse reactions to drugs.
4. No special diet.

Examining this information, he concludes that the likelihood of a drug-induced etiology is remote and can, therefore, be excluded. He then proceeds to the next step.

*Step II.* The pharmacist's next step is to develop a therapeutic goal. Referring to the patient data base, the pharmacist notes that the urinary tract infection is a first occurrence with little or no kidney involvement. On this basis, he selects as his goal curative therapy by sterile urine cultures. Had the patient presented a long history of multiple chronic infections or pyelonephri-

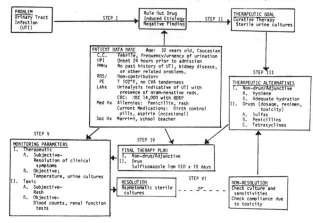

*Figure 2. Diagram of the case example involving urinary tract infection*

tis, it is possible that his therapeutic goal might have been one of symptomatic therapy using the suppression of clinical symptoms as his endpoint. Having established his goal, he proceeds to the next step.

*Step III.* The pharmacist proceeds to review the possible therapeutic alternatives available to him. By virtue of the fact that he has established a therapeutic goal, his options for treatment are automatically narrowed. The therapeutic options utilized in the treatment goals of other types of genito-urinary infections, for example, chronic infections or pyelonephritis, would be excluded, and only those modalities used in the treatment of a first-time acute urinary tract infection would be considered. Following the completion of this step, the pharmacist moves on to his next consideration.

*Step IV.* The pharmacist's next consideration requires a specific decision: From all the available therapeutic options, he must select the final therapy plan most appropriate for this patient. After careful consideration of the pharmacological indications in conjunction with pertinent information from the data base, the pharmacist elects to initiate therapy with sulfisoxazole and the prescribed nondrug adjunctive measures. Having decided upon an appropriate therapy plan, he continues on to the next step.

*Step V.* Following the establishment of an appropriate therapy for the patient, those criteria to be used in monitoring for therapeutic as well as toxic effects of the treatment are determined. It will be necessary to consider both subjective and objective criteria in each case, and from these established parameters determination of the efficacy or nonefficacy of the therapy plan can be made.

# 37 Evaluating Therapeutic Accomplishments

Charles C. Pulliam

The solution to therapeutic dilemmas by making sound therapeutic judgments in a systematic manner is discussed.

"Target selection," "forecasting," and the establishment of "therapeutic endpoints" and "therapeutic strategies" are discussed as requirements for a systematic approach to drug therapy. The selection of specific criteria for evaluating drug therapy is reviewed.

Pharmacy has given emphasis to more patient-oriented aspects of practice in recent years, and in so doing has stressed the value of its contributions to care through monitoring drug therapy. In retrospect, the main focus of attention has been on the detection of adverse drug reactions and the recognition of drug interactions. This has telling implications, because while contributions in this vein are unmistakably in the interest of optimal therapeutic safety and efficacy, there is some evidence that the yield is relatively low considering the energy expended.[1,2]

One can speculate about reasons for emphasis in this direction, but it is most likely that these activities receive primary attention because they can be fulfilled without full participation in the therapeutic decision process. A closer look suggests that it has been more circumstance than intent that has dictated this course. In order to fully monitor drug therapy, i.e., evaluate therapeutic accomplishments, the identification of therapeutic objectives and the means of measuring progress toward those objectives is necessary. The medical record, however, usually contains astoundingly little information regarding a plan for treatment. In fact, it seems remarkably neglected in contrast to the detail and systematic approach given the "history" and "physical examination." In the currently popular (traditional) approach to the write-up of a treatment plan, a therapeutic goal is expressed in very general terms. Clinical experience tends to dictate parameters of evaluation rather than specific characteristics of each case. Consequently, by neglecting to define the results toward which therapy is directed, objectivity in evaluating the progress of therapy and patient response is compromised.

This does not berate the importance or value of detecting an adverse reaction or averting a drug interaction. More implicit than explicit in this approach to monitoring drug use is that it is directed toward the success of therapeutic endeavors. The possibility of a therapeutic failure, however, is far greater than the likelihood of an adverse effect or drug interaction; therefore the scope of monitoring must extend from participation in setting the goal of therapy to assessing the therapeutic outcome.

For several years the concept of therapeutic endpoints has been discussed informally at local and national pharmacy meetings. The idea, while seemingly inherent in the therapeutic decision process, has been exceptionally elusive in practice. In the preceding chapter, Kishi and Watanabe have presented a systematic approach to therapy which develops an outline for participation from identifying the therapeutic goal through assessing the therapeutic accomplishment.[3] This approach provides the orderly, logical pattern which is essential for a thorough and consistent contribution to treatment decisions. It provides the structure for an integrated thought process upon which appropriate action depends.

## Target Selection and Forecasting

Two intellectual exercises that are prerequisites to carrying out this systematic approach to therapy are *target selection* and *forecasting*. They are essential instruments of the process, and the soundness with which they are executed has direct bearing on the outcome of therapy.

*Target selection* is a sorting out of patient problems, both objective and subjective, in order to clarify those aspects of disease which might be altered or prevented by medication. This should be distinguished from both "problem" identification and indication of the "therapeutic endpoint." For example, congestive heart failure as evidenced by a shortness of breath, respiratory rales, ankle edema and cyanosis is a brief sketch of the "problem." In contrast, the *therapeutic targets* would be fluid overload and cardiac output, while "therapeutic endpoints" would be "results toward which therapy is directed,"[3] such as the disappearance of respiratory rales and cyanosis within a specified period of time and diuresis at a designated rate.

Once identified, the targets of treatment provide a reasonable means of limiting the alternatives for therapy to those most appropriate for consideration. Each drug chosen as part of the "final therapeutic plan" should therefore be directed at one of the targets for the purpose of achieving a designated endpoint. A choice of furosemide 80 mg orally each morning would be for fluid overload (directed toward the target) in order to achieve the desired diuresis (toward the endpoint); digitalization followed by daily oral digoxin therapy would be intended to improve cardiac output (toward the target) so as to effect a disappearance of respiratory rales and cyanosis (toward the endpoint). The need to consider potential targets such as hypokalemia should be obvious.

*Forecasting* is an estimate of the probable outcome of therapy for each course of action to be considered. It is based on a projection of several findings-actions-outcome logic sequences, and it is carried out for each target of therapy. Through this disciplined analysis of potential courses of treatment, the possibility of choosing the most appropriate and reasonable endpoint and final plan is enhanced.

By definition, forecasting is a subjective exercise. It takes into account information about the drug, the dynamic characteristics of the disease, the patient's individuality and the availability of resources for executing the plan. It brings into view such otherwise often-ignored factors as the patient's expectations of therapy and the social, cultural and economic influences in his life. Forecasting is the means of drawing together relevant information about each problem so that the relationship of objective data to the patient as an individual is accounted for in determining an endpoint and plan.

### The Therapeutic Endpoint

The cornerstone of the systematic approach to drug therapy is the "therapeutic endpoint." When clearly and concisely identified, it provides an operational base from which to develop a sound plan of treatment. A clear and concise statement of an endpoint should include a specific result which is to be accomplished and a time period in which it should be accomplished. By requiring an explicit statement of *what* is to be accomplished and *when,* a conscious commitment to evaluate the results is almost unavoidable. These can be realistically established once sound target selection and forecasting have been carried out.

Realistic therapeutic endpoints chosen in such a careful and thorough manner are a new asset to drug therapy. Among the several positive benefits the selection of therapeutic endpoints contributes to patient care are its valuable dimension in the problem-oriented medical record (POMR) and its potential for maximizing economies of both effort and cost. Although the "endpoint concept" does not depend on the POMR for application, its worth is most evident in the context of the order and logic in such records. By its explicit nature, a designated endpoint establishes the basis for evaluating the accomplishments of therapy as each problem is assessed. This is very much consistent with the objectives of the POMR.

The potential for economies attributed to the "endpoint concept" is claimed because it promotes greater accuracy in the initial therapeutic effort. An explicit statement of response desired by a specified time facilitates selection of the most appropriate treatment plan and calls for evaluation of progress toward the desired goal. Inadequate doses, excessive doses and refractory conditions are recognized early, and corrective action can be initiated promptly. Savings in both time and expense are thus realized.

In discussing the therapeutic endpoint, Kishi and Watanabe recommended that "in all cases where feasible, the therapy should be directed toward the goal or endpoint of correction of the problem and not simply the correction of symptoms, signs, abnormal studies or laboratory test manifestations of the underlying problem."[3] Practitioners attempting to apply the systematic approach to drug therapy will find this difficult. Only rare conditions exist where the problem is distinctly separate from the symptoms, signs and data manifesting the problem to be treated. The reason for this is that most diagnosis is based on a collection of clinical findings which exist in a characteristic pattern as a reflection of disease. Consequently, it is the change in symptoms, signs and laboratory data which best reflects how well the endpoint is being approached.

The importance of remaining attentive to the dynamic nature of disease received special emphasis from Smith and Melmon in their discussion of conceptual barriers to rational therapeutics. They stressed that the practitioner must "think of a disease as a process with discrete or continuous variables, all subject to potential analysis and all required for appraisal of the state of the disease, therapeutics, and prognosis."[4]

The endpoint reflects a prognosis for therapy while the plan and selection of criteria for evaluating therapy are a strategy for realizing the prognosis. Although the therapeutic endpoint is the cornerstone of the concept, strategy development is the key to bringing it all together, making it a useful tool in patient management. Developing a sound strategy is one of the challenges of the concept and the decisions therein present an important opportunity for exercising therapeutic judgments.

## Therapeutic Strategies

In making therapeutic judgments, the practitioner selects from among several alternatives a logical and appropriate fact (element of strategy in this instance) which will contribute to the therapeutic decision.[5] Well-defined therapeutic strategies have not been a widely applied standard of practice, however, and so reasonable alternatives, particularly with regard to selecting parameters for monitoring drug response in the patient, are only loosely identifed. There are no ordered or patterned means of differentiating among degrees of therapeutic success or failure. In fact, attempts to glean such information from clinical research literature of drug evaluation or therapeutic protocols have been disappointing; such articles have almost uniformly failed to distinguish the stage of disease at the outset of therapy or the various stages of disease reversal through which recovery progressed. The absence of an ordered, widely accepted approach to selecting criteria for evaluating therapeutic accomplishments has been perpetuated by multiple problems, but two resolvable shortcomings seem most apparent: poor standardization and documentation in literature reporting clinical drug trials, and failure to accumulate and analyze collectively data from individual success and clinical experience. It is likely that PSRO legislation will have an impact in this area eventually, but meanwhile, clinical preference sets the standard of practice.[6]

So that sound therapeutic judgments regarding strategy in monitoring drug response can be made, a certain degree of order among the alternative choices of criteria is necessary. Further, adherence to certain basic principles of developing strategy will contribute to consistency in care.

## Selecting Criteria

In examining various criteria for measuring drug effects, it is evident that they can be easily sorted into various objective and subjective findings related to either the drug or the disease or the patient. Sorting the criteria in this manner can provide a means of organizing parameters so that their relative worth in assessing therapeutic progress is evident. As an example, the difficulty in giving certain vivid subjective criteria a quantifiable description (i.e., color changes) might limit their usefulness as a measure of therapeutic success. Listed below are the types of criteria and a brief statement depicting the nature of each type.

    1. Criteria to evaluate drug effects:
       a. Direct effects measured objectively—few such crite-

ria are available, but an assay of plasma concentrations of the drug being evaluated is one example.
       b. Associated effects measured objectively—periodic assay of serum potassium permits an assessment of the hypokalemic response to diuretic therapy.
       c. Associated effects measured subjectively—the degree of orthostatic symptoms reported by a patient taking an antihypertensive agent, for example.
    2. Criteria to evaluate disease alterations or prevention:
       a. Objective changes in basic abnormalities—the changes in blood pressure when treating the hypertensive patient is an example.
       b. Objective changes in associated abnormalities—abnormalities of the fundus which are associated with accelerated hypertension may be followed as a measure of improvement.
       c. Subjective changes in associated abnormalities—a decrease in frequency and severity of headaches that are associated with hypertension is an indicator of a change in the disease.
    3. Criteria to evaluate the patient status:
       a. Objective changes in the signs of patient status—a decrease in body temperature or other objective signs of patient well being are grouped under this heading.
       b. Subjective changes in the symptoms of disease—alteration in the pattern, frequency or severity of pain reflect this type of subjective criteria.

The overlap in classifying criteria this way is inevitable. Differences in subjective changes of disease and subjective changes in patient status are usually difficult to identify; nonetheless, this approach to sorting criteria permits a more appropriate selection of the criteria for assessment of therapeutic progress.

Identifying and sorting the various criteria for evaluation are preliminary steps to the selection of appropriate parameters for monitoring therapy. The selection process is crucial in the development of a strategy; therefore, qualities and characteristics of the criteria must be examined. Among the qualities rendering a particular test valuable in the evaluation of therapy are precision and consistency. Precision is an indicator of the descriptive quality of the test; consistency is an indicator of the reproducibility of the test.

Consider the need to monitor renal function. Creatinine clearance is a precise and consistent measure of renal function because it is accurately descriptive of the glomerular filtration rate and it is easily reproducible since creatinine levels in the serum and urine are influenced by a rather limited number of variables. Blood urea nitrogen (BUN), on the other hand, is less precise and less consistent as a measure of renal function because it lacks descriptive accuracy and its reproducibility is influenced by several variables, including such factors as dietary protein.

The appropriateness of a test as part of the strategy is equally dependent on external factors influencing its value in a given situation. Availability, delay in obtaining results, convenience of measurement and patient acceptance and cooperation are among the many factors which must be considered. Again, consider the need to monitor renal function. In some small hospitals test availability and time required to obtain results are real issues. Many small hospitals have only limited laboratory facilities; while they might be able to measure BUN quickly, quite a few must contract with larger hospitals in their region for tests such as serum creatinine. I am aware of one situation where the reporting delay for creatinine is two to three days. Clearly, the restricted availability and the potential for a 96-hour delay (including the 24-hour urine collection time) makes BUN a more appropriate means of monitoring changes in renal function in this situation. Other factors possibly limiting the appropriateness of creatinine clearance in some settings are the relative inconvenience of collecting a 24-hour urine sample and the necessity to obtain a complete sample (even if the patient is uncooperative). Either problem should be well known to everyone familiar with day-to-day activities of hospital care.

Selecting criteria for treating symptomatic targets provides a special dilemma for developing therapeutic strategies. Symptomatic problems are by definition apparent only to the patient. It is therefore quite clear that the work-up of the patient must elicit concise statements about the character of the problem. Only by description of the prominent features of a symptomatic condition can reasonable and appropriate parameters for following progress be expressed.

Included in the task of selecting laboratory tests and observations to be made, establishment of criteria implies a designation of the frequency that they will be measured so that progress toward the endpoint is appreciated. Tests ordered too frequently are economically inappropriate and inefficient; tests ordered less often than necessary allow for unrecognized toxicities or prolonged nonefficacious therapy.

## Conclusion

Selection of parameters for evaluating therapy, therefore, requires: a quantification of symptomatic targets; consideration of each observation's (1) precision, (2) consistency, (3) availability, (4) reporting delay, (5) measurement convenience and (6) patient acceptance; and a designation of frequency for each observation. As a general expression of the guiding principles for designating appropriate criteria for evaluating therapeutic accomplishments, the following statement is offered: Patients should be characterized as to their physiologic status (identifying aspects of status with potential to alter drug response),[7] and potential susceptibility to adverse drug reactions[8]; criteria of successful therapy should designate the regression of both objective and subjective findings when the endpoint represents a reversal of the disease, or a continuation of negative findings when the endpoint represents preventive therapy; and the reversal or continuation of findings should reflect the natural course of the disease unless acute alterations of problems are felt to be clinically necessary.

Therapeutic dilemmas are encountered often in the care of patients. Their effective and timely solution depends on sound therapeutic judgments made in a systematic approach. The concepts presented here and in the two preceding chapters have provided some guidance for resolving therapeutic dilemmas.[3, 5]

## References

1. Gray, T. K., Adams, L. L. and Fallon, H. J.: Short-Term Intense Surveillance of Adverse Drug Reactions, *J. Clin. Pharmacol. New Drugs 13*:61–67 (Feb.–Mar.) 1973.

2. Puckett, Jr., W. H. and Visconti, J. A.: An Epidemiological Study of the Clinical Significance of Drug-Drug Interactions in a Private Community Hospital, *Amer. J. Hosp. Pharm. 28*:247–253 (Apr.) 1971.

3. Kishi, D. T. and Watanabe, A. S.: A Systematic Approach to Drug Therapy for the Pharmacist, In *Clinical Pharmacy Sourcebook*, pp. 187-190.

4. Melmon, K. L. and Morrelli, H. F. (eds.): Clinical Pharmacology: Basic Principles in Therapeutics, The MacMillan Co., New York, New York, 1972, p. 7.

5. Pulliam, C. C.: Therapeutic Judgments, New York, In *Clinical Pharmacy Sourcebook*, pp. 184-186.

6. Anon.: PSROs and Norms of Care, *JAMA 229*:166-171 (July 8) 1974.

7. Hartshorn, E. A.: Physiological States Altering Response to Drugs, *Drug Intel. Clin. Pharm. 3*:14–20 (Jan.) 1969.

8. Williams, B. O., Eckel, F. M. and Dewey, W. L.: The Need for an Adverse Drug Reaction Prediction and Prevention Program, *Amer. J. Hosp. Pharm. 30*:124–127 (Feb.) 1973.

# 38 Recognition and Management of Secondary Failure to Oral Hypoglycemic Agents

Margaret C. Gebhardt, William R. Garnett, and Charles C. Pulliam

This chapter discusses (1) the thought processes necessary to determine if loss of control by oral hypoglycemic agents is due to drug failure or reversible causes and (2) principles for initiating alternate therapy if drug failure is suspected.

If drug failure is suspected, two general therapeutic alternatives exist: (1) pursue the potential of oral agents and, if they fail, then use insulin; or (2) initiate insulin therapy immediately. There are three successive approaches within the first therapeutic alternative: (1) manipulate the dose of the oral agent currently being used, (2) use another sulfonylurea agent, and (3) combination therapy—a sulfonylurea agent and phenformin.

Standards of diabetic control vary widely among clinicians.[1] These differences are in part influenced by opinions about patient ability to achieve certain therapeutic goals, as ultimately it is the patient's understanding of the goals which determines the relative success of therapy. Regardless of the definition of control, secondary failure to oral hypoglycemic agents is viewed as loss of control following a sustained period of acceptable control on a fixed therapeutic regimen.

Consider the case of R. G., a 55-year-old female with a three-year history of diabetes mellitus, who appeared with an apparent secondary failure to her sulfonylurea therapy. After initially failing to achieve control with diet alone, she achieved a primary therapeutic success with tolbutamide 2.5 g daily and maintained good control on this regimen for more than two years. During the three weeks prior to admission she was unable to remain free of symptoms and excessive glycosuria. She reported having polyuria, polydypsia, weakness and fatigue of increasing severity over the past three weeks while maintaining her usual regimen of medication and diet.

## Reversible Causes of Loss of Control

The dilemma presented by this woman is not an unusual or infrequent therapeutic problem in the middle-aged patient with diabetes mellitus. When secondary failure is suspected, careful effort must be undertaken to rule out reversible causes which may either be corrected by acute management measures or be self-limiting and short-lived. Among the several possible causes for loss of diabetic control which must be considered and assessed in this situation are the following:[1-4]

1. Acute infection
2. Dietary changes (dietary indiscretions)
3. Increase in weight
4. Change in exercise patterns
5. Other medical disorders
6. Pregnancy
7. Emotional stress
8. Addition or deletion of medications
9. Unintentional medication errors
10. Combinations of several factors.

Once these have been ruled out, the possibility of secondary failure to medication can receive an adequate evaluation. A premature diagnosis of secondary failure can prolong the therapeutic efforts to once again achieve control when one of these treatable and correctable causes goes unrecognized.

*Acute Infection.* Infection is one of the leading causes for acute loss of control.[5,6] Endogenous steroids have been implicated as having a role in this effect.[7] It is important to rule out infection early since immediate treatment would probably hasten the return to diabetic control if other causes are not present. Its consideration would include assessment of subjective reports of infectious symptoms (e.g., chills, burning on urination, local tenderness), hematologic studies (e.g., white blood cell count with differential count), urinalysis (e.g., bacteriuria, pyuria) and documenting elevations of body temperature. When an infectious process is documented, its treatment should be judiciously selected to avoid drugs affecting blood glucose, such as the sulfonamides, whenever possible. This would only confound further evaluation while attempting to rule out other causes.

Even if the initial impression is one of infectious process, it should not be assumed that this is the only factor causing the apparent failure in diabetic control. Two or more factors may be simultaneously affecting control; thus, a systematic evaluation of each of the other possibilities must be made.

*Dietary Changes.* Dietary changes, especially an increase in calories which is known as "dietary indiscretion," would be an important early consideration. Detection of dietary changes is not as objective in its evaluation as is identification of an infectious process. A precise patient interview must be conducted—often with the help of or by a dietitian—to establish eating habits and the patient's appreciation of the prescribed diet. In some cases it may be necessary for the patient to keep a diet diary for a few days if he is unable to relate accurately the amount, types, and times of eating. Asking the patient "Are you sticking to your diet?" simply will not give the information necessary to determine dietary indiscretion.

*Increase in Weight.* Weight gain should be considered while evaluating the diet. Obesity is a common cause of diminished response to insulin, and, although the mechanisms proposed are widely debated, it is recognized that an increase in weight will often require an increase in the dose of insulin or oral hypoglycemic agent.

Although at first impression it would seem that weight gain and dietary changes go hand-in-hand, this may not necessarily be so. A person's caloric requirement, like any other aspect of metabolic regulation, is not a static characteristic. The caloric requirement for maintenance of ideal body weight may change with time.

*Change in Exercise Patterns.* A similar effect may be seen if the exercise patterns have changed and calories are not being burned for muscular energy. New jobs, and even new work assignments, should be suspected contributing factors when they are elicited in the history.

*Other Medical Disorders.* Several medical disorders have been reported to aggravate diabetes. These include endocrinopathies (e.g., acromegaly, glucagon excess, hyperthyroidism), liver disease and pheochromocytoma. Other signs and symptoms will determine the appropriateness of a full work-up for these disorders. The point is that such medical disorders must be systematically considered and eliminated as possible contributing factors.

*Pregnancy.* A complex alteration of carbohydrate metabolism occurs during pregnancy, with a resultant decrease in the peripheral effectiveness of insulin and a greater demand for insulin. Contributing to these effects are hormones of both placental origin (e.g., placental lactogen, estrogen, progesterone) and maternal origin (e.g., cortisol) and the placental degradation of insulin.[8] Current labeling requirements recommend against the use of oral hypoglycemic agents during pregnancy because the evidence for teratogenicity is inconclusive, although suggested.[1,9] Thus, ruling out pregnancy is important for two reasons: identifying a possible cause for loss of diabetic control and avoiding possible teratogenic effects of oral agents.

*Emotional Stress.* Emotional stress is a factor which can be evaluated only by patient interview and attention to the patient's subjective behavior.[10] Circumstances that provoke feelings of frustration, excitement, anxiety, loneliness or dejection are frequently accompanied by glycosuria and increased requirements for hypoglycemic medication. This is believed to be caused by an increased release of epinephrine[11,12] and adrenal corticosteroids.[13] The key to effective assessment of this factor depends on determining how these circumstances are perceived by the patient and not just in the identification of stressful conditions. Seemingly insignificant stresses to the interviewer may be perceived as major stresses to the patient.

*Addition or Deletion of Medications.* The addition of nonprescription preparations or prescription agents may alter control. Nonprescription agents containing sympathomimetics may be taken singularly or in combination. With this in mind, a recent history of cold, hay fever, cough, stuffy nose or asthma may alert the clinician to the use and possible abuse of agents such as Dristan, Contac, Neo-Synephrine, Primatine Mist and many others.[14]

Since patients are known to see different physicians for various problems, and may receive therapy for nondiabetic-related disorders, the history should elicit new drugs and disorders. Drugs that have a diabetogenic effect and may aggravate diabetes mellitus include:[15]

1. Contraceptives, oral
2. Corticosteroids
3. Diphenylhydantoin
4. Diuretics
5. Phenothiazines
6. Sympathomimetics
7. Thyroid products.

Drugs may also have an antidiabetic effect. Whereas good control can be achieved while these agents are combined with oral agents, it must be determined if an antidiabetic agent has been suddenly removed from a patient's therapeutic regimen. Drugs that have an antidiabetic effect include:[15]

1. Coumarins
2. Guanethidine
3. Monoamine oxidase inhibitors
4. Phenylbutazone, oxyphenbutazone
5. Salicylates
6. Sulfonamides.

The severity of the diabetes, the dosage of the drug, and the duration of drug use would have to be considered when evaluating a possible drug interaction or drug-induced complication.

*Unintentional Medication Errors.* Inadvertent medication errors also must not be overlooked.[16] Was the prescription for the oral agent dispensed correctly? Does the patient really know which drug is the one for his diabetes? Does he realize the importance of taking it every day at the prescribed times? Has he run out of the medication and not had it refilled due to lack of time or money, misunderstanding or inconvenience? The answers to these and similar questions will provide a useful picture of compliance habits, errors and reliability; frequently they can be determined by having the patient bring his medications to the hospital or clinic. Examination of the bottle and its contents will give clues as to the identity of the drug and dosage directions. A call to his local pharmacist may be helpful in determining how consistently the prescription is being refilled, information which is valuable as an indirect measure of the patient's reliability and compliance pattern.

The above list of "rule out" possibilities for the loss of diabetic control may seem to involve more time and effort than warranted, especially if the final diagnosis is one of secondary failure to an oral hypoglycemic agent, as originally suspected. It is easier to blame the drug, rather than proceed through this list of other causes; but many of the items in the list are reversible in their effects upon diabetic control, so it becomes important to detect these as soon as possible so they can be corrected.

Returning now to the case of R. G., an assessment of the subjective and objective findings at the time of the work-up demonstrated no clear support for any of the factors discussed. There was no evidence of an infectious process. Interview by a dietitian supported her history of no substantial changes in dietary habits. There had been no changes in exercise patterns to suggest decreased caloric requirements. To verify her medication habits, her local pharmacist was consulted since the patient was unable to supply or describe the medicines she had been taking. There was no evidence to suggest that another medical problem was contributing to the dilemma.

Based upon these negative findings, it was felt then that Mrs. G.'s loss of control was due either to a secondary failure to her sulfonylurea agent or to progression of the disease to a more insulin-dependent stage.

Although originally reported to occur most frequently between the fourth and sixth months after initiating therapy, secondary failure is now felt to occur at any time during therapy with oral agents with the most frequent emergence during the third and fourth year. A projected four to eleven percent of the patient population per year develops secondary failure with about 40% of the patient population going out of control in five years.[2]

## Mechanism of Secondary Failure

Although the mechanism of secondary failure is not completely known, several postulations have been made. One theory is that this is a manifestation of progression of disease.[2,17] Another theory suggests that enzyme induction might account for the failure.[18] Also postulated is the theory that the sulfonylureas may act as a hapten by combining with plasma proteins to participate in an antigenic reaction.[19] Each of these theories, however, has been questioned.

## Therapeutic Alternatives

Once the diagnosis of secondary failure to oral agents is likely, therapy must be re-evaluated. Two general therapeutic alternatives exist, and the choice will be strongly influenced by the patient's ability to follow a particular regimen, the degree of metabolic disturbance, and the clinician's experience and interpretation of issues surrounding the use of various oral agents.

The first alternative is to pursue the potential of oral agents and, if they fail, then use insulin. The second course would be to initiate insulin therapy immediately as the final mode of therapy. Outlined briefly, the events may proceed as diagrammed in Figure 1.

Before attempting each step in this "flow pattern," a blood glucose level that renders the patient asymptomatic should be re-established. This may be accomplished by using an oral agent at doses which will probably exceed maintenance doses; or, if metabolic disturbance is sufficiently severe, this may be accomplished reliably and more quickly by a brief period of insulin therapy. Once control is established, the judicious use of oral agents may be sufficient to reach and maintain full diabetic control.

Although intermittent insulin therapy while attempting to regain full control is rational, this procedure has been associated with an increased predisposition to the development of insulin allergy and insulin resistance when insulin is reinstituted at a later date (reported even as late as 20 years after previous insulin therapy).[20,21] This risk is low but nonetheless should be recognized.[22]

Once an asymptomatic state has been re-established, the clinician can then pursue the therapeutic alternatives to establish appropriate maintenance therapy.

*Manipulating Dose of Current Oral Agent.* Seeking further benefit from the oral agents requires that as a first step the clinician manipulate the dose of the sulfonylurea agent currently being used.[4] This means either increasing the dose or changing the way it is being given.[23] With every drug there is a point of maximum benefit beyond which increased dosage shows little additional gain. Package inserts usually give recommended

*Figure 1. Therpeutic alternatives for the suspected diagnosis of secondary failture to oral hypoglycemic agents*

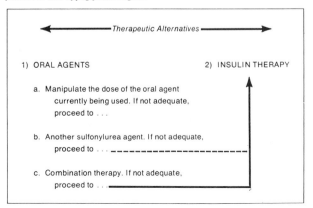

maximal effective doses; however, the experience of one of us (M.C.G.) has shown that in some instances these maximal doses may be exceeded and produce therapeutic results. With the shorter-acting agents (especially tolbutamide), a daily dose could be divided to minimize gastric side effects and to avoid an exagerated peak and valley effect (possibly leading to periods of either hyperglycemia or hypoglycemia).

The patient's response to each change should be watched closely, even daily if necessary. If a satisfactory response (as indicated by improvement in subjective symptoms and lowering of blood glucose) is not obtained within a reasonable time, that therapeutic attempt should be abandoned. "A reasonable time" would be determined by the rate of change in patient status and pharmacokinetic principles. For example, chlorpropamide usually requires five to seven days to reach steady state, so unless there are no early signs of therapeutic response dosage changes should not be made more often than once a week.

*Change to Another Oral Agent.* If the original agent is found to be ineffective, then a change to another oral agent is appropriate. Although the mechanisms of action are thought to be the same for all drugs in this class, there are demonstrable differences in potency and patient response to the various sulfonylurea agents. Many authors have reported the efficacy of changing to another sulfonylurea agent to restore or improve diabetic control.

When changing to a second drug or increasing the dose of the original drug, the patient must be observed for adverse reactions. Most of the side effects of the oral agents (anorexia, nausea, vomiting, epigastric discomfort, weakness, dermatologic reactions) are dose-related or transient; thus, early detection is desirable.

*Combination Therapy.* There is no merit in combining two members of the same drug class; however, since their mechanisms of action are apparently different, a combination of a biguanide (i.e., phenformin) and a sulfonylurea seems to be a reasonable approach. DeLawter and Moss reported a 66% success when phenformin and chlorpropamide were used together for patients who could not be controlled by either drug used alone.

The use of phenformin may be limited, however, by two factors: first, there is concern over the incidence of lactic acidosis associated with the use of this drug, although the etiology of the acidosis may be more rightly associated with the occurance of an hypoxic state or mild to moderate azotemia.[1] Second, intolerable side effects (metallic taste, anorexia, nausea, diarrhea, malaise)[1] often occur before the therapeutic dosage can be reached. Use of the sustained-release product may lessen these effects. Patients may have to learn to tolerate some of these side effects in order to remain on phenformin therapy.

*Insulin Therapy.* The second alternative for the treatment of secondary failure is insulin therapy. This course is mandatory if there is evidence (1) of ketosis, (2) that the diabetes is progressing to a more insulin-dependent stage or (3) that the patient is grossly symptomatic and the blood glucose is elevated to unacceptable levels. Although it may seem simple to make the decision to begin insulin therapy, with this decision goes a grave responsibility to educate the patient in insulin administration, storage, side effects, dosage regulation, aseptic technique, etc. The details of insulin education would warrant an article in itself, so the point to be made here is that serious thought must be given to determine if the patient is a candidate for self-administered insulin therapy. In some instances when oral agents are clearly not indicated, arrangements must be made for someone other than the diabetic to administer the insulin. This necessitates long-term planning and follow-up involving other family members, public health workers, local pharmacists and others.

These approaches for re-establishing control in the face of secondary failure were applied in R.G.'s case. Although she was symptomatic, her blood glucose was not dangerously elevated (the two-hour postprandial level was 220 mg/100 ml) on admission. Laboratory tests demonstrated no evidence of ketoacidosis, and it was felt her disease was not progressing to a more insulin-dependent stage.

Mrs. G.'s admission regimen of 2.5 g tolbutamide daily was already at a level expected to give maximal benefit, so no further manipulation of this agent was attempted. A second sulfonylurea agent was therefore selected; therapy of chlorpropamide 750 mg daily for three days was used to regain a symptom-free state (tolbutamide was discontinued), and a dose of 500 mg daily was found to maintain diabetic control.

Initial evaluation of this therapy one week later showed encouraging results. Mrs. G. was significantly less symptomatic, although her two-hour postprandial blood glucose value was still slightly elevated (155 mg/100 ml). After two weeks of this therapy the two-hour postprandial blood glucose value had improved still further, and Mrs. G. reported no episodes of hypoglycemia or earlier symptoms.

Not withstanding this apparent successful regimen, it should be stressed that patients with clinical manifestations of the type demonstrated by R.G. should be followed after serum glucose levels have been stabilized in order that subsequent modifications of diabetic therapy can be undertaken in a timely fashion.

## Conclusion

Secondary failure in diabetics maintained on oral hypoglycemic agents may occur at any time. All diabetics should be regularly monitored to detect if a re-evaluation of therapy is necessary. This chapter has attempted to (1) establish thought processes to apply in determining if escape from control is due to drug failure or reversible causes and (2) provide guiding principles for initiating alternative therapy if drug failure is suspected.

## References

1. Marble, A., White, P., Bradley, R. F. and Krall, L. P. (eds.): Joslin's Diabetes Mellitus, 11th Edition, Lea and Febiger, Philadelphia, 1971.

2. Campbell, G. D.: Oral Hypoglycemic Agents—Pharmacology and Therapeutics, Academic Press, New York, New York, 1969.

3. Emmer, M., Gordon, P. and Roth, J.: Diabetes in Association with Other Endocrine Disorders, *Med. Clin. N. Amer. 55*: 1057-1064 (July) 1971.

4. Camerini-Davalos, R. A. and Marble, A.: Incidence and Causes of Secondary Failure in Treatment with Tolbutamide. Experience with 2,500 Patients Treated up to Five Years, *JAMA 181*:1-4 (July) 1972.

5. Anon.: Infection and Diabetes, *Brit. Med. J. 3*: 76 (July 13) 1974.

6. Thornton, G. F.: Infection and Diabetes, *Med. Clin. N. Amer. 55*: 931-938 (July) 1971.

7. Bagdade, J. D.: Infections, *In* Diabetes Mellitus: Diagnosis and Treatment, Vol. 3, American Diabetes Association, New York, New York, 1971.

8. Tyson, J. E. and Felig, P.: Medical Aspects of Diabetes in Pregnancy and the Diabetogenic Effects of Oral Contraceptives, *Med. Clin. N. Amer. 55*: 947-959 (July) 1971.

9. Hamwi, G. J. and Seidensticker, J. F.: Therapy: Oral Hypoglycemic Agents, *In* Diabetes Mellitus: Diagnosis and Treatment, Vol. 2, American Diabetes Associations, New York, New York, 1967.

10. Kimball, C. P.: Emotional and Psychosocial Aspects of Diabetes Mellitus, *Med. Clin. N. Amer. 55*: 1007-1018 (July) 1971.

11. Lerner, R. L. and Porte, D.: Epinephrine: Selective Inhibition of the Acute Insulin Response to Glucose, *J. Clin. Invest. 50*: 2453-2457 (Nov.) 1971.

12. Cerasi, E., Luft, R. and Efendic, S.: Effect of Adrenergic Blocking Agents on Insulin Response to Glucose Infusion in Man, *Acta Endocrinologica 69*: 335-346, 1972.

13. Marco, J., Calle, C., Roman, D. et al.: Hyperglucagonism Induced by Glucocorticoid Treatment in Man, *N. Engl. J. Med. 288*: 128-131 (Jan. 18) 1973.

14. Griffenhagen, G. B. and Hawkins, L. L. (eds.): Handbook of Non-Prescription Drugs, American Pharmaceutical Association, Washington, D.C., 1973.

15. Hansten, P. P.: Drug Interactions, 2nd Edition, Lea and Febiger, Philadelphia, Pennsylvania, 1973.

16. Sheldon, J., Anderson, J. and Stoner, L.: Serum Concentration and Urinary Excretion of Oral Sulfonylurea Compounds. Relation to Diabetic Control, *Diabetes 14*: 362-367 (June) 1965.

17. Malins, J.: Clinical Diabetes Mellitus, Eyre and Spottiswoode, London, England, 1968.

18. Burns, J. J.: Implications of Enzyme Induction for Drug Therapy *Amer. J. Med. 37*: 327-331 (Sept.) 1964.

19. Stowers, J. M.: Treatment of Diabetes with Oral Compounds, Disorders of Carbohydrate Metabolism, Pitman, London, England, 1962.

20. Coleman, W. P., Derbes, V. J. and Brown, E. T.: Insulin Allergy, *Ann. Allergy 29*: 383-388 (July) 1971.

21. Lieberman, P., Patterson, R., Metz, R. and Lucena, G.: Allergic Reactions to Insulin, *Amer. Med. Ass. 215*: 1106-1112 (Feb. 15) 1971.

22. Patterson, R., Lucena, G., Metz, R. and Roberts, M.: Reaginic Antibody Against Insulin: Demonstration of Antigenic Distinction Between Native and Extracted Insulin, *J. Immunol. 103*: 1061-1071 (Nov.) 1969.

23. Tittle, C. R. and Kerr, John H.: Treatment of Diabetic Patients with Chlorpropamide after Secondary Failure on Tolbutamide, *Curr. Ther. Research 7*: 297-303 (May) 1965.

24. Tewari, S. N. and Fletcher, R.: Value of Tolazamide ('Tolanas') as an Oral Hypoglycaemic Agent, *Brit. J. Clin. Pract. 21*: 455-460 (Sept.) 1967.

25. Patel, J. C., Dhirawani, M. K. and Doshi, J. C.: Long Term Observations with Oral Hypoglycemic Drugs: Sulphonylureas, Biguanides and Their Combination, *Ind. J. Med. Sci. 24*: 393-403 (July) 1970.

26. Moss, J. M. and DeLawter, D. E.: Long Term Results with Oral Hypoglycemic Drugs, *J. Amer. Geriat. Soc. 21*: 72-76 (Feb.) 1973.

27. DeLawter, D. E. and Moss, J. M.: Twelve Year Experience with Oral Agents in the Treatment of Diabetes Mellitus, *Med. Times 96*: 855-864 (Sept.) 1968.

# 39 The Clinical Pharmacist and the Peptic Ulcer Patient

Gary H. Smith

The role of the pharmacist in providing clinical services to the peptic ulcer patient is discussed.

Diagnosis and treatment of peptic ulcer disease are discussed. Antacid therapy interactions with other drugs are reviewed. Naturally occurring and synthetic anticholinergics, sedatives, and other antiulcer agents also are discussed.

The pharmacist can be of considerable service in the treatment of the peptic ulcer patient. By establishing a medication history and drug profile for each peptic ulcer patient a valuable document will result. The pharmacist can instruct each patient on the proper use of medications and consult with physicians on drug therapy with regard to choice of drugs, possible adverse effects, and possible drug interactions. The pharmacist should also advise the patient as to nonprescription drugs that could possibly be harmful. However, in order for the pharmacist to assume these roles he must have a good understanding of the disease: the clinical signs and symptoms, the diagnostic procedures and the general medical treatment, including drug actions and interactions.

A peptic ulcer is an acute or chronic ulceration or circumscribed defect in any part of the gastrointestinal tract wall that comes in contact with acid and pepsin secreted by the stomach. Since there can be no peptic ulcer without the presence of acid or pepsin, it is sometimes called the "acid-peptic" disease.[1] By definition, one would expect to find most ulcers occurring in the esophagus, stomach or upper part of the duodenum, which is generally the case.[1-4]

The cause of peptic ulcers is still largely unknown, but hypersecretion of acidic gastric juice is an important factor. Emotional, hormonal, endocrine, infectious and vascular contributions must also be considered. "Stress ulcers" are acute erosions in the stomach or duodenum that do not penetrate the muscularis mucosa. They must be considered in patients with sudden onset of upper gastrointestinal bleeding following emotional stress or surgical procedures, or in patients being treated with adrenocorticosteroids and some other drugs. This type of ulcer is not usually caused by hypersecretion of acid and pepsin but these secretions may play an important role.[1-4] Duodenal peptic ulcers are four or five times as common as benign gastric ulcers and occur in men more frequently than women. The men to women ratio is 3:1 to 10:1.[1,4] Gastric ulcers also occur more frequently in males than females in ratios between 2:1 and 4:1. These ratios are closer to one during the years before puberty and after menopause. About one-fifth of the gastric ulcers occur in patients who have had or presently have a duodenal ulcer.[1]

## Signs and Symptoms

The peptic ulcer patient usually has pain. In a duodenal ulcer the pain usually is steady and said to be "gnawing, aching, hunger-like or burning." The pain is usually present one to two hours after meals and is relieved by food or alkali.[1] The pain may also occur during the night, but rarely just prior to breakfast.[1,4] Appetite is usually good and weight remains stable. Vomiting may occur if pain is extremely severe. Sour taste in the mouth and heart burn are usually present. Lower abdominal pain and constipation are also common.[1-4]

The gastric ulcer patient may or may not present the same symptoms as a duodenal ulcer patient. The pain may not be relieved by food. The patient may be nauseated and he may experience gastric distension upon eating. Pain may cover a wider area and there may be more cramping or burning than experienced by the duodenal ulcer patient. Pain at night is not common but may radiate to the back more often than with other peptic ulcers. Also, the gastric ulcer patient may experience anorexia and some weight loss which is not common with duodenal ulcers.[1,2]

Other symptoms may include excessive salivation, diarrhea and anemia due to hemorrhaging.[2]

The physician may use various laboratory tests for a diagnostic work up. These tests may include a gastric acid analysis using either histamine phosphate, betazole or azuresin to determine the amount of gastric hydrochloric acid being secreted by the patient. These tests determine if the patient is secreting an abnormal amount of hydrochloric acid since about 50% of duodenal ulcer patients secrete larger than normal amounts of acid under test conditions.[2] An occult blood test for blood in the stool may also be performed. The most important diagnostic procedure is x-ray of the upper gastrointestinal tract; 95% of the peptic ulcers may be diagnosed by this method alone.[2]

### Treatment

Since there are various causes of peptic ulcers and a wide armamentarium for the treatment of patients, each patient must be evaluated and treated on an individual basis. Only general guidelines which are usually altered to meet individual patient needs, shall be mentioned here.

The main objective in treatment is to remove the cause of the ulcer if possible and to create a condition that enables the ulcer to heal. Rest and relaxation are important in the treatment of peptic ulcers. Since many ulcers may be caused partially by anxiety created at work or home, the patient should be able to stay away from the area that creates anxiety reaction for two or three weeks. Other factors such as diet, proper antacid therapy, and administration of anticholinergic drugs, sedatives and other agents may also be very important.[1-4]

Most peptic ulcer patients are treated on an outpatient basis, but if the ulcer does not heal properly and pain is still present in two weeks, hospitalization may be required.[5] The pharmacist can advise the new peptic ulcer patient about the importance of following prescribed routine. The patient should also be cautioned about taking drugs that could aggravate his condition. Such drugs as xanthine alkaloids, corticosteroids, salicylates, reserpine, corticotropin, phenylbutazone, oxyphenbutazone, indomethacin and potassium chloride have been shown to cause ulcers or even perforation and hemorrhage.[1,4-6] The pharmacist can advise the physician against such drugs and should warn the patient of nonprescription drugs which may be harmful, such as aspirin, caffeine and APC compound. The peptic ulcer patient may be receiving treatment for conditions other than peptic ulcer disease from more than one physician. The pharmacist with the use of the patient drug profiles is in an excellent position to prevent possible drug interactions by communicating with the physicians involved.

### Diet

In the past a great deal of emphasis was placed on the diet for treating peptic ulcers, but controlled studies have not proven that the diet has any clear therapeutic effect.[1,6] However, pain does seem to be relieved by frequent small feedings, as many as five or six per day. The diet should be nutritious, especially for gastric ulcer patients since they are prone to lose weight. Each patient should be evaluated individually and one diet plan will not suffice for all patients. Food which is not tolerated well by the patient should be restricted. Generally, high protein foods are good because they have greater buffering capacity than foods high in carbohydrates and fats. Although proteins stimulate acid secretion, it seems that their buffering capacity outweighs this factor.[1,6,7]

The main dietary restrictions include alcohol, caffeine drinks, pepper and other spices.[4,5,6,13] If the patient is experiencing discomfort from his diet, other restrictions may include roughages, and greasy and fried foods.[1,2] Smoking has been shown to aggravate gastric ulcers and it is recommended that these patients not smoke. However, there is no evidence that smoking irritates duodenal ulcers.[6]

### Antacids

Antacid therapy is a very important part of the treatment of a peptic ulcer patient. Controlling gastric acidity either by buffering or by decreasing secretion is the main clinical objective in ulcer therapy. It has been shown that ulcer patients secrete more acid than normal patients and they do so on a continuous basis rather than intermittently as is the case with normal patients.[8] Gastric $pH$ and secretion can be controlled by antacid therapy and by anticholinergics. The objective of antacid therapy is to elevate the gastric $pH$ to the range between 4 and 5.[9] By elevating the $pH$ to 4 or 5, pepsinogen is inactivated and therefore pepsin is not produced. When the antacid is given one hour after meals, gastric emptying time is delayed, whereas if it is given on an empty stomach, emptying time is shortened. The antacid remains in the stomach longer and less frequent dosing is required when it is given after meals.[10]

As a general rule antacids should be taken at hourly intervals between meals during the day with supplemental doses at night during distress. This dosage varies with the antacid and the patient. In severe cases it may be necessary to administer antacids every hour around the clock.[1,3] The hourly dosage should be maintained until pain is relieved and then reduced to one hour after meals and at bedtime for 90 days.[3] While some claim that it is possible to prolong the elevation of pH by using an anticholinergic in conjunction with antacids, this was not found to be the case in a study by Fordtram et al.[10] Commonly used antacids include aluminum hydroxide, aluminum hydroxide with various magnesium salts (magnesium hydroxide, magnesium trisilicate and magnesium oxide), calcium carbonate, dihydroxyaluminum aminoacetate, hydrated magnesium aluminate and sodium bicarbonate. (A good review of the antacids has been prepared by Penna.[9]) Calcium carbonate is still recognized as the antacid of choice when tolerated. Calcium carbonate elevates gastric pH for a longer period of time than other antacids. Four grams of calcium carbonate taken one hour after meals will elevate gastric pH for more than three hours. Also, calcium carbonate is inexpensive. The problem of side effects may be a limiting factor when using calcium carbonate. The milk alkali syndrome may occur, but is not likely to happen unless large quantities of milk are taken along with calcium carbonate. This combination causes hypercalcemia, systemic alkalosis, azotemia and nephrocalcinosis. The symptoms of the milk alkali syndrome include nausea, vomiting, constipation, anorexia, headaches, mental confusion, weakness, polydypsia and polyuria. They usually occur within one week after starting therapy. Constipation is also a problem with calcium carbonate but may be easily treated by having the patient take a tablespoonful of milk of magnesia at bedtime.[5,6,11,12] The pharmacist should discuss the drug therapy with the ulcer patient and ascertain if any of these side effects have occurred. If these side effects have been noticed by the patient, the pharmacist may suggest an alternate antacid such as aluminum hydroxide. Since it also causes constipation, one of the products with some form of magnesium would be better. Aluminum hydroxide also has the problem of combining with phosphates and causing decreased urinary phosphate and ultimately the phosphate depletion syndrome. This difficulty may not be of any concern in most patients since the diet usually supplies adequate phosphate, but some individuals may have a decreased intake of phosphate or poor absorption.[9,13] When aluminum hydroxide and magnesium are used in a patient with renal failure, magnesium toxicity may

result. Another problem that may result from antacid therapy is excess sodium for patients with congestive heart failure, renal insufficiency or hypertension. A product with low sodium content would be recommended in these situations.

Among the commercially available antacids, hydrated magnesium aluminate (Riopan®) with a sodium content of 2.1 mg/15 ml is the antacid of choice for patients who must restrict their sodium intake. Antacids with larger amounts of sodium should be avoided depending on the patient. Some of these products are: Amphojel® (24.6 mg/15 ml), A.M.T.® (25.5 mg/15 ml), Gelusil® (19.5 mg/15 ml), Maalox® (16.8 mg/15 ml), Rolaids® (53 mg/tablet), Robalate® (28 mg/15 ml) and Titralac® (37 mg/15 ml).[9] Antacids also bind and prevent complete absorption of some orally administered antibiotics, especially the tetracyclines. Patients taking antacids may experience greater or lesser effects from other drugs used for other conditions. Since it is known that an alteration in pH can cause weak bases and weak acids to be in a different state of ionization, one would expect an alteration in the absorption rate of these drugs when taken orally due to an alteration of the pH by the antacid. Since the pH is elevated it would seem logical that increased absorption and an increased blood level may be expected from weak bases such as theophylline, meperidine, amitriptyline, chloroquine, imipramine, quinidine and amphetamine. Decreased absorption and decreased blood levels may be expected of weak acids, such as sulfonamides, penicillin G, nitrofurantoin, nalidixic acid, coumarins and phenobarbital.[14] It will be up to the pharmacist to warn the physician when the potential for these interactions arises.

## Anticholinergics

There is some controversey in the literature as to whether or not anticholinergics are beneficial to the ulcer patient. Because they enhance gastric retention and may lead to gastric dilatation, most evidence supports the belief that anticholinergics should rarely be used by the patient with a gastric peptic ulcer or an obstructing duodenal ulcer.[1-6] In the duodenal ulcer patient, when pain is not adequately relieved by antacids and diet, anticholinergics may be of help. Anticholinergics are said to decrease the motility of the digestive tract and reduce the secretion of hydrochloric acid in the stomach. The extent to which they reduce gastric secretion is controversial, but it appears that some reduction may be measured.[16] Some gastroenterologists believe, however, that the greatest benefit is obtained as a result of decreased gastric emptying time which increases the duration of action of the antacid.[1,3,5,6,15] As mentioned previously, the pH of the stomach may not be prolonged significantly by anticholinergics. Anticholinergics are contraindicated in patients with narrow angle glaucoma or predisposition to glaucoma, urinary bladder-neck obstruction, severe coronary artery disease, gastric ulcer, hiatus hernia, pyloric obstruction, gastric hypomotility, ileus, hemorrhage, prostatic hypertrophy, advanced age, debility, tachycardia, peptic esophagitis, and any gastrointestinal tract obstruction.[1,2,5] They should not be used prior to surgery or gastrointestinal x-ray examination.[5,15] Patients taking anticholinergics should be warned that some nonprescription cold and cough preparations contain anticholinergics and may produce an additive effect with the anticholinergic already being used.

The dose of anticholinergics is established individually by starting with a low dose and then increasing it to obtain the minor side effects, dryness of mouth or blurred vision. Since the secretory effect of the meal is maximal during the first 15 minutes and persists for one hour, and the maximum effect of the anticholinergic is obtained during the second hour after administration, the dose is usually given one hour before meals and at bedtime. A larger dose may be given at bedtime than during the day since higher doses create more side effects and are more readily tolerated at night. Although the dose of anticholinergics is titrated to side effects, no correlation has been demonstrated between the degree of inhibition of gastric secretion and decrease of motility and appearance of side effects.[1,5,6,15]

Since there are a variety of anticholinergic agents, which ones are considered most effective? The quaternary anticholinergics have a greater effect on gastrointestinal motility and secretion with fewer central side effects than the natural alkaloids or tertiary synthetic anticholinergics. The lack of central side effects of the quaternary synthetic anticholinergics results from their inability to cross the blood brain barrier. They do however have a more prolonged action than the natural alkaloids and also possess some ganglionic blocking action. This latter quality is the reason that the quaternary anticholinergics exhibit a greater effect on gastrointestinal activity and are more readily tolerated than other anticholinergics. Tertiary anticholinergics closely resemble the natural alkaloids in ganglionic-blocking properties.[16] Natural alkaloids such as atropine and belladonna are much cheaper and usually are employed if the patient can tolerate the side effects. If synthetics are used, Piper[15] and *The Medical Letter*[6] recommend the use of quaternary products such as propantheline, isopropamide, glycopyrrolate and poldine methylsulfate. Side effects of these drugs include dryness of mouth, blurred vision, urinary retention in patients with prostatic hypertrophy; also, impotence

and postural hypotension may be seen with those anticholinergics having ganglionic blocking action. Photophobia, constipation, nausea, vomiting, heartburn and palpitation may also occur. Other side effects include anhidrosis, precipitation of acute glaucoma, gastrointestinal tract obstruction, formation of viscid bronchial plugs, and hypersensitivity reactions. The nonquaternary type as well as the natural alkaloids may elicit some central effects such as headaches, dizziness, weakness, tremors and mental confusion.[6,15,16] Various drug interactions have also been reported. The clinical significance of these interactions is not clear and more documentation is needed, but the pharmacist should be aware of the possibilities. Antihistamines may create an additive effect with the anticholinergics because many of them have anticholinergic effects themselves.[14] The phenothiazines and the meperidine like analgesics may cause an additive anticholinergic effect.[17,18] Guanethidine, histamine, and reserpine may antagonize any anti-secretory effect the anticholinergics may exert in the dosage used.[19] Antihistamines, meperidine, nitrites, nitrates, tricyclic antidepressants, methylphenidate, procainamide, quinidine, MAO inhibitors and urinary alkalizers may enhance the effects of the anticholinergics.[14,16,20-23] Sympathomimetics may cause increased mydriasis and relaxation of the bronchi.[19] (A good brief compilation of these drug interactions has been prepared by Hartshorn.[24]) The side effects and potential interactions must be well understood by the pharmacist so he may inform the physician when there is a potential for them to occur.

## Other Agents

Since many peptic ulcers occur in patients with emotional problems, some clinicians recommend the use of sedatives as adjunctive therapy with antacids and/or anticholinergics. Although there are many anticholinergic-sedative combination products available, it is the belief of this author that these products should be avoided and that sedatives should be prescribed separately. This procedure will give more flexibility to dosing of both agents. A sedative may not be required for the full duration of the anticholinergic therapy or it may be required for a longer period of time than that anticholinergic drug.

Other anti-ulcer agents have been investigated. Estrogens have been shown to produce remissions of duodenal ulcers, but they generally cause feminization in the male.[6] Carbenoxolone sodium, a licorice derivative commercially available in England, has been tried extensively on an experimental basis in this country. It appears to act as a demulcent, increasing the mucous secretions in the stomach and intestines, therefore protecting the gastrointestinal wall. It is absorbed rapidly and completely from the stomach and excreted in the bile. It has shown great promise, but the side effects of fluid retention and salt retention may make it prohibitive in some patients.[6,25] The side effects have been controlled by thiazide diuretics without impairing the healing properties. When spironolactone was used as a diuretic, however, the healing properties seemed to be impaired.[4,25,26,27]

## Surgery

When medical treatment of peptic ulcer fails, surgical resection of the ulcer is required. Failure of the gastric ulcer to decrease in size by at least 50% in three weeks and to heal completely in six weeks following initiation of therapy is probably an indication for surgery because slow or absent healing may indicate a malignancy or a bad prognosis for medical treatment.[15] Since about 10% of gastric ulcers prove to be due to carcinoma, they are watched very closely for healing.[4] Other indications for surgery are obstruction and perforation and recurrence of either gastric or duodenal ulcers within one year. If a peptic ulcer recurs after two years, surgery may be indicated.[15]

Gastric freezing has also been used for treatment of the peptic ulcer. The results are not very impressive and are no better than those with standard ulcer treatment.[4,11]

## Conclusion

The pharmacist must be aware of the problems associated with the management of the peptic ulcer patient. He must have a good understanding of the patient, his drug, medical and social histories, and must know the methods of treatment before he can recommend appropriate drug therapy. Drug therapy should include an antacid and possibly an anticholinergic. In many cases a sedative may also be necessary. The patient should continue taking his medications for several weeks after the ulcer has healed to avoid rapid recurrence. He should be advised against the use of any ulcerogenic drugs. The pharmacist should emphasize to the patient the importance of following the prescribed therapy when he leaves the clinic or hospital. The patient should be made aware that if he does not follow the prescribed routine, the ulcer could fail to heal or could recur and require surgery.

## References

1. Harrison, T. R. et al.: Principles of Internal Medicine, 6th Edition, McGraw-Hill, New York, New York, 1970, pp. 1444-1453.

2. Lyght, C. E. et al.: The Merck Manual, 11th Edition, Merck, Sharp and Dohme, West Point, Pennsylvania, 1966, pp. 344-346.

3. Conn, H. F.: Current Therapy, Saunders, Philadelphia, Pennsylvania, 1969, pp. 344-346.

4. Brainerd, H., et al.: Current Diagnosis and Treatment, Lange, Los Altos, California, 1970, pp. 313-317.

5. Smith, J. W.: Manual of Medical Therapeutics, J. A. Churchill Ltd., London, England, 1969, pp. 235-246.

6. Anon.: The Medical Treatment of Peptic Ulcer, Med. Letter Drugs Therap. 11:105-107 (Dec.) 1969.

7. Schuster, M. M.: Functional Gastrointestinal Disorders, GP 35:131-138 (Mar.) 1967.

8. Kirsner, J. B.: Controlling Gastric Secretion, Postgrad. Med. 44:76-79 (Nov.) 1968.

9. Penna, R. P.: O-T-C Antacids, J. Amer. Pharm. Ass. NS6:463-465 (Sept.) 1966.

10. Fordtram, J. S. and Coilyns, J. A. H.: Antacid Pharmacology in Duodenal Ulcer: Effect of Antacids on Postcibal Gastric Acidity and Peptic Activity, New Engl. J. Med. 274:921-927 (Apr. 28) 1966.

11. Kirsner, J. B.: Peptic Ulcer: A Review of the Recent Literature on Various Clinical Aspects, Gastroenterology 54: 950-953 (Oct.) 1968.

12. Fordtram, J. S.: Acid Rebound, New Engl. J. Med. 279:900-905 (Oct.) 1968.

13. Zollinger, R. M., et al.: Straight Talk about Peptic Ulcer, Postgrad. Med. 45:160-164 (June) 1969.

14. Anon.: Drug Interactions that Affect Your Patient, Patient Care (Nov.) 1967.

15. Piper, D. W.: Antacid and Anticholinergic Drug Therapy of Peptic Ulcer, Gastroenterology 52:1009-1013 (June) 1967.

16. Goodman, L. S. and Gilman, A. (ed.): The Pharmacologic Basis of Therapeutics, Macmillan, New York, New York, 1965, pp. 521-544 and 900-1007.

17. Warnes, H. et al.: Adynamic Ileus During Psychoactive Medication: A Report of Three Fatal and Five Severe Cases, Canadian Med. Assoc. J. 96:1112 (Apr.) 1967.

18. Meyler, L. and Herxheimer (ed.): Side Effects of Drugs, Vol. VI, Williams and Wilkins, Baltimore, Maryland, 1968.

19. Stuart, D. M.: Drug Metabolism, Part II. Drug Interactions, PharmIndex 10:4-16 (Oct.) 1968.

20. American Hospital Formulary Service, American Society of Hospital Pharmacists, Washington, D.C., 1970.

21. McIver, A. K.: Drug Interactions, Pharm. J. 199:205 (Nov.) 1967.

22. Morrelli, H. F. and Melmon, K. L.: The Clinician's Approach to Drug Interactions, Calif. Med. 109:380 (Nov.) 1968.

23. Sjoqvist, F.: Psychotropic Drugs (2) Interaction Between Monoamine Oxidase (MAO) Inhibitors and Other Substances, Proc. Roy. Soc. Med. 58:967 (Nov.) 1965.

24. Hartshorn, E. A.: Drug Interactions, Autonomic Drugs, Parasympatholytic (Cholinergic Blocking) Agents, Drug Intel. Clin. Pharm. 4:88-89 (Apr.) 1970.

25. McHardy, G.: What is Carbenoxolone Sodium, Gastroenterology 56:818-819 (Apr.) 1969.

26. Watkinson, G.: Treating Ulcer Disease with Carbenoxolone Sodium, Postgrad. Med. 44:92-98 (Nov.) 1968.

27. Cocking, J. B. and MacCaig, J. N.: Healing Related to Duration of Carbenoxolone Theraping, Practitioner 203: 63-66 (July) 1969.

# 40 Digitalis Glycoside Intoxication — A Preventive Role for Pharmacists

Philip P. Gerbino

Various aspects of digitalis glycoside intoxication and the role pharmacists may play in its prevention are discussed.

The clinical manifestations of digitalis glycoside intoxication and the following factors which predispose patients to intoxication are discussed: age; potassium, calcium and magnesium levels; cardiac, renal, pulmonary, thyroid, endocrine and hepatic diseases; nutritional disturbances; and concomitant drug therapy.

Factors which may be useful in evaluating patients with suspected digitalis glycoside intoxication are listed.

Digitalis glycoside intoxication is one of the most common and potentially one of the most serious of today's iatrogenic diseases. Its reported incidence has increased substantially over the past three decades.[1] Estimates from retrospective studies of hospitalized patients taking digitalis glycosides disclosed that 7–20% developed toxicity.[2-7] Mortality in patients in whom intoxication occurred averaged 22% with a range of 7–50%. Mortality as a direct result of cardiac toxicity ranged from 3–21%.[2-7] One study of medical service admissions indicated that 15% of the patients surveyed were taking digitalis glycosides upon admission, and of these, 23% were definitely and 6% possibly digitalis toxic.[7] This total incidence of 29% was confirmed by serial electrocardiograms. Preventive measures must be continuously employed if the incidence of digitalis glycoside intoxication is to be significantly reduced.

The increasing reported incidence of digitalis intoxication is probably due to a multiplicity of factors. Predominant among these are an increasing awareness of the clinical entity, comprehensive surveillance techniques, serial electrocardiography, increased longevity of the population (higher percentage of elderly people, especially with cardiovascular disease) and the use of potent diuretics, corticosteroids or other agents which may induce electrolyte abnormalities.

The following discussion of digitalis glycoside intoxication is presented to pharmacists to assist them in assuming greater responsibility in preventing such problems. A comprehensive presentation of all the predisposing factors and complete clinical manifestations of digitalis glycoside intoxication is reviewed elsewhere.[8]

## Clinical Manifestations

A composite of some of the more frequently reported non-cardiac manifestations of digitalis glycoside intoxication has been compiled by Chung[8] and is presented in Table 1.

Too frequently, patients who have been on maintenance digitalis glycosides for a considerable period of time are seemingly overlooked. Some of the statistics indicating frequency of occurrence of the noncardiac symptoms of digitalis toxicity are certainly impressive.[9] They lead one to believe that no patient taking digitalis glycosides is above suspicion of developing these toxicity symptoms.

In a recent study of 179 patients who were digitalis toxic, 95% complained of acute fatigue, tiredness and muscle weakness with diminished strength; 65% had psychic disturbances in the form of bad dreams, restlessness, agitation, nervousness, drowsiness, fainting, pseudohallucinations and delirium.[10] Anorexia and nausea were present in 80% of the patients while abdominal pain existed in 65%. A high incidence (95%) of visual disturbances was reported. These patients complained of hazy vision, difficulty in reading, glitterings, moving spots and rings, halos, altered color perception and flames of yellow, red, or green with dark spots.[10]

Even though the frequency of some of these general symptoms is high in any chronically ill patient, they should never be viewed as dubious or obscure in origin if a patient is receiving digitalis glycosides. Inquiries to patients maintained on digitalis glycosides in an attempt to elicit if any of these symptoms exist should be done as frequently as possible.

**Table 1. Noncardiac Manifestations of Digitalis Intoxication[8]**

| SYMPTOMS | FREQUENCY | MANIFESTATIONS |
|---|---|---|
| Gastrointestinal | Common | Anorexia, nausea, vomiting, diarrhea, abdominal pain, constipation |
| Neurological | Common | Headache, fatigue, insomnia, confusion, vertigo |
| | Uncommon | Neuralgias (especially trigeminal), convulsions, paresthesias, delirium, psychosis |
| Visual | Common | Color vision, usually green or yellow; colored halos around objects |
| | Uncommon | Blurring, shimmering vision |
| | Rare | Scotomata, micropsia, macropsia, amblyopias (temporary or permanent) |
| Miscellaneous | Rare | Allergic (urticaria, eosinophilia), idiosyncracy, thrombocytopenia, gastrointestinal hemorrhage, and necrosis |

## Predisposing Factors

*Age.* It is well documented that the incidence of digitalis intoxication increases with age disproportionately with the increase of heart disease.[11] There seems to be a narrow margin between therapeutic and toxic levels of digitalis. The therapeutic dose is estimated to be approximately 60% of the toxic dose.[12] This narrow margin may become even further reduced in elderly patients. Digitalis intoxication in the newborn occurs with greater frequency than in older children and is an important cause of accidental poisoning.[13]

Therefore, standard "conventional" maintenance dosages of digitalis glycosides, as set forth by various texts, need periodic reevaluation to be tailored to the individual patient, since cardiac status may change as a function of age.

*Electrolytes. (1) Potassium.* Hypokalemia or hyperkalemia alone can cause cardiac arrhythmias. Potassium depletion will accelerate arrhythmias induced by digitalis glycosides.[14] The potassium concentration in the myocardial cell is most likely the basic factor in the relationship of potassium to digitalis glycoside intoxication. There is no definite correlation between the extracellular potassium level, the severity of cardiac arrhythmias and

the patient's condition, but there is a possibility that the potassium gradient between the intracellular and extracellular fluid plays an important etiological role in digitalis glycoside toxicity.[15] Diuretics (except triamterene and spironolactone) may cause depletion of the intracellular potassium pool, leaving extracellular potassium slightly decreased or within normal limits, thus increasing the susceptibility to digitalis glycoside intoxication.[16] Potassium depletion may also be precipitated by ammonium chloride, corticosteroids, cation exchange resins, cathartics, and excessive diarrhea and vomiting. Infusion of glucose and insulin lowers extracellular potassium. Additional disease states, including Zollinger-Ellison syndrome, salicylate intoxication, respiratory alkalosis, pyloric obstruction, starvation, malabsorption, primary aldosteronism, renal tubular acidosis and sometimes chronic renal failure, are also causes of potassium depletion. Prolonged parenteral hyperalimentation without addition of adequate potassium may also result in serum potassium depletion.

*(2) Calcium.* Calcium and digitalis glycosides have a synergistic effect on myocardial electrophysiology and cardiac contractility. Animal studies have shown that large or toxic doses of digitalis increase both calcium uptake and tissue calcium concentrations, whereas therapeutic doses only increase calcium uptake.[17,18] Even though hypercalcemia enhances digitalis toxicity, this effect is usually only seen with extremely high serum levels of calcium.[19] Parenteral calcium or rapid intravenous infusion of calcium during digitalis glycoside therapy will increase the incidence of arrhythmias and may induce sudden death. Although clinical reports of this interaction are lacking, there appears to be a general consensus that this reaction is clinically significant.[20]

Hypercalcemia occurs in the second and third phases of the milk-alkali syndrome which may result from ingestion of absorbable antacids and has been reported after the administration of estrogens and androgens for the treatment of certain metastatic diseases.[21,22] Disease states, including alkalosis, hyperparathyroidism, bone metastases of malignant disease, parathyroid hormone-secreting tumors of the bronchopulmonary system, hypervitaminosis D, sarcoidosis, multiple myeloma and thiazide diuretic therapy, may also produce hypercalcemia.[23] The significance of the hypercalcemia produced by the above conditions in their relationship to digitalis intoxication remains obscure; however, their presence should render cause for concern.

*(3) Magnesium.* Magnesium ion is known to effect both myocardial contractility and conductivity. Animal studies have shown that hypomagnesemia facilitates digitalis glycoside toxicity. It is felt that loss of magnesium ions will result in loss of intracellular potassium. These observations are clinically significant in view of the fact that many diuretic drugs produce hypomagnesemia[24,25] in addition to potassium depletion; hypomagnesemia can also occur in patients with chronic alcoholism.[26,27]

The many alterations in electrolytes which predispose

a patient to digitalis glycoside toxicity mandate continual monitoring of drugs and awareness of existing disease states which may precipitate electrolyte disturbances. Physicians should always be immediately alerted when it is felt that the hazard of impending electrolyte abnormalities exists.

*Cardiac Disease.* Digitalis glycosides are the primary agents used to treat congestive heart failure and are also useful in the treatment of atrial fibrillation. However, as would be expected, any preexisting or additional heart diseases, conduction defects or serious and bizarre arrhythmias will usually increase the incidence of digitalis intoxication. This seems to be always true in patients who have had a myocardial infarction. It is likely that any increase in the susceptibility to digitalis toxicity relates to the severity of the myocardial infarction and its complications.[28]

The use of digitalis glycosides after acute myocardial infarction has evoked some controversy in the medical literature. Some authors recommend that the dosage of digitalis be reduced by one-third to one-half in patients who have had a myocardial infarction.[29] Others feel that there is a paucity of experimental and clinical evidence supporting the benefits obtained from using digitalis in the treatment of congestive heart failure and cardiomegaly complicating acute myocardial infarction.[28] Nevertheless, when cardiac glycosides are used after acute myocardial infarction, the pharmacist should be aware that the patient may be in a greater risk category for the development of digitalis intoxication and may require reevaluation or reduction of dosage.

*Renal Disease.* The concomitant appearance of congestive heart failure and renal disease is not uncommon. Patients who develop renal failure (either acute or chronic) while taking cardiac glycosides, frequently exhibit digitalis toxicity for many reasons. The two most common are the presence of electrolyte disturbances and prolonged digitalis half-life, resulting in accumulation of the drug. Much work has been done elucidating the alterations in half-lives of cardiac glycosides in patients with renal impairment, and recommendations for dosage schedules for both digoxin and digitoxin in various states of renal failure have been developed.

In patients with reduced creatinine clearance, the excretion of digoxin, which has a normal half-life of 1.5 days, is delayed, and therefore, the maintenance dose requirement may be reduced by up to 40–50%, depending on the degree of renal failure.[9] (See Table 2 for the normal half-lives of digitalis glycosides.) Digitoxin is largely metabolized by the liver and has a half-life of approximately 5.6 days in patients with normal renal function. One of its metabolites is digoxin which is normally excreted by the kidney. The effect of renal failure on decreasing the maintenance requirements of digitoxin seems minimal, probably because digoxin accounts for only a small proportion of the metabolites of digitoxin.[30] One investigator feels that digitoxin might be the cardiac glycoside of choice in uremic patients since the other

**Table 2. Biologic Half-Lives of Digitalis Glycosides in Normal Patients**[43]

| AGENT | HALF LIFE (hrs) |
|---|---|
| Ouabain | 22 |
| Deslanoside | 36 |
| Digoxin | 36 |
| Digitoxin | 136 |

cardiac glycosides are more dependent on the renal excretion for elimination.[30] A complete discussion of digitalis kinetics is beyond the scope of this chapter; however, familiarization with these data is desirable.[31-46]

The pharmacist should establish continual communication with physicians so that he might keep abreast of the degree of renal impairment the patient has incurred. This communication will enable pharmacist consultation, which will assist in the development of accurate digitalis glycoside dosing and monitoring. This might also serve as a stimulus and reminder of the importance of laboratory and clinic visits by the patient.

*Pulmonary Diseases.* There is a high incidence of digitalis intoxication in patients who have chronic pulmonary disease, including pulmonary emphysema, bronchitis, pneumonia and pulmonary embolism. Proposed reasons for this high incidence include unnecessary digitalization, hypoxia, infection and polycythemia.[47,48] In addition to these factors, it is felt that there is an unusual sensitivity to digitalis glycosides in patients with severe and chronic pulmonary disease.[2,49]

There are no guidelines proposed for digitalis dosing in patients with pulmonary diseases.

*Thyroid Disease.* Thyroid disease poses a myriad of problems when trying to maintain patients on digitalis glycosides. Hyperthyroidism causes atrial fibrillation with rapid ventricular responses and also may induce bizarre arrhythmic syndromes. Clinically, doses of digitalis two or three times normal may be needed to control these arrhythmias, thereby increasing the risk of digitalis intoxication. In contrast, hypothyroid patients may require less digitalis than euthyroid patients. One study indicated that regardless of the route of administration, hyperthyroid patients exhibited lower serum levels and hypothyroid patients higher levels of digoxin than did the euthyroid patient.[50]

*Endocrine Disease.* Addison's Disease, Cushing's syndrome, pheochromocytoma, diabetic acidosis, hyperparathyroidism and primary and secondary aldosteronism are all conditions in which multiple electrolyte disturbances can occur. An awareness of the nature of the disturbance and its effect on digitalis glycoside therapy may aid in preventing the development of digitalis toxicity.

*Hepatic Disease.* The high incidence of digitalis glycoside intoxication observed in patients with hepatic disease is probably a result of electrolyte disturbances associated with diuretic therapy.[51] Although it has not been shown clinically, the half-life of digitoxin may be prolonged in patients with various hepatic diseases.[9] Conjecture arises on the effect of hepatic and renal disease on the metabolism of digitoxin. One investigator feels that digitoxin may be the drug of choice in renal disease. Furthermore, he states that the enterohepatic cycling of digitoxin cannot be conclusively proven in man.[30] Cirrhosis of the liver does not change the half-life of digoxin, since this drug is excreted unchanged by the kidney.[52]

*Nutritional Disturbances.* Congestive heart failure is prevalent in many obese patients. A primary reason for obesity might be poor nutritional habits. Congestive heart failure in obese patients is usually associated with edema. Treatment with digitalis glycosides and diuretic agents is usually employed with satisfactory results. However, care must be taken, when therapy is very zealous, to monitor both digitalis dosage and electrolyte levels to prevent toxicity from developing, especially if the patient has been volume depleted rapidly.[53]

Beriberi heart disease caused by thiamine deficiency in chronic alcoholic patients is associated with alcoholic cardiomyopathy[54] and also warrants careful monitoring of therapy to prevent toxicity. Questioning the patient about his dietary habits may often aid in correcting a nutritional problem, as well as detecting if salt restrictions, diet and electrolyte supplementations are being maintained.

*Concomitant Drug Therapy.* If we consider certain facts—digoxin is 80–90% absorbed and digitoxin 100% absorbed from the gastrointestinal tract; digoxin is 23% bound to albumin whereas digitoxin is 97% bound to albumin; digoxin is primarily excreted by the kidney and has a half-life of approximately 36 hours contingent on renal function, whereas digitoxin is excreted by the kidney after liver metabolism to digoxin and enterohepatic cycling, giving a final half-life of about 136 hours contingent on both liver and kidney function—we can predict that drug interactions are likely to occur.

Drugs which affect gastrointestinal absorption (cathartics, neomycin, cholestyramine), enterohepatic circulation (cholestyramine), protein binding (phenylbutazone, tolbutamide, warfarin, sulfadimethoxine, clofibrate), renal excretion by decreasing filtration (guanethidine, methyldopa) and metabolism (phenobarbital, diphenylhydantoin, phenylbutazone) may all theoretically cause alterations in either digoxin or digitoxin serum levels. In the experience of most, these interactions have occurred infrequently and have little clinical significance.

The use of available drug interaction texts in coordination with a patient profile and medication history system, should alert one to the existence of a potential drug-drug interaction. Table 3 is a summary of these interactions. A review by Bigger and Strauss[59] discusses some of these drug interactions and sheds some light on their occurrence, mechanism, and significance

### Table 3. Drug Interactions of Cardiac Glycosides[55–59]

| INTERACTANT | POSSIBLE INTERACTION |
|---|---|
| Hypokalemic drugs[a]<br>Amphotericin B<br>Diuretics<br>Glucose infusion<br>Insulin<br>Cathartics<br>Corticosteroids | Increased digitalis glycoside toxicity on the basis of potassium depletion |
| Oral neomycin | Decreased absorption |
| Cardiac depressants<br>Diphenylhydantoin<br>Quinidine<br>Procainamide<br>Propranolol[a] | Enhanced digitalis effect and bradycardia |
| Phenobarbital | Decreases digitoxin effect on the basis of enzyme induction |
| Reserpine[a] and guanethidine<br>Releasing or affecting catecholamines | Arrhythmias |
| Sympathomimetics (Beta-active)[a]<br>Epinephrine<br>Isoproterenol<br>Ephedrine | Enhanced ectopic pacemaker activity |
| Succinylcholine[a] | Arrhythmias, enhances digitalis effect, shifts potassium |
| Calcium infusions[a] | May precipitate arrhythmias |
| Cholestyramine | 25% reduction of plasma half-life of digitoxin |

[a] Possibly clinically significant.

### Evaluation of the Patient

There are eight generally accepted measures that may be useful in evaluating patients with suspected digitalis glycoside intoxication:[59]

1. A careful history in search of possible predisposing factors
2. Careful questioning of the patient for symptoms of digitalis glycoside toxicity
3. General laboratory evaluation for factors that may alter digitalis glycoside action (serum potassium, renal function tests)
4. Electrocardiogram analysis
5. Plasma digitalis concentrations
6. Calcium and potassium concentrations in the saliva
7. Measurement and computation of total body stores of digitalis (if possible)
8. Observation of arrhythmias when digitalis glycoside is withdrawn.

Most of these measures are very specific and must be initiated by a physician; however, steps 1 and 2 could be performed by a pharmacist.

## Summary

In order to assist in preventing digitalis intoxication the pharmacist must be knowledgeable regarding the clinical manifestations and the predisposing factors to digitalis intoxication. In addition, he must establish a mechanism to monitor the clinical course of the patient. A medication history is always essential and a patient profile must be maintained and used properly, not only to detect if potential drug-drug, drug-disease interactions exist, but also to monitor total drug therapy. The pharmacist must act judiciously as to when and how to alert a physician that the potential of digitalis intoxication exists in one of his patients. He should also supply sufficient data to support this judgment.

These practices along with comprehensive patient education should aid in reducing digitalis intoxication.

## References

1. Friend, D. G.: Cardiac Glycosides, *N. Engl. J. Med.* *266*:88–89, 187–189, 300–302, 402–404 (Jan.-Feb.) 1962.

2. Rodensky, P. L. and Wasserman, F.: Observations on Digitalis Intoxication, *Arch. Internal Med.* *108*:171-188 (Aug.) 1961.

3. Giuffra, L. J. and Tseng, H. L.: Some Clinical Aspects of Digitalis Intoxication, *N.Y. State J. Med.* *52*:581–583 (Mar.) 1952.

4. Sodeman, W. A.: Diagnosis and Treatment of Digitalis Toxicity, *N. Engl. J. Med.* *273*:35–37, 93–95 (July) 1965.

5. Dubnow, M. H. and Burchell, H. B.: A Comparison of Digitalis Intoxication in Two Separate Periods, *Ann Internal Med.* *62*:956-965 (May) 1965.

6. Hurwitz, N. and Wade, O. L.: Intensive Hospital Monitoring of Adverse Reactions to Drugs, *Brit. Med. J.* *1*:531-544 (Mar.) 1969.

7. Beller, G. A. et al.: Digitalis Intoxication, *N. Engl. J. Med.* *284*:989–997 (May) 1971.

8. Chung, E. K.: Digitalis Intoxication, Williams & Wilkins Company, Baltimore, Maryland, 1969, pp. 42-90, 133-157.

9. Melmon, K. L. and Morrelli, H. F.: Clinical Pharmacology, Basic Principles of Therapeutics, Macmillan Company, New York, New York, 1972, p. 191.

10. Ledy, A. H. and Von Enter, C. H. J.: Noncardiac Symptoms of Digitalis Intoxication, *Amer. Heart J.* *83*:149–152 (Feb.) 1972.

11. Dall, J. L.: Digitalis Intoxication in the Elderly Patient, *Lancet 1*:194–195 (Jan.) 1965.

12. Lown, B. and Levine, S. A.: Current Concepts in Digitalis Therapy, Little Brown & Co., Boston, Massachusetts, 1954, p. 36.

13. Herrmann, G. R.: Digitoxicity in the Aged, Recognition, Frequency and Management, *Geriatrics 21*:109–122 (Mar.) 1966.

14. Fowler, R. S. et al.: Accidental Digitalis Intoxication in Children, *J. Pediat. 64*:188–200 (Feb.) 1964.

15. Chung, E. K.: Digitalis Intoxication, Williams & Wilkins Company, Baltimore, Maryland, 1969, p. 133.

16. Mason, D. T. and Zelis, R. et al.: Current Concepts and Treatment of Digitalis Toxicity, *Amer. J. Cardiol. 27*:546–559 (May) 1971.

17. Gersmeyer, G. and Holland, W. C.: Influence of Ouabain on Contractile Force, Resting Tension Ca$^{45}$ Entry and Tissue Ca Content in Rat Atria, *Circ. Res. 12*:620–622 (June) 1963.

18. Lullmann, W. J. and Holland, W. C.: Influence of Ouabain on an Exchangeable Calcium Fraction, Contractile Force, and Resting Tension of Guinea-Pig Atria, *J. Pharmacol. Exp. Ther. 137*:186–192 (Aug.) 1962.

19. Nola, G. T. et al.: Assessment of the Synergistic Relationship Between Serum Calcium and Digitalis, *Amer. Heart J.* *79*:499–507 (Apr.) 1970.

20. Hansten, P. D.: Drug Interactions, Lea & Febiger, Philadelphia, Pennsylvania, 1971, p. 205.

21. Texter, E. C. and Laureta, H. C.: The Milk-Alkali Syndrome, *Amer. J. Dig. Dis. 11*:413–418 (May) 1966.

22. Meyer, L. and Herkheimer, A.: Side Effects of Drugs, Vol. 6, Williams & Wilkins Company, Baltimore, Maryland, and Exerpta Medica Foundation, Amsterdam, Netherlands, 1968, pp. 396-397.

23. Besson, P. B. and McDermott, W.: Cecil-Loeb Textbook of Medicine, 13th ed., W. B. Saunders Company, Philadelphia, Pennsylvania, 1971, pp. 1850-1851.

24. Seller, D. T. et al.: Digitalis Toxicity and Hypomagnesemia, *Amer. Heart J. 79*:57–63 (Jan.) 1970.

25. Smith, W. D. et al.: Magnesium Depletion Induced by Various Diuretics, *J. Okla. Med. Ass. 55*:248 (June) 1962.

26. Heaton, F. W.: Hypomagnesemia in Chronic Alcoholism, *Lancet 2*:802–808 (Oct.) 1962.

27. Frankushen, D. et al.: Significance of Hypomagnesemia in Alcoholic Patients, *Amer. J. Med. 37*:802–812 (Nov.) 1964.

28. Karliner, J. S. and Braunwald, E.: Digitalis Treatment of Acute Myocardial Infarction, *Circulation 45*:891–902 (Apr.) 1972.

29. Marcus, F.: Use of Digitalis in Acute Myocardial Infarction, *Heart Bull. 18*:106–110, 1969.

30. Rasmussen, K. et al.: Digitoxin Kinetics in Patients with Imparied Renal Function, *Clin. Pharmacol. Ther. 13*:6–14 (Jan.-Feb.) 1972.

31. Goodman, L. S. and Gilman, A.: The Pharmacologic Basis of Therapeutics, 4th ed., The Macmillan Company, New York, New York, 1970, pp. 672-708.

32. Doherty, J. E. and Flanigan, W. J. et al.: Tritiated Digoxin: Studies in Human Volunteers, *Circulation 42*:867–873 (Nov.) 1970.

33. Doherty, J. E. et al.: Tritiated Digoxin Excretion in Patients Following Renal Transplantation, *Circulation 37*:865–869 (May) 1968.

34. Doherty, J. E. et al.: Excretion of Tritiated Digoxin, *Circulation 40*:555–561 (Oct.) 1969.

35. Bloom, P. M. and Neld, W. B.: Relation of Excretion of Tritiated Digoxin to Renal Function, *Amer. J. Med. Sci. 251*:133–144 (Feb.) 1966.

36. Doherty J. E.: Studies with Tritiated Digoxin in Anephric Human Subjects, *Circulation 35*:298–302 (May) 1967.

37. Mirkin, B. L.: Drug Therapy in Patients with Impaired Renal Function, *Postgrad. Med. 47*:159–164 (Feb.) 1970.

38. Del Greco, F. et al.: Hemodynamic Studies in Chronic Uremia, *Circulation 40*:87–95 (Jan.) 1969.

39. Reidenberg, M. M.: Renal Function and Drug Action, W. B. Saunders Company, Philadelphia, Pennsylvania, 1971, pp. 48-51.

40. Jelliffe, R. W.: An Improved Method of Digoxin Therapy, *Ann. Internal Med. 69*:703-717 (Apr.) 1968.

41. Jelliffe, R. W. et al.: An Improved Method of Digitoxin Therapy, *Ann. Internal Med. 72*:453-464 (Apr.) 1970.

42. Doherty, J. E. et al.: The Distribution and Concentration of Tritiated Digoxin in Human Tissues, *Ann. Internal Med. 66*:116-124 (Jan.) 1967.

43. Doherty, J. E.: The Clinical Pharmacology of the Digitalis Glycosides: A Review, *Amer. J. Med. Sci. 255*:382–414 (June) 1968.

44. Doherty, J. E. et al.: Tritiated Digoxin Studies in Human Subjects, *Arch. Internal Med. 108*:531-539 (Oct.) 1961.

45. Doherty, J. E. et al.: Studies with Tritiated Digoxin in Renal Failure, *Amer. J. Med. 37*:536-544 (Oct.) 1964.

46. Jelliffe, R. W.: New Developments in Dosage Regimens, *J. Mond. Pharm. 15*:53–78 (Mar.) 1972.

47. Baum, G. L. et al.: Factors Involved in Digitalis Sensitivity in Chronic Pulmonary Insufficiency, *Amer. Heart J. 57*:460–467 (Mar.) 1959.

48. Williams, J. F. et al.: Effect of Acute Hypoxia and Hypercapnic Acidosis on the Development of Acetylstrophanthidin-Induced Arrhythmias, *J. Clin. Invest. 46*:1885–1894 (Mar.) 1968.

49. Drage, C. W.: Respiratory Failure in Chronic Obstructive Lung Disease, *Postgrad. Med. 47*:183–189 (Apr.) 1970.

50. Doherty, J. E. and Perkins, W. H.: Digoxin Metabolism in Hypo- and Hyperthyroidism, *Ann. Internal Med. 64*: 489-500 (Mar.) 1966.

51. Chung, E. K.: Digitalis Intoxication, Williams & Wilkins Company, Baltimore, Maryland, 1969, p. 147.

52. Marcus, F. I. and Kapadia, G. C.: The Metabolism of Tritiated Digoxin in Cirrhotic Patients, *Gastroenterol. 47*:517-524 (Nov.) 1964.

53. Alexander, J. K.: Chronic Heart Disease due to Obesity, *J. Chronic Dis. 18*:895-898 (Oct.) 1965.

54. Evan, W.: Alcoholic Myocardiopathy, *Progr. Cardiovasc. Dis. 7*:151-161 (Sept.) 1964.

55. Hansten, P. D.: Drug Interactions, Lea & Febiger, Philadelphia, Pennsylvania, 1971, pp. 205-207.

56. Hartshorn, E. A.: Handbook of Drug Interactions, Donald E. Francke, Cincinnati, Ohio, 1970, pp. 75-78.

57. Swidler, G.: Handbook of Drug Interactions, Wiley-Interscience, New York, New York, 1971, pp. 79-81.

58. Solomon, H. M. and Abrams, W. B.: Interactions Between Digitoxin and Other Drugs in Man, *Amer. Heart J. 83*:277-280 (Feb.) 1972.

59. Bigger, J. T. and Strauss, H. C.: Digitalis Toxicity: Drug Interactions Promoting Toxicity and the Management of Toxicity, *Sem. Drug Treatment 2*:147-177 (Autumn) 1972.

# 41 Drug Therapy in Terminally Ill Patients

Arthur G. Lipman

The drug treatment of terminally ill patients is reviewed.

The treatment of the major discomforting symptoms of degenerative disease—pain, anxiety, nausea, vomiting, and depression—is reviewed. The use of phenothiazines, anticholinergic drugs, and corticosteroids is discussed. To help patients keep track of their drugs, use of a medication schedule card is recommended.

We live in a society which emphasizes and rewards exhuberant good health. The majority of medical research and care is directed toward the maintenance and regaining of good health whenever possible. But we must also recognize that human life is finite and that an end to each life is as natural as its beginning. When a life is reaching its inevitable end, good care is also very necessary.

In recent years there has been an explosion of literature, symposia and meetings on the topic of death and dying. The inadequacy of terminal care has been documented in Alexander Solzhenitsyn's *The Cancer Ward*[1] and Stewart Alsop's *Stay of Execution.*[2] Professional and lay journals and magazines have included articles and essays on the subject and a national Foundation of Thanatology and *Journal of Thanatology*[3] have been established. Thanatology, defined as the branch of science that treats death in all its aspects,[4] has been unofficially recognized by many as a medical and paramedical discipline.

## Patient Acceptance of Terminal Disease

One of the recognized leaders in thanatology is Dr. Elisabeth Kübler-Ross, author of *On Death and Dying.*[5] In this important documentation of the needs and feelings of terminally ill patients, Dr. Ross has divided the process of adjustment to dying into five stages which follow the initial shock when one learns of the terminality of his or her disease. These stages are:

1. Denial—a buffer period during which the patient prepares his emotional defenses.
2. Anger—a reaction to the seeming "injustice" of the disease.
3. Depression—occurring when denial is no longer a possibility.
4. Bargaining—a brief attempt to postpone the inevitable.
5. Acceptance—the stage at which depression and anger are no longer present and the patient is able to face the fact of his imminent death without emotional distress.

Although we seldom see these stages as distinct periods, an understanding of these reactions helps greatly in becoming aware of patients' feelings and needs during the adjustment period. The acceptance stage is most commonly seen when good symptomatic care is present.

## The Hospice Concept

In 1969 an interdisciplinary study of the needs of the terminally ill was initiated at the Yale-New Haven Medical Center. In 1970 clinical pharmacist involvement in the study was invited.[6] This study group became the basis of Hospice, Inc. Hospice is a private, nonprofit organization providing care for seriously ill patients suffering from chronic degenerative disease and who have limited life expectancies. Hospice presently operates a home care program staffed by medical, nursing, pharmacy, social work, clergy and volunteer personnel and recently began construction on an inpatient facility. Hospice provides for the needs of terminally ill patients that often cannot be met in acute care settings: the need for continuity of comprehensive planned care, the need for patient and family to continue to have control of their lives, the need for symptom management, the need to avoid isolation and conflicting information from various care givers, the need to have open communication and the need to have unnecessary tests and procedures stop. Health care providers need to be supportive and responsibly assist the patient to maintain hope. Patients and families need assistance to maintain their dignity, their humanity and their ability to cope with the crisis of death, with their own life style and with as many aspects of life as possible.[7]

The hospice concept has been successful in a number of centers in Great Britain, but Hospice, Inc. will be the first such organization to provide such comprehensive care in this country. To provide an atmosphere and attitude which makes "death with dignity" most probable, a program of good medical and supportive care with appropriate drug therapy is essential.

## Symptomatic Treatment

Drug therapy in terminal disease will often differ from that used in acute care. In terminal illness many symptoms do not resolve and treatments that are effective in short-term care are of limited value. Patients' metabolic and excretory functions change as disease progresses. Clinical laboratory tests are usually unnecessary and inappropriate; physicians and nurses experienced in good terminal care report these efforts are rarely needed.[8]

Most drug therapy in terminal disease is of a symptomatic nature. Drugs used to achieve cures in other settings are sometimes valuable as palliative agents in dying patients. Lesser illnesses must be treated when they are superimposed on a terminal disease. A toothache hurts just as much when the patient is dying of cancer as when he is otherwise healthy. Major symptoms in which good pharmacological management is essential are pain, nausea and vomiting, constipation, diarrhea, anorexia and the anticholinergic side effects which are often produced by drugs used to manage other symptoms.

*Pain.* This is the major symptom that most people are concerned with when an incurable condition is confirmed. Many don't actually fear death; they fear dying in pain. Severe pain is a problem in only about half of terminal cancer patients. But when pain is present, it may be excruciating. This symptom can be managed without oversedation in nearly all terminal patients.

Pain associated with many chronic degenerative diseases often differs from the acute pain associated with trauma or surgery. Acute pain is often characterized quantitatively as mild, moderate or severe. Chronic pain is better characterized as a continuum from ache to agony (Figure 1). Chronic pain is continually present and, unlike acute pain, does not lessen with time and cannot be rationalized as a necessary part of the healing process or as an important diagnostic parameter. While the aching phase of chronic pain can often be controlled with a mild analgesic, the agony phase usually requires multiple drug management.

Severe chronic pain contains a large psychological component consisting of anxiety and depression as well as the physical component which is seen in acute pain. Both the

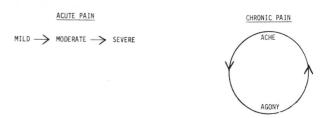

Figure 1. Characterization of pain

psychological and the physical components of severe chronic pain must be treated if the symptom is to be controlled (Figure 2).

The anxiety associated with chronic pain is often due to the patient's knowledge that at a certain time after each analgesic dose is administered the pain will return. The pain does not resolve with time and its return is inevitable. The anticipation of this return causes anxiety which potentiates the physical component of the pain.

Only by preventing the recurrence of the pain can the anxiety about its return be eliminated. This is best achieved by administering each dose of analgesic before the previous dose loses effect. Regularly scheduled analgesic dosing should be instituted and "prn" dosing should be firmly discouraged. Once the pain has reappeared it is far more difficult to control than prior to its reoccurrence. Dr. Cicely Saunders, a leader in developing programs of care for the terminally ill has stated:

> Such pain calls for continuous control, and drugs must be given regularly. Pain itself is the strongest antagonist to analgesia, and it should be kept in constant remission. If treatment anticipates pain, the patient will not anticipate pain and will not continually increase it by fear and tension.[9]

Concurrent use of a phenothiazine tranquilizer such as chlorpromazine has been reported to be effective adjunctive therapy.[10] The tranquilizer provides additive effects to the analgesic plus anxiolytic activity. Benzodiazepines such as chlordiazepoxide may be similarly helpful and may provide nighttime sedation to help with the insomnia which often accompanies chronic pain. The benzodiazepines have not been studied for this purpose, however, while the phenothiazines are in common use.

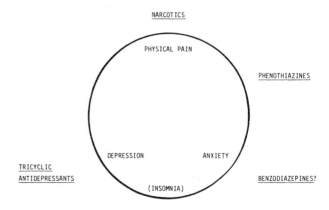

Figure 2. Pharmacologic management of severe chronic pain

Patients with severe chronic pain are often depressed. Reactive depression to the disease is not unexpected and depression was defined as one of Kübler-Ross' stages of dying. This depression is a third component of the agony. Depression is also a common cause of insomnia. Tricyclic antidepressants such as amytriptyline can be an integral part of the management of chronic pain. By giving at least two-thirds or all of the dose at bedtime, we are able to exploit the sedative side effect of tricyclic antidepressants and help relieve the patient's insomnia. With debilitated patients it is necessary to start with smaller doses of these drugs than are normally employed in psychiatric therapy.

Narcotics are nonspecific central nervous system (CNS) depressants. Low doses suppress high CNS centers but higher doses are needed to depress lower centers. Thus, higher doses of narcotics should be required for hypnotic activity than are required for analgesia. When a patient is unable to stay awake due to his narcotic dose, but is still in pain, the problem is often due to a lack of control of the psychological component of his pain. A lower dose of narcotic with antianxiety and antidepressant adjuncts is often more effective than high dose narcotic therapy alone.

Anxiety due to external causes often exacerbates the patient's pain. In 1971, while serving as a visiting clinical pharmacist at St. Christopher's Hospice in London, I met Mrs. E., a 60-year-old lady with metastatic carcinoma of the breast who did not respond to drug therapy for her continuous pain despite high doses of narcotic, chlorpromazine and amytriptyline. It was only after the patient's fifth day in the Hospice that her sister told us that Mrs. E. expressed great fear that her suppurative breast lesion would spread and involve her face. She had requested that her sister help her to kill herself if this occurred. The staff was then able to reassure Mrs. E. that this greatly feared spread would not occur. Only then, when her anxieties were allayed, did the patient respond to treatment of her pain.

Most studies on narcotic analgesics have been performed in patients with acute pain. Commonly used drugs are not always optimal for chronic pain management. Doses which are appropriate for one route of administration are often too high or too low for another due to differences in absorption, distribution and metabolism. Optimal doses of narcotic analgesics for terminal patients usually must be determined by titration of the dose to effect.[11] Average dosage ranges and durations of action are listed in Table 1.

Codeine and its congener oxycodone are not potent analgesics and are often inadequate to control severe chronic pain. Morphine or another potent narcotic analgesic should be considered. Since the analgesic effect is to be maintained continuously, long acting drugs are preferred. As patients' metabolic and excretory functions decline, the duration of action of narcotic analgesics usually increases. Methadone and levorphanol are often effective for as long as eight hours. Meperidine is an effective drug, but must be administered every three hours in doses of

**Table 1. Narcotic Analgesics[a] Used in Terminally Ill Patients**

| DRUG | ROUTE | DOSE (mg) | AVERAGE DURATION OF ACTION (hrs) |
|---|---|---|---|
| Alphaprodine | s.c. | 20–60 | 2–3 |
| (Nisentil) | i.v. | 10–30 | 1–2 |
| Hydromorphone | p.o. | 2–4 | 3–4 |
| (Dilaudid) | p.r. | 3–6 | 3–4 |
| | i.m., s.c. | 3–4 | 3–4 |
| | i.v. | 2–3 | 3–4 |
| Levorphanol | p.o. | 2–3 | 6–8 |
| (LevoDromoran) | s.c. | 2 | 6–8 |
| | i.v. | 2 | 4–6 |
| Meperidine | p.o. | 100–150 | 3 |
| | i.m., s.c. | 75–100 | 3 |
| Methadone | p.o. | 5–15 | 6–8 |
| (Dolophine) | i.m., s.c. | 5–15 | 4–6 |
| Morphine Sulfate | p.o. | 10–20 | 3–4 |
| | i.m., s.c. | 5–15 | 4–6 |
| | i.v. | 5–8 | 3–4 |
| Oxymorphone | p.r. | 2–5 | 4 |
| (Numorphan) | i.m. | 1–1.5 | 4 |

[a] Approximate equianalgesic doses.

100–150 mg orally or 75–100 mg by injection to be effective. Meperidine is commonly given in doses which are too low and administered too seldom.[12] Morphine is commonly thought to be minimally effective orally, but recent work by Twycross in England has shown morphine to be an effective, reliable oral analgesic in severe pain.[13] In all but the most severe pain, oral analgesics are effective as long as the patient is able to absorb orally administered drugs.

Once a patient's pain is controlled, his narcotic requirement usually lessens and he can generally be maintained on a steady dose unless an exacerbation of the disease occurs.[11] Attempts to start with a low dose of narcotic and titrate upward are often ineffective. To achieve pain control initially, a moderately high dose should be administered. This dose should be reduced by small amounts each two to three days (Figure 3). The optimal dose is between the lowest dose with which relief was maintained and the dose at which pain reappears. At this dose, the

*Figure 3. Narcotic dose titration*

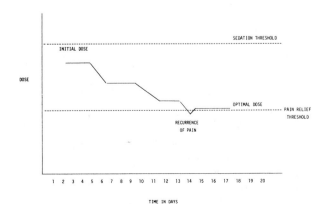

potential for sedation and addiction are minimized. Patients in pain crave relief from pain, not a psychological high from narcotics. Should a patient start to demand seemingly unreasonable amounts of narcotics, it probably means that his pain control is inadequate, not that he is becoming addicted.

*Nausea and Vomiting.* These symptoms are common with many chronic degenerative illnesses and are particularly common with neoplastic diseases. Nausea can be due to the disease itself and to the drugs used to treat the disease and its symptoms (Table 2).

**Table 2. Etiology and Treatment of Nausea and Vomiting in Terminally Ill Patients**

| ETIOLOGY | TREATMENT |
|---|---|
| Disease | Induce remission |
| | Treat at source |
| Antineoplastic drugs | Phenothiazines before treatment |
| Radiation therapy | Phenothiazines before treatment |
| Salicylates | Antacids with salicylate doses |
| Steroids | Antacids with steroid doses |
| Narcotics | Phenothiazines plus antihistamines |
| Uremia | Stop drugs when possible |
| | Dietary control, antiemetics |
| Elevated intracranial pressure | Osmotic diuretics |
| | Glucocorticoids |

When the disease itself is the cause of the problem, treatment must be directed at the source. In gastrointestinal carcinomas, antispasmodics may be of value. Diseases involving the central nervous system often require treatment at several points. A phenothiazine antiemetic such as prochlorperazine plus agents to lower elevated intracranial pressure are indicated.

Administration of a phenothiazine prior to both cancer chemotherapy and radiation therapy is often more effective than giving the antiemetic after the symptoms appear.

Several groups of drugs including salicylates and steroids induce nausea by direct and indirect effects on the gastrointestinal mucosa. Concurrent administration of an antacid with such drugs decreases the direct GI irritation.

Narcotic analgesics appear to induce nausea through both medullary and middle ear mechanisms.[14] When a phenothiazine alone does not adequately control narcotic induced nausea it is wise to administer both a phenothiazine antiemetic and an antihistamine antiemetic such as cyclizine. The more active and ambulant the patient is, the more important the antihistamine which suppresses the vestibular component of the nausea. Intractable nausea and vomiting not infrequently necessitate hospitalization of patients who would otherwise be able to remain at home. This can sometimes be avoided if the patient modifies his normal activities according to his more limited capabilities as the disease progresses. While at St. Christopher's, I met Mrs. R., a 72-year-old lady at the outpatient clinic one Thursday. She had moderately advanced carcinoma of the liver but seemed to be responding well to symptomatic treatment of her pain and nausea and was living a relatively normal life at home. The next Monday,

we were quite surprised to see Mrs. R. being admitted to the hospice complaining of severe nausea and vomiting despite her receiving regularly scheduled doses of prochlorperazine and cyclizine. As she discussed her problem with the staff the next day, Mrs. R. noted that her nausea was most bothersome when she was preparing meals for her husband and herself. He had urged her to allow him to do the cooking, but she wished to maintain as much normality in their lives as possible. At the request of the staff, Mrs. R. agreed to share the task of preparing meals with Mr. R. and a neighbor. She went home two days later with her nausea completely under control and was not seriously troubled by it again for many weeks.

As patients' kidney and liver function fail, drug accumulation occurs. It is, therefore, important to adjust doses of many drugs downward as the patient's metabolic and excretory functions diminish. Acidosis may result in higher narcotic requirements for some patients in their last days. Uremia is a common cause of nausea in advanced terminal disease. Dietary control and elimination of as many drugs as possible is then appropriate. Low doses of antiemetics may be helpful.

### Phenothiazines

Phenothiazine derivatives are useful in managing nausea and anxiety, as sedatives and as adjuncts in pain relief in terminal disease. Differences between the alkylamino and piperazine side chain phenothiazines should be considered when selecting the drug to be used. Piperidine side chain phenothiazines are of limited usefulness as adjuncts in symptomatic control of terminal disease. This group may have a greater anticholinergic effect and offers no advantages over the other two groups (Figure 4).

The propylamino group is more sedating than the piperazine group. This effect may be helpful in agitated, anxious patients who have difficulty sleeping. The piperazine group possesses somewhat greater antiemetic activity and is less sedating; however, it carries a greater potential for extrapyramidal effects.

Methotrimeprazine is a propylamino derivative that possesses profound analgesic activity and may be of value as a narcotic adjunct in refractory pain. This drug is highly sedating, induces significant orthostatic hypotension

*Figure 4. Effects of phenothiazines according to side chains*

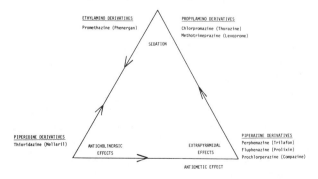

and is available only for intramuscular administration. Ethylamino derivatives such as promethazine are sometimes used as adjuncts to narcotic analgesics. In high doses, these drugs tend to cause CNS excitation and may produce bizarre central nervous effects.

### Anticholinergic Drugs

Several classes of drugs used in symptom management have anticholinergic components (Table 3). This effect is dose related and may often be minimized by back-titrating the doses of the drugs.

Anticholinergic side effects can be particularly troublesome in terminal patients. Dry mouth is uncomfortable and can interfere with verbal communication when a patient finds it very necessary to talk about his feelings. I knew a Mr. C., a 72-year-old man with advanced carcinoma of the stomach who complained of severe dry mouth. He always had a pipe next to his bed, but I'd never seen him smoke it. When I asked if he smoked he replied that he wanted to but didn't think he should since he was ill. I encouraged him to smoke which both made him a little happier and alleviated his dry mouth. Hard, sour candies, chewing gum, or an ice cube to suck on can also be helpful.

Blurred vision can be very disturbing to patients with advanced terminal disease. Time can become very heavy for the patient who is not able to read due to visual anticholinergic effects. Perhaps the most significant anticholinergic induced problem is urinary retention. Urinary catheterization often results in gram-negative infection in debilatated patients. Management of urinary retention with bethanechol is greatly preferred to catheterization. Constipation is a common problem in many patients and is exacerbated by narcotics. Anticholinergic effects may worsen this problem. Dietary management and cathartics are often necessary.

### Corticosteroids

Corticosteroids are valuable symptomatic agents in advanced terminal disease. They have an initial euphoriant effect which contributes greatly to the patient's sense of well being, and they cause some weight gain which is comforting both to the debilitated patient and his visitors.

Corticosteroids contribute to pain relief through antiinflammatory activity. Recent studies of corticosteroids in cancer indicate the need for lower narcotic doses to control pain in patients receiving corticosteroids than in patients not receiving them concurrently.[16] Resolution of weakness and relief of dyspnea have also been attributed to corticosteroid therapy in terminal patients. Lessening of hypercalcemia may be accomplished by corticosteroids. Hypercalcemia has been implicated in pain, anorexia, nausea, weakness and lethargy.[15–17] Due to concurrent hypoalbuminemia, hypercalcemia is not always evident from serum calcium determinations in severely ill patients.[16]

The potential benefits of corticosteroids in terminal cancer patients greatly outweigh the potential risks. The effect of corticosteroids in terminal cancer patients was documented by Schell in 280 cancer patients who received corticosteroids and 235 who did not (Table 4). A broad range of neoplasms was included. Postmortem examinations were performed on all patients and the history, physical examination, laboratory studies and clinical course of each patient were reviewed. Only in the incidence of gastrointestinal ulcer did the corticosteroid recipients show a higher incidence of adverse effects.[18,19]

Administration of corticosteroids to terminal patients has been shown by Twycross to increase survival time (Figure 5). Four hundred and twelve patients with a prognosis of less than 13 weeks received corticosteroids while 421 similar patients did not. During the first four days after admission 12% of the corticosteroid recipients died compared to 27% of the non-recipients. Forty-six percent of the corticosteroid recipients lived for more than 28 days compared to 24% of those not receiving corticosteroids. Both differences are highly statistically significant ($p < 0.001$).[15]

### Table 3. Drugs with Anticholinergic Components

| DRUG GROUP | USES |
| --- | --- |
| Phenothiazines | Narcotic adjuncts<br>Sedatives<br>Antianxiety agents |
| Tricyclic antidepressants | Antidepressants |
| Antihistamines | Antiemetics<br>Symptomatic agents |
| Anticholinergic agents | Antisecretory agents<br>GI hypermotility |

### Table 4. Effects of Steroids in Terminal Cancer Patients Upon Autopsy[19]

| | STE- ROIDS[a] | NO STE- ROIDS[b] | STATISTICAL ANALYSIS[c] |
| --- | --- | --- | --- |
| Gastrointestinal effects | | | |
| Ulcer, active | 10.0% | 3.0% | significant $p < 0.01$ (3.14) |
| Ulcer, complicated | 5.0% | 0.9% | significant $p < 0.01$ (2.59) |
| Esophagitis | 3.6% | 3.0% | N.S. (0.42) |
| Active infection | | | |
| Pulmonary (not TB) | 62.0% | 65.0% | N.S. (0.70) |
| Tuberculosis | 0.7% | 1.3% | N.S. (0.69) |
| Pyelonephritis | 15.0% | 15.0% | N.S. (0) |
| Endocarditis | 1.4% | 0.4% | N.S. (1.15) |
| Diabetic complications | — | — | N.S. (0) |
| Pulmonary embolism | 13.6% | 11.2% | N.S. (0.82) |

[a] 280 patients.
[b] 235 patients.
[c] Significant if $\geq 2.58$, binomial distribution, two-tailed $p = 0.01$.

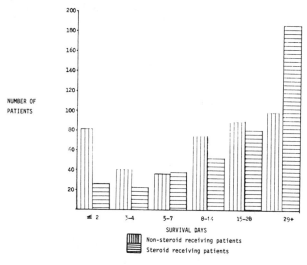

*Figure 5. Comparative histogram of patient survival according to Twycross*

Thus, corticosteroids appear to have both specific and nonspecific benefits in the management of terminal illness. Corticosteroids may improve both the quality and quantity of the life remaining to a patient with a terminal prognosis.

## Medication Schedule Cards

Patients with terminal disease often receive several drugs concurrently. Emotional stress on the patient and his family may result in confusion about administration of medications. A medication scheduling card can help alleviate this problem (Figure 6). Such a card contains spaces for the names of each drug, the time that each dose should be taken and additional comments. The same form may be used for a patient to check off the times at which he actually takes his medication each day.

## Psychedelic Drugs

In the past five years, research into the role that psychedelic agents may play in helping patients to accept their terminal illnesses has been conducted.[19-21] Hallucinogens have been used as adjuncts to psychotherapy. Results of this work appear similar to results of the hospice approach to terminal disease in which psychedelic agents are not employed. In both approaches, open honest communication with the patients and excellent social support are provided. This communication and support appear to be major factors in successful encounters with terminal disease.

## Conclusion

Multiple drug therapy is often appropriate for symptomatic management of terminal disease. Polypharmacological approaches resulting in drug-induced symptoms must be avoided. The changing metabolic state of patients with advanced disease usually necessitates frequent dose adjustments. Whenever additional medication is prescribed, potential interactions and adverse effects in a patient whose metabolic functions are already compromised must be considered.

Patients with terminal illnesses have drug therapy needs which differ from those of individuals with acute illnesses. An understanding of the social and psychological needs of terminal patients is necessary for proper management of symptoms. Appropriate drug therapy resulting in symptomatic relief can profoundly alter the character of terminal illness, allowing a patient to die in peace and with dignity.

*Figure 6. Patient medication schedule card*

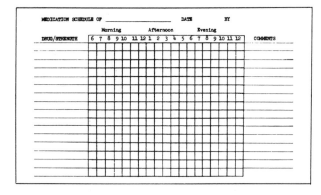

## References

1. Solhzenitsyn, A.: The Cancer Ward, Dell Publishing Co., New York, New York, 1968.
2. Alsop, S.: Stay of Execution, Lippincott, Philadelphia, Pennsylvania 1974.
3. *The Journal of Thanatology,* published by the Foundation of Thanatology, 630 West 168th Street, New York 10032.
4. Stedman's Medical Dictionary, 21st ed., Williams and Wilkins, Baltimore, Maryland, 1966.
5. Kübler-Ross, E.: On Death and Dying, MacMillan, New York, New York, 1969.
6. McCart, G., Lipman, A. et al.: Care of the Dying Patient, an Interdisciplinary Approach, presented at the 6th Annual Midyear Clinical Meeting, American Society of Hospital Pharmacists, Washington, D.C., 1971.
7. Dobihal, E. F.: Presentation to the State of Connecticut Commission on Hospitals and Health Care, May 10, 1974.
8. Saunders, C.: St. Christopher's Hospice, London, personal communication.
9. Saunders, C.: The Management of Terminal Illness, Hospital Medicine, London, 1967.
10. Twycross, R.: The Use of Diamorphine in the Management of Terminal Cancer, *J. Thanatology 2*:733–743 (Summer–Fall) 1972.
11. Twycross, R.: Clinical Experience with Diamorphine in Advanced Malignant Disease, *Int. J. Clin. Pharmacol. 9*:184–198 (3) 1974.
12. Marks, R. and Sachar, E.: Undertreatment of Medical Inpatients with Narcotic Analgesics, *Ann. Internal Med. 78*: 173-181 (Feb.) 1973.
13. Anon.: Strong Analgesics by Mouth, *Drug Ther. Bull. 12:* 61–62 (Aug. 2) 1974.

14. Jaffe, J.: Narcotic Analgesics *In* Goodman, L. and Gilman, A. (eds.): The Pharmacologic Basis of Therapeutics, MacMillan, New York, New York, 1970, p. 244.

15. Anon.: Glucocorticosteroids in Terminal Cancer, *Drug Ther. Bull. 12*:63–64 (Aug. 2) 1974.

16. Twycross, R.: Personal unpublished observations.

17. Watson, L.: Diagnosis and Treatment of Hypercalcemia, *Brit. Med. J., 2*:150–152, 1972.

18. Schell, H. W.: The Risk of Adrenal Corticosteroid Therapy in Far Advanced Cancer, *Amer. J. Med. Sci. 252*:641, 1966.

19. Schell, H. W.: Adrenal Corticosteroid Therapy in Far Advanced Cancer, *Geriatrics 27*:131–141, (Jan.) 1972.

20. Grof, S., Pahnke, W. et al.: Psychedelic Drug Assisted Psychotherapy in Patients with Terminal Cancer, unpublished report, Maryland Psychiatric Research Center, 1971.

21. Richards, W., Grof, S. et al.: LSD-assisted Psychotherapy and the Human Encounter with Death, *J. Transpersonal Psychol. 4*:121–150 (2) 1972.

# 42 Drugs in the Production of Direct Coombs' Test Positivity

Philip D. Hansten

False-positive direct Coombs' test results induced by drugs are discussed.

The mechanism of penicillin-, complement-, methyldopa-, and cephalothin-type effects are reviewed. Drugs producing such effects may include penicillin, quinidine, quinine, isoniazid, chlorpropamide, phenylbutazone, chlorpromazine, phenytoin, aminosalicylic acid, melphalan, methyldopa, mephenamic acid, levodopa, phenacetin, cephalosporins, ethosuximide, hydralazine, mephenytoin, procainamide, streptomycin, sulfonamides, and tetracycline. The clinical implications of this effect are reviewed. Pharmacists should be aware of this effect in order to function effectively in providing drug information to other health professionals.

Immunology is a subject which is important to the understanding of nearly all facets of medicine. Drug allergy, infectious disease, organ transplantation, neoplastic disease, autoimmune diseases, and many other areas intimately involve immunological mechanisms. In most cases, the remarkable ability of the human body to distinguish between its own tissues and the endless number of foreign substances to which it is subjected works effectively and appropriately. However, some drugs, infecting organisms, and other factors may induce these intricate defensive mechanisms to exert their effects in a way which is detrimental to the individual. Some examples of this phenomenon include glomerulonephritis, possible lupus erythematosus and rheumatoid arthritis, Hasimoto's thyroiditis, and autoimmune hemolytic anemia.[1] It is this last area, namely immunological mechanisms directed against erythrocytes that will be discussed here.

## The Direct Coombs' Test

The direct Coombs' test, also called the direct antiglobulin test, is essentially a measure of the coating of erythrocytes with antibodies (globulins), although complement and other serum proteins on red cells may also yield positive results. This test is useful in the diagnosis of erythroblastosis fetalis in which a sensitized Rh negative mother has transmitted antibodies to the infant's circulation resulting in destruction of fetal erythrocytes. Investigation of hemolytic transfusion reactions is another use for the direct antiglobulin test. Finally, the differential diagnosis of hemolytic anemias may involve the use of the direct antiglobulin test to determine if immune mechanisms are involved.

The basis for the detection of globulins on the erythrocytes involves the addition of an antihuman globulin serum to the sample of erythrocytes, followed by agglutination of the globulin-coated cells. Agglutination is the sign of a positive direct Coombs' test. The antihuman globulin is acquired by injecting laboratory animals with human serum, causing the animals to produce antibodies to human serum proteins. These antibodies (antihuman globulin), when added to human globulin-coated erythrocytes, result in the agglutination (Figure 1). Excellent discussions of the principles and uses of the Coombs' test can be found in a number of sources.[2-5]

*Figure 1. Diagrammatic illustration of a positive direct Coombs' test (direct antiglobulin test)*

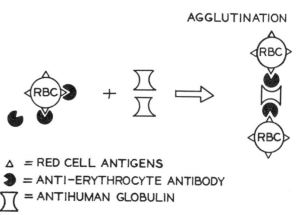

AGGLUTINATION

△ = RED CELL ANTIGENS
❱ = ANTI-ERYTHROCYTE ANTIBODY
⧖ = ANTIHUMAN GLOBULIN

## Effect of Drugs

It is well established that drugs may be involved in the production of positive direct Coombs' tests,[6-11] but the mechanisms involved are still under investigation. It has become obvious that the mechanisms are different for different drugs, and the following four types have been proposed:

1. Penicillin type
2. Complement type ("innocent bystander")
3. Methyldopa type
4. Cephalothin type.

With penicillin G,[12-15] the drug is firmly bound to the erythrocyte and large doses of drug are required to elicit positive direct Coombs' tests. This penicillin bound to the erythrocyte may evoke the production of immunoglobulins to the penicillin, and in a small number of patients the immunologic reactions result in red cell destruction (hemolytic anemia) (Figure 2).

*Figure 2. The penicillin type of drug-induced direct Coombs' test positivity*

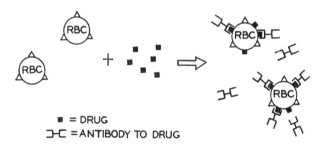

The complement or "innocent bystander" mechanism involves the combination of the drug with drug antibody. In this type, the drug and its antibody appear to have a greater affinity for each other than does the drug for the red cell membrane. The drug-antibody complex subsequently binds to the erythrocyte, activating the complement mechanism with resultant cell lysis or coating of the cell with complement proteins (Figure 3). Erythrocytes thus coated may be destroyed more readily by the reticuloendothelial system. This same mechanism is thought to occur with

*Figure 3. The complement ("innocent bystander") type of drug-induced Coombs' test positivity*

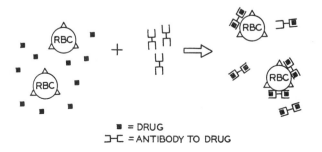

platelets, which may result in thrombocytopenia. The drug is the primary target for the immunological response, with the erythrocyte or platelet being injured secondarily, thus the term "innocent bystander." Some of the drugs which are thought to produce Coombs' positive tests by this mechanism include quinidine,[6,8,9] quinine,[6,8,9] isoniazid,[16] chlorpropamide,[17] and possibly phenylbutazone, chlorpromazine, diphenylhydantoin, aminosalicylic acid and melphalan.[7,9]

The positive Coombs' tests produced by methyldopa are quite intriguing and have been studied by several investigators.[18-25] While the two mechanisms described above involve immune mechanisms, the methyldopa type appears to result from an autoimmune phenomenon. The antibodies produced are not directed toward the drug, but rather react with specific red cell antigens on the patient's own cells. The immunoglobulins (IgG type) on the erythrocytes appear to be directed toward the erythrocyte Rh antigens. Perhaps methyldopa alters the biosynthesis of the antigens in the Rh system (Figure 4-A) or affects the immune mechanisms of the body so that the Rh antigens appear to be "foreign" (Figure 4-B). In accord with these hypotheses, the positive direct Coombs' tests usually develop only after several months of methyldopa therapy and usually remain for several months following discontinuation of methyldopa. Some of the other drugs which appear to produce direct Coombs' positive tests by this mechanism include mephenamic acid[26] and possibly levodopa[27-30] and phenacetin.[31]

*Figure 4. Two possible mechanisms for the methyldopa type of drug-induced direct Coombs' test positivity*

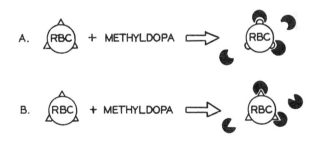

△ = "NORMAL" RED CELL ANTIGENS
○ = RED CELL ANTIGENS ALTERED BY METHYLDOPA
◗ = ANTIBODIES PRODUCED AGAINST "METHYLDOPA-INDUCED" ANTIGENS
◖ = ANTIBODIES PRODUCED AGAINST "NORMAL" RED CELL ANTIGENS

The direct Coombs' test positivity induced by cephalosporin antibiotics[15,32-34] is also quite interesting in that the mechanism appears to be nonimmunologic. It is thought that cephalosporins combine with pre-existing serum proteins and this cephalosporin-protein complex attaches to the red cell. When antihuman globulin is added to the red blood cells (as in the Coombs' test) agglutination of the erythrocytes occurs yielding a positive result (Figure 5). Cephalosporins alone have not been shown to produce a hemolytic anemia along with the positive direct Coombs' tests.

In addition to the drugs involved in the above four mechanisms, a number of other drugs have been implicated in the production of positive direct Coombs' tests (with or without hemolytic anemia) for which mechanisms are obscure or have not been proposed. It is interesting to note that many of the drugs which may induce or exacerbate systemic lupus erythematosus (SLE)[35] have appeared to be involved in positive direct antiglobulin tests. However, this is not surprising since patients with SLE often have positive direct Coombs' tests, and both the disease and the test involve immunological mechanisms. Some of the drugs implicated in the production of both positive direct Coombs' tests and SLE include the following:

1. Aminosalicylic acid
2. Diphenylhydantoin
3. Ethosuximide
4. Hydralazine
5. Isoniazid
6. Mephenytoin
7. Methyldopa
8. Penicillin
9. Phenylbutazone
10. Procainamide
11. Streptomycin
12. Sulfonamides
13. Tetracycline.

## Clinical Implications

What is the clinical significance of this discussion to the specific patient? First, hemolytic anemia may result from the same events that produce the positive direct Coombs' test. This anemia may be severe, and it is important to identify and discontinue the offending drug in an effort to reverse the anemia. Secondly, drug-induced direct Coombs' positive tests in the absence of hemolytic anemia may result in diagnostic confusion unless the physician is aware that the finding is drug-related. Also, crossmatching of blood can be confused in

*Figure 5. The cephalosporin type of drug-induced Coombs' test positivity*

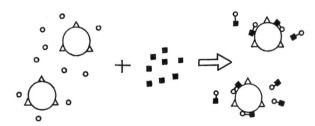

o = PRE-EXISTING SERUM PROTEINS
■ = DRUG (CEPHALOSPORIN)
o-■ = DRUG-PROTEIN COMPLEX

such patients since the direct Coombs' test may be part of the minor crossmatch. Finally, investigations of drug-induced positive direct Coombs' tests, especially the methyldopa type, are leading to a better understanding of diseases involving autoimmunity such as idiopathic autoimmune hemolytic anemia.

With the information on drug-induced Coombs' positive tests at hand, the hospital pharmacist can make a number of contributions. He should try to disseminate the information via a pharmacy newsletter or similar publication. Personal discussions with laboratory personnel on this topic are mutually beneficial. The information should also be used in the pharmacist's adverse drug reaction detection system. For example, upon finding a patient with unexplained anemia who is receiving one of the drugs implicated above, one might want to check to see if the physician had ordered a direct Coombs' test. Finally, since drug-induced Coombs' test positivity may result in diagnostic confusion and disruption of laboratory precedures, these effects should be considered when monitoring patients for drug effects on clinical laboratory results.

## Conclusion

Understanding of the production of positive direct Coombs' tests by drugs can be important in the evaluation of adverse drug reactions and the influence of drugs on clinical laboratory results. The pharmacist should be aware of these effects in order to function effectively in providing drug information to other health professionals.

## References

1. Boyd, W.: A Textbook of Pathology, 8th Ed., Lea & Febiger, Philadelphia, Pennsylvania, 1970, p. 142-184.
2. Bove, J.R.: Coombs' (Antiglobulin) Test, *JAMA 200*: 459 (May 8) 1967.
3. Bohnen, R. F., Ultmann, J. E., Gorman, J. G., Farhangi, M. and Scudder, J.: The Direct Coombs' Test: Its Clinical Significance—Study in a Large University Hospital, *Ann. Internal Med.* 68:19-32 (Jan.) 1968.
4. Davidsohn, I. and Henry, J. B.: Todd-Sanford, Clinical Diagnosis by Laboratory Methods, 14th ed., W. B. Saunders Company, Philadelphia, Pennsylvania, 1969, pp. 343-344.
5. Levinson, S. A. and MacFate, R. P.: Clinical Laboratory Diagnosis, 7th ed., Lea & Febiger, Philadelphia, Pennsylvania, 1969, pp. 853-855.
6. Croft, J. D., Jr., Swisher, S. N., Jr., Gilliland, B. C., Bakemeier, R. F., Leddy, J. P. and Weed, R. I.: Coombs'-Test Positivity Induced by Drugs—Mechanisms of Immunologic Reactions and Red Cell Destruction, *Ann. Internal Med.* 68:176-187 (Jan.) 1968.
7. Beutler, E.: Drug-Induced Hemolytic Anemia, *Pharmacol. Rev.* 21:73-103 (Mar.) 1969.
8. Anon.: Drugs and the Coombs' Antiglobulin Test (editorial), *New Engl. J. Med.* 277:157-158 (July 20) 1967.
9. Pirofsky, B.: Autoimmunization and the Autoimmune

Hemolytic Anemias, Williams and Wilkins Company, Baltimore, Maryland, 1969.

10. Worlledge, S. M.: Drug-Induced Haemolytic Anemia With an Immunologial Mechanism, In de C. Baker, S. B. and Tripod, J. (eds.): Sensitization to Drugs, Proceedings of the European Society for the Study of Drug Toxicity, Vol. 10, Exerpta Medica Foundation, Amsterdam, Netherlands, 1969, pp. 19-26.

11. Battett, O., Jr.: Hematologic Diseases, In Moser, R. H. (ed.): Diseases of Medical Progress: A Study of Iatrogenic Disease, Charles C. Thomas, Springfield, Illinois, 1969, pp. 298-360.

12. Swanson, M. A., Chanmougan, D. and Schwartz, R. S.: Immunohemolytic Anemia Due to Antipenicillin Antibodies—Report of a Case, New Engl. J. Med. 274:178-181 (Jan. 27) 1966.

13. Petz, L. D. and Fudenberg, H. H.: Coombs'-Positive Hemolytic Anemia Caused by Penicillin Administration, New Engl. J. Med. 274:171-178 (Jan. 27) 1966.

14. Roy, R. B., Doris, L. and Beanlands, D. S.: Positive Direct Coombs' Test Without Hemolytic Anemia, Attributed to Penicillin Therapy, Can. Med. Assoc. J. 99:321-326 (Aug. 17) 1968.

15. Nesmith, L. W. and Davis, J. W.: Hemolytic Anemia Caused by Penicillin—Report of a Case in Which Antipenicillin Antibodies Cross-Reacted with Cephalothin Sodium, JAMA, 203:27-30 (Jan. 1) 1968.

16. Robinson, M. G. and Foadi, M.: Hemolytic Anemia With Positive Coombs' Test—Association With Isoniazid Therapy, JAMA 208:656-658 (Apr. 28) 1969.

17. Logue, G. L., Boyd, A. E., III, Rosse, W. F.: Chlorpropamide-Induced Immune Hemolytic Anemia, New Engl. J. Med. 283:900-904 (Oct. 22) 1970.

18. Mackay, I. R., Cowling, D. C., Hurley, T. H.: Drug-Induced Autoimmune Disease: Haemolytic Anaemia and Lupus Cells After Treatment With Methyldopa, Med. J. Australia 2:1047-1050 (Dec. 7) 1968.

19. Anon: Methyldopa and Haemolytic Anaemia (Leading Article), Lancet II:151-152 (July 16) 1966.

20. Louis, W. J., Doyle, A. E., Jerums, G. and Kincaid-Smith, P.: Methyldopa and Haemolytic Anemia, Med. J. Australia 2:104-106 (July 15) 1967.

21. Sherman, J. D., Love, D. E. and Harrington, J. F.: Anemia, Positive Lupus and Rheumatoid Factors With Methyldopa—A Report of Three Cases, Arch. Internal Med. 120:321-326 (Sept.) 1967.

22. Klapper, M. S. and Noto, T. A.: Positive Direct Antiglobulin Reactions and Methyldopa, Alabama J. Med. Sci. 5:421-427 (Oct.) 1968.

23. de Torregrosa, M. V., Bulls, A. G. and Rivera, A. A. C.: Coombs'-Positive Drug-Induced Hemolytic Anemia, Amer. J. Clin. Pathol. 53:490-493 (Apr.) 1970.

24. Distenfeld, A., Florita, C. and Gelfand, M. L.: Hemolytic Anemia Induced by Alpha-Methyldopa, N. Y. State J. Med. 70:570-573 (Feb. 15) 1970.

25. LoBuglio, A. F. and Jandl, J. H.: The Nature of the Alpha-Methyldopa Red-Cell Antibody, New Engl. J. Med. 276:658-665 (Mar. 23) 1967.

26. Scott, G. L., Myles, A. B. and Bacon, P. A.: Autoimmune Haemolytic Anaemia and Mefenamic Acid Therapy, Brit. Med. J. 3:534-535 (Aug. 31) 1968.

27. Cotzias, G. C.: Metabolic Modification of Some Neurologic Disorders, JAMA 210:1255-1262 (Nov. 17) 1969.

28. Cotzias, G. C., Papavasiliou, P. S.: Autoimmunity in Patients Treated With Levodopa (Letter), JAMA 207:1353-1354 (Feb. 17) 1969.

29. LoBuglio, A. F., Masouredis, S. P., Pisciotta, A. V., Papavasiliou, P. S. and Cotzias, G. C.: Characteristics of Red Cell Autoantibodies Induced by L-Dopa, Clin. Res. 17:333 (Apr.) 1969.

30. Beutler, E.: L-Dopa and Favism, Blood 36:523-525 (Oct.) 1970.

31. Hart, M. N. and Mesara, B. W.: Phenacetin Antibody Cross-Reactive with Autoimmune Erythrocyte Antibody, Amer. J. Clin. Pathol. 52: 695-701 (Dec.) 1969.

32. Molthan, L., Reidenberg, M. M. and Eichman, M. F.: Positive Direct Coombs' Tests Due to Cephalothin, New Engl. J. Med. 277:123-125 (July 20) 1967.

33. Gralnick, H. R., Wright, L. D., Jr. and McGinnis, M. H.: Coombs' Positive Reactions Associated With Sodium Cephalothin Therapy, JAMA 199:725-726 (Mar. 6) 1967.

34. York, P. S., Landes, R. R. and Seay, L. S.: Coombs' Positive Reactions Associated With Cephaloridine Therapy (Letter), JAMA 206:1086 (Oct. 28) 1968.

35. Hansten, P. D.: Drug Induced Systemic Lupus Erythematosus, Hosp. Formulary Management 4:27 (Aug.) 1969.

36. Livingston, S., Rodriguez, H., Greene, C. A. and Pauli, L. L.: Systemic Lupus Erythematosus—Occurrence in Association With Ethsuximide Therapy, JAMA 204:731-732 (May 20) 1968.

37. FDA Reports of Suspected Adverse Reactions to Drugs, 1967, No. 670301-053-00201 (Ethosuximide).

# 43 Significance of Drug-Altered Laboratory Test Values

Gary W. Cripps, Domingo R. Martinez, R. Allan Gilliam, and Thomas J. Caldwell

Drug alteration of clinical laboratory test values was studied in 100 adult, general medicine service patients to determine the value of routine pharmacist monitoring of patient records to detect this potential drug-related problem.

Data were collected prospectively on the total number of laboratory tests ordered, the number of tests that could be potentially altered by the patient's drug therapy, and the number of altered tests attributed to drug therapy.

Of 1,405 laboratory tests ordered, 45 were altered by drug therapy. Of these 45, 16% were false alterations (none of which resulted in clinically significant problems), and 84% were true alterations (none of which resulted in invalid clinical conclusions).

It is concluded that it is not necessary for pharmacists to routinely and comprehensively monitor all patients for potential drug-altered laboratory test values. However, this service should be provided on request from physicians, and pharmacists should still utilize laboratory test values for evaluating therapeutic efficacy and detecting adverse effects.

Clinical services provided by pharmacists have recently begun to take on greater importance as an approach to improved health care. One such clinical pharmacy service is monitoring drug therapy through the use of patient profiles. This involves the detection, correction and/or prevention of many possible drug-related problems. One example of such a drug-related problem is drug alteration of clinical laboratory test values. In developing comprehensive clinical services at the University of Tennessee–City of Memphis Hospital, we became involved with this particular problem and found that a great deal of our patient-monitoring time was consumed in efforts to detect and correct potential problems related to drug-altered laboratory test values. We began to wonder if these efforts were worthwhile in terms of the patient's health care. Would it be better to spend this time dealing with other types of drug-related problems, counseling patients concerning their discharge medications, or some other clinical service? To answer this question we first turned to the literature. There are many publications citing numerous potential drug-laboratory test alterations[1-12] but only a few dealing with occurrence or significance,[13-16] and none of these fully answered our questions. Therefore, in order to determine the extent to which the time and efforts of our pharmacists spent on this particular problem were beneficial, we undertook a project to determine the occurrence and significance of drug-altered lab values in 100 general medicine patients.

## Background

The major applications of clinical laboratory tests include (1) making or confirming a diagnosis, (2) aid in following the progress of a particular patient, (3) assistance with drug and dosage selection, (4) evaluation of drug efficacy, (5) detection of adverse drug effects and (6) detection of various physiological abnormalities and imbalances.

Drugs can alter laboratory test values in one of two ways: False alterations via technical interference; and true alterations reflecting a drug's normal pharmacological or toxic effects (in other words, a drug-induced physiological change).

The results of a falsely altered laboratory test value can be a wrong diagnosis, the unnecessary use of a drug, the use of an inappropriate dose, and/or a poor conception of the patient's progress or response to his drug therapy. True alterations reflecting a drug's pharmacological or toxic effects can be expected or unexpected, desired or undesired, and can lead to an invalid conclusion which in turn can produce clinical problems; or they can lead to valid conclusions and appropriate corrective measures if necessary.

Falsely altered laboratory test values that produce significant problems can lead to one of several courses of action:

1. Discontinue the drug (if possible) and conduct the laboratory test.

2. Employ a different analytical procedure in the test (some drugs may interfere with only one of several procedures for doing a particular test).
3. Use a different laboratory test with which the drug does not interfere but which provides the same physiological evaluation.
4. Conduct the test in the presence of the drug, and judge the results with an awareness of the possible false alteration.
5. Change the drug product to one that doesn't interfere but provides the same therapeutic benefit.

## Methodology

One hundred adult general medicine patients were monitored for drug-altered laboratory test values with the aid of a patient monitoring profile. Patients were selected from only two of six medicine services. Each patient was followed for his entire period of hospitalization, and it required slightly over three months to collect the initial data. Although various patient characteristics were not quantitated, casual observation by the pharmacists monitoring the patients indicated the usual mixture of ages, sexes, disease states, etc. on a general medicine service.

A laboratory test value was considered to be altered if it fell outside the normal limits according to hospital standards, or if the physician considered a particular value for an individual patient to be abnormal. This prospective monitoring coupled with a discussion of each potential problem with the medical staff produced the initial data. However, each patient's monitoring profile and chart were also reviewed retrospectively for further classification, analysis, and/or correlation of data. Various literature sources were used to aid in the detection and verification of laboratory tests that could potentially be altered by a patient's drug therapy.[1-12] Once a potential alteration was detected it was followed up to determine if an alteration actually occurred, and if it produced a clinically significant problem. If a problem resulted, the pharmacist assisted in solving it and documented the problem, its apparent mechanism, and its solution.

## Results

The average number of drugs for each patient during his hospital stay was 10.4, and the average number of different laboratory tests performed on each patient was 14.1. The laboratory tests most frequently cited as being potentially altered by drugs were blood urea nitrogen, serum electrolytes, white cell count and serum glucose. A laboratory test was counted as one test regardless of how many times it was repeated on a particular patient. The most frequently cited types of drugs in terms of potential for altering laboratory test values were diuretics, salicylates, penicillins and corticosteroids. Table 1 shows the results of the combined data from the 100 patients. The 38 true alterations reflecting a drug's pharmacologi-

### Table 1. Combined Data for 100 Adult General Medicine Patients

| | |
|---|---|
| 1. Total number of different laboratory tests performed | 1,405 |
| 2. Number of laboratory tests that had the potential to be altered by the patient's drug therapy | 383 |
| 3. Breakdown of item #2 (383 tests) | |
|   a. Not altered | 232 |
|   b. Altered—attributed primarily to disease, diet, etc. | 106 |
|   c. Altered—attributed to drug therapy | 45 |
| 4. Breakdown of item #3-c (45 tests) | |
|   a. Drug alteration a true reflection of pharmacological or toxic effects | 38 |
|     (1) Resulted in invalid conclusions and/or inappropriate or unnecessary corrective measures | 0 |
|     (2) Resulted in valid conclusions and proper corrective measures when necessary | 38 |
|   b. Drug alteration a false technical interference | 7 |
|     1. Produced a clinically significant problem | 0 |
|     2. Did not cause a clinically significant problem | 7 |

cal or toxic effects were subdivided into those which were expected and undesired (30) and those which were unexpected and undesired (8). Whether a particular result or effect is expected or unexpected would, of course, vary with different physicians. Obviously these true alterations were sometimes indicative of adverse drug effects that were significant and required corrective measures. However, in no instances were secondary problems detected which were due to invalid conclusions drawn from the truly altered values. True alterations which were both expected and desired, such as alteration of prothrombin time due to warfarin or changes in blood sugar due to hypoglycemics, were not considered or tabulated as alterations in this study.

Of the seven false alterations that could have caused problems, none were found to do so, either because the physicians were aware of the alteration, had other laboratory test values available which were contradictory to the altered value, or ignored the alteration. These false alterations were:

1. & 2. Two false positive Coombs tests attributed to cephalothin.
3. A 3$^+$ Guaiac test attributed to ferrous sulfate.
4. An elevated urinary catecholomines attributed to methyldopa.
5. A bromsulphalein retention test which was delayed until the blood sample for a serum creatinine determination had been taken.[a]
6. A falsely elevated urinary protein attributed to penicillin.
7. A transiently elevated serum glutamic oxaloacetic transaminase value attributed to ampicillin and/or methyldopa.

[a] This situation did not involve the actual occurrence of a false alteration of a laboratory test value. It is included in the tabulation because it represented a situation where a predictable interference was very likely based on the physician's original orders. The interference did not occur because it was prevented when a staff physician suggested the possible problem, and this was verified and documented by the pharmacist, resulting in a change in the original orders. Therefore, secondary problems were avoided through prevention rather than through drawing valid conclusions after the interference had occurred.

**Table 2. Analysis of Drug-Altered Laboratory Test Data**

| CATEGORY | % TOTAL LAB TESTS (1405) PERFORMED | % LAB TESTS (383) WITH POTENTIAL TO BE ALTERED | % LAB TESTS (45) ALTERED BY DRUG THERAPY |
|---|---|---|---|
| 1. Laboratory tests (383) with potential to be altered | 27.3 | — | — |
| 2. Laboratory tests (45) altered due to drug therapy | 3.2 | 11.8 | — |
| a. False alteration (7) | | | |
| (1) Produced clinically | 0.5 | 1.8 | 15.6 |
| significant problem (0) | 0.0 | 0.0 | 0.0 |
| b. True alteration (38) | | | |
| (1) Invalid conclusion | 2.7 | 9.9 | 84.4 |
| drawn (0) | 0.0 | 0.0 | 0.0 |

Table 2 shows the relationship between the various categories of data. It is very interesting to note that although 27.3% of the laboratory tests performed had the potential to be altered by the patient's drug therapy, only 3.2% were actually altered by drug therapy. Of this 3.2%, only 0.5% were false alterations, none of which produced clinically significant problems; and 2.7% were true alterations, none of which lead to invalid conclusions.

## Discussion

Several factors possibly contributed to the very low incidence of invalid conclusions and secondary problems found in this study. These included an active patient monitoring program by pharmacists, a strict formulary program, the presence of a medical teaching program in which all patient medications are discussed and reviewed by the medical team, inservice education programs to familiarize the patient care team with the problem (a preventive measure) and the availability of drug information services. The pharmacy and medical staffs agreed that the low incidence of secondary problems due to invalid conclusions drawn from drug-altered laboratory test values was not primarily a result of pharmacy monitoring efforts, but reflected a naturally low incidence and significance of these types of problems.

We felt that this conclusion warranted a decreased emphasis on drug-altered laboratory test values as far as our pharmacist's monitoring efforts were concerned.

As a part of our routine monitoring efforts, we still detect the more common potential problems and follow through on them; in addition, any physician who is concerned about the relationship between a particular laboratory test value and the patient's drug therapy can request information on the matter from the hospital's drug information center or request a pharmacist to take a close look at the problem.

Retrospective evaluation of patient records indicate that there has been little, if any, change in the occurrence and significance of drug-altered laboratory test value problems since we decreased our emphasis on monitoring for this particular drug-related problem. We feel that we have this problem in better perspective and are handling it adequately for our particular institution. The reallocation of our monitoring time and activities has helped us make greater strides in the detection, correction and prevention of other types of drug-related problems.

## Conclusions

The results indicated that none of the false alterations and none of the true alterations led to clinically significant problems or invalid conclusions. This, coupled with the fact that only 3.2% of all laboratory tests ordered (and only 11.8% of those tests which could potentially be altered) were actually altered due to drug therapy, provided the basis for the following conclusions:

1. It is not necessary to routinely and comprehensively monitor all patients for all potential drug-altered laboratory test values. Informing the medical staff about those problems which might commonly occur would appear to prevent most of the problems from occurring.
2. This service can and should be performed upon request, or some of the more common significant problems can be detected as a part of regular screening procedures for drug-related problems.
3. The pharmacist's time might be better spent on other aspects of patient monitoring and counseling or other clinical functions.
4. Laboratory test values should still be utilized by the pharmacist in his patient monitoring efforts to assist with:
   a. Detecting adverse drug effects. (Eight of the truly altered values in this study helped confirm or detect adverse drug effects, but valid conclusions and appropriate corrective measures resulted each time.)
   b. Following the patient's diagnosis, progress and treatment.
   c. Evaluating therapeutic efficacy.

### References

1. Elking, Sister M. P. and Kabat, H. F.: Drug Induced Modifications of Laboratory Test Values, *Amer. J. Hosp. Pharm.* 25:485–519 (Sept.) 1968.

2. Wirth, W. A. and Thompson, R. L.: The Effect of Various Conditions and Substances on the Results of Laboratory Procedures, *Amer. J. Clin. Pathol. 43*:579–590 (June) 1965.

3. Christian, D. G.: Drug Interferences with Blood Chemistry Determinations, *Amer. J. Clin. Pathol. 54*:118-142 (July) 1970.

4. Hicks, J. T.: Drugs Affecting Laboratory Values, *Hosp. Form Manage. 2*:19–21 (Dec.) 1967.

5. Hopkins, L. E.: Introduction to Clinical Laboratory Test Interactions, *Hosp. Pharm. 6*:30–32 (Aug.) 1971.

6. Cross, F. C., Canada, A. T. and Davis, N. M.: The Effects of Certain Drugs on the Results of Some Common Laboratory Diagnostic Procedures, *Amer. J. Hosp. Pharm. 23*:234–239 (May) 1966.

7. Garb, S.: Clinical Guide to Undesirable Drug Interactions and Interferences, Springer Publishing Company, New York, New York, 1971.

8. Garb, S.: Laboratory Tests in Common Use, 4th ed., Springer Publishing Company, New York, New York, 1966.

9. Hartshorn, E. A.: Handbook of Drug Interactions, Don E. Francke, Cincinnati, Ohio, 1970.

10. Hansten, P. D.: Drug Interactions, Lea & Feibger, Philadelphia, Pennsylvania, 1971.

11. Hansten, P.: The Effects of Drugs on Common Clinical Laboratory Procedures, *In* Meyers, F. H., Jawetz, E. and Goldfien, A. (eds.): Review of Medical Pharmacology, Lang Medical Publications, Los Altos, California, 1968 pp. 647-663.

12. Young, D. S., Thomas, D. W., Friedman, R. B. and Pestaner, L. C.: Effects of Drugs on Clinical Laboratory Tests, *Clin. Chem. 18*:1041–1303 (Oct.) 1972.

13. Munzenberger, P. and Sister Emmanuel: The Incidence of Drug-Diagnostic Interferences in Outpatients, *Amer. J. Hosp. Pharm. 28*:786–791 (Oct.) 1971.

14. Ellinoy, B. J., Schuster, J. S., Yatsgo, J. C. and Rosenthal, L. W.: Pharmacy Audit of Patient Health Records—Feasibility and Usefulness of a Surveillence System, *Amer. J. Hosp. Pharm. 29*:749–754 (Sept.) 1972.

15. Bouchard, V. E., Bell, S. E., Freedy, H. R., and Duffy, Sister M. G.: A. Computerized System for Screening Drug Interactions and Interferences, *Amer. J. Hosp. Pharm. 29*:564–569 (July) 1972.

16. Van Peenen, H. J. and Files, J. B.: The Effect of Medication on Laboratory Test Results, *Amer. J. Clin. Pathol. 52*:666-670 (Dec.) 1969.

# 44 Practical Pharmacokinetic Techniques for Drug Consultation and Evaluation I: Use of Dosage Regimen Calculations

G. E. Schumacher

This chapter discusses the use of dosage regimen calculations as a facet of drug evaluation that can be implemented by the pharmacist.

The tetracycline and penicillin antibiotics are used as examples to illustrate and corroborate the application of these calculations in drug evaluation and consultation. Methods for determining the dosage regimen are presented for a variety of situations: (1) when the blood level must remain above a minimum concentration, (2) when both a minimum blood concentration and the dosing interval are stipulated, (3) when only an average blood concentration is desired during a dosing interval, and (4) when the blood level must remain within a minimum and maximum concentration. These methods are applied to the readily available clinical literature on the tetracyclines and penicillinase-resistant penicillins. An analysis of the data facilitates the comparison of the derivations in terms of dosage, frequency of administration, and durability of the blood level.

Twice daily dosing of tetracycline is shown to be as efficacious in maintaining blood levels as the administration of various newer derivatives, using the qualifications imposed in this study. Among the penicillinase-resistant penicillins, dicloxacillin is shown to be as effective for maintaining blood levels as cloxacillin and oxacillin, yet dicloxacillin may be administered at a smaller dose and less frequently than the other derivatives.

These examples emphasize the value of performing relatively simple calculations to determine dosage regimens useful in comparing a series of closely related drugs.

In recent years, colleges of pharmacy have introduced courses in biopharmaceutics and pharmacokinetics intended to strengthen the practitioner's knowledge of factors that influence the design of dosage forms, their bioavailability upon administration, and the time-course of drug activity. Another goal includes the application, by practitioners, of pharmacokinetic techniques in the evaluation, interpretation, and clarification of drug data and the clinical literature. There is scant evidence to substantiate this endeavor, however. Few practical applications of pharmacokinetic techniques have appeared in the clinical literature.

There is some justification for the trepidation in translating theory to practice, however. Sound pharmacokinetic analyses of drug data are only achieved when studies are designed with this goal in mind. In order for the pharmacist to generate pharmacokinetic interpretations of drug data and the clinical literature, he must rely on clinical studies which usually provide inadequate data for comprehensive evaluation.

Despite these reservations, some practical pharmacokinetic techniques can be utilized by the pharmacist, with qualifying approximations and assumptions, as a contribution to improving drug therapy. This chapter demonstrates the use of dosage regimen calculations as another, as yet undeveloped, facet of drug evaluation which can be implemented by the pharmacist. For although the formal theory of dosage regimen calculations has appeared in the literature,[1-6] no emphasis has been placed on using these calculations mainly as an index of comparison. The tetracycline and penicillin groups of antibiotics provide a rich source of data useful in the illustration and corroboration of dosage regimen calculations in drug evaluation and consultation.

## Estimating the Dosage Regimen

The basic principles of pharmacokinetics have been collated in a number of recent textbooks.[7-10] A knowledge of the fundamental theories presented in these references is accepted as a requisite to the full appreciation of the applications and limitations of the dosage regimen calculations employed in this chapter.

The application of pharmacokinetic techniques in the determination of the dosage schedule stems from the insight of several investigators[1-6] who have shown that the administration of equal doses of a drug at equal dosage intervals results in the accumulation of

drug in the body if the dosage interval is less than the time required for elimination of a single dose from the system. Since the time required to eliminate a drug is at least six-fold greater than its biological half-life, it is apparent that accumulation is commonplace in therapy. Blood levels increase with successive doses until a plateau, or equilibrium, state is reached in which the maximum and minimum blood levels are constant during successive dosing intervals. This process is illustrated for intravenous administration in Figure 1. Using pharmacokinetic techniques, it is possible to estimate a dosage regimen which will yield a desired set of maximum and minimum levels and to determine a loading dose which will achieve the plateau after the first dose.

Equations 1 and 2 are used to predict the maximum and minimum blood levels attained after multiple dosing by the intravenous route, based on information obtained from a single dose study:

*Figure 1. Drug accumulation resulting from intravenous administration of repeated maintenance doses at equal time intervals (● represents blood level resulting from loading dose designed to achieve $C_{max}$ during first dose, ▲ represents blood level resulting from initial dose equal to maintenance doses)*

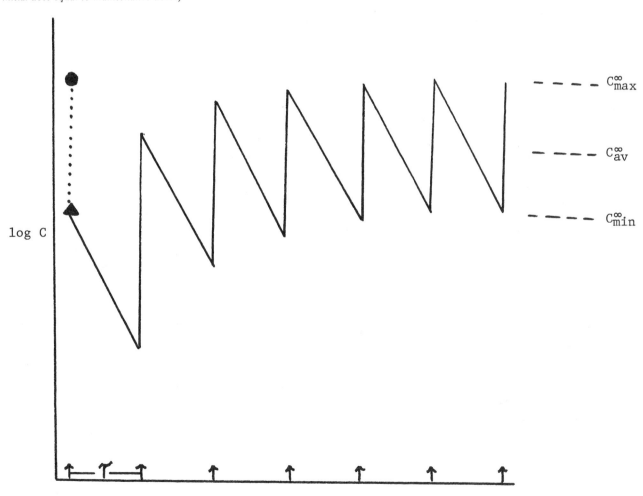

$$C\,_{max}^{\infty} = \frac{C_o'}{1 - 10^{-0.3\tau/t_{1/2}}} \qquad (1)$$

$$C\,_{min}^{\infty} = \frac{C_o'\,10^{-0.3\tau/t_{1/2}}}{1 - 10^{-0.3\tau/t_{1/2}}} \qquad (2)$$

$C\,_{max}^{\infty}$, $C\,_{min}^{\infty}$ = maximum and minimum blood levels achieved at equilibrium after repeated dosing

$C_o'$ = blood level at time zero after the first intravenous dose as extrapolated from the terminal linear portion of the blood level-time plot

$\tau$ = dosing interval

$t_{1/2}$ = biological half-life (elimination half-life) of the drug in the body

For extravascular administration, of which the oral route is most common, the equations are more complex due to an absorption phase. The equations can be simplified, however, and used to estimate plateau levels if the half-life for absorption is much less than that for elimination, which is the case with most drugs:

$$C\,_{max}^{\infty} = \frac{C_o\,10^{-0.3\,t_a/t_{1/2}}}{1 - 10^{-0.3\tau/t_{1/2}}} \qquad (3)$$

$$C\,_{min}^{\infty} = \frac{C_o\,10^{-0.3\tau/t_{1/2}}}{1 - 10^{-0.3\tau/t_{1/2}}} \qquad (4)$$

$C_o$ = apparent blood level at time zero after the first oral dose as extrapolated from the terminal linear portion of the post-absorption phase of the blood level-time plot

$t_a$ = time required for absorption of a single dose

The determination of these parameters is depicted in Figure 2 for the administration of a single oral dose. In Figure 2a, the clinical blood level data have been converted to log values. A least squares line of best fit, as discussed in most books on statistical analysis, should be drawn through the terminal data points and extrapolated to zero time. As noted, slope represents the absolute value, ignoring the sign, of the

*Figure 2. Determination of dosage regimen parameters $C_0$, $C_0'$, and $t_{1/2}$ for oral administration*

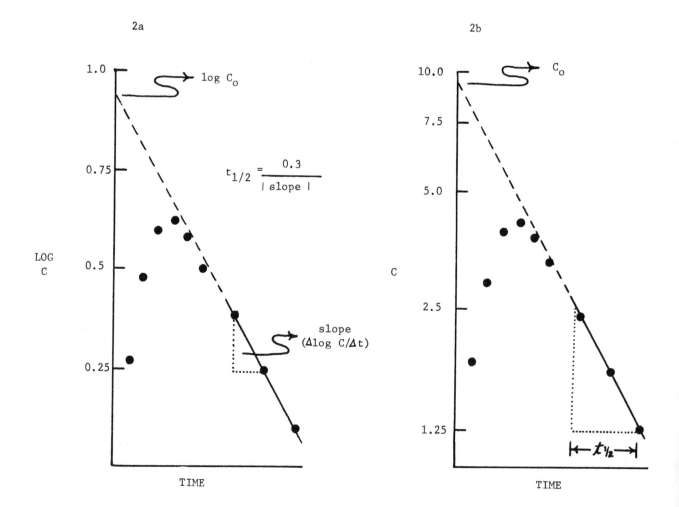

change in the log of the blood level during a given time interval, $\Delta \log C/\Delta_t$. In Figure 2b, the clinical blood level data have not been converted to log values but have been plotted directly onto semi-log graph paper. The same operations are performed in this treatment as noted above.

## Limitations of the Technique

The techniques illustrated in Figure 2 and applied in equations 1-4 are readily handled by the pharmacist. It is important to realize, however, some of the assumptions, approximations, and pitfalls implicit in this procedure:

1. The technique used in Figure 2 assumes that a one-compartment open kinetic model, in which distribution of drug between blood and tissues is instantaneous, best fits the data. It is more common, however, for the distributive phase of the drug to require a finite time to reach equilibrium, as characterized by the two-compartment open kinetic model.[7-10] Yet, unless blood samples are taken at very frequent intervals during the early stage after iv administration, and this is an uncommon procedure in most clinical studies that the pharmacist will use, the data will appear to be best fitted by using the one-compartment approach as shown in Figure 2. Furthermore, the distributive phase following oral administration may be obscured by the absorption phase if blood samples are used. Fortunately, Wagner and Metzler[11] have shown that the application of simple one-compartment techniques to most two-compartment data does not jeopardize the application of Equations 1-4.

2. The parameters $C_o$, $C_o'$, and $t_{1/2}$ are generated from the terminal linear portion of the blood level curve after distribution equilibrium between blood and tissues has been achieved and, in the case of extravascular administration, absorption has ceased. When the pharmacist has access to a thorough single dose study in which the blood level has been monitored until the drug has been almost completely eliminated, it is not difficult to determine the biological half-life from the terminal portion of the blood level-time curve. In most clinical studies, however, the blood level has not been followed as long as is necessary to insure the determination of terminal data points. This forces the pharmacist to accept the latter points of the study in question as terminal, and the technique of Figure 2 is performed, even though the data may not truly represent postdistributive and postabsorption data. As noted by van Rossum[12] and Gibaldi and Weintraub,[13] this usually results in underestimating the $t_{1/2}$. In addition, extrapolation of $C_o$ and $C_o'$ is generally overestimated under these conditions. Fortunately, $C_o$, or $C_o'$, and $t_{1/2}$ oppose each other in Equations 1-4 and this decreases the error involved in improper assessment. In general, the significance of this type of error is not great when comparing a series of similar drugs, as suggested in this paper, because their pharmacokinetic characteristics are similar. In terms of estimating a dosage regimen, however, the practical consequence of this type of error is administration of the drug more frequently than necessary.

3. When it is desirable to predict $C_{max}^{\infty}$ upon oral administration, as noted in Equation 3, it becomes necessary to assess the time required for absorption

of the drug, $t_a$. While techniques for determining this parameter are available in the literature,[7-10] the pharmacist can often render an estimate that will not introduce a serious error. Since absorption ceases at some time after the peak blood level has been achieved, $t_{max}$, it is often reasonable to assess the time for absorption, $t_a$, as twice that required for appearance of the peak blood level ($t_a \sim 2\ t_{max}$), if $t_{max}$ appears to be four hours or less. This suggests an additional approximation in the determination of $t_{max}$ because the clinical literature rarely presents data which have been sampled frequently enough to assess this value. In practice, $t_{max}$ must usually be taken as the time for attainment of the highest blood level reported after a single dose. Fortunately, a rough estimate of $C_{max}$ is generally all that is required to insure the calculation of a dosage regimen that achieves a maximum level well below the estimated value.

4. Equations 3 and 4 are approximations of the true values.[6] They may be used, however, when certain rather conservative restrictions are observed. If absorption time, $t_a$, is estimated to be completed in at least six hours ($t_{max} \leqslant 3$ hours), the dosage interval, $\tau$, is chosen at least as great as $t_a$, and the biological half-life is at least four times that of the absorption half-life (as estimated by $t_a/5$), then no serious error is introduced in the estimation of $C_{max}^{\infty}$ and $C_{min}^{\infty}$. These constraints are generally observed with most drugs. When they are violated, however, it will readily appear upon evaluating the single dose data as in Figure 2.

5. Equations 3-5 and 8-11 in this chapter assume that the provisions in #4 above are observed.

6. It is assumed that the $t_{1/2}$ and the volume of distribution of the drug are not altered during the course of treatment. If the half-life has been accurately determined, as discussed above, these parameters usually remain constant.

## Dosage Regimen Calculations as a Guide To Evaluating the Tetracycline Antibiotics

The tetracycline family of antibiotics provides an opportunity for applying dosage regimen calculations as one parameter of the comparative evaluation of these drugs. Blood level data abstracted from the clinical paper of Steigbigel et al.[14] on the absorption and excretion of various tetracyclines are recorded in Table 1. This paper is more informative for calculating the regimen than many clinical papers because it monitors single dose blood levels for a longer period than is common in the literature. Infrequent sampling by the investigators during the first few hours, however, necessitates an estimate of $t_{max}$ and $t_a$. Furthermore, although plotting the data as in Figure 2 suggests that a two-compartment kinetic model is appropriate, infrequent sampling also makes it necessary, but acceptable, to apply the one-compartment treatment of Figure 2, as discussed previously. The 24- and 48-hour data points were used to describe the linear portion of the terminal segment of the blood level curve in the case of demeclocycline, methacycline and minocycline. For tetracycline and doxycycline, approximations were made in describing the linear plot. Based

Table 1. Single Dose Blood Levels Resulting From Oral Administrations of Various Tetracyclines[14]

| DERIVATIVE | DOSE | BLOOD LEVEL ($\mu$g/ml) | | | | |
|---|---|---|---|---|---|---|
| | | 2 hr | 4 hr | 8 hr | 24 hr | 48 hr |
| Tetracycline | 0.5 g | 2.88 | 3.25 | 1.97 | 0.53 | <0.03 |
| Demeclocycline | 0.3 g | 0.97 | 1.74 | 1.68 | 0.53 | 0.17 |
| Methacycline | 0.3 g | 2.10 | 2.40 | 1.85 | 0.56 | 0.16 |
| Doxycycline | 0.15 g | 1.49 | 1.28 | 1.21 | 0.44 | 0.23 |
| Minocycline | 0.15 g | 2.19 | 1.85 | 1.40 | 0.53 | 0.19 |

on the technique illustrated in Figure 2, $C_o$ and $t_{1/2}$ values were determined as recorded in Table 2. The $t_{1/2}$ values obtained by this method vary by less than 15% from the more accurate data recorded by Doluisio and Dittert[15] in their studies of tetracyclines during the plateau state. The $C_o$ values that were estimated in Table 2, as opposed to those obtained by graphical analysis of the data, were calculated on the basis of the pharmacokinetic observation that $C_o$ is approximately proportional to the dose. [3,16]

The relationship of blood level to therapeutic effect depends upon the type of drug being used. For pharmacodynamic drugs, the pharmacological response may often be related to the blood level even though the site of action is usually in some tissue and not in the blood. The onset of response is denoted by a minimum effective concentration in blood while a maximum level is set below the concentration producing toxic responses. For a few drugs, the pharmacological response is not related to the blood level.

For antibiotic therapy, however, there appears to be no consensus among clinicians regarding the maintenance of a minimum blood level of antibiotic as opposed to the "peak and valley" effect in which blood levels may fall below some minimum level during dosage intervals. For bacteriostatic drugs like the tetracyclines, however, it is usually considered

desirable to maintain a minimum level of drug in the blood as an index of adequate diffusion of drug into tissues.[4,5,15,17] Although there is no quantitative relationship between blood and specific tissue levels,[15,18] investigators have shown that maintenance of a minimum blood level does provide a rough gauge of adequate penetration of tetracyclines to many tissues.[18-20]

With this in mind, $C_{min}^\infty$ can be fixed as the minimum inhibitory concentration (MIC) of the tetracycline derivative *in blood* for a given organism. If MIC values in blood serum are unavailable but data in protein-free broth or agar are published, as is often the case, then an estimate of the blood values may be obtained by dividing the latter values by the fraction of drug which is free (not bound to proteins) in blood.[21] Many clinicians circumvent this problem by seeking blood levels that exceed broth-agar MIC values by fivefold;[22-24] when protein binding exceeds 80%, however, this guide may seriously underestimate the required blood level. The estimated MIC data recorded in Table 2 were obtained by doubling the MIC values in 50% serum as reported in the literature.[14] A $C_{min}^\infty$ value of 1.6 $\mu$g/ml was used for all tetracyclines in this chapter, despite slight variations in MIC values, because these variations are less than the potential errors in the determination of MIC data in blood.

Some methods for estimating the dosage regimen may now be illustrated. A variety of comparative regimens are possible depending upon the variables chosen. For example, the blood level range during therapy may be stipulated by fixing $C_{max}^\infty$ and $C_{min}^\infty$ values. Under these conditions, the dose and dosing interval are variables to be calculated. Another method fixes $C_{min}^\infty$ and the dosing interval, leaving the dose to be calculated. Five common methods are presented below.

Table 2. Data Used in Calculating the Dosage Regimens for the Various Tetracyclines

| DERIVATIVE | DOSE (g) | $C_o$ ($\mu$g/ml) | $t_{1/2}$ (hours) | MIC[b] IN BROTH[14] ($\mu$g/ml) | MIC[c] IN BLOOD ($\mu$g/ml) | % PROTEIN BOUND IN SERUM[25] |
|---|---|---|---|---|---|---|
| Tetracycline | 0.5 | 3.9 | 9.5 | 0.068 | 0.8 | 55 |
| Tetracycline | 0.25 | 1.95[a] | 9.5 | 0.068 | 0.8 | 55 |
| Demeclocycline | 0.3 | 1.6 | 15.0 | 0.039 | 1.6 | 75 |
| Demeclocycline | 0.15 | 0.8[a] | 15.0 | 0.039 | 1.6 | 75 |
| Methacycline | 0.3 | 2.0 | 13.0 | 0.025 | 0.8 | 78 |
| Methacycline | 0.15 | 1.0[a] | 13.0 | 0.025 | 0.8 | 78 |
| Doxycycline | 0.15 | 1.2 | 19.0 | 0.048 | 0.8 | 82 |
| Doxycycline | 0.1 | 0.8[a] | 19.0 | 0.048 | 0.8 | 82 |
| Minocycline | 0.15 | 1.5 | 15.0 | 0.011 | 1.6 | 85[a] |
| Minocycline | 0.1 | 1.0 | 15.0 | 0.011 | 1.6 | 85[a] |

[a]Estimated as discussed in the text.

[b]Streptococcus 98.

[c]Estimated from the MIC broth data of reference 14 as discussed in the text

Method A: Fixed Dose and $C_{min}^{\infty}$, Variable $\tau$ and $C_{max}^{\infty}$

To calculate the oral dosing interval, $\tau$, Equation 4 is rearranged to yield Equation 5.

$$\tau = 3.32\, t_{1/2} \log (1 + C_o/C_{min}^{\infty}) \qquad (5)$$

Using a 0.5 g tetracycline dose and the data of Table 2 as an example:

$$\tau = (3.32)(9.5) \log (1 + 3.9/1.6) = 16.9 \text{ hours}$$

As illustrated in Figure 1 and discussed previously, $C_{max}^{\infty}$ and $C_{min}^{\infty}$ will not be reached after the first dose unless the drug is completely eliminated from the body prior to administration of the second dose. Many investigators[4-6,17] have defined a rough index of the amount of accumulation that results from giving equal doses of drug at regular intervals, $\tau$, which applies if the interval is at least as great as the time for absorption, $t_a$, as is usually the case.

$$A = \frac{M^{\infty}}{D} = \frac{1}{1 - 10^{-0.3\tau/t_{1/2}}} \qquad (6)$$

$A$ = accumulation resulting from repeated dosing, D, at regular intervals, $\tau$
$M^{\infty}$ = maximum amount of drug in the body after reaching the plateau level
$D$ = maintenance dose

Equation 6 may be used to calculate the loading dose, D*, that will achieve plateau levels after the first dose, as shown in Figure 1. The use of a loading dose is particularly important for drugs with long half-lives. Since it takes approximately five half-lives for a drug to achieve the plateau, or equilibrium state, it may take days to reach equilibrium for drugs with long half-lives but only hours for drugs with short half-lives. The tetracyclines have long half-lives which make them candidates for administering a loading dose. The penicillins, to be discussed later, have half-lives that are usually less than the dosing interval. Since these agents do not accumulate in blood, the administration of a loading dose is usually wasteful and unnecessary. Equation 7 defines the ratio of loading dose to maintenance dose as equal to the amount of accumulation resulting from maintenance doses.

$$\frac{D^*}{D} = \frac{1}{1 - 10^{-0.3\tau/t_{1/2}}} \qquad (7)$$

D* = loading dose

Applying the tetracycline example to Equation 7:

$$\frac{D^*}{0.5 \text{ g}} = \frac{1}{10^{-0.3(16.9/9.5)}}$$
$$D^* = 0.7 \text{ g}$$

Thus one estimate of a dosage regimen for tetracycline, as generated by Equations 5 and 7, yields a loading dose of 0.7 g followed by maintenance doses of 0.5 g every 17 hours.

Representative regimens for the other tetracyclines, using this method and the data recorded in Table 2, are shown in Table 3.

Method B: Fixed $\tau$ and $C_{min}^{\infty}$, Variable Dose and $C_{max}^{\infty}$

As noted in Table 3, Method A often results in irregular dosing intervals. Equation 4 may be rearranged to enable the calculation of a dose when $\tau$ and $C_{min}^{\infty}$ are fixed.

$$\log (1 + C_o^2/C_{min}^{\infty}) = \tau/3.32\, t_{1/2} \qquad (8)$$

Inserting the tetracycline data from Table 2, using $\tau$ and $C_{min}^{\infty}$ of 12 hours and 1.6 $\mu$g/ml, respectively:

$$\log (1 + C_o^2/1.6) = 12/(3.32)(9.5)$$
$$C_o^2 = 2.24 \; \mu\text{g/ml}$$

$C_o^2$ represents the extrapolated zero time value, as

**Table 3. Dosage Regimens Calculated for the Various Tetracyclines[a]**

| | METHOD A | | | METHOD B | | | METHOD C | | |
|---|---|---|---|---|---|---|---|---|---|
| DERIVATIVE | LOADING DOSE (g) | MAIN-TENANCE DOSE (g) | $\tau$ (hr) | LOADING DOSE (g) | MAIN-TENANCE DOSE (g) | $\tau$ (hr) | LOADING DOSE (g) | MAIN-TENANCE DOSE (g) | $\tau$ (hr) |
| Tetracycline | 0.70 | 0.50 | 16.9 | 0.49 | 0.29 | 12 | 0.41 | 0.21 | 9.5 |
| | 0.46 | 0.25 | 10.9 | | | | | | |
| Demeclocycline | 0.60 | 0.30 | 15.0 | 0.52 | 0.22 | 12 | 0.60 | 0.30 | 15.0 |
| | 0.45 | 0.15 | 8.8 | | | | | | |
| Methacycline | 0.54 | 0.30 | 15.2 | 0.46 | 0.22 | 12 | 0.48 | 0.24 | 13.0 |
| | 0.39 | 0.15 | 9.1 | | | | | | |
| Doxycycline | 0.35 | 0.15 | 15.3 | 0.31 | 0.11 | 12 | 0.40 | 0.20 | 19.0 |
| | 0.30 | 0.10 | 11.1 | | | | | | |
| Minocycline | 0.30 | 0.15 | 14.3 | 0.28 | 0.12 | 12 | 0.32 | 0.16 | 15.0 |
| | 0.26 | 0.10 | 10.4 | | | | | | |

[a]Based on $C_{min}^{\infty}$ = 1.6 $\mu$g/ml.

shown in Figure 2, for the oral maintenance dose, $D^2$, administered every 12 hours in order to maintain a $C_{min}^{\infty}$ of 1.6 $\mu$g/ml. Since $C_0$ is proportional to $D$, and a dose of 0.5 gm was shown to yield a $C_0$ value of 3.9, as shown in Table 2:

$$\frac{C_0^2}{C_0} = \frac{D^2}{D} \tag{9}$$

$$\frac{2.24}{3.90} = \frac{D^2}{0.5}$$

$$D^2 = 0.287 \text{ g}$$

The loading dose, $D^*$, is calculated with Equation 7 as before. Estimated regimens for the tetracyclines, using this method, and the data recorded in Table 2, are shown in Table 3.

## Method C: Fixed $\tau = t_{1/2}$, Fixed $C_{min}^{\infty}$, Variable Dose and $C_{max}^{\infty}$

Krüger-Thiemer[4,5] has suggested a convenient approximation of the dosage regimen which has been corroborated with a number of sulfonamides.[26] As noted in Equation 7, when the dosing interval is taken as the biological half-life of the drug ($\tau = t_{1/2}$), the loading dose becomes fixed at twice the maintenance dose. To use this approximation, the data in Table 2 are converted through use of Equation 10. Utilizing the tetracycline data as before:

$$\frac{C_{min}}{C_0} = \frac{D^2}{D} \tag{10}$$

$$\frac{1.6}{3.9} = \frac{D^2}{0.5}$$

$$D^2 = 0.205 \text{ g}$$

$$D^* = 2D^2 = 0.410 \text{ g}$$

This convenient method, suggesting a tetracycline loading dose of 0.41 g followed by 0.21 g maintenance doses given every 9.5 hours, often yields awkward dosage intervals, because $\tau = t_{1/2}$. Thus it suffers the same limitations as Method A.

Estimated regimens for the various tetracyclines are recorded in Table 3.

## Method D: Fixed $C_{min}^{\infty}$ and $C_{max}^{\infty}$, Variable Dose and $\tau$

When drug toxicity is a problem, it is possible to stipulate a blood level range by fixing $C_{min}^{\infty}$ and $C_{max}^{\infty}$. Equations 3 and 4 are rearranged to yield Equation 11.

$$\tau = (3.32 \, t_{1/2} \log C_{max}^{\infty}/C_{min}^{\infty}) + t_a \tag{11}$$

The maintenance and loading doses are then calculated through the sequential use of Equations 8, 9 and 7. This method has not been used in this paper, however, because an estimation of $C_{max}^{\infty}$ using Equation 3 demonstrated that none of the regimens generated with Methods A, B and C resulted in toxic blood levels.

## The Choice of Methods

The various regimens recorded in Table 3 demonstrate that a number of dosage schedules can be developed depending upon which parameters are held constant during the calculations. Method B presents the most practical procedure for comparative evaluations because the relative doses of a series of derivatives can be assessed under conditions of fixed $C_{min}^{\infty}$ and $\tau$. Method A is useful for evaluating the durability of blood levels in a series of related drugs. Method D is chosen when the use of Equation 3 suggests that toxic blood levels may result from the use of Methods A, B and C.

The estimation of dosage regimens, therefore, provides another index of the comparative efficacy of a family of drugs in addition to the usual parameters such as potency, toxicity, tissue distribution, speed of onset, duration of response, and others. As the next few paragraphs will indicate, certain differences in the tetracyclines only appear upon an analysis of this type.

In Table 4, the various tetracycline regimens recom-

## Table 4. Comparison of Calculated and Recommended Dosage Regimens for the Various Tetracyclines

| DERIVATIVE | CALCULATED[a] | | | RECOMMENDED[b] | | |
| | LOADING DOSE (g) | MAIN-TENANCE DOSE (g) | $\tau$ (hr) | LOADING DOSE (g) | MAIN-TENANCE DOSE (g) | $\tau$ (hr) |
|---|---|---|---|---|---|---|
| Tetracycline | 0.50 | 0.25 | 12 | — | 0.25-0.50 | 6 |
| Demeclocycline | 0.45 | 0.15 | 8 | — | 0.15 | 6 |
| Methacycline | 0.45 | 0.15 | 8 | — | 0.15 | 6 |
| Doxycycline | 0.30 | 0.10 | 12 | 0.2[c] | 0.1 | 24 |
| Minocycline | 0.30 | 0.10 | 12 | 0.2 | 0.1 | 12 |

[a]Adjusted from the regimens recorded in Table 3 in order to conform to commercially available dosage forms.
[b]Manufacturer's recommendations.
[c]As 0.1 g q12h x 2.

mended by the manufacturer have been compared to representative regimens gleaned from the calculations in Table 3 in which the latter schedules have been adjusted to conform to commercially available dosage forms. By comparing the regimens in Table 4, as well as those calculated with Method B in Table 3, some differences in the durability of the blood levels of the various tetracyclines are apparent.

Accepting the many limitations and approximations of this technique, the stipulation of a higher $C_{min}^{\infty}$ than imposed by many investigators, and the use of blood levels as an index of tissue levels and distribution, the calculated and recommended regimens for demeclocycline, methacycline and minocycline compare favorably, as shown in Table 4. Relating the schedules for doxycycline, however, suggests that once a day dosing may be too conservative. On the other hand, tetracycline dosage may be excessive. Other investigators[15,27] have also suggested that the dosing interval for tetracycline may be too frequent.

It is apparent upon comparing the calculated regimens for the various tetracyclines in Table 4, as well as those obtained with Method B in Table 3, that twice daily dosing with 0.25-0.50 g of tetracycline compares favorably with other tetracycline derivatives based upon the provisions of this chapter. Although tetracycline is less potent in a protein-free medium than the newer compounds, it is also less bound to proteins, resulting in a smaller diminution of activity in blood, as shown in Table 2. The possibility of decreasing the frequency of dosing with tetracycline, making it comparable to the schedules of the other derivatives, is an important economic as well as therapeutic consideration. Tetracycline may well be as efficacious and less expensive than the newer tetracycline derivatives. Further corroboration of the prognostic significance of estimating dosage regimens in general, and the observations concerning tetracycline dosing in particular, are found in the work of Holvey et al.[24,28] These investigators, in a nonpharmacokinetic study, demonstrated the efficacy of twice a day dosing with tetracycline as well as the durability of its blood levels in relation to other derivatives.

Three more reservations should be noted for the use of blood levels in estimating dosage regimens:

1. As stated previously, blood levels are not an absolute index of tissue distribution although this parameter has been used by clinicians, undoubtedly will continue to be employed, and may even be appropriate as a tacit guide to tissue penetration and therapeutic efficacy. As illustrated with the penicillins in the next section, however, it is not possible to relate the blood level to the total amount of drug in the body without knowledge of the volume of distribution of the drug.
2. The $C_0$ values used in the dosage regimen calculations are a function of dietary habits, physical activity, and other patient characteristics. The values obtained in this chapter were generated from blood

level data[14] which were generally higher than observed in other studies for similar doses, [15,24,28] although no major differences in study protocol were apparent.
3. The $C_{min}^{\infty}$ value of 1.6 µg/ml is a conservative estimate for most susceptible pathogens. For some gram-negative and gram-positive organisms, a greater $C_{min}^{\infty}$, and therefore a larger dose, may be necessary.
4. For urinary tract infections, and in patients with renal insufficiency, other factors must also be considered in the choice of derivatives. For urinary tract infections, the derivatives with the greater renal clearance, such as tetracycline and oxytetracycline, are preferred. In cases of renal insufficiency, the derivatives with low renal clearances, such as doxycycline and minocycline, are favored.

## Dosage Regimen Calculations as a Guide to Evaluating the Penicillin Antibiotics

The various lactamase-stable penicillin derivatives offer an opportunity to demonstrate still another method for estimating the dosage regimen as a guide to comparative evaluation. Since the penicillins possess biological half-lives of an hour or less,[29-31] and their attainment of peak blood levels upon oral administration exceeds one hour,[32-34] one of the constraints placed upon the use of Equations 3-11 has been violated; the biological half-life is probably not at least four times as great as the absorption half-life. Furthermore, since oral dosage regimens generally provide for only two to four administrations daily, it is impractical to stipulate $C_{min}^{\infty}$ levels for antibiotics with such short half-lives because the drug will undoubtedly fall below this value during the dosing interval. In these situations, it is more reasonable to estimate dosage regimens which will provide for an average blood level, $C_{av}^{\infty}$, during dosage intervals, as shown in Figure 1. For bactericidal antibiotics like the penicillins, this procedure is even advantageous because short periods of sub-$C_{min}^{\infty}$ levels are considered desirable for maximum bactericidal activity.[22,23]

## Method E: Fixed $C_{av}^{\infty}$, Variable $\tau$ or Dose

Wagner[27] has developed a method for estimating the dosage regimen which is independent of absorption half-life and the choice of pharmacokinetic model,[13] as long as elimination occurs from the blood-containing compartment, as is usually the case.

$$D = \frac{\tau V C_{av}^{\infty}}{1.44 \, f t_{1/2}} \tag{12}$$

$$\tau = \frac{1.44 \, f D t_{1/2}}{V C_{av}^{\infty}} \tag{13}$$

f = fraction of dose, D, absorbed from single dose administration

V = volume of distribution of drug in the body

$C_{av}^{\infty}$ = average blood level achieved during a dosage interval, $\tau$, once plateau levels are attained

This method is somewhat more difficult to apply than the previous methods because the fraction of dose absorbed and the volume of distribution, parameters often unavailable in the clinical literature and values that vary with the method of calculation, must be known. Techniques for obtaining these data are readily available in the literature.[7-10] In using the previous methods, wherein $C_o$ was obtained as shown in Figure 2, the fraction of dose absorbed and the volume of distribution were components of the $C_o$ term, as shown in Equation 14, and did not have to be measured independently.

$$C_o = \frac{fD}{Vx} \qquad (14)$$

$$x = \left[ \frac{t_{1/2}{}^{*}}{t_{1/2}} - 0.7 \right]$$

$t_{1/2}{}^{*}$ = absorption half-life
$t_{1/2}$ = biological half-life (elimination half-life)

The various parameters needed to utilize Equations 12 and 13 are recorded in Table 5. Although the primary indication for the use of the lactamase-stable penicillins is in the treatment of infections resulting from lactamase-secreting staphylococci, these penicillins are commonly employed against other gram-positive organisms. For this reason, regimens were estimated for treating representative staphylococcal and streptococcal infections. The same $C_{av}^{\infty}$ parameter was chosen for all of the penicillins, despite slight variations in the MIC values for the compounds, because these variations are less than the potential errors in the determination of MIC values in blood.

The various regimens, as calculated using Equation 12 and recommended by the manufacturer, are shown in Table 6. Once again, these estimates provide unique information regarding the comparative efficacy of a group of similar compounds. From the viewpoint of

the parameters in Table 5, dicloxacillin may need to be administered in ⅔ and ⅓ the daily doses of cloxacillin and oxacillin, respectively. Whereas, the manufacturer's recommendations appear appropriate for infections due to relatively sensitive organisms, like many strains of streptococci, the regimens may be too conservative for lactamase-secreting staphylococci.

The high regimens calculated for nafcillin are, in part, a function of its relatively large volume of distribution in the body, as shown in Table 5. This points up another consideration in the interpretation of dosage regimen calculations. Although the blood level has been used in this chapter, and by many clinicians, as an index of tissue distribution, the blood level does not yield an indication of the total amount of drug in the body unless the volume of distribution is also known. These factors are related, using a one-compartment model, through Equation 15.

$$A = CV \qquad (15)$$

A = amount of drug in the body
C = concentration of drug in the blood

Once plateau levels have been achieved using the regimens calculated for staphylococcal infections in Table 6, the average amount of drug in the body at any given moment is 66, 76, 91 and 189 mg of dicloxacillin, cloxacillin, oxacillin and nafcillin, respectively, using Equation 15. If the amount of drug in the body is used as a parameter in calculating the regimen, then reducing the nafcillin dosage by three-fold, yielding an average body content of 63 mg, results in similar amounts of the various derivatives in the body. This suggests that some modification in the estimation of dosage regimens may be necessary when there are large differences in the volumes of distribution of similar drugs. These same considerations apply to regimens estimated with the methods discussed previously. The significance of the volume of distribution in pharmacokinetics is discussed in the literature[7-10,36] and is an important consideration in designing the dosage regimen. The choice of the blood level or the amount of drug in the body as the basis for either estimating the dosage regimen or comparing similar drugs, however, depends upon the locus of the infection and the pharmacokinetic parameters that are available.

### Table 5. Data Used in Calculating the Dosage Regimens for the Various Penicillins

| DERIVATIVE | MIC IN BLOOD FOR STAPH.[a] ($\mu$g/ml) | $C_{av}^{\infty}$ FOR STAPH. ($\mu$g/ml) | MIC IN BLOOD FOR STREP.[b] ($\mu$g/ml) | $C_{av}^{\infty}$ FOR STREP. ($\mu$g/ml) | f[34] | V[31] (liters) |
|---|---|---|---|---|---|---|
| Dicloxacillin | 6.2 | 7.0 | 2.0 | 2.0 | 0.80 | 9.4 |
| Cloxacillin | 7.0 | 7.0 | 1.8 | 2.0 | 0.77 | 10.8 |
| Oxacillin | 5.4 | 7.0 | 1.3 | 2.0 | 0.67 | 13.0 |
| Nafcillin | 5.0[c] | 7.0 | 1.0 | 2.0 | 0.50[c] | 27.0 |

[a]Estimated from lactamase-producing strains of *Stapholococcus aureus*.[35]
[b]Estimated from group A hemolytic streptococci.[21,35]
[c]Estimated from various studies.

Table 6. Dosage Regimens for the Various Penicillins[a]

| DERIVATIVE | STAPH. INFECTIONS | | STREP. INFECTIONS | | | |
| | $\tau = 6$ hrs | ADJUSTED[b] | $\tau = 8$ hrs | $\tau = 12$ hrs | ADJUSTED[b] | RECOMMENDED[c] |
|---|---|---|---|---|---|---|
| Dicloxacillin | 0.49 g | 0.50 g q6h | 0.19 g | 0.28 g | 0.25 g q12h | 0.125-0.25 g q6h |
| Cloxacillin | 0.66 g | 0.75 g q6h | 0.26 g | 0.38 g | 0.25 g q8h | 0.25 -0.50 g q4-6h |
| Oxacillin | 1.40 g | 1.50 g q6h | 0.54 g | 0.81 g | 0.50 g q8h | 0.25 -0.50 g q4-6h |
| Nafcillin | 2.87 g | 2.00 g q4h | 1.09 g | 1.64 g | 1.00 g q8h | 0.25 -0.50 g q4-6h |

[a]Based on $C_{av}^{\infty} = 7.0$ μg/ml and 2.0 μg/ml for staphylococcal and streptococcal infections, respectively.
[b]Adjusted in order to conform to commercially available dosage forms.
[c]Manufacturer's recommendations.

Accumulation, as estimated by Equations 6 and 7, probably does not occur upon repeated administration of the penicillins due to the short half-life of the compounds in comparison to the relatively long dosing interval. For this reason, no loading dose has been suggested in Table 6. Equation 7 can be used with Method E, however, to determine a loading dose where appropriate.

It should be noted that the estimation of dosage regimens by Methods A-E will be modified in uremic patients due to a decrease in the biological half-life. To compensate for this effect, the dosage interval should be prolonged.

## Dosage Regimen Calculations for Intravenous Administration

Some of the limitations that apply to use of Equations 3-11 for oral administration, resulting from the existence of an absorption phase, are not applicable to Equations 1 and 2 for intravenous administration. Assuming that $C_o'$ values have been obtained with reasonable accuracy, as shown in Figure 2, the use of Equations 1, 2, and 5-11 results in reliable estimates of the dosage regimen for intravenous administration. Equations 12 and 13 may also be used assuming complete absorption. Since no estimates of the amount of drug absorbed and the time for absorption are necessary for intravenous dosing, these regimens are more accurate than oral schedules.

## Conclusions

The tetracycline and penicillin antibiotics have been used to demonstrate the application of dosage regimen calculations in drug evaluation and consultation. Emphasis has been placed on the use of these calculations as one of the parameters of efficacy in comparing a series of closely related drugs. When reliable assumptions and approximations can be applied to the data, however, the calculations may be used to estimate optimum dosage schedules.

## References

1. Boxer, G. and Jelinek, V.: Streptomycin in the Blood: Chemical Determinations After Single and Repeated Intramuscular Injections, *J. Pharmacol. Exp. Ther.* 92:226, 1948.
2. Dost, F.: Der Blutspiegel, Arbeitsgemeinschaft Medizinischer Verlage G.M.B.A., Leipzig, Germany, 1953.
3. Swintosky, J. et al.: Sulfaethylthiadiazole IV: Steady State Blood Concentration and Urinary Excretion Data Following Repeated Oral Doses, *J. Amer. Pharm. Ass. (Sci. Ed.)* 47:753, 1958.
4. Krüger-Thiemer, E.: Dosage Schedule and Pharmacokinetics in Chemotherapy, *J. Amer. Pharm. Ass. (Sci. Ed.)* 49:311, 1960.
5. Krüger-Thiemer, E.: Formal Theory of Drug Dosage Regimens, *J. Theor. Biol.* 13:212, 1966.
6. Wiegand, R. et al.: Multiple Dose Excretion Kinetics, *J. Pharm. Sci.* 52:268, 1963.
7. Swarbrick, J.: Current Concepts in the Pharmaceutical Sciences: Biopharmaceutics, Lea & Febiger, Philadelphia, Pennsylvania, 1970.
8. Wagner, J.: Biopharmaceutics and Relevant Pharmacokinetics, Drug Intelligence Publications, Hamilton, Illinois, 1971.
9. Gibaldi, M.: Introduction to Biopharmaceutics, Lea & Febiger, Philadelpia, Pennsylvania, 1971.
10. Notari, R.: Biopharmaceutics and Pharmacokinetics: An Introduction, Marcel Dekker, New York, New York, 1971.
11. Wagner, J. and Metzler, C.: Prediction of Blood Levels after Multiple Doses from Single-Dose Blood Level Data: Data Generated with Two-Compartment Open Model Analysed According to the One-Compartment Open Model, *J. Pharm. Sci.* 58:87, 1969.
12. Van Rossum, J., *In* Ariens, E. (ed.): Drug Design, Vol. 1, Academic Press, New York, New York, 1971, ch. 7.
13. Gibaldi, M. and Weintraub, H.: Some Considerations as to the Determination and Significance of Biological Half-Life, *J. Pharm. Sci.* 60:624, 1971.
14. Steigbigel, N. et al.: Absorption and Excretion of Five Tetracycline Analogues in Normal Young Men, *Amer. J. Med. Sci.* 255:296, 1968.
15. Doluisio, J. and Dittert, L.: Influence of Repetitive Dosing of Tetracyclines on Biological Half-Life in Serum, *Clin. Pharmacol. Ther.* 10:690, 1969.
16. Dost, F., *In* Raspé, G. (ed.): Advances in the Biosciences-5, Pergamon Press, London, England, 1970, pp. 137-144.
17. Dettli, L., *In* Raspé G. (ed.): Advances in the Biosciences-5, Pergamon Press, London, England, 1970, pp. 39-54.
18. Schach von Wittenau, M. and Delahunt, C.: The Distribution of Tetracyclines in Tissues of Dogs After Repeated Oral Administration, *J. Pharmacol. Exp. Ther.* 152:164, 1966.
19. Kelly, R. and Kanegis, L.: Metabolism and Tissue Distribution of Radioisotopically Labeled Minocycline, *Toxicol. Appl. Pharmacol.* 11:171, 1967.
20. Racz, G.: Tissue Concentration of Antibiotic Following Oral Doses of Tetracycline Phosphate Complex, *Curr. Ther.*
21. Kunin, C.: Clinical Pharmacology of the New Penicillins, *Clin. Pharmacol. Ther.* 3:166, 1966.

22. Garrod, L. and O'Grady, F.: Antibiotic and Chemotherapy, 2nd ed., E. & S. Livingstone, Edinburgh, Scotland, 1968, ch. 14.

23. Weinstein, L., *In* Goodman, L. and Gilman, A. (eds.): The Pharmacological Basis of Therapeutics, Macmillan, 4th ed., New York, New York, 1970, ch. 57.

24. Olon, L. and Holvey, D.: Evaluation of Tetracycline Phosphate Complex, Demethylchlortetracycline HCl, and Methacycline HCl, *Clin. Med.* 75:33, 1968.

25. Schach von Wittenau, M. and Yeary, R.: The Excretion and Distribution in Body Fluids of Tetracyclines After Intravenous Administration to Dogs, *J. Pharmacol. Exp. Ther.* 140:258, 1963.

26. Krüger-Thiemer, E. and Bunger, P.: The Role of the Therapeutic Regimen in Dosage Design, *Chemotherapia 10:* 61, 1965.

27. Wagner, J.: Drug Accumulation, *J. Clin. Pharmacol.* 7:84, 1967.

28. Holvey, D. et al.: Serum Concentrations and Recovery in Urine of Four Tetracycline Analogues, *Curr. Ther. Res.* 12:536, 1970.

29. Gibaldi, M. et al.: Serum Levels of Penicillins: A Pharmacokinetic View, *In* Hobby, G. (ed.): Antimicrobial Agents and Chemotherapy-1968, American Society of Microbiology, Ann Arbor, Michigan, 1969, pp. 378-381.

30. Dittert, L. et al.: Pharmacokinetic Interpretation of Penicillin Levels in Serum and Urine After Intravenous Administration, *In* Hobby, G. (ed.): Antimicrobial Agents and Chemotherapy-1969, American Society of Microbiology, Ann Arbor, Michigan, 1970, pp. 42-48.

31. Standiford, H. et al.: Clinical Pharmacology of Carbenicillin Compared with Other Penicillins, *J. Inf. Dis.* 122S:59, 1970.

32. Doluisio, J. et al.: Pharmacokinetic Interpretation of Dicloxacillin Levels in Serum After Extravascular Administration, *In* Hobby, G. (ed.): Antimicrobial Agents and Chemotherapy-1969, American Society of Microbiology, Ann Arbor, Michigan, 1970, pp. 49-55.

33. Sutherland, R. et al.: Flucloxacillin, A New Isoxazolyl Penicillin, Compared with Oxacillin, Cloxacillin, and Dicloxacillin, *Brit. Med. J.* 4:455, 1970.

34. Modr, Z. and Dvoracek, K., *In* Raspé, G. (ed.): Advances in the Biosciences-5, Pergamon Press, London, England, 1970, pp. 219-230.

35. Hammerstrom, C. et al.: Clinical, Laboratory and Pharmacological Studies of Dicloxacillin, *In* Hobby, G. (ed.): Antimicrobial Agents and Chemotherapy-1966, American Society of Microbiology, Ann Arbor, Michigan, 1967, pp. 69-74.

36. Benet, L. and Ronfeld, R.: Volume Terms in Pharmacokinetics, *J. Pharm. Sci.* 58:639, 1969.

# 45 Practical Pharmacokinetic Techniques for Drug Consultation and Evaluation II: A Perspective on the Renal-impaired Patient

G. E. Schumacher

The general quantitative relationships between drug plasma concentrations, elimination pathways, the extent of renal impairment, and dosage regimen modifications in patients with renal impairment are reviewed.

Two methods of modifying dosage regimens for patients with renal impairment, using pharmacokinetic calculations, are discussed. One method is based on average plasma concentration and the other is based on maximum plasma concentration.

It is generally not necessary to consider reducing the normal dose or prolonging the normal dosage interval for drugs eliminated up to 25% by excretion, or for drugs excreted 50% until renal function is abolished, or for drugs excreted 75% until renal function is reduced to one-third of normal, or for drugs excreted 90% until renal status declines to less than one-half of normal.

It is concluded that an appreciation by the pharmacist of the mechanisms by which drugs are eliminated by the body will result in a more intuitive grasp of dosage regimen theory and better guidelines for modifying dosage regimens during renal impairment.

Dosage regimens for patients with renal impairment have come under scrutiny in recent years resulting in a proliferation of publications by physicians,[1-10] pharmacists,[11] and pharmaceutical scientists[12,13] citing recommendations for modifying normal regimens as renal function diminishes. Beginning with the work of Kunin,[14] who should be credited with developing in clinicians an awareness of the need for regimen modifications,[10] over 100 clinical studies have assessed various aspects of the influence of renal impairment on dosage.[1,2,5,7] Most of these studies have used the basic pharmacokinetic principles best summarized in the reviews of Wagner,[12] Dettli,[15,16] and Jelliffe.[17,18]

Most of the reviews on modified dosing, with the exception of those by Wagner and Dettli, are characterized by a tabular presentation relating the degree of renal impairment to an appropriate prolongation of the normal dosing interval. While this approach is essential for rapid consultation and monitoring, it places undue reliance on assessing only the regimens of drugs reported in tables, masks the underlying principles used to develop the tables, and fails to provide the clinician with basic techniques for approaching the regimen modifications of drugs in general. Furthermore, there appears to be no treatment in the literature of the general quantitative relationships between drug plasma concentrations, elimination pathways, the extent of renal impairment and dosage regimen modifications. This chapter examines these latter considerations with the goal of enhancing pharmacy input into drug therapy through a greater appreciation of the principles associated with modifying dosage regimens.

## General Principles

The reader is referred to the reviews of Wagner[12] and Dettli[15,16] for a more extensive treatment of some of these principles. Most drugs are cleared from the plasma by both renal and nonrenal mechanisms, although a few drugs are removed essentially by only one of these processes. These mechanisms contribute to the overall elimination rate constant as follows (see appendix for explanation of symbols):

one compartment open model: $K = k_{nr} + k_r$ \qquad (1)

two compartment open model: $\beta = k_{nr} + k_r$ \qquad (2)

Since the rate constant for excretion of unchanged drug ($k_r$) is related to the creatinine clearance, which is an easily measured clinical laboratory parameter, by a proportionality constant (a) that is a function of the ratio of the renal clearances of drug to creatinine ($Cl_d/Cl_{cr}$),

$$k_r = (a)(Cl_{cr}) \qquad (3)$$

the overall elimination rate constant is expressed in terms of the creatinine clearance as follows,

$$K = k_{nr} + (a)(Cl_{cr}) \qquad (4)$$

The recognition by the clinician of the relationship described in Equation 4 is particularly fortuitous because it indicates that a plot of K vs. $Cl_{cr}$ will be a straight line with an intercept for anuric patients ($Cl_{cr} = 0$) representing the nonrenal elimination rate constant ($k_{nr}$), as shown in Figure 1. It is the awareness of this linearity between K and $Cl_{cr}$ that leads to the potential for greater utilization of clinical data for estimating modifications in dosage regimens. By plotting existing and future literature data as shown in Figure 1, and fitting a least-squares line through the data points, it is possible to predict an elimination rate constant ($K_{ri}$) for patients with any degree of renal impairment ($Cl_{cr} < 100$ ml/min). Since no such linearity exists between the half-life ($t_{1/2}$) and creatinine clearance, all equations and data will be presented here in terms of the overall elimination rate constant. The conversion of half-life data to K data is accomplished by using Equation 5.

$$K = 0.693/t_{1/2} \qquad (5)$$

There are two common methods used for modifying dosage regimens for patients with renal impairment:

1. Method of average plasma concentration ($C^\infty av_n = C^\infty av_{ri}$)
   a. Maintaining dose but prolonging dosage interval
   b. Maintaining dosage interval but decreasing dose
   c. Decreasing dose plus prolonging dosage interval
2. Method of maximum plasma concentration ($C^\infty max_n = C^\infty max_{ri}$)
   a. Maintaining dose but prolonging dosage interval
   b. Maintaining dosage interval but decreasing dose

To employ the method of average plasma concentration, in which the goal is to maintain the average steady-state plasma level during the dosage interval for the patient in normal and impaired renal function, Equation 6 of Wagner et al.[19] is employed:

$$C_{av}^\infty = \frac{fD}{VK\tau} = \left(\frac{f}{V}\right)\left(\frac{D}{K\tau}\right) \qquad (6)$$

In order to maintain the goal of $C^\infty av_n = C^\infty av_{ri}$, making the fair assumption that f and V remain constant for each dose of a multiple dose regimen,

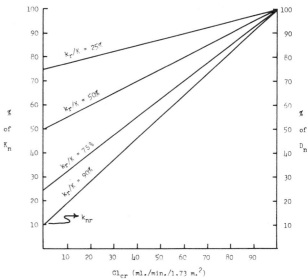

Figure 1. Determination of overall elimination rate constant or dose as a function of creatinine clearance

$$\left[\frac{D}{K\tau}\right]_n = \left[\frac{D}{K\tau}\right]_{ri} \qquad (7)$$

Maintaining $D_n = D_{ri}$, and rearranging Equation 7, results in Equation 8,

$$\frac{\tau_n}{\tau_{ri}} = \frac{K_{ri}}{K_n} \quad \text{(when } D_n = D_{ri} \text{ and } Cav_n^\infty = Cav_{ri}^\infty) \qquad (8)$$

Maintaining $\tau_n = \tau_{ri}$, and rearranging Equation 7, leads to Equation 9,

$$\frac{D_{ri}}{D_n} = \frac{K_{ri}}{K_n} \quad \text{(when } \tau_n = \tau_{ri} \text{ and } Cav_n^\infty = Cav_{ri}^\infty) \qquad (9)$$

Altering both dose and dosage interval, while rearranging Equation 7, produces Equation 10,

$$\frac{D_{ri}\tau_n}{D_n\tau_{ri}} = \frac{K_{ri}}{K_n} \quad \text{(when } Cav_n^\infty = Cav_{ri}^\infty) \qquad (10)$$

Equations 8–10 suggest that the goal of maintaining an average plasma concentration is achieved by altering the dose, dosage interval, or both, by the ratio $K_{ri}/K_n$, while keeping the appropriate variables constant. The use of Equation 8, in which the normal dose is used at a prolonged dosage interval, results in a greater difference between maximum and minimum plasma concentrations during the dosage interval ($C^\infty max - C^\infty min$) than the use of Equation 9, in which a reduced dose is employed at the normal dosage interval. The significance of this observation in therapy depends on the minimum and maximum concentrations in plasma that are appropriate for a given drug. Equation 10 is employed when the modifications achieved with Equations 8 and 9 yield awkward dosage intervals or doses, respectively; using Equation 10 allows the clinician to balance off a reduced dose and prolonged interval until reasonable and practical values are achieved.

To employ the method of maximum plasma concentration, in which the goal is to replace enough dose per dosage interval to reestablish the same maximum plasma concentration for the patient in normal and impaired renal function, Equation 11 is employed, assuming that a one-compartment model is adequate to describe the multiple dose kinetics. Although the equation is exact for intravenous administration, it represents a reasonable approximation for the renal impaired patient using oral therapy.

$$D_\tau = D_0 \cdot 10^{-0.43K\tau} \qquad (11)$$

Based on Equation 11, the dose (D) to be replaced at the beginning of each dosage interval is calculated using Equation 12.

$$D = D_0 - D_\tau \qquad (12)$$

In order to maintain the goal of $C^\infty max_n = C^\infty max_{ri}$, without altering the replacement dose in normal or renal impaired status ($D_n = D_{ri}$), it can be shown using Equations 11 and 12 that the prolongation of the normal dosage interval is calculated using Equation 8.

Alternately, to maintain the normal dosage interval ($\tau_n = \tau_{ri}$), while reducing the dose, Equation 13 is employed.

$$\frac{D_{ri}}{D_n} = \frac{1 - 10^{-0.43K_{ri}\tau}}{1 - 10^{-0.43K_n\tau}} \qquad (13)$$

$$(\text{when } \tau_n = \tau_{ri} \text{ and } \overset{\infty}{C}max_n = \overset{\infty}{C}max_{ri})$$

As before, fluctuations in plasma concentration during the dosage interval are less when using Equation 13 than Equation 8, because prolonging the dosage interval always increases the fluctuation.

In order for clinicians to employ Equations 8, 9, 10 and 13, it is first necessary to cast data from clinical studies in the form of Figure 1, using a least-squares regression line. Then, using the patient's creatinine clearance as an index of kidney function ($k_r$) specifically and drug clearance from the plasma in general, as indicated in Equation 4, a vertical line is drawn to the regression line followed by a horizontal line to the K axis, to estimate $K_{ri}$ for the patient. After determining $K_n$ in the same manner ($Cl_{cr} = 100$ ml/min), Equations 8, 9, 10 and 13 are used as appropriate to meet the goals of the clinician.

Some practitioners prefer to estimate renal status by using serum creatinine ($Cr_s$) measurements because of the greater ease of obtaining this value as compared to creatinine clearance. Since the use of creatinine clearance leads to a better graphical presentation of data, and the accuracy of estimating K data at low creatinine clearance values is much greater than K data at corresponding high serum creatinine values, it is best to express $Cr_s$ data in terms of $Cl_{cr}$. To effect this conversion, the older equations of Jelliffe[20] have been frequently used but they are least accurate at high $Cr_s$ values in which dosage adjustments are most critical. As a practical guide for patients aged 25–50 years and weighing 60–80 kg, the clinician is more accurate at the critical high $Cr_s$ values by using the rough approximation that $Cl_{cr}$ is related to the reciprocal of $Cr_s$ in a linear fashion.[21]

$$Cl_{cr}(\text{ml/min}) = \frac{100}{Cr_s(\text{mg}/100 \text{ ml})} \qquad (14)$$

Since the relationship between these two parameters is truly not linear, however, the most accurate method of conversion employs a mathematical assessment of the patient's creatinine output ($Cl_{cr}$ = creatinine output/$Cr_s$) which is a function of sex, age, and weight. Rapid and accurate methods for converting serum creatinine to creatinine clearance data, using an estimate of creatinine output, have now been developed.[22,23]

Finally, the reader is referred to the variety of shorthand procedures that have been developed by some practitioners, with varying degrees of accuracy and flexibility, as a rapid guide to modifying dosage regimens.[24-27] Examples of the technique outlined in this chapter are also available.[12,28-30]

## Relationships between Plasma Concentration, Metabolism, Renal Status and Dosage Regimen

An examination of Equations 8, 9, 10 and 13 suggests that any impairment of renal function ($K_{ri} < K_n$) should result in a modification of the normal drug dosage regimen. It is reasonable to question, however, under what conditions is it really necessary to make alterations in the regimen. To address this question, some of the variables that influence the results achieved by employing the above equations have been evaluated below.

As mentioned previously, Figure 1 has been constructed by employing Equation 4. It is apparent from this equation that the overall elimination rate constant (K) is an additive function of the excretion ($k_r$) and nonrenal ($k_{nr}$) elimination rate constants. Drugs that rely on excretion of unchanged drug ($k_r$) more than on nonrenal mechanisms ($k_{nr}$) such as metabolism, fecal excretion, etc., for overall elimination are more dependent on healthy kidney function than those drugs utilizing nonrenal elimination as the major clearance mechanism. To evaluate the influence of varying dependence on renal and nonrenal elimination patterns, Figure 1 has been constructed for prototype drugs whose ratios of renal/nonrenal elimination are 90%/10%, 75%/25%, 50%/50% and 25%/75%.

The following assumptions are observed in evaluating the data:

1. Declining renal status does not result in a compensatory alteration in the nonrenal elimination mechanism for the drug; $k_{nr}$ remains constant as the patient's $Cl_{cr}$ decreases.
2. Declining renal status does not result in a change in the steady-state volume of distribution of the drug in the body; $V_{ss}$ remains constant as the patient's $Cl_{cr}$ decreases.
3. Declining renal status does not result in a change in other factors normally contributing to the plasma concentration of the drug such as the fraction of drug absorbed (f), enterohepatic recycling, tubular secretion, and tubular reabsorption.
4. Metabolism of the drug results in the formation of inactive or only very weakly active by-products.
5. The pharmacological response of the drug is a function of the plasma concentration.

To construct Figure 1, a creatinine clearance of 100 ml/min was taken to represent normal kidney function and was associated with a normal overall elimination rate constant ($K_n$). A creatinine clearance less than 100 ml/min was then taken as an indication of an impaired overall elimination rate constant ($K_{ri}$). Alternately, the creatinine clearance value in Figure 1 can be viewed as a percentage of normal renal function (e.g., $Cl_{cr}$ of 50 ml/min represents 50% of normal renal function). The $K_{ri}$ values obtained at various $Cl_{cr}$ values from Figure 1 were then used in Equations 8, 9 and 13 to assess the influence of impaired renal function on dosage regimens.

Equation 9 was used to calculate the data shown in Table 1 and depicted in Figure 1. Since the percent decrease in normal dose for the renal impaired patient ($D_{ri}/D_n \times 100$) is directly proportional to the percent decrease in normal overall elimination rate constant ($K_{ri}/K_n \times 100$), as shown in Equation 9, Figure 1 can be used to relate either $D_{ri}$ or $K_{ri}$ to $Cl_{cr}$. To arrive at the data in Table 1 and Figure 1, the normal dosage interval and the normal average steady-state plasma concentra-

tion were maintained for the renal impaired patient ($\tau_n = \tau_{ri}$ and $C^\infty av_n = C^\infty av_{ri}$), as required by Equation 9. As expected, the data in Table 1 support the expectation that for a given degree of renal impairment, the need to reduce the dose is greatest for drugs exhibiting the greater dependence on excretion ($k_r$) as an elimination pathway; the more important metabolism or other nonrenal means of elimination is for a drug, the less the need for decreasing the dose in renal impairment. As shown in Table 1 for example, in patients with severe renal impairment ($Cl_{cr} \leq 10$ ml/min, or $Cr_s \geq 10$ mg/100 ml) the dose is reduced to 77%, 55%, 32% and 19% of the normal dose when excretion constitutes 25%, 50%, 75% and 90%, respectively, of the overall elimination process. The serum creatinine values were obtained from the creatinine clearance values by using Equation 14, although, as stated previously, these estimations of $Cr_s$ represent only an approximation for illustrative purposes since a more accurate assessment must account for patient variables such as age, weight and sex.

Although a reduction in dose for renal impaired patients while maintaining the normal dosage interval results in smaller plasma concentration fluctuations than prolonging the dosage interval while maintaining the normal dose, the awkward doses calculated by using the former method may sometimes represent a greater burden to the nursing staff than the use of the latter method. Since most tabular presentations of dosage regimen modifications have emphasized the latter method, Equation 8 was used to calculate the data shown in Table 2 and Figure 2. Once again, analogous to the data in Table 1, the data support the expectation that for a given degree of renal impairment, the need to prolong the dosage interval is greatest for drugs exhibiting the greater dependence on excretion of unmetabolized drug as an elimination pathway. For example, in patients with severe renal impairment, the dosage interval is prolonged 129%, 182%, 308% and 526% of the normal dosage interval when excretion constitutes 25%, 50%, 75% and 90%, respectively, of the overall elimination process.

Since the use of Equations 8 and 9 to generate the data in Tables 1 and 2 presupposes the goal of maintaining the same average steady-state plasma concentration in the patient during normal and impaired renal function ($C^\infty av_n = C^\infty av_{ri}$), it is appropriate to inquire into the fate of $C^\infty av$ if no modifications in dosage regimen follow a decline in renal function. Rewriting Equation 6 as,

$$C\overset{\infty}{a}v \ K \ = \ \frac{fD}{V\tau} \qquad (15)$$

and assuming no change in fD, V and $\tau$ values for normal and renal impaired status, then,

$$\frac{C\overset{\infty}{a}v_n}{C\overset{\infty}{a}v_{ri}} \ = \ \frac{K_{ri}}{K_n} \ (\text{when } D_n \ = \ D_{ri} \text{ and } \tau_n \ = \ \tau_{ri}) \qquad (16)$$

#### Table 1. Percent of Normal Dose in Relation to Renal Function[a]

| $k_r/K$[b] | CREATININE CLEARANCE (ml/min) | | | |
| | 50 | 25 | 10 | 0 |
| | or SERUM CREATININE (mg/100 ml)[c] | | | |
| | 2 | 4 | 10 | ∞ |
|---|---|---|---|---|
| 25% | 87%[a] | 81% | 77% | 75% |
| 50% | 75% | 62% | 55% | 50% |
| 75% | 62% | 44% | 32% | 25% |
| 90% | 55% | 32% | 19% | 10% |

[a] Expressed as percent of normal dose used in patients with normal renal function ($Cl_{cr}$ = 100 ml/min), when the normal dosage interval is maintained, as obtained by Figure 1 and Equation 9.
[b] Expressed as percent of overall elimination rate constant contributed by rate constant for excretion of unmetabolized drug; this approximates the percent of drug excreted by the kidney in unmetabolized form.
[c] Estimated by using Equation 14.

## Table 2. Percent of Normal Dosage Interval or Percent of Normal Average Plasma Concentration in Relation to Renal Function[a]

| | CREATININE CLEARANCE (ml/min) | | | |
| | 50 | 25 | 10 | 0 |
| | or | | | |
| | SERUM CREATININE (mg/100 ml)[c] | | | |
| $k_r/K$[b] | 2 | 4 | 10 | $\infty$ |
|---|---|---|---|---|
| 25% | 114%[a] | 123% | 129% | 133% |
| 50% | 133% | 160% | 182% | 200% |
| 75% | 160% | 233% | 308% | 400% |
| 90% | 182% | 308% | 526% | 1000% |

[a] Expressed as percent of normal dosage interval used in patients with normal renal function ($Cl_{cr}$ = 100 ml/min), when the normal dose is maintained, as obtained by Figures 1 and 2 and Equation 8. Alternately, expressed as percent of normal average plasma concentration ($C^\infty av_n$) when the normal dose and the normal dosage interval are maintained, as obtained by Figures 1 and 2 and Equation 16.
[b] Expressed as percent of overall elimination rate constant contributed by rate constant for excretion of unmetabolized drug; this approximates percent of drug excreted by the kidney in unmetabolized form.
[c] Estimated by using Equation 14.

A perusal of Equations 16 and 8 suggests that changes in $C^\infty av$ with impaired renal function will be the same as the alterations in the dosage interval when the appropriate variables required of the two equations are held constant. For this reason, the data in Table 2 and Figure 2 may also be used to evaluate elevations in $C^\infty av_n$ when dosage regimen modifications are not observed. Again, as expected, the increase in $C^\infty av$ for a given degree of renal impairment will be greatest for drugs exhibiting the greater dependence on excretion of unmetabolized drug when no alteration in dose or dosage interval is effected.

*Figure 2. Determination of average plasma concentration or dosage interval as a function of creatinine clearance*

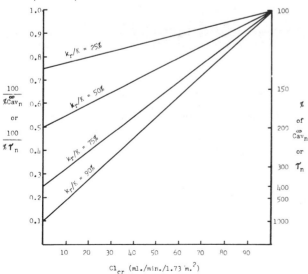

The data in Tables 1 and 2 are summarized in Tables 3 and 4. As examples of use of these tables, no modifications of dosage regimens are generally anticipated for drugs excreted up to 25% in unmetabolized form, even in anuric patients; for drugs excreted 50% in unmetabolized form, it should generally not be necessary to halve the normal dosage or double the normal dosage interval until kidney function ceases; for drugs excreted 75% and 90%, it should generally not be necessary to reduce the normal dosage to 1/3 or triple the normal dosage interval until kidney status declines to 1/10 and 1/4 of normal, respectively. Practical applications of these general principles may be observed by consulting any of the various tables in the literature for dosage regimens.[1,3,4,7,9]

It is also possible to compile data similar to Tables 1–4 by using Equations 8 and 13 when the goal of the clinician is to replace enough dose per dosage interval to reestablish the same maximum plasma concentration for the patient in normal and impaired renal function. Space limitations and the realization of trends similar to those presented in Tables 1–4 limit the presentation of the data, however.

It is important to recognize the potential limitations inherent in some of the assumptions asserted above to develop the data in Tables 1–4. Although it was assumed that there was no compensatory alteration in the nonrenal elimination rate constant for drugs during renal impairment, examples of such a compensatory mechanism have been reported.[5,31] Although it was assumed that there was no decrease in the steady-state volume of distribution ($V_{ss}$), which is the most important of the vol-

## Table 3. Relationship of Creatinine Clearance to Dosage Regimen Modifications[a]

| | $2 \times C^\infty av_n$[b] | $3 \times C^\infty av_n$ | $4 \times C^\infty av_n$ | $5 \times C^\infty av_n$ |
| | or | | | |
| | $2 \times \tau_n$[c] | $3 \times \tau_n$ | $4 \times \tau_n$ | $5 \times \tau_n$ |
| | or | | | |
| $k_r/K$[e] | $1/2 \times D_n$[d] | $1/3 \times D_n$ | $1/4 \times D_n$ | $1/5 \times D_n$ |
|---|---|---|---|---|
| 25% | — | — | — | — |
| 50% | 0[a] | — | — | — |
| 75% | 33 | 10 | — | — |
| 90% | 44 | 25 | 17 | 11 |

[a] Expressed as creatinine clearance value at which column heading occurs (see b, c and d below).
[b] Expressed as proportional increase in normal average plasma concentration, when the normal dose and dosage interval are maintained, as obtained by Figures 1 and 2 and Equation 16.
[c] Expressed as proportional increase in normal dosage interval, when the normal dose is maintained, as obtained by Figures 1 and 2 and Equation 8.
[d] Expressed as proportional decrease in normal dose, when the normal dosage interval is maintained, as obtained by Figure 1 and Equation 9.
[e] Expressed as percent of overall elimination rate constant contributed by rate constant for excretion of unmetabolized drug; this approximates percent of drug excreted by the kidney in unmetabolized form.

**Table 4. Relationship of Serum Creatinine to Dosage Regimen Modifications[a]**

| $k_r/K^e$ | $2 \times C^\infty \, av_n^b$ or $2 \times \tau_n^c$ or $1/2 \times D_n^d$ | $3 \times C^\infty \, av_n$ $3 \times \tau_n$ $1/3 \times D_n$ | $4 \times C^\infty \, av_n$ $4 \times \tau_n$ $1/4 \times D_n$ | $5 \times C^\infty \, av_n$ $5 \times \tau_n$ $1/5 \times D_n$ |
|---|---|---|---|---|
| 25% | — | — | — | — |
| 50% | ∞ | — | — | — |
| 75% | 3.0[a] | 10.0 | — | — |
| 90% | 2.3 | 4.0 | 5.9 | 9.1 |

[a] Expressed as serum creatinine value at which column heading occurs (see b,c and d below). Values estimated from creatinine clearance values by using Equation 14.
[b] Expressed as proportional increase in normal average plasma concentration, when the normal dose and dosage interval are maintained, as obtained by Figure 1 and Equation 16.
[c] Expressed as proportional increase in normal dosage interval, when the normal dose is maintained, as obtained by Figure 1 and Equation 8.
[d] Expressed as proportional decrease in normal dose, when the normal dosage interval is maintained, as obtained by Figure 1 and Equation 9.
[e] Expressed as percent of overall elimination rate constant contributed by rate constant for excretion of unmetabolized drug; this approximates percent of drug excreted by the kidney in unmetabolized form.

ume terms in relating the average plasma concentration to the average amount of drug in the body during multiple dosing at the steady-state,[32,33] an example of a significant decrease in $V_{ss}$ has been reported for digoxin.[34] The practical consequence of assuming no change in $V_{ss}$ when it indeed has decreased during renal impairment would be the estimation of a larger modified dose ($D_{ri}$) than is actually needed. Lastly, it is possible that the assumption that no changes occur during renal impairment to other factors contributing to the plasma concentration of the drug may be invalid for a few drugs.

## Conclusions

The data in Tables 1–4 draw fundamental relationships between the plasma concentrations of drugs, their elimination pathways, their dosage regimens and renal status. Despite the reservations and cautions inherent in the various assumptions used to derive the data, general patterns relating to the modification of dosage regimens during renal impairment are clearly evident. In Tables 3 and 4, for instance, it is apparent that the need to modify dosage regimens is not just an inherent consequence of renal impairment but is also a function of the proportional increase in plasma concentration of drugs that can be tolerated by patients. Within the assumptions and limitations of the data, it appears that alterations in dosage regimens are rarely of consequence for drugs eliminated up to 25% by excretion; drugs eliminated up to approximately 50% by excretion will not generally

reach a two-fold elevation in the normal average plasma concentration until the patient is anuric; even drugs greatly dependent on elimination by excretion ($k_r/K_n$ = 90%) will not usually double in normal average plasma concentration until the patient's renal status declines to less than 50% of normal. Other fundamental relationships are apparent: It is generally not necessary, within the assumptions and limitations of the data, to even consider reducing the normal dose or prolonging the normal dosage interval for drugs eliminated up to 25% by excretion, or for drugs excreted 50% until renal function is abolished, or for drugs excreted 75% until renal function is reduced to one-third of normal, or for drugs excreted 90% until renal status declines to less than one-half of normal.

These and other patterns suggest a challenge for the clinically oriented pharmacist: A greater attention to, and appreciation of, the mechanisms by which drugs are eliminated by the body will result in a more intuitive grasp of dosage regimen theory, better guidelines for modifying dosage regimens during renal impairment, and greater input into the drug therapy of patients.

### References

1. Bennett, W. M., Singer, I. and Coggins, C. H.: Guide to Drug Usage in Adult Patients with Impaired Renal Function: A Supplement, *JAMA 223*:991, 1973.
2. Bailey, G. L.: Hemodialysis: Principles and Practice, Academic Press, New York, New York, 1972.
3. Kunin, C. M.: Antibiotic Usage in Patients with Renal Impairment, *Hosp. Pract.* 7:141, 1972.
4. Hatch, S. E., Johnson, J. G. and Lee, S.: A Guide to Drug Therapy in Renal Failure, *Res. Staff Phys.* 18:31 (June) 1972.
5. Reidenberg, M. M.: Renal Function and Drug Action, W. B. Saunders Co., Philadelphia, Pennsylvania, 1971.
6. O'Grady, F.: Antibiotics in Renal Failure, *Brit. Med. Bull.* 27:142, 1971.
7. Bennett, W. M., Singer, I. and Coggins, C. H.: A Practical Guide to Drug Usage in Adult Patients with Impaired Renal Function, *JAMA 214*:1468, 1970.
8. Bulger, R. J. and Petersdorf, R. G.: Antimicrobial Therapy in Patients with Renal Insufficiency, *Postgrad. Med.* 47:160, 1970.
9. Mirkin, B. L.: Drug Therapy in Patients with Impaired Renal Function, *Postgrad. Med.* 47:159, 1970.
10. Kunin, C. M.: A Guide to Use of Antibiotics in Patients with Renal Disease, *Ann. Internal Med.* 67:151, 1967.
11. Giusti, D. L.: A Review of the Clinical Use of Antimicrobial Agents in Patients with Renal and Hepatic Insufficiency, I. The Penicillins, *Drug Intel. Clin. Pharm.* 7:62, 1973.
12. Wagner, J. G.: Theory and Practice of Adjusting Dosage of Drugs on the Basis of Endogenous Creatinine Clearance or Serum Creatinine Conentration, *In* Biopharmaceutics and Relevant Pharmacokinetics, Drug Intelligence Publications, Hamilton, Illinois, 1971, ch. 28.
13. Mayersohn, M.: Dosage Regimen Calculations in Patients with Renal Insufficiency, *Can. J. Hosp. Pharm.* 24:215, 1971.
14. Kunin, C. M. and Finland, M.: Restrictions Imposed on Antibiotic Therapy by Renal Failure, *Arch. Internal Med.* 104:1030, 1959.
15. Dettli, L., Spring, P. and Ryter, S.: Multiple Dose Kinetics and Drug Dosage in Patients with Kidney Disease, *Acta Pharmacol. Toxicol.* 29 (*suppl.*):211, 1971.
16. Dettli, L.: Multiple Dose Elimination Kinetics and Drug Accumulation in Patients with Normal and with Impaired Kid-

ney Function, *In* G. Raspé (ed.) : Advances in Biosciences-5, Pergamon Press, London, England, 1970, pp. 39-54.

17. Jelliffe, R. W.: New Developments in Drug Dosage Regimens, *J. Mondial Pharmacie 15*:53, 1972.

18. Jelliffe, R. W.: An Improved Method of Digoxin Therapy, *Ann. Internal Med. 69*:703, 1968.

19. Wagner, J. G. et al.: Blood Levels of Drug at the Equilibrium State After Multiple Dosing, *Nature 207*:1301, 1965.

20. Jelliffe, R. W.: Estimation of Creatinine Clearance When Urine Cannot be Collected—An Aid to Adjusting Dosage to Impaired Renal Function, *Lancet 1*:975, 1971.

21. Kassirer, J. P.: Clinical Evaluation of Kidney Function-Glomerular Function, *N. Engl. J. Med. 285*:385, 1971.

22. Siersback-Nielson, K. et al.: Rapid Evaluation of Creatinine Clearance, *Lancet 1*:1133, 1971.

23. Jelliffe, R. W. and Jelliffe, S. M.: A Computer Program for Estimation of Creatinine from Unstable Serum Creatinine Levels, Age, Sex, and Weight, *Math. Biosc. 14*:17, 1972.

24. Gingell, J. C. and Waterworth, P. M.: Dose of Gentamicin in Patients with Normal Renal Function and Renal Impairment, *Brit. Med. J. 2*:19, 1968.

25. Jelliffe, R. W.: Administration of Digoxin, *Dis. Chest 56*:56, 1969.

26. Cutler, R. E. and Orme, B. M.: Correlation of Serum Creatinine Concentration and Kanamycin Half-Life, *JAMA 209*:539, 1969.

27. McHenry, M. C. et al.: Gentamicin Dosages for Renal Insufficiency, *Ann. Internal Med. 74*:192, 1971.

28. Dettli, L., Spring P. and Habersang, R.: Drug Dosage in Patients with Impaired Renal Function, *Postgrad. Med. J. 46* (suppl.):32, 1970.

29. Chan, R. A., Benner, E. J. and Hoeprich, P. D.: Gentamicin Therapy in Renal Failure: A Nomogram for Dosage, *Ann. Internal Med. 76*:773, 1972.

30. Bechtol, L. D.: Therapy with Cephaloridine in Renal Impairment, *Curr. Therap. Res. 14*:790, 1972.

31. Letteri, J. M. et al.: Diphenylhydantoin Metabolism in Uremia, *N. Engl. J. Med. 285*:648, 1971.

32. Perrier, D. and Gibaldi, M.: Relationship Between Plasma or Serum Drug Concentration and Amount of Drug in the Body at Steady State Upon Multiple Dosing, *J. Pharmacokin. Biopharm. 1*:17, 1973.

33. Jusko, W. J. and Gibaldi, M.: Effects of Change in Elimination on Various Parameters of the Two-Compartment Open Model, *J. Pharm. Sci. 61*:1270, 1972.

34. Reuning, R. H., Sams, R. A. and Notari, R. E.: Role of Pharmacokinetics in Drug Dosage Adjustment, I. Pharmacologic Effect Kinetics and Apparent Volume of Distribution of Digoxin, *J. Clin. Pharmacol. 13*:127, 1973.

## Appendix of Symbols

| | |
|---|---|
| $K$ | Apparent first order rate constant for overall elimination of drug by the body using a one-compartment open model. |
| $K_n$ and $K_{ri}$ | Apparent K value for patients with normal and impaired renal function, respectively. |
| $k_r$ | Apparent first order rate constant for renal excretion of unmetabolized drug. |
| $k_{nr}$ | Sum of apparent first order rate constants for nonrenal elimination of drug. |
| $\beta$ | Apparent first order rate constant for overall elimination of drug by the body using a two-compartment open model. |
| $\tau_n$ and $\tau_{ri}$ | Dosage interval for patients with normal and impaired renal function, respectively. |
| $D_n$ and $D_{ri}$ | Dose for patients with normal and impaired renal function, respectively. |
| $D_o$ and $D_\tau$ | Amount of drug in the body, expressed in terms of dose, at the beginning and end of the dosage interval, respectively. |
| $C^\infty av_n$ and $C^\infty av_{ri}$ | Average concentration of drug in the plasma of patients with normal and impaired renal function, respectively, during the dosage interval once the steady-state (equilibrium) has been achieved. |
| $C^\infty_{max}$ and $C^\infty_{min}$ | Maximum and minimum concentrations of drug in the plasma of patients, respectively, during the dosage interval once the steady-state (equilibrium) has been achieved. |
| $V$ | Apparent volume of distribution of drug in the body. |
| $V_{ss}$ | Apparent volume of distribution of drug in the body as measured at the instant that the rate of change of the amount of drug in the tissue compartment is zero for the two-compartment open model. |
| $Cl_{cr}$ and $Cl_d$ | Renal clearance of creatinine and drug, respectively. |
| $a$ | Ratio of renal clearance of drug to renal clearance of creatinine $(Cl_d/Cl_{cr})$. |
| $Cr_s$ | Serum or plasma concentration of creatinine. |
| $t_{1/2}$ | Half-life for loss of drug from plasma. |
| $f$ | Fraction of dose which is absorbed. |

# 46 Practical Pharmacokinetic Techniques for Drug Consultation and Evaluation III: Psychotherapeutic Drugs as Prototypes for Illustrating Some Considerations in Pharmacist-generated Dosage Regimens

G. E. Schumacher and J. Weiner

Two practical techniques for evaluating and developing dosage regimens are discussed, and four prototype psychotherapeutic drugs are used to illustrate applications and restrictions of these techniques as they relate to reassessing published clinical data and traditional dosage regimens.

The two techniques used for estimating dosage regimens are the average plasma concentration method and the superposition method. In addition, the half-life method is discussed.

Lithium illustrates the relative simplicity in predicting dosage regimens for drugs cleared from the body almost exclusively by excretion. The use of nortriptyline data illustrates the potential for using the methods for estimating regimens to suggest modified dosage regimens worthy of clinical trial. The use of diazepam data shows some of the dangers in estimating regimens when plasma concentration versus therapeutic response data are vague and when a marked variation in interstudy pharmacokinetic parameters exists. Chlorpromazine is an example of drugs for which the prediction of dosage regimens is highly speculative because of poor correlation between drug plasma concentration and pharmacologic response.

The literature suggests an increasing involvement of pharmacists in monitoring, evaluating and developing drug dosage regimens.[1-8] Although initial interest has been directed toward antibiotics, cardiac glycosides and antiarrhythmics, the psychotherapeutic drugs represent a therapeutic category that can serve as a prototype for illustrating some techniques and limitations in developing pharmacist-generated dosage regimens. With this observation in mind, an ongoing study has been initiated to reassess the dosage regimens for psychotherapeutic drugs by using therapeutic response and pharmacokinetic data gleaned from the clinical literature. Study goals are to (1) examine the practicality of using published clinical data to reassess, and modify where appropriate, psychotherapeutic drug dosage regimens (2) evaluate the ability of the pharmacist to interpret the literature and develop the regimens; (3) use the modified regimens to initiate clinical studies evaluating the impact of the new schedules on drug side effects, costs and patient compliance with prescribed regimens; and (4) use these drugs as examples of the techniques, cautions and limitations observed in evaluating and developing dosage regimens in general.

Goal (4) is the subject of this chapter. Two practical techniques for evaluating and developing dosage regimens are discussed, and four prototype psychotherapeutic drugs are used to illustrate applications and restrictions of these techniques as they relate to reassessing published clinical data and traditional dosage regimens.

A few general papers on the pharmacokinetic and

pharmacologic properties of the psychotherapeutic drugs have been published.[9-12] Any attempt to evaluate and develop dosage regimens for these drugs, as for most other therapeutic categories, requires an appreciation of the interrelationship between the pharmacokinetic and pharmacologic response factors depicted in Figure 1. As suggested by this schematic representation, in order for the pharmacist to assess and predict dosage regimens on the basis of plasma concentration versus pharmacological response data, it is necessary to assume that there is a direct and predictable relationship between dose and plasma concentration as well as between plasma concentration and response. Substantial interpatient variation in absorption (pathway 1), poor correlation between plasma concentration and response (pathway 2) and biotransformation of the drug to pharmacologically active metabolites (pathways 4 and 5) seriously compromise the ability of the pharmacist to assess and predict dosage regimens without benefit of specific additional clinical trials designed to evaluate the significance of these complications.

The clinical and pharmacological literature on four prototype psychotherapeutic drugs, lithium, nortriptyline, diazepam and chlorpromazine, was evaluated. These drugs represent therapeutic as well as pharmacokinetic prototypes; they differ in (1) their therapeutic applications and in (2) their pharmacokinetic and predictability of therapeutic response profiles.

1. Lithium,[13-20] an antimanic drug, illustrates the *relative* simplicity in predicting dosage regimens for drug cleared from the body almost exclusively by excretion (included in pathway 3). Pathway 1 is not a significant problem because the drug is almost completely absorbed from tablets and capsules, and interpatient variation in absorption is not great. The drug is not metabolized (pathway 4) so this presents no complications. Interpatient variation in elimination (pathway 3) is marked but not nearly as great as the variation attending drugs that are metabolized as well as excreted. Lastly, there is a good correlation between drug plasma concentration and pharmacological response (pathway 2). Thus the important variables are pathways 1, 2 and 3.
2. Nortriptyline,[21-31] an antidepressant drug, is representative of the potential problems associated with predicting dosage regimens for drugs cleared from the body primarily by metabolism. Interpatient variation in elimination patterns for drugs cleared partially or completely by metabolism is generally much greater than that observed for drugs cleared primarily by excretion because metabolism is often under genetic control, enzyme production varies markedly among individuals and other drugs may stimulate or inhibit synthesis of the metabolizing enzymes. Furthermore, enzyme saturation may occur with increases in dose resulting in an alteration in elimination profiles. Fortunately, nortriptyline metabolites are very weak or inactive so that pathway 5 is not a consideration. Drug absorption from solid dosage forms is good and interpatient variation is not excessive. There is a reasonable correlation between plasma concentration and response. The clinical literature suggests that the important variables, pathways 1, 2, 4 and 6, do yield to reasonable predictions of dosage regimens.
3. Diazepam,[32-38] an antianxiety drug, demonstrates the cautions associated with predicting dosage regimens for drugs that generate pharmacologically active metabolites (pathways 4 and 5). Furthermore, neither the comparative activity of diazepam and its metabolites nor the relationship between the plasma concentration range and desired therapeutic responses is well defined; although pathway 2 appears to be operative, the concentration vs. therapeutic response profile has not been clarified in the literature. Fortunately, drug absorption from solid dosage forms is optimum and interpatient variation is not marked. Thus, the important variables are pathways 1-6.
4. Chlorpromazine,[39-44] an antipsychotic drug, is an example of drugs for which the prediction of dosage regimens is highly speculative due to the poor correlation between drug plasma concentration and pharmacologic response (pathway 2). Since pathway 2 is a precept for developing dosage regimens based on drug plasma concentrations, the potential for reassessing regimens for these types of drugs is limited.

It is important to point out that the accuracy of estimation of most dosage regimens based on drug plasma concentration as a reference is a function of the degree of interpatient variation in (1) pathway 1, drug absorption; (2) pathways 3 and 4, drug clearance from the plasma; and (3) the volume of distribution of the drug. The latter parameter is not indicated in Figure 1, but drug diffusion out of the plasma and into other extracellular fluids, intracellular fluids and tissues is a variable in patients. Therefore, the four drugs used in this study are all subject to variation in these parameters but, in addition, nortriptyline, diazepam and chlorpromazine exhibit complications in other pathways depicted in Figure 1, as noted above.

**Techniques for Estimating Dosage Regimens**

There are three general methods available to practitioners for estimating dosage regimens:

1. Half-life method
2. Average plasma concentration method
3. Superposition method.

In using the half-life method, the practitioner applies the pharmacokinetic observation that when a drug is dosed on its half-life ($\tau = t_{1/2}$) the plasma concentration accumulates until the maximum and minimum plasma concentrations of drug at the steady state ($C_{max}^{\infty}$ and $C_{min}^{\infty}$) are approximately twice as great as the respective concentrations ($C_{pk}$ and $C_{\tau}$) achieved after a single dose of the drug; in other words, $C_{max}^{\infty}/C_{pk}$ and $C_{min}^{\infty}/C_{\tau}$

*Figure 1. Schematic representation of selected factors influencing plasma concentration of drugs and pharmacologic effects*

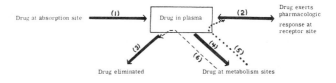

are expected to be roughly 2. This is observed in Figure 2 for a hypothetical drug dosed on its half-life. Given the plasma concentration versus time profile for a single dose of drug and an approximation of the drug's half-life, the practitioner can estimate the maximum and minimum steady-state plasma concentrations when the drug is administered at a dosage interval approximating the half-life. In terms of a dosage regimen, if the plasma concentration versus time profile for a single dose appears to yield an appropriate pharmacologic/therapeutic response over the chosen dosage interval, then the single dose represents the loading dose ($D_l$) and one-half of the loading dose is administered as a maintenance dose ($D_m$) at a dosage interval of every half-life. Alternately, if the plasma concentration versus time profile for the single dose is subtherapeutic but the predicted twofold accumulation upon repetitive dosing on the half-life does achieve suitable plasma concentrations, then the loading dose is estimated as twice the amount of drug used for the single dose study and the maintenance dose represents the amount of drug used for the single dose study. The limitation in using this method to estimate dosage regimens is the restriction of a dosage interval approximating the half-life.

In this study the average plasma concentration and superposition methods were used to predict steady state plasma concentrations and design dosage regimens. The equations for employing the average plasma concentration method,[45-47] as developed by Wagner,[46] are given below (see appendix for explanation of symbols):

$$C_{av}^{\infty} = \frac{fD_m}{V\beta\tau} = \frac{1.44\ fD_m t_{1/2}}{V\tau} \qquad (1)$$

$$C_{av}^{\infty} = \frac{(AUC/d)D_m}{\tau} \qquad (2)$$

The practitioner may employ Equation 1 when f, V, and $\beta$ are available from the literature; the best estimates of dosage regimens and blood levels are achieved when f, V, and $\beta$ represent the average values from a number of studies.[3,4] Then one of the three remaining variables, $C_{av}^{\infty}$, $D_m$ and $\tau$, is calculated by assigning values to the other two variables. For example, if the practitioner knows the desired average plasma concentration and the dosage interval, then the maintenance dose may be calculated. When one or more of the f, V and $\beta$ parameters are unavailable but the area under the plasma concentration versus time curve (AUC) is given or can be estimated, then it is possible to use Equation 2 (since $AUC/d = f/V\beta$) to estimate dosage regimens. For example, the predicted average plasma concentration can be calculated once the area under the curve is obtained and the maintenance dose and dosage interval are fixed by the practitioner. Studies comparing the accuracy of predictions of the average plasma concentration when using Equation 1 versus Equation 2 do not seem to have been published, but intuition suggests that, when given the option, Equation 2 may yield the more accurate predictions; AUC is the only experimental variable required for Equation 2 whereas three variables, f, V and $\beta$, are

needed for Equation 1. Furthermore, the values obtained for f, V and $\beta$ vary with the method of pharmacokinetic analysis and computations used. The reader is referred to the literature for a more rigorous treatment of the application of Equations 1 and 2.[45-47]

As seen in Figure 2, Equations 1 and 2 yield an estimate of the average plasma concentration but no predictions, other than intuitive estimates, of the maximum and minimum plasma concentrations achieved during each dosage interval. When it is necessary to obtain these estimates, either for drugs in which a therapeutic plasma concentration range has been determined or a toxic concentration is known, the maximum and minimum plasma concentrations may be obtained by using the superposition method. The reader is referred to the work of Westlake[48,49] for a more complete discussion of this method. As shown in Figures 2 and 3, the superposition method is based on the pharmacokinetic observation that the plasma concentration versus time profile for each successive dose of a multiple dose regimen (e.g., 10 mg q6h) may be layered or superimposed on the plasma concentration of drug remaining just prior to administering each dose. Thus the maximum and minimum plasma concentrations achieved at the steady state can be estimated by using data observed from a single dose of the drugs as follows:

$$C_{max}^{\infty} = C_{pk} + \frac{C_{\tau}10^{-0.3t_{pk}/t_{1/2}}}{1 - 10^{-0.3\tau/t_{1/2}}} = C_{pk} + \frac{C_{\tau}10^{-0.43\beta t_{pk}}}{1 - 10^{-0.43\beta\tau}} \qquad (3)$$

$$C_{min}^{\infty} = C_{\tau} + \frac{C_{\tau}10^{-0.3\tau/t_{1/2}}}{1 - 10^{-0.3\tau/t_{1/2}}} = C_{\tau} + \frac{C_{\tau}10^{-0.43\beta\tau}}{1 - 10^{-0.43\beta\tau}} \qquad (4)$$

The data required for employing Equations 3 and 4, as shown in Figure 3, include (1) the peak plasma concentration and time of achieving the peak ($C_{pk}$ and $t_{pk}$, respectively) during administration of a single dose, (2) the half-life ($t_{1/2}$) or elimination rate constant ($\beta$) as obtained from the linear regression line fitted to the terminal single dose plasma concentration data and (3) the plasma concentration just prior to administering the second dose ($C_{\tau}$), as predicted from the regression line. Sometimes it becomes necessary to propose a dose for a dosage regimen which differs from the literature dose. To convert plasma concentration data from the literature dose to predicted plasma concentration data for the proposed new dose, in order to supply new $C_{pk}$ and $C_{\tau}$

*Figure 2. Accumulation profile for a drug dosed on its half-life*

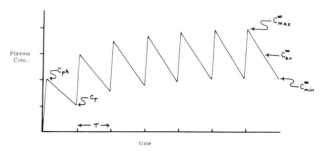

*Figure 3. Obtaining parameters for the superposition method*

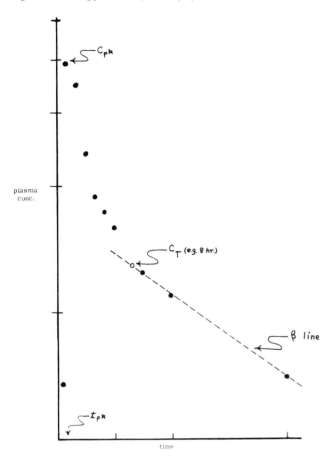

**Table I. Data Used to Generate Dosage Regimens for Nortriptyline[a]**

| PARAMETER[b] | UNITS | SAMPLE SIZE | SAMPLE MEAN | 95% CONFIDENCE INTERVAL[c] |
|---|---|---|---|---|
| $\beta$ | hours$^{-1}$ | 6 | 0.0277 | 0.0182–0.0372 |
| $t_{1/2}$ | hours | 6 | 26.9 | 18.4–35.4 |
| AUC | ng/ml/hr | 6 | 1668 | 924–2394 |
| $V_{ss}$ | liters/kg | 6 | 15.7 | 10.1–21.3 |
| f | — | 3 | 0.64 | 0.42–0.85 |
| $t_{pk}$ | hours | 6 | 5.6 | 3.5–7.7 |
| $C_{pk}$ | ng/ml | 6 | 44.4 | 31.4–56.9 |
| $C_6^d$ | ng/ml | 6 | 35.9 | 28.5–43.3 |
| $C_{12}^d$ | ng/ml | 6 | 30.6 | 22.9–38.3 |
| $C_{24}^d$ | ng/ml | 6 | 22.4 | 14.8–30.0 |

[a] Data taken from references 21 and 22 using a dose of 1 mg/kg.
[b] See appendix for explanation of symbols.
[c] It is conjecture whether the confidence interval or the tolerance interval is the more appropriate statistic. The common practice of reporting the confidence interval has been used.
[d] Plasma concentrations at 6, 12 and 24 hours as predicted by the least squares regression line for the $\beta$ elimination phase.

values at the various dosage intervals by using the regression line provided for each subject. A therapeutic plasma concentration range of 50–150 ng/ml was chosen because it appears to be achieving a growing acceptance despite some controversy in the literature.[25-31] We applied a 95% confidence interval to each parameter by using the standard statistical technique.

Predicted steady state plasma concentration data resulting from various dosage regimens are shown in Table 2. The first three entries show the estimated $C_{max}^\infty$, $C_{min}^\infty$ and $C_{av}^\infty$ values resulting from a *daily* dose of 1.43 mg/kg administered q.d., b.i.d. and q.i.d., respectively. The data suggest that this standard daily dose maintains plasma concentrations well within the therapeutic goal of 50–150 ng/ml whether given as a single daily dose or in increments throughout the day. Reducing the daily dose to 0.71 mg/kg q.d. does not maintain plasma concentrations within the therapeutic range. In order to calculate the 95% confidence interval about the predicted $C_{max}^\infty$ and $C_{min}^\infty$ values, the data from the confidence interval for each parameter shown in Table 1 were used. The interpretation applied to the confidence interval about the predicted $C_{max}^\infty$ and $C_{min}^\infty$ range is that 95% of the $C_{max}^\infty$ and $C_{min}^\infty$ values calculated from data obtained in studies conducted similarly to that of Alexanderson et al.[21,22] should yield values falling within the 95% confidence interval reported in Table 2. The confidence interval is a useful guide to the practitioner in assessing the potential variability in the calculated estimates. This variability stems from interpatient variation in absorption, distribution and elimination.

Appraising the predictions shown in Table 2 in another way, a dose of 100 mg q.d., 50 mg b.i.d., or 25 mg q.i.d. in patients of average body weight should yield steady state plasma concentration versus time profiles that are maintained within the therapeutic goal of 50–150 ng/ml. A dose of 50 mg q.d. would be expected to be less effective. We expect the 100 mg h.s. dose to maintain patients as effectively as the traditional q.i.d. regimen

data for Equations 3 and 4, the literature dose data are scaled up or down by using Equation 5:

$$\frac{D^2}{D^1} = \frac{C_{pk}^2}{C_{pk}^1} = \frac{C_\tau^2}{C_\tau^1} \qquad (5)$$

In using Equations 3 and 4 for the superposition method it is only necessary to assess $t_{1/2}$ or $\beta$ and utilize the reported plasma concentration data for a single dose. On the other hand, to use Equations 1 or 2 for the average plasma concentration method, it is necessary to obtain various parameters such as f, V, $t_{1/2}$, $\beta$ or AUC.

### Nortriptyline Dosage Regimens

A growing body of literature suggests that psychotherapeutic drugs with long half-lives may be candidates for once-daily administration in contrast to their traditional t.i.d. and q.i.d. regimens.[50-56] These modified regimens are expected to decrease side effects, decrease prescription and drug administration costs and increase patient compliance with prescribed regimens. Nortriptyline, with a half-life of approximately one day, was evaluated with a view to proposing less frequent administration of the drug. The data of Alexanderson et al.,[21,22] as shown in Table 1, were used as a basis for predicting modified regimens; parameters such as $\beta$, $t_{1/2}$, V, AUC, f, $C_{pk}$ and $t_{pk}$ were provided by their studies. We obtained $C_\tau$

**Table 2. Predicted Steady State Plasma Concentration Data for Nortriptyline Resulting From Various Dosage Regimens**[a]

| DOSE (mg/kg) | DOSE/70 kg (mg) | $\tau$ (hr) | MEAN ESTIMATES | | | $C_{min}^{\infty} - C_{max}^{\infty}$ RANGE BASED ON 95% CONFIDENCE INTERVAL[e] (ng/ml) |
|---|---|---|---|---|---|---|
| | | | $C_{max}^{\infty}$ (ng/ml)[b] | $C_{min}^{\infty}$ (ng/ml)[c] | $C_{av}^{\infty}$ (ng/ml)[d] | |
| 1.43 | 100 | 24 | 120 | 66 | 88 | 36–195 |
| 0.71 | 50 | 12 | 97 | 77 | 88 | 45–170 |
| 0.36 | 25 | 6 | 88 | 88 | 88 | 50–162 |
| 0.71 | 50 | 24 | 60 | 33 | 44 | 18–97 |

[a] Based on data in Table 1; adjusted for appropriate dose using Equation 5.
[b] Calculated using Equation 3.
[c] Calculated using Equation 4.
[d] Calculated using Equation 1.
[e] See footnote c in Table 1.

and, in addition, to reap the benefits of once-daily administration as discussed above.

Choosing the superposition method, in which $C_{max}^{\infty}$ and $C_{min}^{\infty}$ values are calculated for each proposed regimen, or the average plasma concentration method, in which a $C_{av}^{\infty}$ value is computed, is probably not a critical consideration for a drug like nortriptyline with a long half-life and a relatively generous therapeutic plasma concentration range. The less mathematically rigorous average plasma concentration method, in choosing a therapeutic goal of $C_{av}^{\infty} = 75$–$100$ ng/ml, is probably as appropriate for predictions as the superposition method, which employed a therapeutic range of 50–150 ng/ml. Other considerations also influence the choice of methods such as the concern for toxicity or therapeutic ineffectiveness resulting from plasma concentrations above and below the therapeutic range, respectively, and the availability of clinical data such as f, V, $\beta$, AUC, etc.

### Lithium Dosage Regimens

Reassessing lithium dosage regimens was performed mainly as an exercise in demonstrating methods and because the drug serves as a pharmacokinetic prototype, as discussed previously. Dosage regimens for lithium are individualized on the basis of routine monitoring of plasma concentrations to a much greater extent than is the practice for nortriptyline. There is a general consensus that individual dosage regimens should be titrated to

**Table 3. Data Used to Generate Dosage Regimens for Lithium**[a]

| PARAMETER[b] | UNITS | SAMPLE SIZE | SAMPLE MEAN | 95% CONFIDENCE INTERVAL[c] |
|---|---|---|---|---|
| $\beta$ | hours$^{-1}$ | 4 | 0.0838 | 0.0196–0.057 |
| $t_{1/2}$ | hours | 4 | 19.2 | 9.6–28.8 |
| $t_{pk}$ | hours | 6 | 1.33 | 0.74–1.92 |
| $C_{pk}$ | mEq/liter | 6 | 0.260 | 0.212–0.308 |
| $C_8$[d] | mEq/liter | 6 | 0.079 | 0.054–0.104 |
| $C_{12}$[d] | mEq/liter | 6 | 0.067 | 0.047–0.087 |
| $C_{24}$[d] | mEq/liter | 6 | 0.043 | 0.031–0.055 |

[a] Data taken from references 13 and 14 using an average dose of 3.47 mg/kg.
[b] See appendix for explanation of symbols.
[c] See footnote c in Table 1.
[d] Plasma concentrations at 8, 12 and 24 hours as predicted by the least squares regression line for the $\beta$ elimination phase.

maintain patients within a therapeutic plasma concentration range of 1.0–2.0 mEq/liter for the acute phase of manic-depressive disorder and 0.4–1.2 mEq/liter for the maintenance phase or prophylaxis.[15,16,18-20]

The data of Caldwell et al.,[13-14] as shown in Table 3, were used as a basis for predicting plasma concentration and dosage regimens; $C_{pk}$ and $t_{pk}$ values were provided by their studies while we calculated $\beta$, $t_{1/2}$ and $C_{\tau}$ values from the plasma concentration versus time data provided for each patient.[14] Predicted steady state plasma concentration data resulting from various dosage regimens are shown in Table 4. The sevenfold range in the 95% confidence interval for the predicted $C_{max}^{\infty}$ and $C_{min}^{\infty}$ values is important to note.

**Table 4. Predicted Steady State Plasma Concentration Data for Lithium Resulting From Various Regimens**[a]

| DOSE (mg/kg) | DOSE/70 KG (mg) | $\tau$ (hr) | MEAN ESTIMATES | | $C_{min}^{\infty} - C_{max}^{\infty}$ RANGE BASED ON 95% CONFIDENCE INTERVAL[d] (mEq/liter) |
|---|---|---|---|---|---|
| | | | $C_{max}^{\infty}$ (mEq/liter)[b] | $C_{min}^{\infty}$ (mEq/liter)[c] | |
| 4.29 | 300 | 8 | 0.67 | 0.37 | 0.18–1.26 |
| 4.29 | 300 | 12 | 0.53 | 0.23 | 0.12–0.90 |
| 8.57 | 600 | 8 | 1.36 | 0.76 | 0.36–2.53 |
| 8.57 | 600 | 12 | 1.08 | 0.46 | 0.24–1.79 |
| 17.14 | 1200 | 24 | 1.61 | 0.35 | 0.21–2.26 |

[a] Based on data in Table 1; adjusted for appropriate dose using Equation 5.
[b] Calculated using Equation 3.
[c] Calculated using Equation 4.
[d] See footnote c in Table 1.

For example, although the $C_{max}^{\infty}$ and $C_{min}^{\infty}$ estimates of 0.67 mEq/liter and 0.37 mEq/liter for a regimen of 4.29 mg/kg q8h (corresponding to 300 mg q8h in patients of average weight) suggest appropriate maintenance therapy, the confidence interval shows that for some groups the $C_{max}^{\infty}$ value resulting from this regimen may really be as great as 1.26 mEq/liter while for other groups the $C_{min}^{\infty}$ value may be as low as 0.18 mEq/liter, a value that is too low for effective treatment. $C_{max}^{\infty}$ and $C_{min}^{\infty}$ estimates based on a regimen of 8.57 mg/kg (corresponding to 600 mg in patients of average weight) q8h or q12h do not appear to yield markedly different plasma concentration versus time profiles. This suggests that patients maintained satisfactorily on the 600 mg q8h regimen may perhaps achieve a satisfactory response on the 600 mg q12h regimen. Although the $C_{max}^{\infty}$ and $C_{min}^{\infty}$ estimates resulting from a dose of 17.14 mg/kg (corresponding to 1200 mg in patients of average weight) administered just once daily are interesting, and perhaps worthy of some consideration, the confidence interval suggests the potential for toxicity in some groups of patients. Based on these observations, some thought to evaluating b.i.d. and q.d. regimens, in contrast to the traditional t.i.d. regimen, appears worthy, and the possibility of initiating clinical trials with these regimens is under consideration here.

## Diazepam Dosage Regimens

Reassessing diazepam dosage regimens illustrates some of the pitfalls, in addition to those already cited, that await the practitioner interested in evaluating dosage regimens. For one thing, despite the widespread utilization of the drug there appear to be no published studies relating plasma concentrations to appropriate antianxiety, anticonvulsant and muscle relaxant re-

sponses. Secondly, the chief metabolite of diazepam, desmethyldiazepam, is appreciably active in itself and achieves similar concentrations to diazepam at the steady state; this complicates the estimation of dosage regimens based on plasma concentration versus response data since two species contribute to the therapeutic effect. Thirdly, as will be shown in Table 6, the estimated $C_{av}^{\infty}$ values vary more than threefold depending on the method of calculation and the pharmacokinetic analysis used. One reasonable approach to estimating a clinically effective plasma concentration to serve as a therapeutic goal, in the absence of published data, is to substitute the pharmacokinetic parameters from various studies and the usual dosage regimens into Equations 1 or 2 in order to calculate an average plasma concentration. Based on the common regimens for employing diazepam as an antianxiety agent, daily doses of 15–40 mg, therapeutically effective average plasma concentrations probably fall within a $C_{av}^{\infty}$ range of 200–1000 ng/ml of diazepam. Furthermore, since as illustrated schematically in Figure 1, diazepam concentrations in plasma may be assumed to represent an index of desmethyldiazepam concentrations (and thus an index of overall pharmacological response), it is a reasonable approach to estimate dosage regimens based on plasma concentrations and pharmacokinetic parameters for diazepam alone.

Data from three separate studies, Kaplan et al.,[32] Berlin et al.[33] and van der Kleijn,[34] as shown in Table 5, were used as a basis for predicting average plasma concentrations. The estimates of $C_{av}^{\infty}$ resulting from a regimen of 0.143 mg/kg (corresponding to 10 mg in patients of average weight) q8h are recorded in Table 6. The first three entries represent the use of Equation 1 which utilizes the f, V, $\beta$ or $t_{1/2}$ data gleaned from the three studies. Although the estimated $C_{av}^{\infty}$ values calculated from the data of each of the three studies varies from 410–730 ng/ml this range is included within the 95% confidence interval for each of the three estimates. The variation in

**Table 5. Data Used to Generate Dosage Regimens for Diazepam**

| PARAM-ETER[a] | UNITS | SAMPLE SIZE | SAMPLE MEAN | 95% CONFIDENCE INTERVAL[b] |
|---|---|---|---|---|
| $\beta^c$ | hours$^{-1}$ | 4 | 0.0235 | 0.0087–0.0383 |
| $\beta^d$ | hours$^{-1}$ | 7 | 0.0184 | 0.0138–0.0230 |
| $\beta^e$ | hours$^{-1}$ | 9 | 0.0367 | 0.0208–0.0526 |
| $t_{1/2}^c$ | hours | 4 | 32.4 | 11.7–53.1 |
| $t_{1/2}^d$ | hours | 7 | 39.6 | 30.2–49.0 |
| $t_{1/2}^e$ | hours | 9 | 22.8 | 15.0–30.6 |
| $V^c$ | liter/kg | 4 | 1.86 | 1.51–2.22 |
| $V_{ss}^d$ | liter/kg | 7 | 1.62 | 1.25–1.99 |
| $V_{ss}^e$ | liter/kg | 9 | 0.66 | 0.37–0.95 |
| $AUC^c$ | $\mu$g/hr/ml | 4 | 2.27 | 1.46–3.08 |
| $f^c$ | — | 4 | 1.00 | 0.75–1.25 |

[a] See appendix for explanation of symbols.
[b] See footnote c in Table 1.
[c] Data taken from reference 32 using an average dose of 0.132 mg/kg.
[d] Data taken from reference 33 using an average dose of 0.079 mg/kg.
[e] Data taken from reference 34 using an average dose of 0.141 mg/kg.

**Table 6. Predicted Steady State Plasma Concentration Data for Diazepam Using Data From Various Studies**

| DOSE (mg/kg) | DOSE/ 70 kg (mg) | $\tau$ (hr) | MEAN ESTIMATE $C_{av}^{\infty}$ (ng/ml) | 95% CONFIDENCE INTERVAL[a] $C_{av}^{\infty}$ (ng/ml) |
|---|---|---|---|---|
| 0.143 | 10 | 8 | 730[b] | 270–2300[b] |
| 0.143 | 10 | 8 | 600[c] | 290–1040[c] |
| 0.143 | 10 | 8 | 410[d] | 160–1360[d] |
| 0.143 | 10 | 8 | 300[e] | 190–410[e] |
| 0.143 | 10 | 8 | 1040[f] | — |

[a] See footnote c in Table 1.
[b] Calculated using Equation 1 and the mean parameters in Table 5, as taken from the data of van der Kleijn et al.[34]
[c] Calculated using Equation 1 and the mean parameters in Table 5, as taken from the data of Berlin et al.[33]
[d] Calculated using Equation 1 and the mean parameters in Table 5, as taken from the data of Kaplan et al.[32]
[e] Calculated using Equation 2 and the mean parameters in Table 5, as taken from the data of Kaplan et al.[32]
[f] The mean of the individual $C_{av}^{\infty}$ values calculated using Equation 1, as taken from the data of van der Kleijn et al.[34]

estimated $C_{av}^{\infty}$ values is a function of the twofold and threefold variation in $\beta$ and V values, respectively, observed in the three studies, as shown in Table 5. This illustrates the substantial interstudy variation in pharmacokinetic parameters which the practitioner may encounter. For a drug like diazepam, with an apparently generous, although poorly defined, range of therapeutic plasma concentrations, a wide interstudy variation in pharmacokinetic parameters may not jeopardize the estimation of plasma concentrations and dosage regimens. However, for drugs with narrow therapeutic indices, e.g., cardiac glycosides, antiarrhythmics, etc., the problem is significant.

The fourth entry in Table 6 represents the use of Equation 2, which employs only AUC data, to estimate a $C_{av}^{\infty}$ value. Note the not unexpected variation in $C_{av}^{\infty}$ values calculated from Equations 1 and 2, based on data obtained from the same group of patients; Equations 1 and 2 yield $C_{av}^{\infty}$ values of 410 and 300 ng/ml, respectively, using the data provided by the study of Kaplan et al.[32] The use of three pharmacokinetic variables in Equation 1 as opposed to one variable in Equation 2 not only invites a variation in the results but also suggests an explanation for the wider confidence interval resulting from the use of Equation 1.

The last entry in Table 6 uses data from the study of van der Kleijn,[34] as does the first entry. In both cases Equation 1 was used to estimate $C_{av}^{\infty}$ values, but the estimate of 730 ng/ml is the result of inserting the mean f, V, and $\beta$ values, as shown in Table 5, into the equation whereas the estimate of 1040 ng/ml represents the mean value of the individual $C_{av}^{\infty}$ values calculated for each patient. It is important for the practitioner to acknowledge the potential variation in results achieved by using these two methods of estimation.

Lastly, it is valuable to note from an inspection of Equation 1 that a regimen of 15 mg q 12 h or b.i.d. would be expected to yield the same $C_{av}^{\infty}$ value as a regimen of 10 mg q8h or t.i.d., although postadministration sedation may be greater from the former regimen. This very property may be put to therapeutic advantage for patients controlled on a regimen of 15 mg daily, for example; 15 mg q.d. should yield the same $C_{av}^{\infty}$ value as 5 mg q8h or t.i.d.

**Summary and Conclusion**

This study suggests, as have others,[1,3-5,7] that pharmacists are capable of interpreting the clinical literature and applying basic pharmacokinetic principles to the reassessment of traditional dosage regimens for drugs. Lithium, nortriptyline, diazepam and chlorpromazine were chosen for this study because they represent therapeutic and pharmacokinetic prototypes which are useful for illustrating the applications and restrictions of practical dosage regimen theory as utilized by pharmacists. The use of nortriptyline data, specifically, shows the potential for using the various methods for estimating regimens to suggest modified dosage regimens worthy of clinical trial. The use of diazepam data illustrates some

of the pitfalls in estimating regimens when plasma concentration versus therapeutic response data are vague and when a marked variation in interstudy pharmacokinetic parameters exists. The goals sought by increased pharmacy input into reassessing traditional dosage regimens are increased patient response to treatment, decreased side effects, prescription and drug administration costs and increased patient compliance with prescribed regimens.

**References**

1. Schumacher, G.: Practical Pharmacokinetic Techniques for Drug Consultation and Evaluation I: Use of Dosage Regimen Calculations, In *Clinical Pharmacy Sourcebook*, pp. 226-236.
2. Schumacher, G.: Practical Pharmacokinetic Techniques for Drug Consultation and Evaluation II: A Perspective On the Renal Impaired Patient, In *Clinical Pharmacy Sourcebook*, pp. 237-243.
3. Levy, R. and Smith, G.: Dosage Regimens of Antiarrhythmics I: Pharmacokinetic Properties. In *Clinical Pharmacy Sourcebook*, pp. 291-297.
4. Levy, R. and Smith, G.: Dosage Regimens of Antiarrhythmics II: Applications, In *Clinical Pharmacy Sourcebook*, pp. 298-302.
5. Giusti, D. and Hayton, W.: Dosage Regimen Adjustment in Renal Impairment, *Drug Intel. Clin. Pharm.* 7:382, 1973.
6. Torosian, G. et al.: Hazards of Bromides in Proprietary Medication, *Amer. J. Hosp. Pharm.* 30:716–718 (Aug.) 1973.
7. Niebergall, P. et al.: Potential Dangers of Common Drug Dosing Regimens, In *Clinical Pharmacy Sourcebook*, pp. 308-313.
8. Jackson, E. A. and McLeod, D. C.: Pharmacokinetics and Dosing of Antimicrobial Agents in Renal Impairment, Part I, *Amer. J. Pharm.* 31: 36–52 (Jan.) 1974.
9. Usdin, E.: Absorption, Distribution and Metabolic Fate of Psychotropic Drugs, *Psychopharmacol. Bull.* 6:4, 1970.
10. Sjoqvist, F.: A Pharmacokinetic Approach to Depression, *Int. Pharmacopsychiat.* 6:147, 1971.
11. Curry, S.: Plasma Levels of Psychotropic Drugs and Their Possible Significance in Therapeutics, *J. Hosp. Pharm.* 20:308, 1971.
12. Gardos, G. and Cole, J.: The Importance of Dosage in Antipsychotic Drug Administration—A Review of Dose-Response Studies, *Psychopharmacologia* 29:221, 1973.
13. Caldwell, H. et al.: A Pharmacokinetic Analysis of Lithium Carbonate Absorption From Several Formulations in Man, *J. Clin. Pharmacol.* II:349, 1971.
14. Westlake, W.: In Swarbrick, J. (ed.): Current Concepts in the Pharmaceutical Sciences: Dosage Form Design and Bioavailability, Lea & Febiger, Philadelphia, Pennsylvania, 1973, pp. 174-178.
15. Cooper, T. et al.: The 24-Hour Serum Lithium Level as a Prognosticator of Dosage Requirements, *Amer. J. Psychiat.* 130:601, 1973.
16. Wren, J.: Lithium Carbonate: Dosage, Serum Levels and Toxicity, *J. Maine Med. Ass.* 63:146, 1972.
17. Sedvall, G. et. al.: Individual Differences in Serum Levels of Lithium in Human Subjects Receiving Fixed Doses of Lithium Carbonate: Relation to Renal Lithium Clearance and Body Weight, *Pharmacologia Clinica* 2: 231, 1970.
18. Prien, R. et al.: Relationship Between Serum Lithium Level and Clinical Response in Acute Mania Treated with Lithium, *Brit. J. Psychiat.* 120:409, 1972.
19. Schou, M.: Pharmacological and Clinical Problems of Lithium Prophylaxis, *Brit. J. Psychiat.* 116:615, 1970.
20. Fry, D. and Marks, V.: Value of Plasma Lithium Monitoring, *Lancet* 1:886, 1971.
21. Alexanderson, B.: Pharmacokinetics of Nortriptyline in Man after Single and Multiple Oral Doses: The Predictability of Steady State Plasma Concentrations From Single-Dose Plasma Level Data, *Europ. J. Clin. Pharmacol.* 4:82, 1972.
22. Alexanderson, B. et al.: The Availability of Orally Administered Nortriptyline, *Europ. J. Clin. Pharmacol.* 5:181, 1973.
23. Anderson, B. and Sjoqvist, F.: Individual Differences in the Pharmacokinetics of Monomethylated Tricyclic Antidepres-

sants: Role of Genetics and Environmental Factors and Clinical Importance, *Ann. N. Y. Acad. Sci.* 179:739, 1971.

24. Sjoqvist, F. et al: Pharmacokinetics and Biological Effects of Nortriptyline in Man, *Acta Pharmacol. Toxicol.* 29: 255 (Suppl. 3) 1971.

25. Asberg, M. et al.: Correlation of Subjective Side Effects with Plasma Concentrations of Nortriptyline, *Brit. Med. J.* 4:18, 1970.

26. Asberg, M. et al.: Relationship Between Plasma Level and Therapeutic Effect of Nortriptyline, *Brit. Med. J.* 3:311, 1971.

27. Burrows, G. et al.: Plasma Concentration of Nortriptyline and Clinical Response in Depressive Illness, *Lancet* 2:619, 1972.

28. Sorenson, P. et al.: Plasma Nortriptyline Levels in Endogenous Depression, *Lancet* 1:113, 1973.

29. Rifkin, A. et al.: Plasma Nortriptyline Levels in Depression, *Lancet* 1:1258, 1973.

30. Gruvstad, M.: Plasma Levels of Antidepressants and Clinical Response, *Lancet* 1:95, 1973.

31. Braithwaite, R. et al.: Clinical Significance of Plasma Levels of Tricyclic Antidepressant Drugs in the Treatment of Depression, *Lancet* 1:556, 1973.

32. Kaplan, S. et al.: Pharmacokinetic Profile of Diazepam in Man Following Single Intravenous and Oral and Chronic Oral Administrations, *J. Pharm. Sci.* 62: 1789 (Nov.) 1973.

33. Berlin, A. et al.: Determination of Bioavailability of Diazepam in Various Formulations From Steady State Plasma Concentration Data, *Clin. Pharmacol. Ther.* 13:733, 1972.

34. Van der Kleijn, E.: Pharmacokinetics of Distribution and Metabolism of Ataractic Drugs and an Evaluation of the Site of Antianxiety Activity, *Ann. N. Y. Acad. Sci.* 179:115, 1971.

35. Van der Kleijn, E. et al.: Pharmacokinetics of Diazepam in Dogs, Mice and Humans, *Acta Pharmacol. Toxicol.* 29:109 (Suppl. 3) 1971.

36. De Silva, A. et al.: Blood Level Distribution Patterns of Diazepam and Its Major Metabolites in Man, *J. Pharm. Sci.* 55:692, 1966.

37. Randall, L. et al.: Pharmacology of the Metabolites of Chlordiazepoxide and Diazepam, *Curr. Ther. Res.* 7:590, 1965.

38. Schallek, W. et al.: Recent Developments in the Pharmacology of the Benzodiazepines, *Adv. Pharmacol. Chemother.* 10:120, 1972.

39. Sakalis, G. et al.: Physiologic and Clinical Effects of Chloropromazine and Their Relationship to Plasma Level, *Clin. Pharmacol. Ther.* 13:931, 1972.

40. March, J. et al.: Interpatient Variation and Significance of Plasma Levels of Chlorpromazine in Psychotic Patients, *J. Med.* 3:146, 1972.

41. Curry, S.: Chlorpromazine: Concentrations in Plasma, Excretion in Urine and Duration of Effect, *Proc. Roy. Soc. Med.* 64:285, 1971.

42. Curry, S. et al.: Factors Affecting Chlorpromazine Plasma Levels in Psychiatric Patients, *Arch. Gen. Psychiat.* 22:209, 1970.

43. Curry, S. et al.: Chlorpromazine Plasma Levels and Effects, *Arch. Gen. Psychiat.* 22:289, 1970.

44. Huang, C. and Kurland, A.: Chlorpromazine Blood Levels in Psychotic Patients, *Arch. Gen. Psychiat.* 5: 509, 1961.

45. Wagner, J.: Biopharmaceutics and Relevant Pharmacokinetics, Drug Intelligence Publications, Hamilton, Illinois, 1972.

46. Wagner, J. et al.: Blood Levels of Drug at the Equilibrium State after Multiple Dosing, *Nature* 207:1301, 1965.

47. Sawchuck, R.: The Plateau Principle in Drug Therapy, *Minn. Pharm.* 27:10 (Mar.) 1973.

48. Westlake, W.: Problems Associated with Analysis of Pharmacokinetic Models, *J. Pharm. Sci.* 60:882, 1971.

49. Westlake, W.: *In* Swarbrick, J. (ed.): Current Concepts in The Pharmaceutical Sciences: Dosage Form Design and Bioavailability, Lea & Febiger, Philadelphia, Pennsylvania, 1973, pp. 172-174.

50. Mendelo, J. and Digiacamo, J.: The Treatment of Depression with a Single Daily Dose of Imipramine Pamoate, *Amer. J. Psychiat.* 130:1022, 1973.

51. Prien, R. et al.: Intermittent Pharmacotherapy in Chronic Schizophrenia, *Hosp. Comm. Psychiat.* 24:317, 1973.

52. DiMascio, A.: Psychotropic Drug Overuse: An Examination of Prescription Practices, *Mass. J. Ment. Health* 2:23, 1972.

53. Chien, C. and DiMascio, A.: Clinical Effects of Various Schedules of Medication. *Behavioral Neuropsychiat.* 3:5 (Apr.) 1971.

54. Saraf, K. and Klein, D.: The Safety of a Single Daily Dose Schedule for Imipramine, *Amer. J. Psychiat.* 128:115, 1971.

55. Brophy, J.: Single Daily Doses of Neuroleptic Drugs, *Dis. Nerv. Syst.* 30:120, 1969.

56. Hrushka, M. et al.: Therapeutic Effects of Different Modes of Chlorpromazine Administration, *Dis. Nerv. Syst.* 27:522, 1966.

## Appendix of Symbols

| | |
|---|---|
| $\beta$ | Apparent first order rate constant for overall elimination of drug by the body. |
| $t_{1/2}$ | Half-life for loss of drug from plasma $(0.693/\beta)$. |
| f | Fraction of dose that is absorbed. |
| V | Apparent volume of distribution of drug in the body. |
| $V_{ss}$ | Apparent volume of distribution of drug in the body as measured at the instant that the rate of change of the amount of drug in the tissue compartment is zero for the two compartment open model. |
| AUC | Area under the plasma concentration vs. time curve for administration of single dose of drug from $t = 0$ to $t = \infty$. |
| $C_{max}{}^{\infty}$, $C_{av}{}^{\infty}$ and $C_{min}{}^{\infty}$ | Maximum, average and minimum concentrations of drug in the plasma of patients, respectively, during the dosage interval once the steady state (equilibrium) has been achieved. |
| $C_{pk}$ | Maximum concentration of drug in the plasma of patients during the administration of a single dose. |
| $C_{\tau}$ | Concentration of drug in the plasma of patients immediately before administration of the second dose, as predicted by the least-squares regression line for the $\beta$ elimination phase. |
| $C(\tau + t_{pk})$ | Concentration of drug in the plasma of patients at time equal to $\tau + t_{pk}$, as predicted by the least-squares regression line for the $\beta$ elimination phase. |
| $\tau$ | Dosage interval. |
| $t_{pk}$ | Time for achievement of maximum concentration of drug in the plasma of patients during the administration of a single dose. |
| $D_l$ and $D_m$ | Loading dose and maintenance dose of drug, respectively, used in dosage regimens. |
| d | Dose of drug used to generate AUC data. |

# 47 Practical Pharmacokinetic Techniques for Drug Consultation and Evaluation IV: Gentamicin Blood Level Versus Time Profiles of Various Dosage Regimens Recommended for Renal Impairment

G. E. Schumacher

The gentamicin blood level vs. time profiles of various dosage regimens recommended for renal impairment were reassessed by applying pharmacokinetic techniques to the patient data in the clinical literature.

Eight dosage regimen modifications were tested in eight prototype cases of renal impairment (serum creatinine range of 0.9–12.0 mg/100 ml and creatinine clearance range of 5–100 ml/min/1.73 m$^2$) using simulated blood level vs. time profiles generated from the known pharmacokinetic parameters for gentamicin. Employing a one-hour intravenous infusion at dosages and dosing intervals recommended by the various methods, significant differences were observed in the various blood level vs. time profiles. Methods recommending shorter dosing intervals (every 24 hours and less) generally resulted in a greater percent duration of the dosing interval above the selected "effective response concentration" (ERC) of a 4 μg/ml blood level and a markedly shorter duration of sub-ERC blood levels. Methods based on creatinine clearance as an index of renal function generally achieved greater percent duration of the dosing interval above the ERC and lesser duration of blood levels below this value than methods based on serum creatinine.

In 30 years of antibiotic therapy we have yet to clarify the relationship between blood levels and therapeutic response; the significance of peak levels and the duration of supra-inhibitory and sub-inhibitory antibiotic concentrations as they influence effectiveness is unresolved. While it is unlikely that these questions will be fully answered by direct clinical study, some investigators are seeking answers indirectly through animal experiments, in vitro studies and the application of pharmacokinetic theory to existing clinical data.

I have chosen the retrospective pharmacokinetic approach for evaluating gentamicin dosage regimens because this antibiotic has a number of properties that make it an excellent candidate for this type of analysis:

1. Gentamicin has a narrow therapeutic index that imposes severe restrictions on the range of useful blood level versus time profiles.

2. It is eliminated from the body almost completely by renal excretion (nonrenal elimination is minimal) which makes dosage and the blood level versus time profiles highly dependent on kidney function.

3. An ample body of literature on the pharmacokinetics of gentamicin has been published.

4. Some in vitro and in vivo data on blood levels in relationship to therapeutic effectiveness have been reported.

For years clinicians have suggested that safe and effective dosage regimens of gentamicin should yield blood levels of 2–12 μg/ml depending on bacterial sensitivity.[1–6] Yet it has not been clear whether the peak blood level, the average blood level or the total blood level versus time profile should be maintained within this range.

Some clarification is provided in recent studies, however. Klastersky,[7] in an elegant study using gentamicin and other antibiotics for septicemia and both wound and respiratory infections, noted that clinical success was 67%

and >80% when the peak blood level exceeded the minimum inhibitory concentration by fourfold and eightfold, respectively. Others have looked even more directly at the relationship between blood levels and therapeutic outcome. Riff and Jackson,[8,9] in studying gentamicin specifically in a limited number of patients, found that regimens insuring peak concentrations of 4 μg/ml and above eliminated Pseudomonas in all patients except those who had poor host defense mechanisms; peak concentrations below 4 μg/ml were generally ineffective. Noone[10] observed that 84% of the patients with gram-negative septicemia, urinary tract infections and wound infections responded to regimens insuring peak blood levels of 5 μg/ml of gentamicin or more while pneumonia required peaks of 8 μg/ml or more. Hewitt[11] concurred that peak blood levels of 4 μg/ml or greater are probably necessary for effective treatment although he cautioned that this would be difficult to verify. Finally, some in vitro studies of bacterial growth rates suggest that continuous exposure of Pseudomonas to blood levels of 4 μg/ml or more for greater than one hour is generally necessary for substantial inhibition of growth.[12-14]

In view of these observations, it appears that gentamicin represents one of the very few antibiotics for which some initial data have been collected on the relationship between blood levels and therapeutic outcome. Peak blood levels appear to have a bearing on clinical success, but no data have yet been reported on the relationship between effectiveness and the duration of supra-inhibitory and sub-inhibitory blood levels. Until more definitive information is acquired, it seems appropriate to designate a peak blood level of 4 μg/ml as the "effective response concentration" that must be achieved to yield a high degree of antimicrobial effectiveness with gentamicin. Based on these observations, many clinicians are now recommending that gentamicin dosage regimens, except for urinary tract infections, be initiated at 5–8 mg/kg/day for the first day followed by maintenance therapy of 3–4.5 mg/kg/day in patients with normal renal function.[4,8,10,11,15,16]

Because of the constraints placed on gentamicin dosage due to the drug's narrow therapeutic index and high dependence on renal excretion, patients with renal impairment will rapidly accumulate blood levels to potentially toxic concentrations if normal dosage regimens are maintained. These properties have resulted in the development of a number of specific nomograms, formulas and computer programs for modifying gentamicin dosage regimens during various stages of renal impairment.[1-4,19,20] Furthermore, general methods for modifying dosage regimens can be applied to gentamicin.[21-26] No comparative evaluation of these various methods has been reported, however.

Using the published pharmacokinetic studies on gentamicin,[17,27-34] the objectives of this study were:

1. To determine if a pharmacist can evaluate the existing clinical literature, interpret the heterogeneous in vitro

and in vivo studies and then apply basic pharmacokinetic principles in order to reassess the quality of gentamicin dosage regimens.
2. To determine if significant differences exist in the blood level versus time profiles for the various dosage regimens of gentamicin recommended for patients with impaired renal function.
3. To introduce the concept of an "effective response concentration" as a new factor to be considered when evaluating the blood level versus time profiles of gentamicin.
4. To demonstrate general techniques for comparing various dosage regimens.

## Methodology

Several limitations were imposed on this study:

1. Since intramuscular blood level versus time profiles for varying degrees of renal impairment are not available in the literature, it was not practical to use the superposition method[40-42] to estimate maximum and minimum blood levels. Therefore, a one-hour intravenous infusion of gentamicin was assumed. This is not impractical because: (a) this route of administration is recommended for patients in shock, with edema, severe burns, hemorrhagic disorders and for patients receiving anticoagulant therapy and hemodialysis[31,32,35,36] and (b) the qualitative interpretation of the results will not differ for intramuscular administration.
2. An average half-life of 2.1 hours and an average volume of distribution of 0.20 liters/kg were chosen for patients with normal renal function; excretion of the drug was chosen as 98%. This represents the mean values for the various results reported in the literature.[1,17,27-33]
3. The volume of distribution was assumed to remain constant during declining renal function and there is some justification for this in the literature, although the matter is unresolved.[5,33]
4. A one-compartment pharmacokinetic model was employed.
5. An "effective response concentration" (ERC) of 4 μg/ml was selected as a working guide on the basis of the studies cited previously.[8-11]

Table 1 shows the eight prototype cases evaluated in this study. For each case the serum creatinine value was fixed (in order to demonstrate a wide range of renal function from normal to severely impaired) and the corresponding creatinine clearance value was estimated using the calculations of Jelliffe[37] which account for age and sex in converting serum creatinine to creatinine clearance. Only in case D was the patient's weight considered in estimating creatinine clearance by using the equation of Jelliffe[38] or the nomogram of Siersback-Nielsen.[39] The estimated half-life values were calculated using the method of Schumacher[23] or the equation of Giusti and Hayton[24], normal half-life and creatinine clearance values were taken as 2.1 hours and 100 ml/min/1.73 m², respectively. Renal excretion was assumed to be the route of elimination for 98% of the gentamicin.

There are nine methods used to modify dosage regimens for gentamicin during renal impairment (see Table 2):

1. Modifications based on serum creatinine.
   a. Cutler[19]
   b. McHenry[2]

## Table 1. Prototype Cases Used For Evaluating the Various Gentamicin Dosage Regimens

| CASE | ESTIMATED CREATININE CLEARANCE[a] (ml/min/1.73 M²) | FIXED SERUM CREATININE (mg/100 ml) | ESTIMATED HALF-LIFE[c] (hr) | AGE (yr) | LEAN WEIGHT (kg) | SEX |
|---|---|---|---|---|---|---|
| A | 5 | 12 | 30.4 | 70 | 70 | M |
| B | 10 | 5 | 18.0 | 70 | 60 | F |
| C | 18 | 5 | 10.7 | 30 | 70 | M |
| D | 23[b] | 5 | 8.6 | 30 | 70 | M |
| E | 30 | 3 | 6.7 | 30 | 70 | M |
| F | 45 | 2 | 4.6 | 30 | 70 | M |
| G | 58 | 1 | 3.6 | 70 | 70 | M |
| H | 100 | 0.9 | 2.1 | 30 | 70 | M |

[a] Estimated from the fixed serum creatinine value by using the equations of Jelliffe[37]; patient weight is not a factor in these equations.

[b] In this case only, the value was estimated from the fixed serum creatinine value by using the equations of Jelliffe[38]; patient weight is a factor in these equations.

[c] Estimated by using the method of Schumacher[23] or the equation of Giusti and Hayton.[24]

## Table 2. Methods Used for Modifying Gentamicin Dosage Regimens[a]

1. Chan[3]: Loading dose of 1.7 mg/kg; maintenance doses from a nomogram in the published paper.

2. Cutler-1[19]: Loading dose of 2.0 mg/kg; maintenance doses of 1.0 mg/kg every 4 $Cr_s$.

3. Cutler-2[19]: Loading dose of 2.0 mg/kg; maintenance doses of 2.0 mg/kg every 9–12 $Cr_s$.

4. Devine[20]: Loading dose (mg/kg) $= 1.04 + Cl_{cr}/180$ for $Cl_{cr}$ of 15 ml/min or less or $1.07 + Cl_{cr}/250$ for $Cl_{cr}$ of 16 ml/min and greater; maintenance dose (mg/kg) $= -0.80 (Cl_{cr}/100)^2 + 2.05 (Cl_{cr}/100) - 0.21 + 0.034 (\tau)$.

5. Gingell[1]: Loading dose of 1.1 mg/kg; maintenance doses from a table in the published paper.

6. Half-life[25]: Loading dose of 1.7 mg/kg; maintenance doses of approximately one-half of the loading dose administered at a convenient dosing interval close to the half-life during renal impairment.

7. Jelliffe[17]: Loading and maintenance doses provided by computer-based input variables such as blood level desired, dosing interval desired, renal status, age, weight and sex.

8. McHenry[2]: Loading dose of 1.1 mg/kg; maintenance doses of 1.1 mg/kg every 8 $Cr_s$.

9. Schumacher[23] and Giusti[24]: (a) $\tau_{ri}$ method—normal loading dose of 1.7 mg/kg at a dosing interval prolonged over the normal in proportion to the increase in half-life value.
(b) $D_{ri}$ method—normal dosing interval of eight hours with maintenance doses decreased from the normal dose of 1.7 mg/kg in proportion to the increase in half-life values; loading dose calculated from the maintenance dose using equations in the cited references.

[a] In applying these methods to the individual cases in Table 1, the calculated dosing interval was adjusted to the nearest realistic and convenient interval.

2. Modifications based on creatinine clearance.
   a. Chan[3]
   b. Devine[20]
   c. Gingell[1]
   d. Schumacher[23] Giusti[24] Wagner[22]
   e. Half-life[25]
3. Modifications based on serum creatinine or creatinine clearance.
   a. Jelliffe[17,18]

As shown in Table 2, the methods of Cutler, McHenry, Chan, Gingell and Devine stipulate the dosage to be used. The method of Jelliffe calculates the dosage on the basis of the blood level desired by the clinician; concentrations of 5 μg/ml and 8 μg/ml were chosen as variables. The half-life method and the method of Schumacher, Giusti and Wagner modify dosage on the basis of the "normal" dose chosen by the clinician; a dose of 1.7 mg/kg every eight hours (5.1 mg/kg/day) was selected on the basis of the observations cited previously.[4,8,10,11,15,16]

Seven parameters were evaluated in this study in order to compare the blood level versus time profiles resulting from the use of the various methods for modifying dosage regimens:

1. The 24-hour dose (dose administered during the first 24-hour interval).
2. The 96-hour dose (dose administered during subsequent 96-hour intervals).
3. $C^{\infty}_{max}$ (maximum blood level achieved during each dosing interval at the steady-state).
4. $C^{\infty}_{min}$ (minimum blood level achieved during each dosing interval at the steady-state).
5. % > ERC (percent of each dosing interval in which the steady-state blood level exceeds the "effective response concentration" [ERC] of 4 μg/ml).
6. Hours of $\tau$ sub-ERC (continuous hours of each dosing interval in which the steady-state blood level is less than the ERC of 4 μg/ml).
7. Intensity factor (product of $[C^{\infty}_{max}/ERC]$ times % > ERC).

The parameters recorded in Tables 3–11 were calculated as follows (see Appendix for explanation of symbols):

1. The peak blood level achieved at the end of the first one-hour intravenous infusion was calculated using Equation 1:

$$C_{pk} = \frac{1.44 R_o t_{1/2}}{V}(1 - 10^{-0.3/t_{1/2}}) \qquad (1)$$

2. The trough blood level achieved at the end of the first dose (just prior to administration of the second intravenous infusion) was calculated using Equation 2:

$$C_\tau = C_{pk}10^{-0.3(\tau - 1)/t_{1/2}} \qquad (2)$$

3. The maximum blood level achieved during the steady-state was calculated using the superposition method,[40–42] as shown in Equation 3:

$$C^\infty_{max} = C_{pk} + \frac{C_\tau 10^{-0.3 tpk/t_{1/2}}}{1 - 10^{-0.3\tau/t_{1/2}}} \qquad (3)$$

4. The minimum blood level achieved during the steady-state was calculated using Equation 4:

$$C^\infty_{min} = C^\infty_{max}10^{-0.3(\tau - 1)/t_{1/2}} \qquad (4)$$

5. The percent of each dosing interval in which the steady-state blood level exceeded the ERC (% > ERC) was calculated using Equations 5 and 6:

$$t_{ERC} = 3.32 t_{1/2}\log(C^\infty_{max}/4.0) \qquad (5)$$

$$\% > ERC = (t_{ERC}/\tau) \times 100 \qquad (6)$$

6. The intensity factor was calculated using Equation 7:

$$\text{Intensity Factor} = (C^\infty_{max}/4.0) \times (\% > ERC) \qquad (7)$$

7. The continuous hours of each dosing interval in which the steady-state blood level was less than the ERC was calculated using Equation 8:

$$\text{Hours of } \tau \text{ sub-ERC} = \tau\text{-}t_{ERC} \qquad (8)$$

## Results

The data in Table 3 give some indication of the parameters to be expected when various doses of gentamicin are given every eight hours to patients with normal renal function. The "traditional" dosage regimen of 1 mg/kg every eight hours yields estimated $C^\infty_{max}$ values just above the ERC value of 4 µg/ml and the ERC is exceeded

**Table 3. Parameters Obtained for Various Doses of Gentamicin When Renal Function is Normal[a]**

| REGIMEN[b] (every eight hours) | ESTI-MATED[c] $C^\infty_{max}$ (µg/ml) | ESTI-MATED[c] $C^\infty_{min}$ (µg/ml) | % OF $\tau^c$ > ERC | HOURS OF $\tau^c$ SUB-ERC | INTEN-SITY[c] FACTOR |
|---|---|---|---|---|---|
| 2.0 mg/kg | 9.1 | 0.9 | 31 | 5.5 | 71 |
| 1.5 mg/kg | 6.8 | 0.7 | 20 | 6.4 | 34 |
| 1.0 mg/kg | 4.5 | 0.5 | 4 | 7.6 | 5 |

[a] Half-life of 2.1 hours, volume of distribution of 0.20 liter/kg, $Cl_{cr} = 100$ ml/min/1.73 m²; case H is a representative example.
[b] Intravenous infusion of one hour.
[c] See methodology for explanation of parameters.

for only 4% of the eight-hour dosing interval. It is not surprising that some clinicians are recommending increased doses because 1.5 mg/kg and 2.0 mg/kg, both every eight hours, increase the duration of blood levels above the ERC to 20% and 31% of the dosing interval, respectively. Although a dose of 2.0 mg/kg every eight hours achieves an average $C^\infty_{max}$ value of 9.1 µg/ml, which is well within the therapeutic range, a few patients will obviously achieve higher and potentially toxic blood levels at this dose.

As shown in both Table 2 and the preceding discussion of methods, the various approaches to modifying dosage regimens for gentamicin during renal impairment use either the serum creatinine or the creatinine clearance as the index of renal function.

The methods of Cutler[19] and McHenry[2] use fixed doses with dosing intervals computed by multiplying the stable serum creatinine value by a constant. Despite the great popularity of these methods, and their admitted impact on decreasing toxicity with gentamicin, I, along with others, have been skeptical of their use because serum creatinine is a most indirect index of kidney function. Similar serum creatinine values in patients of different sex, weight or age can represent markedly different levels of renal function (see cases B, C and D of Table 1). Yet, the methods of Cutler and McHenry do not account for these factors. In addition, serum creatinine as an index of renal function is least accurate when kidney function is most impaired. Yet, this is when modifications in dosage regimens are most critical.

Creatinine clearance is recognized as a much more accurate index of renal function and it does account directly for sex, weight and age. This parameter is used to modify regimens in the guidelines of Gingell[1] and the nomogram of Chan.[3] Devine and other clinical pharmacists at the University of Michigan[20] have developed calculations, as yet unpublished, using creatinine clearance. Schumacher[23] and Giusti,[24] working independently, developed the same general method for adjusting dosage regimens based on creatinine clearance which is applicable to gentamicin. Wagner's method,[22] which is similar to Schumacher's and Giusti's, also employs creatinine clearance. These methods fix either the dose or the dosing interval while varying the other parameter as a function of the impaired creatinine clearance. Finally, Jelliffe developed a nomogram[18]

**Table 4. Parameters Obtained for Case B[a]**

| METHOD[b] | DOSE[c] 24 hr (mg/kg) | DOSE[c] 96 hr (mg/kg) | ESTIMATED[c] $C^\infty_{max}$ ($\mu$g/ml) | ESTIMATED[c] $C^\infty_{min}$ ($\mu$g/ml) | % OF $\tau$[c] > ERC | HOURS OF $\tau$[c] SUB-ERC |
|---|---|---|---|---|---|---|
| Cutler-2 (q. 48 hr) | 2.0 | 4.0 | 11.6 | 1.9 | 59 | 20 |
| McHenry (q. 48 hr) | 1.1 | 2.2 | 6.4 | 1.0 | 26 | 35 |
| Gingell (q. 48 hr) | 1.1 | 2.2 | 6.4 | 1.0 | 26 | 35 |
| Chan (q. 8 hr) | 2.4 | 4.1 | 6.3 | 4.8 | 100 | 0 |

[a] See Table 1; fixed $Cr_s$ = 5, estimated $Cl_{cr}$ = 10 ml/min/1.73 m², estimated $t_{1/2}$ = 18 hours, female, 60 kg, age 70.
[b] See Table 2 for dosage guidelines.
[c] See methodology for explanation of parameters.

which fixes the dosing interval while varying the dose based on serum creatinine or creatinine clearance. Jelliffe's computer program[17] predicts the dose based upon the clinician's choice of dosing interval and desired peak blood level.

Table 4 presents some data for case B—a 70-year-old female patient with a fixed serum creatinine of 5 mg/100 ml, an estimated creatinine clearance of 10 ml/min/1.73m², and an estimated half-life of 18 hours. The most popular methods of modifying gentamicin dosage regimens are included for comparison. Observe the following:

1. During the first 24 hours, and any subsequent 96-hour interval, the Chan and Cutler methods recommend twice the dose of the McHenry and Gingell methods.
2. Both the Cutler and McHenry methods modify regimens on the basis of serum creatinine values. Yet, at the identical value, Cutler provides for twice the dose of McHenry.
3. Although both methods are based on serum creatinine values, the Cutler method, as a result of the larger dose, yields twice the maximum blood level and twice the percent of dosing interval above the ERC as does the McHenry method.
4. Although the estimated maximum blood levels achieved by the methods of Chan, McHenry and Gingell are similar, the percent of the dosing interval above the ERC is markedly different. Assessing peak blood levels alone as an outcome criterion may be misleading.
5. The methods of Chan and Cutler provide for administering the same dose per interval but there is a fourfold difference in the ERC values. Administering appropriate small doses every eight hours generally sustains blood levels above the ERC longer than larger doses at less frequent intervals. Chan maintains supra-ERC values for the entire dosing interval.
6. All four methods achieve peak blood levels above the ERC of 4 $\mu$g/ml. However, the ERC values of quite different. In fact, the ERC value for the methods of McHenry and Gingell is probably marginal at best, especially in view of the following discussion of sub-ERC values.
7. The hours of sub-ERC, which denotes the number of continuous hours at sub-effective concentrations, is most

likely an important criterion. While the Chan method yields no hours below the ERC, the Cutler, McHenry and Gingell methods yield sub-ERC values of 20–35 hours during each dosage interval. This value of 1–1½ days of each dosage interval at sub-effective concentrations seems of probable concern.

Table 5 shows data for case D—a 30-year-old male patient, again with a fixed serum creatinine of 5 mg/100 ml, an estimated creatinine clearance of 23 ml/min/1.73 m², and an estimated half-life of 8.6 hours. This case was chosen to illustrate the potential changes in results which occur when the same serum creatinine of 5 mg/100 ml yields greater than a twofold increase in creatinine clearance (23 versus 10 ml/min/1.73 m²), as a result of changes in sex, age and weight. Even converting serum creatinine to creatinine clearance by using equations[37] which consider sex and age, but not weight, yields an increase in creatinine clearance from 10 to 18 ml/min/1.73 m², as shown in cases B and C, respectively, of Table 1. The methods based on serum creatinine as the index of renal function, such as those of Cutler and McHenry, will not yield a change in their dosage recommendations but the methods based on creatinine clearance will lead to an increase in dosage. Observe the following in Table 5:

1. Chan provides for considerably more gentamicin over the first 24-hour and subsequent 96-hour intervals than Gingell, Cutler and McHenry. Indeed, Chan recommends more than three times the dose of McHenry.
2. The more frequently administered doses, resulting from the Gingell and Chan methods based on creatinine clearance, sustain markedly shorter sub-ERC values than the less frequently administered doses of Cutler and McHenry based on serum creatinine; once again, the Chan method yields a significantly greater supra-ERC value than that shown by the other methods.

The two cases (B and D), in which the serum creatinine values did not change but the estimated creatinine clear-

**Table 5. Parameters Obtained for Case D[a]**

| METHOD[b] | DOSE[c] 24 hr (mg/kg) | DOSE[c] 96 hr (mg/kg) | ESTIMATED[c] $C^\infty_{max}$ ($\mu$g/ml) | ESTIMATED[c] $C^\infty_{min}$ ($\mu$g/ml) | % OF $\tau$[c] > ERC | HOURS OF $\tau$[c] SUB-ERC |
|---|---|---|---|---|---|---|
| Cutler-2 (q. 48 hr) | 2.0 | 4.0 | 9.8 | 0.2 | 24 | 36 |
| McHenry (q. 48 hr) | 1.1 | 2.2 | 5.4 | 0.1 | 9 | 44 |
| Gingell (q. 24 hr) | 1.1 | 4.4 | 6.2 | 1.0 | 25 | 18 |
| Chan (q. 8 hr) | 3.0 | 7.6 | 6.3 | 3.6 | 77 | 2 |

[a] See Table 1; fixed $Cr_s$ = 5, estimated $Cl_{cr}$ = 23 ml/min/1.73 m², estimated $t_{1/2}$ = 8.6 hours, male, 70 kg, age 30.
[b] See Table 2 for dosage guidelines.
[c] See methodology for explanation of parameters.

ance and thus the degree of renal impairment and the estimated half-life did change, are summarized in Table 6. The data illustrate the potential concern for regimen modifications based on serum creatinine rather than creatinine clearance. The Chan and Devine methods, as well as others based on creatinine clearance, have compensated for improved renal function in case D by increasing their dosage recommendations (see Tables 4 and 5) while the Cutler and McHenry methods do not provide for dosage alterations. In general, this results in greater supra-ERC periods and less duration of sub-ERC blood levels for methods based on creatinine clearance. Although some of these observations are the result of the shorter dosing intervals for the Chan and Devine methods, the Cutler and McHenry methods force a prolonged dosage interval due to their dependence on serum creatinine as the determinant of the length of the interval. Furthermore, the ability of methods based on creatinine clearance to compensate for changes in renal function, although the serum creatinine remains unchanged (as shown in cases B and D), results in the maintenance of high supra-ERC and low sub-ERC values, while the methods based on serum creatinine yield lower supra-ERC values and higher sub-ERC values for case D compared to case B. In fact, the low supra-ERC value for the McHenry method in case D and the high sub-ERC values for the Cutler and McHenry methods in both cases B and D seem of concern.

Table 7 is presented to examine some of the relationships between peak blood levels, duration above the ERC, sub-ERC periods and the intensity factor. The comparative influence of peak blood levels versus duration of time above the ERC is speculative and unresolved. Many investigators consider both factors to be important and complementary.[8,12,21,43] From a pharmacokinetic viewpoint, in terms of achieving appropriate tissue concentrations of antibiotic, I concur with the importance of both factors. A high blood level may compensate for only a modest duration above the ERC. Conversely, a long duration above the ERC may compensate for an adequate but not high blood level. Therefore, a rough guide to the influence of both factors may be obtained by computing an intensity factor which considers both the magnitude of the peak blood level and the duration of the level above the ERC. It is important to note that the quantitative

value of the intensity factor has no particular meaning and can only be judged qualitatively in comparing other dosage regimens. Furthermore, although the concept of an intensity factor was developed for this study, its clinical significance is unknown and has not been tested in clinical situations. Observe the following in Table 7:

1. The three methods were chosen to represent (a) dosage regimen modifications based on serum creatinine and creatinine clearance, (b) varying dosing intervals and (c) varying dosages. The ratio of 24-hour and 96-hour dosages recommended by the various methods is approximately 1:2:3 for the methods of McHenry, Cutler-1 and Chan, respectively.
2. Although the McHenry method does achieve a peak concentration above the ERC with each dose, the duration of supra-ERC concentrations and the intensity factor may be inadequate. Furthermore, a prolonged period of 43 hours of sub-ERC blood levels is observed during each dosage interval.
3. Although the methods of Cutler-1 and Chan achieve similar peak blood levels, the more frequent dosing of Chan results in a considerably greater percent of each dosage interval above the ERC, therefore a greater intensity factor, and fewer hours at sub-ERC; there is simply more drug at supra-ERC levels for a longer period of time using the Chan method.
4. In order to attach some significance to the numerical value of the intensity factor, observe that in Table 3 values greater than 30 are achieved in patients with normal renal function receiving dosage regimens of 1.5 mg/kg or greater every eight hours. Yet, under these circumstances the continuous hours of concentrations at sub-ERC levels is less than seven. It may be necessary to achieve higher intensity factor values in patients with renal impairment who are administered regimens stipulating less frequent dosing intervals because, as observed in Table 7, a substantial number of hours at sub-ERC levels may occur.
5. The above observations are largely the result of variations in the dosage and frequency of dosing used in the three methods; Chan > Cutler > McHenry.

The Cutler method has two variations, both of which yield similar dosage over 96-hour intervals but differ in the frequency of administering the dose; as shown in Table 2, both Cutler-1 and Cutler-2 methods use loading doses of 2.0 mg/kg but whereas Cutler-1 provides maintenance doses of 1.0 mg/kg at dosing intervals simulating one half-life (as estimated from the serum creatinine value) Cutler-2 provides maintenance doses of 2.0 mg/kg at intervals simulating three half-lives. A comparison of

## Table 6. Comparing Parameters Obtained for Cases B and D[a]

| METHOD[b] | % OF $\tau$[c] >ERC | | HOURS OF $\tau$[c] SUB-ERC | | ESTIMATED[c] $C^{\infty}_{max}$ ($\mu$g/ml) | |
|---|---|---|---|---|---|---|
| | B | D | B | D | B | D |
| Cutler-2 (q. 48 hr) | 59 | 24 | 20 | 36 | 11.6 | 9.8 |
| McHenry (q. 48 hr) | 26 | 9 | 35 | 44 | 6.4 | 5.4 |
| Devine (q. 8 hr) | 100 | 47 | 0 | 4 | 5.2 | 5.2 |
| Chan (q. 8 hr) | 100 | 77 | 0 | 2 | 6.3 | 6.3 |

[a] See Table 1 for characteristics of the individual cases.
[b] See Tables 2, 4 and 5 for dosage guidelines.
[c] See methodology for explanation of parameters.

## Table 7. Parameters Obtained for Case C[a]

| METHOD[b] | ESTIMATED[c] $C^{\infty}_{max}$ ($\mu$g/ml) | % OF $\tau$[c] >ERC | HOURS OF $\tau$[c] SUB-ERC | INTENSITY[c] FACTOR |
|---|---|---|---|---|
| McHenry (q. 48 hr) | 5.5 | 11 | 43 | 15 |
| Cutler-1 (q. 24 hr) | 6.1 | 29 | 17 | 44 |
| Chan (q. 8 hr) | 6.4 | 100 | 0 | 160 |

[a] See Table 1; fixed $Cr_s$ = 5 mg/100 ml, estimated $Cl_{cr}$ = 18 ml/min/1.73 m², estimated $t_{1/2}$ = 10.7 hours, male, 70 kg, age 30.
[b] Doses calculated using guidelines in Table 2: First 24-hour doses of 1.1, 2.0, and 2.8 mg/kg for McHenry, Cutler-1 and Chan, respectively; subsequent 96-hour doses of 2.2, 4.0 and 6.5 mg/kg for McHenry, Cutler-1 and Chan, respectively.
[c] See methodology for explanation of parameters.

these two variations for cases A, C and E, spanning a range of creatinine clearance values of 5–30 ml/min/1.73 m$^2$, is shown in Table 8. No outstanding differences are noted except for the lower sub-ERC values for the Cutler-1 method. The higher $C^\infty_{max}$ values achieved by the Cutler-2 method results in a greater intensity factor value for cases C and E; in fact, the Cutler-2 method yields greater intensity for five of the seven cases studied. Although it is not possible to conclude that one variation is superior to the other on the basis of the parameters obtained in the study, the lower sub-ERC values for the Cutler-1 variation may be an important criterion.

As suggested by the Cutler-1 method, another general approach to modifying dosage regimens is to administer maintenance doses which are one-half of the loading dose at a dosing interval close to the estimated half-life of the drug for a given degree of renal impairment.[25] This method is based on the pharmacokinetic principle that blood levels similar to the peak and trough concentrations obtained from a loading dose may be achieved by providing one-half of this dose at a dosing interval of one half-life. As observed in Table 8 for the Cutler-1 method, however, when the estimate of the half-life is based on the serum creatinine value, which does not account for variables influencing the half-life such as age, weight and sex, long intervals at sub-ERC levels can be expected. The use of the half-life principle when based on creatinine clearance, however, is more satisfactory, as shown in Table 9.

Table 9 compares the half-life method for cases A, C and E with the popular Chan and McHenry methods. This method compares quite favorably with the method of Chan and appears markedly superior to the McHenry method. Since in cases A, B and C the half-life method provides for practical dosage intervals of every 24 hours, every 12–24 hours and every 12 hours, respectively, this method offers a good alternative to the Chan method for clinicians who are reluctant to dose gentamicin on an every-eight-hour basis during severe renal impairment. When the estimated half-life is less than the "normal" dosing interval (every eight hours for gentamicin), as observed for cases E, F and G, the normal dosing interval is used but the maintenance dose is increased to greater than one-half the loading dose.

Table 10 shows data which herald concern for using the method of Schumacher,[23] Giusti,[24] Wagner,[22] Tozer[26] and Dettli.[25] As noted in Table 2, each of these investigators have advocated the method of modifying dosage regimens in which either the dose is reduced or the dosing interval

**Table 9. Comparing Parameters Obtained for Cases A, C and E Using Various Methods**[a]

| METHOD | ESTIMATED[b] $C^\infty_{max}$ (µg/ml) | | | % OF $\tau$[b] >ERC | | | HOURS OF $\tau$[b] SUB-ERC | | |
|---|---|---|---|---|---|---|---|---|---|
| | A | C | E | A | C | E | A | C | E |
| Half-life[c] | 9.4 | 8.0 | 7.2 | 100 | 100 | 70 | 0 | 0 | 2 |
| Chan[d] | 6.8 | 6.4 | 6.8 | 100 | 100 | 70 | 0 | 0 | 2 |
| McHenry[e] | 6.1 | 5.5 | 5.7 | 20 | 11 | 16 | 77 | 43 | 20 |

[a] See Table 1 for characteristics of the individual cases.
[b] See methodology for explanation of parameters.
[c] As shown in the guidelines of Table 2, approximately one-half of the loading dose of 1.7 mg/kg was administered at convenient dosing intervals close to the half-life; the dosing interval for cases A, C and E was every 24 hours, every 12 hours and every 8 hours, respectively.
[d] Doses calculated using guidelines in Table 2: Loading dose of 1.7 mg/kg; maintenance doses of 0.23 mg/kg, 0.54 mg/kg, and 0.80 mg/kg every 8 hours for cases A, C and E, respectively.
[e] Doses calculated using guidelines in Table 2: Loading and maintenance doses of 1.1 mg/kg administered every 96 hours, every 48 hours, and every 24 hours for cases A, C and E, respectively.

is prolonged in direct proportion to the increase in half-life observed in renal impairment; in so doing, the objective of maintaining the same average steady-state blood level ($C^\infty_{av}$) in normal and renal-impaired states is achieved. In using this method, however, the reduced dose ($D_{ri}$) given at the normal dosing interval is considerably less than the normal dose given at a prolonged dosing interval ($\tau_{ri}$); although the same average blood level will be achieved by these two variations the $D_{ri}$ alternative obviously achieves lower $C^\infty_{max}$ and supra-ERC values than the $\tau_{ri}$ alternative. As shown in Table 10, the ERC exceeds the $C^\infty_{max}$ values for the $D_{ri}$ method when creatinine clearance values are less than 23 ml/min/1.73 m$^2$. Thus for an antibiotic like gentamicin which has an effective response concentration, and this parameter has not been characterized for most antibiotics, the "$C^\infty_{av}$ method" has limitations when kidney function falls to less than 30% of normal. Both alternatives suffer limitations: the $D_{ri}$ alternative yields sub-effective blood levels while the $\tau_{ri}$ alternative achieves effective blood levels but suffers long periods of sub-ERC levels. This previously unreported limitation of this method, which has achieved wide acceptance, warrants further investigation with other drugs. Actually, the Chan method is a form of the $D_{ri}$ alternative but it is effective because it is designed to reach its full "normal" dosage at a creatinine clearance of 70 ml/min/1.73 m$^2$ whereas the general method[22–24,26] does not reach full dosage until a creatinine clearance of

**Table 8. Comparing Parameters Obtained for Cases A, C and E Using Variations of the Cutler Method**[a]

| METHOD[b] | ESTIMATED[c] $C^\infty_{max}$ (µg/ml) | | | % OF $\tau$[c] >ERC | | | HOURS OF $\tau$[c] SUB-ERC | | | INTENSITY[c] FACTOR | | |
|---|---|---|---|---|---|---|---|---|---|---|---|---|
| | A | C | E | A | C | E | A | C | E | A | C | E |
| Cutler-1 | 7.4 | 6.1 | 6.6 | 57 | 29 | 44 | 21 | 17 | 7 | 105 | 44 | 73 |
| Cutler-2 | 10.5 | 10.0 | 10.3 | 36 | 30 | 40 | 77 | 33 | 14 | 95 | 75 | 103 |

[a] See Table 1 for characteristics of the individual cases.
[b] Doses for the first 24 hours and subsequent 96 hours, as calculated using the guidelines in Table 2, are similar for both methods.
[c] See methodology for explanation of parameters.

**Table 10. Comparing Parameters Obtained for Cases A, B, D and F Using Methods Designed to Achieve the Same Average Blood Level in Patients with Normal and Impaired Renal Function**[a]

| METHOD | ESTIMATED[b] $C^\infty_{max}$ ($\mu$g/ml) | | | | % OF $\tau^b$ >ERC | | | | HOURS OF $\tau^b$ SUB-ERC | | | |
|---|---|---|---|---|---|---|---|---|---|---|---|---|
| | A | B | D | F | A | B | D | F | A | B | D | F |
| Schumacher[c]—$D_{ri}$ | 3.5 | 3.7 | 4.2 | 4.9 | 0 | 0 | 14 | 23 | all[e] | all[e] | 7 | 6 |
| Schumacher[d]—$\tau_{ri}$ | 8.9 | 8.9 | 9.6 | 9.4 | 30 | 30 | 47 | 51 | 84 | 51 | 13 | 6 |

[a] See Table 1 for characteristics of the individual cases.
[b] See methodology for explanation of parameters.
[c] Using the guidelines in Table 2, all doses administered at the normal dosing interval of every eight hours. Loading doses of 0.72 mg/kg, 0.8 mg/kg, 0.90 mg/kg and 1.2 mg/kg for cases A, B, D and F, respectively, as calculated from the maintenance doses using equations in the cited references[23,24]; maintenance doses of 0.12 mg/kg, 0.20 mg/kg, 0.42 mg/kg and 0.78 mg/kg for cases A, B, D and F, respectively.
[d] Using the guidelines in Table 2, loading and maintenance doses of 1.7 mg/kg administered every 120 hours, every 72 hours, every 24 hours, and every 12 hours for cases A, B, D and F, respectively.
[e] Blood levels are sub-ERC for the entire dosing interval.

100 ml/min/1.73 m²; thus a higher dose, for any given creatinine clearance value, is recommended by the Chan method as compared to the general method.

Finally, the Jelliffe computer program for gentamicin was evaluated. The Jelliffe method assumes a volume of distribution of 14.3% whereas 20% (0.2 liters/kg) was chosen for this study. Therefore, the dosages recommended by the computer were entered in Equation 1 using the 20% volume of distribution value used throughout the study. This decreased the $C^\infty_{max}$ values obtained in Equation 3 compared to the values predicted by the computer. As shown in Table 11, using desired maximum blood levels of 5 $\mu$g/ml and 8 $\mu$g/ml as input variables, the results were less satisfactory than for some other methods. Requesting a maximum blood level of 5 $\mu$g/ml yielded $C^\infty_{max}$ values that were sub-therapeutic for all cases studied (only cases B, D and E are reported here) due to the

greater volume of distribution assumed in this study. Requesting a maximum blood level of 8 $\mu$g/ml achieved $C^\infty_{max}$ values that exceeded the ERC although substantial periods of sub-ERC levels were observed for every 24-hour schedules. Although this method was superior to the Cutler and McHenry methods it does appear inferior to some of the other methods discussed. Unless further studies corroborate Jelliffe's assumption of a 14% volume of distribution, some adjustment in the data upon which the computer program is based seems appropriate.

**Conclusions**

The objectives of this study have been achieved: (1) Dosage regimens for gentamicin have been reassessed by a pharmacist using basic pharmacokinetic principles; (2) significant differences do exist in the blood level versus time profiles for the various dosage regimens of gentamicin recommended for patients with impaired renal function; and (3) a general technique has been presented for comparing various dosage regimens for drugs.

Although this study evaluated various gentamicin dosage regimens the conclusions reached probably have general application:

1. Most methods recommended for modifying gentamicin dosage regimens during renal impairment achieve peak steady-state blood levels that exceed the "effective response concentration" of 4 $\mu$g/ml. The percent duration of the dosing interval above the ERC varies markedly for the methods, however, as does the duration of sub-ERC blood levels. These variations probably have therapeutic significance.
2. Shorter dosing intervals generally promote a greater percent duration of the dosing interval above the ERC and a markedly shorter duration of sub-ERC blood levels.
3. Methods based on creatinine clearance as an index of renal function generally achieve greater percent supra-ERC values and lesser duration of sub-ERC values than methods based on serum creatinine. The latter methods are less desirable because (a) they are not as responsive to changes in renal function as methods based on creatinine clearance and (b) they recommend unduly long dosing intervals during moderate to severe renal impairment.
4. The widely recommended method of decreasing the dosage or increasing the dosing interval in proportion to the prolongation of the half-life during renal impairment may have marked limitations when a specific blood level must be achieved for some portion of the dosing interval.

**Table 11. Parameters Obtained for Cases B, D and E Using Computer-assisted Dosage Regimens Developed by Jelliffe**[a]

| MAXIMUM[b] BLOOD LEVEL RE-QUESTED ($\mu$g/ml) | $\tau$ (hours) | ESTIMATED[c,d] $C^\infty_{max}$ ($\mu$g/ml) | | | % OF $\tau^c$ >ERC | | | HOURS OF $\tau^c$ SUB-ERC | | |
|---|---|---|---|---|---|---|---|---|---|---|
| | | B | D | E | B | D | E | B | D | E |
| 8[e] | q 24 h | 5.8 | 5.8 | 5.8 | 40 | 19 | 15 | 14 | 19 | 20 |
| 8[f] | q 8 h | — | — | 5.8 | — | — | 45 | — | — | 4 |
| 5[g] | q 24 h | 3.6 | 3.6 | 3.6 | 0 | 0 | 0 | all[h] | all[h] | all[h] |

[a] See Table 1 for characteristics of the individual cases.
[b] Required input to computer.
[c] See methodology for explanation of parameters.
[d] Estimated blood levels do not match requested blood levels because computer program is based on a volume of distribution of 0.14 liter/kg whereas 0.20 liter/kg was used in this study; computer results were adjusted for this difference.
[e] To achieve the requested level, computer recommends loading doses of 1.2 mg/kg followed by maintenance doses every 24 hours of 0.72 mg/kg, 1.04 mg/kg and 1.13 mg/kg for cases B, D and E, respectively.
[f] To achieve the requested level, computer recommends a loading dose of 1.2 mg/kg followed by maintenance doses every 8 hours of 0.69 mg/kg for case E.
[g] To achieve the requested level, computer recommends a loading dose of 0.75 mg/kg followed by maintenance doses every 24 hours of 0.45 mg/kg, 0.65 mg/kg, and 0.71 mg/kg for cases B, D and E, respectively.
[h] Blood levels are sub-ERC for the entire dosing interval.

## References

1. Gingell, J. and Waterworth, P.: Dose of Gentamicin in Patients with Normal Renal Function and Renal Impairment, *Brit. Med. J.* 2:19 (Apr. 6) 1968.

2. McHenry, M. et al.: Gentamicin Dosages for Renal Insufficiency, *Ann. Internal Med.* 74:192 (Feb.) 1971.

3. Chan, R. et al.: Gentamicin Therapy in Renal Failure: A Nomogram for Dosage, *Ann. Internal Med.* 76:773, 1972.

4. Mawer, G. et al.: Prescribing Aids for Gentamicin, *Brit. J. Clin. Pharmacol.* 1:45, 1974.

5. Christopher, T. et al.: Gentamicin Pharmacokinetics During Hemodialysis, *Kidney Internat.* 6:38, 1974.

6. Giusti, D.: A Review of the Clinical Use of Antimicrobial Agents in Patients with Renal and Hepatic Insufficiency III: The Aminoglycosides, *Drug Intel. Clin. Pharm.* 7:540, (Dec.) 1973.

7. Klastersky, J. et al.: Antibacterial Activity in Serum and Urine as a Therapeutic Guide in Bacterial Infections, *J. Infect. Dis.* 129:187, 1974.

8. Riff, L.: Pseudomonas Bacteremia: Evaluation of Factors Influencing Response to Therapy, *Acta Path. Microbiol. Scand. B.* 81:79 (suppl. 241), 1973.

9. Jackson, G. and Riff, L.: Pseudomonas Bacteremia: Pharmacologic and Other Bases for Failure of Treatment with Gentamicin, *J. Infect. Dis.* 124:185 (suppl.), 1971.

10. Noone, P. et al.: **Experience in Monitoring Gentamicin Therapy During Treatment of Serious Gram-Negative Sepsis,** *Brit. Med. J.* 1:477, 1974.

11. Hewitt, W.: Reflections on the Clinical Pharmacology of Gentamicin, *Acta Path. Microbiol. Scand. B.* 81:151 (suppl. 241), 1973.

12. Zagar, Z.: Kinetics of Antibacterial Inhibition Power of Ampicillin, Cloxacillin, Carbenicillin, and Gentamicin at Changing Concentration Similar to that in the Body Fluids, *In* Hejzlar, M. (ed.): Advances in Antimicrobial and Antineoplastic Chemotherapy, Vol. I/2, University Park Press, Baltimore, Maryland, 1972, pp. 715-717.

13. Helm, E. and Stille, W.: Kinetics of Bactericidal Action of Carbenicillin, Gentamicin and Polymixin B Against Pseudomonas Aeruginosa, *In* Hejzlar, M. (ed.): Advances in Antimicrobial and Antineoplastic Chemothrapy, Vol. I/2, University Park Press, Baltimore, Maryland, 1972, pp. 719-722.

14. Rubenis, M. et al.: Laboratory Studies on Gentamicin, *In* Sylvester, J. (ed.): Antimicrobial Agents and Chemotherapy, American Society of Microbiology, Ann Arbor, Michigan, 1964, pp. 153-156.

15. Darrell, J.: Gentamicin in Urinary Infection, *Brit. Med. J.* 4:427, 1972.

16. Wise, R. and Reeves, D.: Gentamicin Dosage, *Brit. Med. J.* 4:732, 1972.

17. Jelliffe, R. et al.: Computer Assistance for Gentamycin Therapy, *Clin. Res.* 18:137, 1970.

18. Jelliffe, R.: Nomograms for Gentamycin Dosage, 1971, available from University of Southern California School of Medicine Business Office, Los Angeles.

19. Cutler, R. et al.: Correlation of Serum Creatinine Concentration and Gentamicin Half-life, *JAMA* 219:1037, 1972.

20. Devine, B. et al.: College of Pharmacy, University of Michigan, Ann Arbor, personal communication, 1974.

21. Kruger-Thiemer, E.: Dosage Schedule and Pharmacokinetics in Chemotherapy, *J. Amer. Pharm. Ass. (Sci. Ed.)* 49:311, 1960.

22. Wagner, J.: Biopharmaceutics and Relevant Pharmacokinetics, Drug Intelligence Publications, Hamilton, Illinois, 1971, ch. 28.

23. Schumacher, G.: Practical Pharmacokinetic Techniques for Drug Consultation and Evaluation II: A Perspective on the Renal Impaired Patient, In *Clinical Pharmacy Sourcebook*, pp. 237-243.

24. Giusti, D. and Hayton, W.: Dosage Regimen Adjustment in Renal Impairment, *Drug Intel. Clin. Pharm.* 7:382, 1973.

25. Dettli, L.: Drug Dosage in Patients With Renal Disease, *Clin. Pharmacol. Ther.* 16:274 (Part II), 1974.

26. Tozer, T.: Nomogram for Modification of Dosage Regimens in Patients with Chronic Renal Function Impairment, *J. Pharmacokin. Biopharm.* 2:13, 1974.

27. Modr, Z. and Dvoracek, K.: Contribution to the Pharmacokinetics of Gentamicin in Man, *In* Hejzlar, M. (ed.): Advances in Antimicrobial and Antineoplastic Chemotherapy, University Park Press, Baltimore, Maryland, 1972, pp. 925-929.

28. Modr, Z. et al.: Pharmacokinetics of Gentamicin After Repeated Administration, *In* Hejzlar, M. (ed.): Advances in Antimicrobial and Antineoplastic Chemotherapy, University Park Press, Baltimore, Maryland, 1972, pp. 163-165.

29. Gyselynck, A. et al.: Pharmacokinetics of Gentamicin: Distribution and Plasma and Renal Clearance, *J. Inf. Dis.* 124:70 (suppl.), 1971.

30. Regamey, C. et al.: Comparative Pharmacokinetics of Tobramycin and Gentamicin, *Clin. Pharmacol. Ther.* 14:396, 1973.

31. Simon, V. et al.: Pharmacokinetic Studies of Tobramycin and Gentamicin, *Antimicrob. Ag. Chemother.* 3:445, 1973.

32. Rodriguez, V. et al.: Gentamicin Sulfate Distribution in Body Fluids, *Clin. Pharmacol. Ther.* 11:275, 1970.

33. Wilson, T. et al.: Elimination of Tritiated Gentamicin in Normal Human Subjects and in Patients with Severely Impaired Renal Function, *Clin. Pharmacol. Ther.* 14:815, 1973.

34. Kaye, D.: The Unpredictability of Serum Concentrations of Gentamicin: Pharmacokinetics of Gentamicin in Patients with Normal and Abnormal Renal Function, *J. Inf. Dis.* 130:150, 1974.

35. Korner, B.: Gentamicin Therapy Administered by Intermittent Intravenous Injections, *Acta Path. Microbiol. Scand. B.* 81:15 (suppl. 241), 1973.

36. Buhl-Nielsen, A. and Elb, S.: The Use of Gentamicin Intravenously, *Acta Path. Microbiol. Scand. B.* 81:23 (suppl. 241), 1973.

37. Jelliffe, R.: Creatinine Clearance: Bedside Estimate, *Ann. Internal Med.* 79:604, 1973.

38. Jelliffe, R. and Jelliffe, S.: A Computer Program for Estimation of Creatinine Clearance from Unstable Serum Creatinine Levels, by Age, Sex, and Weight, *Math. Biosc.* 14:17, 1972.

39. Siersback-Nielsen, K. et al.: Rapid Evaluation of Creatinine Clearance, *Lancet* 1:1133, 1971.

40. Westlake, W.: Problems Associated with Analysis of Pharmacokinetic Models, *J. Pharm. Sci.* 60:882, 1971.

41. Schumacher, G. and Weiner, J.: Practical Pharmacokinetic Techniques for Drug Consultation and Evaluation. III: Psychotherapeutic Drugs as Prototypes for Illustrating Some Considerations in Pharmacist-generated Dosage Regimens, In *Clinical Pharmacy Sourcebook*, pp. 244-251.

42. Wagner, J.: Relevant Pharmacokinetics of Antimicrobial Drugs, *Med. Clin. N. Amer.* 58:479, 1974.

43. Rolinson, G.: The Significance of Protein of Antibiotics In Vitro and In Vivo, *In* Waterson, A. (ed.): Recent Advances in Medical Microbiology, Little, Brown & Co., Boston, Massachusetts, 1967, pp. 254-283.

## Appendix of Symbols

| | |
|---|---|
| ERC | Effective response concentration; concentration of drug in the blood (blood level) that must be achieved for some portion of the dosing interval in order to expect effective therapy for the majority of patients infected with microorganisms sensitive to the antimicrobial drug. |
| $t_{ERC}$ | Time during the dosing interval at which the concentration of drug in the blood (blood level) falls to the ERC. |
| $t_{1/2}$ | Half-life for loss of drug from the blood. |
| $t_{pk}$ | Time for achievement of maximum concentration of drug in the blood (blood level) during the administration of a single dose. |

$C_{pk}$ — Maximum concentration of drug in the blood (blood level) during the administration of a single dose.

$C_{\tau}$ — Concentration of drug in the blood (blood level) immediately before administration of the second dose, as predicted by the least-squares regression line for the elimination phase.

$C^{\infty}_{max}$, $C^{\infty}_{av}$, $C^{\infty}_{min}$ — Maximum, average and minimum concentrations of drug in the blood (blood level), respectively, during the dosing interval once the steady-state (equilibrium) has been achieved.

$\tau$ — Dosing interval.

$V$ — Apparent volume of distribution of drug in the body.

$R_0$ — Rate of drug administration during intravenous infusion.

$Cl_{cr}$ — Creatinine clearance.

$Cr_s$ — Serum creatinine.

$D_{ri}$ and $\tau_{ri}$ — Reduced dose and prolonged dosing interval, respectively, during renal impairment.

# 48 Pharmacokinetics and Dosing of Antimicrobial Agents in Renal Impairment, Part I

Eric A. Jackson and Don C. McLeod

The dosing considerations of antimicrobial agents when used in patients with renal impairment are discussed extensively.

Criteria for establishing the degree of renal impairment are given, and the relationship between serum creatinine and creatinine clearance is discussed. The drugs covered in this chapter are the penicillins, the cephalosporins, the tetracyclines, antifungal agents (amphotericin, flucytosine, and griseofulvin), the polymyxins, and the aminoglycosides.

Many antimicrobial agents are eliminated from the body primarily by being excreted unchanged in the urine. The drug may reach the urine by glomerular filtration or by renal tubular secretion. Some of the filtered or secreted drug may undergo tubular reabsorption back into the blood. The penicillins, for example, are removed by both glomerular filtration and tubular secretion, whereas vancomycin is removed only by glomerular filtration. Some of these drugs exhibit dangerous toxicities and the margin between effective and toxic serum levels may be small. These drugs need special consideration when being given to patients with renal disease. In the absence of adequate dosing information on the use of drugs in patients with renal impairment, it is not surprising that grave toxicities have been encountered in hundreds of patients. The pharmacokinetics of many drugs have not been well studied in renal impairment, and dosing guidelines are empirical. The pharmacokinetics of some agents are well known, and dosing guidelines are more scientifically established.

Of the several previous reviews on the use of antibiotics in renal impairment,[1-5] the work of Kunin is outstanding. This chapter borrows freely from his work and that of other authors, but certain aspects do differ. More antimicrobial agents are reviewed here than in previous works, and each drug is discussed in detail when possible. Effective and toxic serum levels, adverse effects, renal excretion, and dosage regimens are discussed. Commentary on the effects of dialysis and hepatic dysfunction is included on many drugs when data are available. The tables should not be used without reading the discussion and referring to original articles in some cases. Serum half-lives presented are often averages, and this fact should be considered in unusual patients. Clinical judgment and observation are still imperative because of the physiological variability of patients. Guidelines presented are intended to be safe but not dogmatic.

## Estimation of Severity of Renal Impairment

The Council on the Kidney in Cardiovascular Disease of the American Heart Association has established criteria for evaluating the severity of renal disease,[6] but the drug literature does not generally follow these recently established guidelines. Creatinine, a normal metabolic by-product, is freely and completely filtered by the glomerulus and accumulates in the body in direct proportion to the degree of impairment of the glomerular filtration rate (GFR). Creatinine clearance ($C_{cr}$) is a universally accepted means of estimating the GFR. The $C_{cr}$ is somewhat difficult to obtain since an accurate 24-hour urine volume must be collected, and several methods exist to estimate the $C_{cr}$ from the serum creatinine ($S_{cr}$) level. The $S_{cr}$ is more useful than blood urea nitrogen (BUN) in estimating the degree of renal impairment.

Creatinine production decreases with age, is higher in men than women, and decreases per unit weight with increasing fat stores. Jelliffe[7] has developed a simplified formula for bedside use which allows for sex differences in creatinine production as follows:

$$\text{For men—} \quad C_{cr} = 100/S_{cr} - 12 \tag{1}$$
$$\text{For women—} \quad C_{cr} = 80/S_{cr} - 7 \tag{2}$$

$$C_{cr} = \text{ml/min/150 lbs}$$
$$S_{cr} = \text{mg/100 ml}$$

From data now available from computerized programs developed to estimate $C_{cr}$ from $S_{cr}$, Jelliffe has recommended another formula for adults 20–80 years old with stable $S_{cr}$.[8] The formula is for male patients; for females, 90% of the $C_{cr}$ value is used for the conversion of $S_{cr}$ to $C_{cr}$.

$$C_{cr} = \frac{98 - 16 \dfrac{(Age - 20)}{20}}{S_{cr}} \qquad (3)$$

$C_{cr}$ is in ml/min/1.73 m² body surface area; age is the patient's age in years (from 20 to 80), rounded to the nearest 10 years; and $S_{cr}$ is in mg/100 ml. For example, consider a 77-year-old woman whose stable $S_{cr}$ level is 1.0 mg/100 ml. Start with her age, rounding it to 80 years. That minus 20 is 60, which divided by 20 is 3. Three times 16 is 48; 98 minus 48 is 50, which, divided by the $S_{cr}$ value, yields 50. Because the patient is a woman, 90% of 50 yields an estimated $C_{cr}$ of 45 ml/min/ 1.73 m² body surface area.

Since $S_{cr}$ values may fluctuate, an average of two $S_{cr}$ levels is a more accurate means of determining $C_{cr}$. Those readers desiring a more thorough treatment of the relationship between $S_{cr}$ and $C_{cr}$ should refer to Jelliffe's model of creatinine kinetics.[7] Figure 1 is a nomogram developed by Siersback-Nielson et al.[9] which allows the estimation of $C_{cr}$ from the $S_{cr}$ taking into consideration age, sex and weight. Results with this nomogram closely approximate Jelliffe's methods.

A normal $C_{cr}$ in the adult is 100 ml/min ± 20 ml, and this generally corresponds to a $S_{cr}$ of 1.4 mg/100 ml of serum or less. A $S_{cr}$ above 12 mg/100 ml is associated with a $C_{cr}$ of <4 ml/min and indicates essentially no kidney function. The patient could be said to be oliguric (little urine flow) if not anuric (no urine flow). Table 1 categorizes the various degrees of renal impairment and denotes the corresponding $S_{cr}$ and $C_{cr}$ ranges.

Generally, a $C_{cr}$ of 50 ml/min indicates a GFR about 50% of normal, a $C_{cr}$ of 25 ml/min indicates a GFR about 25% of normal, etc. Theoretically, the serum $t_{1/2}$ of a drug totally eliminated by glomerular filtration and not reabsorbed should increase by a factor of two with a $C_{cr}$ of 50 ml/min, by a factor of four with a $C_{cr}$ of 25 ml/min, by a factor of ten with a $C_{cr}$ of 10 ml/min, etc. The pharmacokinetics of most drugs are not this simple, although those of vancomycin approach it. Most drugs undergo some metabolism, biliary excretion, tubular reabsorption, or tubular secretion and do not conform to this simple analysis.

### The Penicillins

The penicillins are among the least toxic of all antibiotics, and even though they accumulate in the serum during renal impairment, only small dosing adjustments are needed. The penicillins are primarily excreted un-

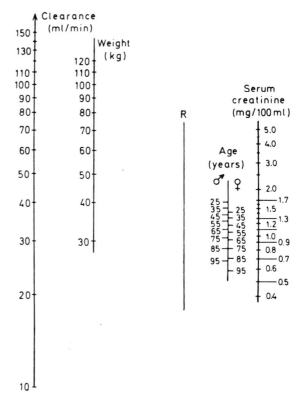

*Figure 1. Nomogram for rapid evaluation of endogenous creatinine clearance—with a ruler, join weight to age, keep ruler at crossing point of line marked R; then move the right hand side of the ruler to the appropriate serum creatinine value and read the patient's clearance from the left side of the nomogram*[9]

changed in the urine. About 10–25% of a penicillin dose is metabolized by the liver, and in severe uremia the liver plays an important role in penicillin elimination. Hypersensitivity reactions represent the major adverse effect of the penicillins, but massive doses have caused neurotoxicity and convulsions.[10-12] Hyperkalemia and hypernatremia (depending on the salt used) may also occur with large doses, particularly in renal impairment.

*Penicillin G.* The pharmacokinetics of penicillin G in renal impairment has been studied by Kunin and Maxwell[13] and by Plaut et al.[14] Penicillin G has a normal serum $t_{1/2}$ of 0.5 hour. Kunin and Maxwell report an anuric $t_{1/2}$ of 7–10 hours, and they observed one anuric patient with severe liver damage in which the $t_{1/2}$ was 30.5 hours. Plaut et al. studied ten azotemic patients and ten normal patients and found a logarithmic relationship between rising penicillin serum $t_{1/2}$ and inulin clearance (Figure 2). With massive penicillin G doses

**Table 1. Categorization of Renal Impairment Based on Serum Creatinine and Creatinine Clearance**

| DEGREE OF RENAL FAILURE | CREATININE CLEARANCE ($C_{cr}$) (ml/min) | APPROXIMATE SERUM CREATININE ($S_{cr}$) (mg/100 ml) |
|---|---|---|
| Normal | >80 | 1.4 |
| Mild | 50–79 | 1.5–1.9 |
| Moderate | 10–49 | 2.0–6.4 |
| Severe | <10 | >6.4 |
| Anuric | 0 | >12 |

Figure 2. *Relationship between penicillin $t_{1/2}$ and glomerular filtration rate as measured by inulin clearance*[12]

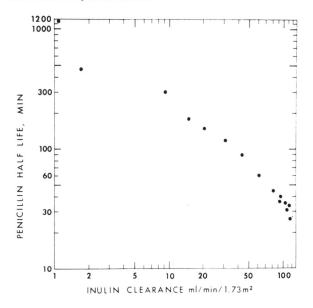

(40–100 million units/day) neurotoxicity and hyperkalemia are definite problems in severe renal impairment. Penicillin G potassium injection contains 1.7 mEq K+ per million units. Neurotoxicity incidence would be greater with concomitant liver disease. Penicillin G dosage should be changed only in severe renal impairment, and a dosing interval of 8–12 hours should be sufficient. Penicillin is bound about 50% to serum proteins, and Schreiner[15] states that hemodialysis reduces penicillin G serum levels, but no quantitative information is given.

*Carbenicillin.* Hoffman et al.[16] studied carbenicillin and found a normal $t_{1/2}$ of one hour and an anuric $t_{1/2}$ of 10–15 hours (Figure 3). With both anuria and liver damage the $t_{1/2}$ may be prolonged to 20 hours or more. Eighty percent or more of an intravenous carbenicillin dose is excreted unchanged in the urine, whereas about 40–43% of an oral dose is recovered in the urine. The values for urinary recovery after an oral dose are based on the work of Wallace et al.[17] They reported an average

Figure 3. *Relationship between creatinine clearance and the serum $t_{1/2}$ of carbenicillin after a single 2-g intravenous dose*[16]

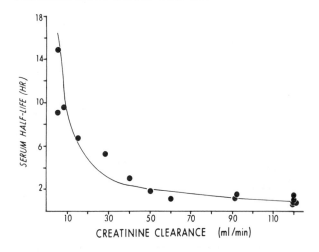

of about 34% recovery, but apparently did not consider that the 500 mg dose of carbenicillin indanyl ester contains only 382 mg of carbenicillin base. When the oral dose of the base is divided by the urinary recovery (mg of base), a value of 40–43% is obtained. Apparently only about 50% of the oral carbenicillin formulation is absorbed. Oral carbenicillin is indicated only for urinary tract infections caused by sensitive strains of *Pseudomonas* and *Proteus. The Medical Letter.*[18] quoting an article by Cox to be published in the *Journal of Infectious Diseases,* states that patients with a $C_{cr} < 14$ ml/min do not excrete orally administered carbenicillin in a concentration sufficient to inhibit sensitive organisms.

The minimum inhibitory concentration (MIC) for most strains of susceptible organisms ranges from 10–50 μg/ml, however, some *Pseudomonas* strains require serum levels of 200–400 μg/ml. It is necessary to give 4–5 g every four hours by continuous i.v. infusion over two hours to maintain blood levels greater than 100 μg/ml. Carbenicillin is not nephrotoxic and is particularly useful in systemic *Pseudomonas* infections when impaired renal function is also present (gentamicin is nephrotoxic and ototoxic). Whelton et al.[19] report that severe renal disease markedly decreases the penetration of carbenicillin into the renal parenchyma. They stress the importance of maintaining elevated serum levels in order to achieve therapeutic levels in the urine and renal tissue.

As with other penicillins, carbenicillin may cause neurotoxicity when given in massive doses (50 g or more over a two-day period). One gram of disodium carbenicillin contains 4.7 mEq of sodium. Obviously, large doses would cause problems with patients requiring sodium restriction. Carbenicillin has been reported to cause hemorrhage due to a disturbance in platelet function. Waisbren et al.[20] have reviewed the several reported cases and warn that this excessive bleeding is more likely to occur with renal impairment and very high serum levels.

The drug is poorly removed by peritoneal dialysis. Hemodialysis is very efficient in reducing carbenicillin blood levels, causing a 50–70% decrease in $t_{1/2}$. The specific dosage adjustments in Table 2 are suggested by Hoffman et al.[16] for patients with renal or hepatic diseases, or both, who have systemic infections caused by *P. aeruginosa.*

*Ampicillin.* Ampicillin has activity against many gram-negative as well as gram-positive bacteria, and the MIC for susceptible organisms may range from 1–8 μg/ml. An early study by Reudy[21] reported a normal serum $t_{1/2}$ of 0.5 hours and an oliguric $t_{1/2}$ of 11–15 hours. Lee and Hill[22] observed that a marked increase in the incidence of side effects (mostly skin rashes) occurs when ampicillin is given in standard doses to patients with severe chronic renal failure. Decreasing the daily dose to 500 mg or less causes the rash to disappear. Jusko et al.[23] studied the elimination kinetics of ampicillin in normal and anephric patients. They found two phases in the elimination of ampicillin from the serum. The first

## Table 2. Proposed Dosage of Carbenicillin for Extraurinary Tract Infections by *Pseudomonas aeruginosa*

| CREATININE CLEARANCE (ml/min) | DOSAGE |
|---|---|
| >30 ± hepatic dysfunction | 4–5 g every 4 hr |
| 10–30 | 2–4 g every 6–12 hr |
| <10 | 2 g every 12 hr |
| <10 + hepatic dysfunction | 2 g every 24 hr |
| Intermittent hemodialysis | 2 g after each dialysis |

short phase represents renal and hepatic elimination plus distribution in various body compartments. The second and major phase represents continued elimination of the drug and has a serum $t_{1/2}$ of 1.3 hours normally, and goes as high as 20 hours in the anephric patient (Figure 4). Jusko et al. found an average of 92% of the i.v. ampicillin dose unchanged in the urine. After an oral dose, 20–65% of the dose may be recovered unchanged. Nonrenal removal mechanisms, i.e., metabolism and biliary excretion, account for only 8% of the ampicillin dose. Ampicillin is bound about 20% to plasma proteins; peritoneal dialysis does not significantly decrease serum levels.[21] Hemodialysis has been shown to reduce the anuric serum $t_{1/2}$ of 20 hours down to about five hours.[23] Due to the wide margin of safety with ampicillin only minor dosage adjustments are indicated.

*Figure 4. Plasma concentrations of ampicillin as a function of time in an anephric patient; data were observed during a period of nondialysis (□) and during hemodialysis where blood samples were collected from the artificial kidney inflow (●) and outflow (○); broken line shows comparative data from normal subjects, and all lines were fitted by computer least-square regression; the data were normalized for a 500-mg dose of ampicillin and 1.73 m² body surface area[23]*

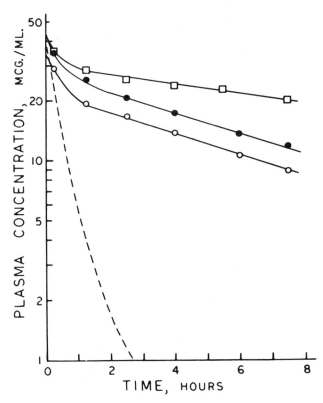

*Hetacillin.* Hetacillin has no antimicrobial action and owes its activity to its hydrolysis product, ampicillin. Jusko et al.[23] have compared the kinetics of hetacillin and ampicillin in normal and anephric patients. The $t_{1/2}$ of the conversion of hetacillin to ampicillin is 12 min, and the overall elimination kinetics can be considered to be the same as for ampicillin. Dosing modifications in renal impairment are the same as those for ampicillin. Hetacillin has no therapeutic advantage over ampicillin.

There are five penicillin derivatives currently in use because they possess antimicrobial activity against penicillinase-producing staphylococci. All of these are clinically effective, but there are certain important differences. These penicillin derivatives are methicillin, dicloxacillin, cloxacillin, nafcillin, and oxacillin.

*Methicillin.* This drug was the first penicillinase-resistant penicillin, but is has some disadvantages when compared to the other derivatives. Methicillin cannot be given orally, and it occasionally produces an allergic interstitial nephritis which causes impaired renal function. Several studies have reported this nephrotoxicity.[24-26] In addition, it is not very active on a relative weight basis and requires relatively high serum levels to reach the MIC. About 70% of a dose of methicillin is excreted in the urine. The normal serum $t_{1/2}$ for methicillin is 0.5 hour and may be as high as four hours in the anuric patient. Liver dysfunction may further prolong the serum $t_{1/2}$ of methicillin. Although the drug is bound only about 39% to serum proteins,[27] hemodialysis is not very effective in lowering serum levels.[28] As with the other penicillins, slight dosage adjustments are indicated in renal impairment.

*Dicloxacillin.* Dicloxacillin is now available in the United States in both oral and injectable forms. Dicloxacillin is well absorbed from the gut and produces serum levels almost twice as high as cloxacillin, oxacillin, or nafcillin.[29-30] It also has a lower in vitro MIC than these other drugs. However, dicloxacillin is more highly bound to serum proteins (96%),[27] and this may reduce its relative greater activity when compared to cloxacillin, nafcillin, and oxacillin.[29] Dicloxacillin has a normal serum $t_{1/2}$ of 0.7 hour and an anuric $t_{1/2}$ of about one hour.[29] Thus dicloxacillin is not significantly retained in renal impairment and can be dosed normally even when severe renal impairment exists. The degree of liver dysfunction reported thus far with the use of dicloxacillin has only slight effects on the serum $t_{1/2}$.[31-32] The drug is not removed significantly by peritoneal dialysis or hemodialysis.[31-32]

*Cloxacillin.* Cloxacillin is a congener of oxacillin and is available only in oral forms. It is well absorbed from the gut and is bound about 94% to serum proteins.[27] It has a normal serum $t_{1/2}$ of 0.5 hour and an anuric $t_{1/2}$ of 0.8 hour.[29] Even in severe renal impairment dosage adjustment is not critical, although an increased dosage interval has been recommended as with the other penicillins. Liver disease has little if any effect on the serum $t_{1/2}$ of cloxacillin. Due to the high degree of protein binding, dialysis should have very little effect on the elimination rate of this drug.

*Oxacillin.* Oxacillin is available in both oral and parenteral forms. It is bound about 95% to serum proteins[27] and has a normal serum $t_{1/2}$ of less than 0.5 hour. In the anuric patient the serum $t_{1/2}$ has been reported from 0.5–1 hour.[28-29] As with the other penicillins, only slight dosage modifications are suggested in severe renal failure and in hepatic dysfunction. Hemodialysis does not significantly remove oxacillin.[27]

*Nafcillin.* Nafcillin is available in both oral and parenteral forms. The oral formulation is absorbed somewhat erratically from the gut.[33] The parenteral form has the advantage of being stable for 24 hours when reconstituted. Nafcillin is 89% bound to serum proteins, and about 30% of a parenteral dose is recovered unchanged in the urine.[27] The normal serum $t_{1/2}$ is about 1.0 hour. As much as 90% of a dose of nafcillin is excreted in the bile, and thus liver disease may increase the serum $t_{1/2}$ of nafcillin. Once excreted in the bile the drug may be reabsorbed and still exert activity. An anuric serum $t_{1/2}$ has not been found in the literature, but the serum $t_{1/2}$ probably does not increase significantly. Although specific references are lacking, it seems that hemodialysis would not be effective in reducing nafcillin serum levels due to the high percentage of serum protein binding.

## Cephalosporins

The cephalosporins are extensively prescribed because of their relative lack of toxicity and their spectrum which includes gram-positive cocci, penicillinase-producing staphylococci, and many gram-negative bacilli. Although there is some cross allergenicity between penicillin and the cephalosporins, many penicillin-sensitive patients can safely receive the cephalosporins. Since the kidney is the major route of cephalosporin elimination, all the presently available derivatives accumulate in renal impairment, and dosage adjustments are particularly important in severe impairment. The toxicity potential is low, except for cephaloridine which is nephrotoxic at high serum levels. Concomitant liver dysfunction may result in additional accumulation of the cephalosporins and could necessitate greater dosage reduction, although definitive studies are lacking.

*Cephalothin.* The pharmacokinetics of cephalothin in renal impairment has been studied by several workers.[34-40] In the normal patient about one-third of a dose of cephalothin given i.v. is desacetylated by the liver enzymes to *o*-desacetylcephalothin,[39] a metabolite which has about one-fifth of the antibacterial activity of cephalothin. Several studies have shown that the normal serum $t_{1/2}$ of cephalothin is about 0.5 hour. Tuano et al.[35] have found that 55% of a cephalothin dose is recovered unchanged in the urine and that the desacetylated metabolite contributes a small additional amount of antimicro-

bial activity. Kabins and Cohen[39] have shown that in the azotemic patient the elimination of cephalothin is biphasic or curvilinear (Figure 5). In 12 severely azotemic patients with a $C_{cr} < 5$ ml/min, they found the serum antibiotic activity to have a $t_{1/2}$ of 2.8 ± 0.9 hours during the first eight hours after a dose. During the 8–24-hour period after a single dose, the $t_{1/2}$ was 12 ± 4 hours. After cessation of multiple doses of cephalothin in severely azotemic patients, the elimination rate is monophasic and a $t_{1/2}$ of about 18 hours exists. In this same study, 69% of the dose (as measured by activity) was recovered in the urine of normal patients, whereas only about 2.5% was found in the urine of the severely azotemic patients. Yamasaku et al.[37] have also reported a biphasic elimination rate for cephalothin. They found a serum activity $t_{1/2}$ of 4.6 hours in the first nine hours and one of about 16 hours over the 9- to 72-hour period. Kirby et al.[38] studied the elimination rate of cephalothin in uremic patients after a multiple-dosing steady state was reached, and they found a serum activity $t_{1/2}$ of three hours in the early stage and 12–18 hours in the later stage of elimination. Several studies have shown that hemodialysis reduces the $t_{1/2}$ of cephalothin to about three hours in the anuric patient.[34,37,38] Peritoneal dialysis is not as efficient as hemodialysis but does remove a small percent of the serum level.[36,37]

Most gram-positive coccal infections require 1 μg/ml for inhibition. These levels are easily reached in the serum of patients with renal impairment, and except in almost complete renal failure these levels are obtained many times over in the urine. Cephalothin direct toxicity is of a low order and the drug can be safely used, with proper dosage adjustments, in renal impairment. There have been several reports of nephrotoxicity with cephalothin. In most reports it was used concurrently with other nephrotoxic drugs, i.e., kanamycin, gentamicin, colistin, and amphotericin B. In most cases there was also preexisting renal disease. Hansten[40] has briefly reviewed these

*Figure 5. Cephalothin decay in vivo after a single 1-g intravenous dose in three patients; $C_{cr}$, creatinine clearance; $t_{1/2}$ serum cephalothin half-life[39]*

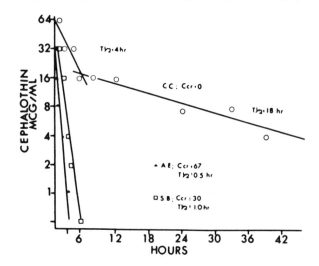

reports and recommends caution in the use of cephalothin with aminoglycosides in renally-impaired patients. A positive direct Coombs' test is frequently encountered and rarely hemolytic anemia. The drug may be dosed normally except in severe renal impairment, where the usual dose should be given every 8–12 hours rather than every four hours. During hemodialysis a 1-g dose at the beginning and end of the dialysis has been recommended.[41] During peritoneal dialysis a dose every 6–12 hours has been recommended by Perkins et al.[36]

*Cephaloridine.* Cephaloridine has been shown in numerous cases to be nephrotoxic.[42-48] Linsell et al.[42] have observed substantial quantities of hyaline casts in the urine of normal patients given a total of 6 g of cephaloridine daily. Foord[43] has noted that nephrotoxicity of cephaloridine was associated with serum levels above 160 µg/ml, while Winchester and Kennedy[49] recommend that 80 µg/ml should not be exceeded. Dodds and Foord[44] have shown that the use of potent diuretics such as furosemide may enhance the nephrotoxicity of cephaloridine. Concomitant use of other nephrotoxic drugs, particularly in the elderly, may be especially dangerous. Existing renal impairment, of course, sets the stage for toxic accumulation of cephaloridine unless proper dosage adjustments are made.

Cephaloridine undergoes less hepatic metabolism than cephalothin, although a significant portion of the dose is inactivated by nonrenal mechanisms. Cephaloridine has a normal serum $t_{1/2}$ of about 1.5 hours, a value about three times that of the other cephalosporins and the penicillins. In the anuric patient the serum $t_{1/2}$ is about 20 hours. [34-38,50] Figure 6 illustrates the changing $t_{1/2}$ of cephaloridine in relation to $C_{cr}$. Cephaloridine is bound to serum proteins only slightly, and hemodialysis is effective in removing the drug. Several studies have shown the serum $t_{1/2}$ to be about 3–4 hours with hemodialysis,[34,37,38] and one study found a $t_{1/2}$ of 8–9 hours on peritoneal dialysis.[34]

In the patient with normal renal function a dose of 500 mg-1 g may be given every 6–12 hours. In mild renal impairment, this interval should be every 8–12 hours; in moderate impairment, every 12–24 hours; and in severe renal impairment, every 24–48 hours. Due to the absence of nephrotoxicity with cephalothin and cephazolin, cephaloridine should be avoided with or without preexisting renal impairment.

*Cephalexin.* This drug has the advantage of oral administration as compared to cephalothin, cephazolin, and cephaloridine. Other than hypersensitivity, no serious adverse effects have been reported to date. Cephalexin is useful for systemic and urinary tract infections and has a spectrum similar to the other cephalosporins. Serum levels up to 12 µg/ml are needed for some gram-positive organisms, and the MIC for some gram-negative organisms may be 30 µg/ml. Kunin and Finkelburg[52] have reported that as much as 98% of a dose of cephalexin is recovered unchanged in the urine within six hours.

Lindquist et al.[52] found that cephalexin has a normal serum $t_{1/2}$ of 0.9 hour and an anuric $t_{1/2}$ of 30 hours or more (Figure 7). Bailey et al.[53] have reported similar pharmacokinetics in renal impairment. Kunin and Finkelburg found a urinary recovery of 100% of a cephalexin dose in one uremic patient, but Bailey et al. report that about 37% of a dose is recovered in 48 hours from patients with a $C_{cr}$ < 10 ml/min. Therapeutic concentrations for most susceptible urinary pathogens are maintained until the $C_{cr}$ is 2.5 ml/min or less.[4] Lindquist et al.[52] have recommended a dosing interval of 8–12 hours with a $C_{cr}$ of 16–30 ml/min, 24 hours with a $C_{cr}$ of 5–15 ml/min and 48–60 hours with a $C_{cr}$ of 0–4 ml/min. Kabins et al.[54] have recommended an initial loading dose of 1 g with a $C_{cr}$ of 10–33 ml/min. They suggest a loading dose of 500 mg followed by 250 mg every 48 hours with a $C_{cr}$ < 10 ml/min. These loading doses seem

*Figure 7. Correlation between cephalexin half-life ($t_{1/2}$) and creatinine clearance*[52]

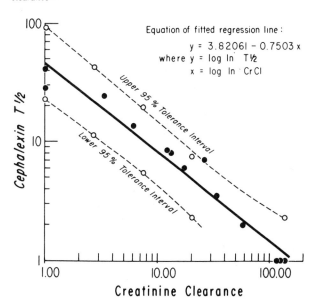

*Figure 6. Relationship between renal function, as expressed by creatinine clearance, and half-life of cephalothin and cephaloridine in serum after a single 500-mg intramuscular injection; each point represents a subject in whom both determinations were made*[34]

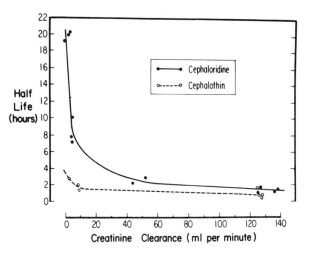

warranted in order to achieve and maintain adequate serum levels in renal impairment.

Hemodialysis effectively removes cephalexin. One study[52] found that the serum $t_{1/2}$ was 6.3 hours on hemodialysis and 30.8 hours without dialysis. A 500-mg dose at the end of dialysis resulted in serum levels of 3–6 $\mu$g/ml prior to the next dialysis. Hemodialysis (12 hours) removed 75% of a dose of cephalexin given at the beginning of dialysis. Bailey et al.[53] have reported a serum $t_{1/2}$ of 4.5 hours during hemodialysis. Yamasaku et al.[37] found that peritoneal dialysis was not nearly as efficient as hemodialysis in removing cephalexin; peritoneal dialysis removed the drug at a rate similar to a $C_{cr}$ of 16 ml/min.

*Cephaloglycin.* Cephaloglycin is another orally administered cephalosporin, but it has no important advantages over the more versatile cephalexin. Cephaloglycin is indicated only for urinary infections, whereas cephalexin is useful for both systemic and urinary infections. Peak serum levels of cephaloglycin are inadequate to treat systemic infections, but the drug is concentrated adequately in the urine.[55] Cephaloglycin is more active in an acidic urine than a neutral or alkaline one, while cephalexin activity is not altered by changes in urine $p$H.[56] In one study on the use of cephaloglycin in renally-impaired patients, the authors found that patients with a $C_{cr}$ as low as 20 ml/min could excrete a urine concentration of 20 $\mu$g/ml. The authors postulated that patients with severely reduced renal function can still achieve bactericidal urine concentrations of cephaloglycin.[57] These authors reported an anuric $t_{1/2}$ of 14 hours and a normal serum $t_{1/2}$ of four hours. The latter figure is incorrect since cephaloglycin is rapidly eliminated similarly to cephalexin, and thus the anuric serum $t_{1/2}$ may also be incorrect.

*Cephacetrile.* This is an investigational cephalosporin which accumulates in renal impairment similar to the other cephalosporins. It is allegedly not nephrotoxic as is cephaloridine. Nissenson et al.[58] studied 15 patients whose renal function ranged from normal to anephric. All subjects received a dose of 20 mg/kg, and the normal subjects received cephacetrile via a constant infusion pump at a rate of 400–500 mg/hour for three hours. The average serum concentration at the end of three hours was 22 $\mu$g/ml and was reached within one hour after initiating the infusion. The mean serum $t_{1/2}$ was $1.3 \pm 0.3$ hours in the normal subjects. An average of 88% of the dose was recovered unchanged in the urine. In patients with a $C_{cr} < 1$ ml/min, the cephacetrile serum $t_{1/2}$ was $23.7 \pm 5.9$ hours. Hemodialysis decreased the mean serum $t_{1/2}$ to $4.7 \pm 0.7$ hours, a decrease of 70%. Exact dosage modifications are not suggested in the article, but appear to be on the order of those for cephaloridine.

*Cephazolin.* Cephazolin is a recently marketed parenteral cephalosporin which may be administered i.m. or i.v. Kirby and Regamey[59] compared the pharmacokinetics of cephazolin to those of cephaloridine, cephalothin, and cephalexin in healthy adults. After i.m. and i.v. injections, the serum concentration of cephazolin was twice as high as that of cephaloridine and four times as high as that of cephalothin. An i.v. infusion of 500 mg of cephazolin over a 20-minute period gave a peak level of 118 $\mu$g/ml, as compared with 70 $\mu$g/ml after a 1-g dose of cephalothin. The serum $t_{1/2}$'s for cephazolin, cephaloridine, and cephalothin were 1.8, 1.1, and 0.5 hour, respectively. Corresponding renal clearances were 64 ml/min/1.73 m$^2$, 125 ml/min/1.73 m$^2$, and 274 ml/min/1.73 m$^2$. Almost 100% of the dose of cephazolin was recovered in the urine within 24 hours. Protein binding of cephazolin was 86% and the apparent volume of distribution was 10 liters/1.73 m$^2$.

Craig et al.[60] have studied the kinetics of cephazolin in normal and uremic patients. In healthy adults given equivalent doses of cephazolin and cephalothin, cephazolin serum levels exceeded those of cephalothin by four- to six-fold, and concentrations of free cephazolin were three times higher. Serum protein binding of cephazolin was 84% while that of cephalothin was 65%. The normal serum $t_{1/2}$ of cephazolin was 1.9 hours and was as long as 35 hours in severe uremia. High urine concentrations of cephazolin were obtained even in patients with a $C_{cr}$ as low as 10 mg/min.

Levinson et al.[61] have studied the kinetics of cephazolin in renal impairment. The mean serum $t_{1/2}$ was 2.2 hours with $C_{cr}$ of 26 ml/min, 12.0 hours with $C_{cr}$ of 12–17 ml/min, and 56.6 hours with a $C_{cr} < 5$ ml/min. Hemodialysis lowered the serum $t_{1/2}$ to 8.8 hours in patients with a $C_{cr} < 5$ ml/min. Peritoneal dialysis had little effect on the serum $t_{1/2}$. McCloskey et al.[62] found a mean serum $t_{1/2}$ of 6.5 hours during hemodialysis of seven patients. They administered a 500 mg i.v. dose of cephazolin prior to dialysis, and found that dialysis removed 138 mg of drug. Prior to the next dialysis the serum level of cephazolin was 8–10 $\mu$g/ml, a sufficient level for most susceptible bacteria. They recommend a single dose prior to each dialysis with no additional drug after dialysis. Rein et al.[63] have reported an anuric cephazolin $t_{1/2}$ of 42 hours. In more severe degrees of renal impairment, half the usual dose approximately every $t_{1/2}$ should prove sufficient.

Cephazolin appears to be a promising addition to the cephalosporin antibiotics. It provides higher and more prolonged levels of free drug, while being as active microbiologically as cephalothin. It apparently does not possess the nephrotoxicity of cephaloridine and can be given i.m. It should replace cephaloridine in practice, and it may replace cephalothin. Definitive studies in cases of meningitis are needed to allow a good comparison with cephazolin.

### The Tetracyclines

There are eight tetracycline derivatives in current use in the United States, and considerable data are available on their use in renal impairment. Tetracycline, oxytetracycline, methacycline, rolitetracycline, and probably demeclocycline accumulate if dosed normally in renal impairment, and grave toxicity is possible. Doxycycline and chlortetracycline do not accumulate when dosed normally in renal impairment, but chlortetracycline may cause a large increase in the blood urea nitrogen. There is conflicting data on the status of minocycline use in renal impairment.

The tetracyclines are generally effective in serum levels of 4 $\mu$g/ml or less. The tetracyclines are often thought to be nontoxic, but severe complications may result when serum levels are above 12 $\mu$g/ml. Pregnant women or mothers with newborns are particularly prone to acute fatty liver and pancreatitis even when given normal amounts of tetracyclines. Often there is concomitantly unrecognized nephrotoxicity.[64,65] Outdated, degraded tetracycline has produced a Fanconi-like syndrome with renal tubular damage.[66] It has also been noted that the concurrent use of tetracycline and methoxyflurane may result in serious impairment of renal function.[67] Tetracyclines have an antianabolic effect and will normally cause a rise in blood urea nitrogen, but not serum uric acid and creatinine.[68]

*Tetracycline.* With preexisting azotemia, tetracycline can cause a greatly increased level of blood urea nitrogen, acidosis, electrolyte imbalance, and even death.[69] Increased sodium excretion with resulting hypovolemia may result. Serum levels of 12 $\mu$g/ml or more can produce acidosis, hyperphosphatemia, and further increases in blood urea nitrogen in the azotemic patient, and levels of 16 $\mu$g/ml can be hepatotoxic. George and Evans[70] have shown that in uremic patients tetracycline also causes a rise in $S_{cr}$ and a fall in $C_{cr}$. A rise in BUN is often accompanied by renal function deterioration which is potentially lethal. Diuretics will accentuate the rise in BUN. Kunin et al.[71] studied the accumulation of tetracycline in renal impairment and found that the serum $t_{1/2}$ may increase from 6–8 hours in the normal patient to at least 110 hours in anuric patients (Figure 8). Hem-

odialysis resulted in a 14–17% decrease in tetracycline serum levels in three patients. Kunin et al. recommend that in mild renal impairment tetracycline can be dosed normally with appropriate checks on blood urea nitrogen, acid-base balance, and electrolyte balance. In moderate renal impairment the dosing interval should be every 24–48 hours while in severe impairment the drug should be dosed every 48–96 hours.

*Oxytetracycline.* Oxytetracycline possesses the same liabilities as tetracycline in renal impairment. Two cancer patients treated with oxytetracycline apparently died from toxicity due to drug accumulation. One died after reaching serum levels of 12.8 $\mu$g/ml and the other after reaching levels of 15 $\mu$g/ml.[72] A German study[73] has reported that oxytetracycline accumulates like tetracycline in renal impairment, and a New Zealand study[74] has shown that uremia is increased by the drug. Fabre et al.[75] have shown that the usual serum $t_{1/2}$ of about nine hours will increase to 48–66 hours in the anuric patient. Figure 9 relates the serum $t_{1/2}$ of oxytetracycline to the $S_{cr}$ rather than the $C_{cr}$. Oxytetracycline has no important advantages over tetracycline and can be avoided in the normal or renally-impaired patient. Using the methods of Dettli et al.,[4] guidelines for dosage in renal impairment can be estimated from Figure 9. Merier et al.[76] have shown that oxytetracycline is easily dialyzable. Hemodialysis cleared the blood at a rate of 60 ml/min, and the serum $t_{1/2}$ was reduced from about 54 hours to 12 hours.

*Methacycline.* Fabre et al.[77] of Geneva have studied the dosing of methacycline in renal impairment. For adult patients with normal renal function, 300 mg of methacycline every 12 hours maintains a fairly constant serum level of about 2 $\mu$g/ml. After three-day therapy in a group of patients with an average $C_{cr}$ of 23 ml/min, the serum levels were an average of 2.6 times greater than in normal patients. From the data obtained, the authors recommend a normal dosing when $C_{cr}$ is > 40 ml/min, a 300 mg dose every 24 hours with a $C_{cr}$ of 20–40 ml/min, a dose every 48 hours between 10–20 ml/

*Figure 8. Relationship of half-life of tetracycline in serum following an intravenous dose to the renal function as reflected in the creatinine clearance* [71]

*Figure 9. Serum half-life of oxytetracycline as a function of blood creatinine levels (regression curve and confidence limits p = 0.05)* [75]

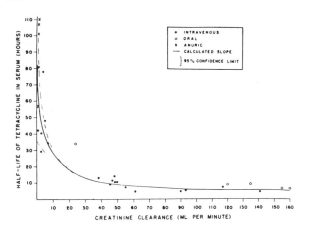

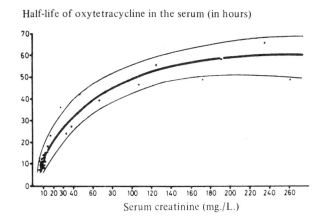

Half-life of oxytetracycline in the serum (in hours)

Serum creatinine (mg./L.)

min, every 72 hours between 5–10 ml/min, and every 96 hours in anuria.

*Minocycline.* This is a new tetracycline derivative which has not been well studied in renal impairment. One report by Bernard et al.[78] indicates that the drug accumulates in the manner of tetracycline in renal impairment. In normal patients they found the serum $t_{1/2}$ to be about 13 hours, whereas eight patients with renal impairment had a $t_{1/2}$ of 18–68 hours. The higher $t_{1/2}$ was observed with a $C_{cr}$ of 3 ml/min. This finding is somewhat surprising since the authors found that only 6% of a minocycline dose is normally recovered unchanged in the urine. Two more recent studies, one by Lang[79] and the other by McHenry and Wagner,[80] report findings different from those of Bernard et al. Both of these studies found no significant change in overall elimination of minocycline in uremic patients as compared to patients with normal renal function. Lang reported a normal serum $t_{1/2}$ of 12–16 hours, similar to that reported by Bernard et al. George et al. of Australia[81] have reported a significant increase in blood urea nitrogen in eight renally-impaired patients receiving oral minocycline for four days. The average increase in blood urea nitrogen was 51 mg/100 ml. The maximum serum levels were normal in four of the patients, mildly elevated in three, and very high in one (12 µg/ml). The kinetics of minocycline may not be predictable in renal impairment, for reasons unknown. Minocycline should not be used in renal impairment until more definitive studies are performed.

*Demeclocycline.* One study has shown that demeclocycline further increases the blood urea nitrogen in the uremic patient,[74] but other studies in renal impairment have not been located. Demeclocycline is probably the most photosensitizing tetracycline derivative, and it possesses no important advantages over tetracycline. It can be avoided in the patient with normal renal function and should not be used in any degree of renal impairment.

*Rolitetracycline.* One study on the use of rolitetracycline in renal impairment has been located, and the serum $t_{1/2}$ increased from 12 hours in the normal patient to 35 hours in the anuric patient.[82] It has no distinguishing advantages over tetracycline and should be avoided in renal impairment.

*Chlortetracycline.* Of the eight tetracycline derivatives, doxycycline and chlortetracycline are unique in their pharmacokinetics during renal impairment. Kunin et al.[71] have studied the serum levels of chlortetracycline in normal and renally-impaired patients. In renal impairment the serum $t_{1/2}$ of chlortetracycline does not increase. Even in anuria, the serum $t_{1/2}$ for chlortetracycline did not exceed 11 hours, the normal being about seven hours. Chlortetracycline is unstable in serum and alkaline aqueous solutions,[83] and it is also not normally excreted as rapidly in the urine as tetracycline. There are reports of its sequestration in the liver.[84] Whereas Kunin et al.[71] have recommended no dosing modifica-

tions in renal impairment, Shils[85] has reported that chlortetracycline increased the blood urea nitrogen from 80 to 160 mg/100 ml in a patient with advanced renal disease receiving 250 mg twice daily for six days. If dosing adjustments are made to prevent the increase in uremia, subtherapeutic serum levels will result. Thus chlortetracycline cannot be recommended for patients with renal impairment.

*Doxycycline.* Doxycycline is a relatively new tetracycline and its pharmacokinetics in renal impairment has been well studied, particularly in several French, German, and Swiss studies. Fabre et al.[86] first observed that the serum $t_{1/2}$ of doxycycline is not increased in renal impairment. Several other studies[87-92] confirmed this initial work of Fabre et al. Whereas tetracyclines as a group exert an antianabolic effect and increase blood urea nitrogen, doxycycline has been found to have no significant effect on blood urea nitrogen.[74] The lack of accumulation in renal impairment has also been confirmed in the i.v. use of doxycycline.[89] Doxycycline may thus be dosed in renal impairment at its usual maintenance dose without fear of toxicity. Doxycycline is bound 80–90% to serum proteins, and is not significantly removed by hemodialysis.[91-92] The serum $t_{1/2}$ for doxycycline varies from 13–22 hours in the various studies reported. It is generally recognized that doxycycline is the longest acting of the tetracyclines. For a good comparative pharmacokinetic study of several tetracycline analogs, the work of Doluisio and Dittert[93] should be read.

In summary, all of the tetracycline derivatives except doxycycline and chlortetracycline, and perhaps minocycline, accumulate in renal impairment, and all except doxycycline will greatly increase blood urea nitrogen. Grave toxicity can result if serum levels exceed 12 µg/ml with the various tetracyclines. For patients with normal renal function requiring a tetracycline antibiotic, tetracycline hydrochloride is the drug of choice due to its low cost and general effectiveness. In renal impairment, doxycycline either orally or i.v. may be very useful for systemic infections particularly if renal status is not well known and the physician is not knowledgeable in dosing adjustments for tetracycline. For urinary tract infections, particularly in renal impairment, doxycycline has the disadvantage of low urinary excretion when compared to tetracycline. In renal impairment doxycycline is dosed in the usual way and does not accumulate, does not significantly increase blood urea nitrogen, and has shown no toxicity.

## Antifungals

*Amphotericin.* Amphotericin has been the mainstay of therapy for systemic fungal infections during the past 15 years. Nephrotoxicity and hypokalemia are the two major factors limiting the amount of amphotericin B that may be administered to patients.[94] Hypokalemia is the most characteristic and widely recognized complication of amphotericin B therapy and this can be corrected with oral potassium supplements. About 80% of patients receiving the drug experience some degree of nephrotoxicity, and the danger is particularly great when there is prior renal impairment. Both glomerular and tubular lesions are common. The damage is usually reversible if the total dose is less than 5 g, but is frequently irreversible above this amount.[95] Renal tubular acidosis also commonly occurs.[96] An early sign of impending renal damage is a rise in urine $pH$ of at least 0.5 unit. The usual dose employed has been an i.v. injection once daily, but alternate day dosing has proven to be better tolerated by the patient. Renal toxicity is apparently about the same on each regimen.[97]

The pharmacokinetics of amphotericin B is apparently quite complicated. Bindshadler and Bennett[97] have studied the serum, urine, and cerebrospinal fluid levels after i.v. infusions on both daily and alternate day therapy. Included in the study were 17 patients, three of whom were renally-impaired. The i.v. infusions were over a four-hour period, and "peak" levels were measured immediately after the infusion and "valley" levels just prior to the next infusion. At the end of the infusion only about 10% of the dose is accounted for in the serum. Assuming an equal concentration in extracellular body water, no more than 40% of the dose is in this body compartment. Urinary excretion accounts for only 2–5% of the dose; thus, a large portion of the injection is apparently inactivated or stored by some mechanism. Traces of amphotericin B can be detected in the urine up to two months after a dose,[98] and some of the drug remains in the tissues up to a year after therapy.[99] Bindshadler and Bennett[97] found that doses up to 90 mg on alternate days gave higher peak serum levels than doses up to 45 mg daily, but that the valley serum levels were similar. The drug did not tend to accumulate after repeated doses. In the patients with renal impairment, the peak serum levels tended to correlate positively with increasing serum creatinine; however, renal impairment did not increase the valley serum levels. Preexisting renal disease had no consistent effect upon either excretion of amphotericin B or plasma concentrations of the drug. To avoid nephrotoxicity with the use of amphotericin B, the smallest and least frequent doses that are effective should be used. The prediction of the exact regimen needed does not seem possible from available data.

*Flucytosine.* This is a new antifungal effective in many cases of crytococcosis and candidiasis. In the United States, the drug is available only in oral form and the usual dose is 50–150 mg/kg/day divided into four doses. Flucytosine is well absorbed from the gut and about 90% of the dose is recovered unchanged in the urine.[100] Less than 4% of the dose is metabolized.[101] A 2-g dose in adults produces peak serum levels of 30–40 μg/ml. Flucytosine is 48–49% bound to serum protein and is removed by hemodialysis. An early study[100] reported the serum $t_{1/2}$ for two patients with renal impairment. Ex-

trapolation of the data on semi-log paper indicates that the normal serum $t_{1/2}$ is about three hours and the anuric serum $t_{1/2}$ is 2–3 days. A subsequent study by Schönebeck reports a normal serum $t_{1/2}$ of 2.9 hours and an anuric serum $t_{1/2}$ of 70 hours (Figure 10).[101] The manufacturer's package insert suggests a dose of 50 mg/kg/day in renal impairment, but there is no basis for this advice and the great range of renal impairment is ignored. The chief toxicity of flucytosine has been a reversible bone marrow suppression. It appears that there is no nephrotoxicity. In a patient with normal renal function, a maintenance dose every six hours (two half-lives) produces no toxic accumulation of drug. To maintain a dose approximately every second $t_{1/2}$ in renal impairment, the following schedule is suggested:[102]

| $C_{cr}/1.73 M^2$ | $T_{1/2}$ (hr) | $K_e$ | Dose Recommended |
| --- | --- | --- | --- |
| 100 ml/min | 2.9 | .24 | 12–35 mg/kg/6 hours |
| 50 ml/min | 5.8 | .12 | 12–35 mg/kg/12 hours |
| 10 ml/min | 23.1 | .03 | 12–35 mg/kg/48 hours |
| 0 ml/min | 70 | .01 | 12–35 mg/kg/6 days |

When the $C_{cr}$ is 10 ml/min or less, half the usual dose given every half-life may prevent subtherapeutic serum levels from being present for extended periods of time. For example, with a $C_{cr}$ of 10 ml/min a dose of 6–18 mg/kg/24 hours may maintain more optional serum levels than a larger dose every two days.

*Griseofulvin.* Griseofulvin is given orally to treat mycotic infections of the skin, hair, and nails due to Micros-

*Figure 10. $k_e$ in relation to creatinine clearance, $C_{cr}$; the point where the line intersects the ordinate ($C_{cr} = 0$) is $k_{nr}$, i.e., the portion of 5-fluorocytosine that is eliminated by extrarenal routes[101]*

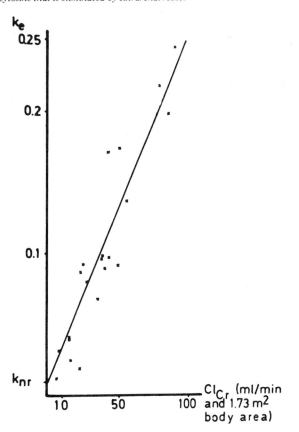

porum, Trichophyton, and Epidermophyton. Less than 1% of a dose of griseofulvin is recovered in the urine, most being found in the feces due to biliary excretion and poor absorption. Griseofulvin can cause albuminuria and cylindruria, but there is no evidence of it causing a decreased GFR. With such a low degree of urinary excretion, there is no reason to suspect complications if used in patients with renal impairment.[103]

### Polymyxins

*Polymyxin B.* Polymyxin B is a cationic polypeptide detergent which is useful against many gram-negative infections. It is very poorly absorbed when given orally or applied to the surface of burns. About 60% of an i.m. dose can be recovered in the urine within three days of the dose. Concentrations up to 100 $\mu$g/ml are found in the urine after usual doses.[103] Polymyxin B can produce azotemia, respiratory paralysis through neuromuscular blockade, and a decrease in the GFR. Parenteral doses of 2.5 mg/kg/day frequently cause proteinuria, cylindruria, and hematuria. With doses above 3 mg/kg/day, azotemia frequently develops and the GFR diminishes. These effects are reversible if treatment is short. In patients with normal renal function, the administration of 2.2 mg/kg/day is not accompanied by significant nephrotoxicity. Patients with mild or moderate renal impairment should receive 1–1.5 mg/kg/day for 5–10 days. Those with severe renal impairment should receive two or three normal doses to achieve adequate serum and tissue levels, and then doses should be stopped or sharply reduced.[104] The serum $t_{1/2}$ in normal patients is about 4.4 hours, while in the oliguric patient it may be 35 hours or so.[4]

*Colistin.* This is a polypeptide antibiotic similar to polymixin B. It is available as colistin sulfate for oral use and as sodium colistimethate for parenteral use. Colistin sulfate is not appreciably absorbed following oral administration and is used only for infections of the gastrointestinal tract caused by susceptible organisms. The remainder of this discussion concerns only the parenteral form of colistin. Colistimethate is excreted primarily by glomerular filtration. Urine levels of the active antibiotic are considerably higher than serum levels. Because of the relatively low serum concentration, colistimethate is more effective against urinary tract infections than against systemic infections. It is used primarily for urinary tract infections caused by susceptible strains of *Pseudomonas aeruginosa* and other susceptible gram-negative organisms. Most strains of *Proteus* are resistant. The normal serum $t_{1/2}$ of colistimethate is 1.5 hours, and the anuric $t_{1/2}$ is greater than 10 hours.[105] In normal individuals, 60–75% of colistimethate is recovered in the urine. The dosage interval must be increased for colistimethate in all stages of renal impairment. McKay and Kaye[105] have suggested a single 2 mg/kg dose when anuria is present. Although protein binding is

low for colistimethate, hemodialysis does not appreciably lower blood levels. There are conflicting reports on the effectiveness of peritoneal dialysis in decreasing serum levels.[105-107]

Patients with normal renal function receiving daily colistimethate doses greater than 5 mg/kg may develop neurotoxicity and nephrotoxicity.[108] Patients 50 years and older are more susceptible to nephrotoxicity and should receive daily doses no larger than 2.5–3 mg/kg. Neurotoxicity caused by colistimethate is most commonly characterized by parasthesias; but severe CNS symptoms, including convulsions and coma, are seen in uremic patients.

### Aminoglycosides

*Streptomycin.* Streptomycin has been in clinical use since 1945 and several years passed before the danger of ototoxicity in renal impairment was well understood. The Second Edition of *The Pharmacologic Basis of Therapeutics* in 1955 warned about the danger of serum accumulation in renal impairment, but subsequent articles indicated that this advice was not applied in practice.[109,110] A total dose as small as 3 g in three days has been known to produce vestibular damage.[109] The nephrotoxic symptoms may not appear until 3–4 weeks after cessation of therapy, and this fact may complicate recognition of streptomycin overdose.[110] Kunin and Finland[13] were the first to describe well the elimination kinetics of streptomycin. Streptomycin is about 34% bound to serum proteins and glomerular filtration clears 30–70 ml of blood per minute. They found the normal serum $t_{1/2}$ to be 2–3 hours, and in one woman with a urine output of about 210 ml daily, the $t_{1/2}$ went as high as 110 hours. In mild renal impairment, the maintenance dose (1 g usually) should be given once daily. In moderate renal impairment a dose every 2–3 days should be sufficient, and in severe impairment a dose every 3–4 days is sufficient. Streptomycin can be effectively removed by hemodialysis.[110]

*Gentamicin.* This drug is potentially nephrotoxic and ototoxic, and its use should be reserved for serious infections caused by susceptible organisms resistant to safer antibiotics. The drug is almost completely eliminated by the kidneys and accumulates in all degrees of renal impairment. During the first few days of therapy, only about 40% of the administered dose is recovered in the urine. After this, the amount recovered in the urine each day is about the same as the dose given. Gentamicin binding to serum proteins cannot be demonstrated under controlled conditions.[111] The normal serum $t_{1/2}$ is about two hours,[112] and the anuric $t_{1/2}$ may reach 67 hours. The therapeutic serum level for gentamicin is 4–8 $\mu$g/ml. A serum level $\geq$ 12 $\mu$g/ml and/or prolonged therapy (> 10 days) are associated with nephrotoxicity and damage to the vestibular and auditory portions of the eighth cranial nerve. Previous administration of other ototoxic drugs, such as streptomycin or kanamycin, may redispose to gentamicin toxicity. Potent diuretics, such as ethacrynic acid and furosemide, may enhance ototoxicity.

McHenry et al.[113] have reported the relationship between the serum creatinine concentration and the serum $t_{1/2}$ of gentamicin (Figure 11). Cutler et al.[114] combined their data with that of McHenry et al. to produce another plot (Figure 12) of serum creatinine versus drug $t_{1/2}$. They recommend the following formula to estimate the serum $t_{1/2}$ of gentamicin from the serum creatinine level: $t_{1/2}$ (hrs) = 4 × serum creatinine (mg/100 ml). McHenry et al. suggest dosing 1–1.3 mg/kg every second $t_{1/2}$ during renal impairment to prevent accumulation. They have experienced clinical success with such a regimen despite periods of subtherapeutic serum levels. Using their recommendation, an 80-kg man with a serum creatinine of 4.0 would be dosed as follows:

Dose = 80 kg × 1.0 mg/kg = 80 mg
$t_{1/2}$ = 4 × $S_{cr}$ = 4 × 4 = 16 hours
Dosing interval = 16 × 2 = 32 hrs
Schedule = 80 mg every 32 hrs

This dosage schedule may not be optimal when the $t_{1/2}$ is 24 hours or more since periods of several hours lapse with subinhibitory serum levels and the dosage administration schedule is difficult to follow. More effective serum levels may be achieved by giving half the loading dose every $t_{1/2}$.

Cutler et al. suggest giving a loading dose of 2 mg/kg every third $t_{1/2}$. Therefore the empirical dosing interval would be 12 × serum creatinine. In severe renal failure, such a schedule would result in even greater periods of subtherapeutic serum levels than the schedules suggested by McHenry et al. Cutler et al. do offer an alternative, however, in the form of the nomogram shown in Figure 13. This nomogram is not very useful if the serum creatinine is more than 5 mg/100 ml. The nomogram is

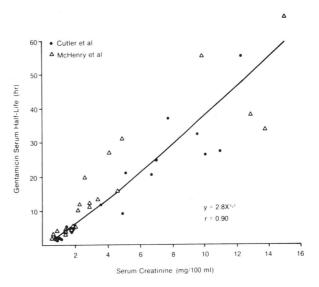

*Figure 12. Correlation of gentamicin sulfate half-life and serum creatinine concentration (combined data)[114]*

used to calculate the gentamicin dose to be given every eight or 12 hours. Assuming a 2 mg/kg loading dose, the proper dose for either an 8- or 12-hour interval can be determined if the patient's weight and serum creatinine are known. A loading dose of 2 mg/kg is about twice the recommended dose of 1–1.3 mg/kg and should be used only in life-threatening infections, and this nomogram should only be used in such conditions. Chan et al.[115] have also developed a nomogram (Figure 14) designed to maintain safe, inhibitory gentamicin levels of 3–8 μg/ml. Their nomogram regimen is based on the elimination constant ($K_2$) for eight-hour periods. During hemodialysis Chan et al. recommend giving 1 mg/kg initially, then a small sustaining dose, calculated from the nomogram, every eight hours. The loading dose of 1.7 mg/kg suggested by Chan et al. is somewhat higher than the recommended dose of 1–1.3 mg/kg. However, in severe infections such doses are justified. Chan et al. reported clinical success in 17 patients with renal failure and life-threatening infections. The gentamicin serum

*Figure 11. Relationship of serum half-life of gentamicin to serum creatinine concentration in 24 patients[113]*

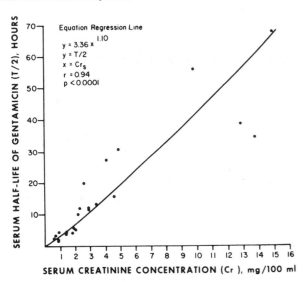

*Figure 13. Nomogram for calculating interval gentamicin sulfate dose if loading dose and serum creatinine concentration are known; for example, an 80-kg patient receiving 160-mg loading dose (2 mg/kg) with serum creatinine concentration of 10 mg/100 ml should receive 20 mg every eight hours[114]*

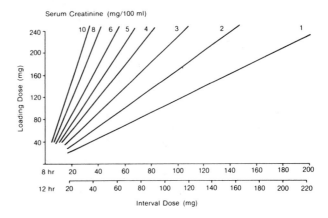

Figure 14. Dosage nomogram for patients with renal failure; to use the nomogram regimen, a loading dose of gentamicin, 1.7 mg/kg body weight, is administered; the sustaining dose is determined by passing a line perpendicular from the patient's $C_{cr}$ value to the point where it intercepts the sloping line ($K^2$ versus the $C_{cr}$) on the nomogram; from the point of intercept, a horizontal line intersects the dose schedule, on the right side; this dose should be given every eight hours for steady-state therapy[115]

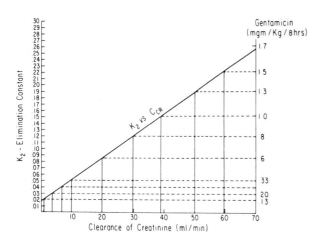

Figure 15. Using serum creatinine concentration as a determinant of renal function, Cutler and Orme derived a regression equation for kanamycin half-life: y (half-life) = 2.8 + 2.5x (serum creatinine concentration); when this equation is plotted, one sees a straight-line relationship of drug half-life to serum creatinine concentration[3]

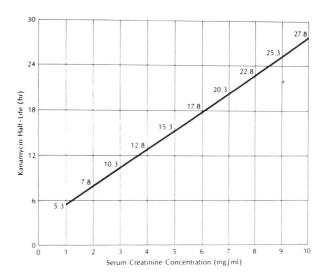

levels stayed in the 3–8 μg/ml range, and there were no cases of toxicity.

Both of the nomograms vary the maintenance dose administered while keeping a rather short and constant dosing interval. This results in less serum level fluctuations. This is similar, as far as serum levels are concerned, to the idea of giving half the loading dose every $t_{1/2}$ rather than a full dose every other $t_{1/2}$. Of the several dosing recommendations, that of Chan appears to be the soundest in theory. The reader is reminded that in patients with changing renal function it is necessary to calculate the dose and schedule periodically during therapy. Also, the dosing schedules determined by these formulas and nomograms should be checked when possible by obtaining serum gentamicin levels.

*Kanamycin.* As with other aminoglycosides, kanamycin is an extremely toxic antibiotic and its use should be restricted to serious infections caused by susceptible organisms that are resistant to safer antibacterial agents. The drug is excreted rapidly and almost completely by the kidneys and accumulates in all degrees of renal impairment. Nearly all of a parenteral dose is excreted in the urine within 6–9 hours. The normal serum $t_{1/2}$ is 3–5 hours and may reach 84 hours[116] in severely azotemic patients. Using the data of Cutler and Orme,[117] Kunin[3] plotted a graph (Figure 15) showing an essentially linear relationship between kanamycin serum $t_{1/2}$ and serum creatinine concentration.

Therapeutic serum levels are 10–30 μg/ml. Normally peak serum levels should not exceed 30 μg/ml to avoid the nephrotoxic and ototoxic (both auditory and vestibular) effects of kanamycin. Parenteral daily doses should not exceed 15 mg/kg or a total daily dose of 1.5 g regardless of the patient's weight. A total of 20 g for the entire course of treatment should not be exceeded. The inci-

dence of ototoxicity and nephrotoxicity is increased with previous or concomitant administration of other ototoxic and nephrotoxic drugs and with increased age. Dehydration increases the chance of nephrotoxicity. Kanamycin given orally is poorly absorbed, but the small amount absorbed, about 0.6%,[118] can accumulate in azotemic patients taking large doses as a bowel preparation.

The approximate serum $t_{1/2}$ for kanamycin in uremic patients can be determined empirically by multiplying the serum creatinine by no more than five and no less than three.[116] The most widely accepted formula as determined by Cutler and Orme[117] is as follows: $t_{1/2}$ (hrs) = 3 × serum creatinine (mg/100 ml). Their kinetic analysis predicts that a loading dose of 7 mg/kg repeated every third $t_{1/2}$ will result in therapeutic, nontoxic serum levels in patients with renal failure. It should be pointed out that during severe renal failure, when the $t_{1/2}$ is prolonged to several days, dosing every third $t_{1/2}$ can result in extended periods of subtherapeutic serum levels. Less fluctuation in the maximum and minimum serum levels can be achieved by giving 3.5 mg/kg of kanamycin every $t_{1/2}$ after an initial 7 mg/kg loading dose. This should produce no accumulation of the antibiotic provided the $t_{1/2}$ is calculated accurately. In the anuric patient a single 7 mg/kg loading dose should give adequate serum levels for the entire treatment period.

Mawer et al.[119] have developed a nomogram (Figure 16) for determining dosage schedules of kanamycin that are applicable to patients with all degrees of renal impairment. The nomogram takes into account renal function (as determined by serum creatinine), age, sex and body weight and is designed to give a therapeutic serum concentration of 10–30 μg/ml two hours after each dose. If the patient is severely oliguric, the dose schedule should be obtained by joining with a straight line the

*Figure 16. Nomogram for calculating kanamycin dosage in renal impairment; join with a straight line the serum-creatinine concentration appropriate to the sex on scale A and the age on scale B; mark the point at which the straight line cuts line C; join with a straight line the mark on line C and the body weight on scale D; mark the points at which this line cuts the dosage line L and M; The loading dose (mg) is written against the marked part of line L; the maintenance dose (mg) and the appropriate interval (hours) between doses are written against the marked part of line M[116]*

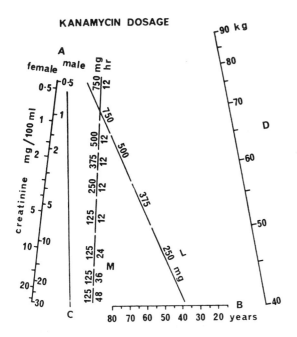

glycoside which may possess greater activity against *Pseudomonas* than does gentamicin. The pharmacokinetics of tobramycin is remarkably similar to that of gentamicin. Regamy et al.[121] did a comparative study of the two drugs in four healthy adult volunteers. Mean peak blood levels after a one-hour infusion of 100 mg were 4.86 $\mu$g/ml for gentamicin and 4.61 $\mu$g/ml for tobramycin. A steady state was obtained with an infusion rate of 30 mg/hour, and during the third hour the serums levels were 3.90 $\mu$g/ml for gentamicin and 3.83 $\mu$g/ml for tobramycin. When the infusions were stopped the blood levels declined according to first order kinetics; a $t_{1/2}$ of 2.0 hours for gentamicin and 2.15 hours for tobramycin were calculated. Eighty-one percent of the gentamicin dose and 88% of the tobramycin dose were recovered unchanged in the urine within 24 hours. Regamy et al. report that under physiologic conditions of temperature and *p*H there is no serum protein binding of tobramycin or gentamicin. The renal clearance of the two drugs was about 95% of the $C_{cr}$.

Lockwood and Bower[122] found the serum $t_{1/2}$ of tobramycin to be the same as that of gentamicin in patients with similar renal function. The values ranged from two hours in normal volunteers to 53.4 hours in anephric patients. Both drugs were readily removed from the serum by the Kiil artificial kidney, with a 70% reduction in serum level during a 12-hour dialysis. Apparently, tobramycin will require dosage adjustments in renal impairment very similar to those required for gentamicin.

lowest point on line C to the body weight on scale D. For example, a 70-year-old, 70-kg male with a serum creatinine of 4 mg/100 ml should receive a loading dose of approximately 450 mg and a maintenance dose of 200 mg every 12 hours according to the nomogram. Using the equation of Cutler and Orme,[117] the same patient would receive 500 mg every 36 hours.

Dose = 7 mg/kg × 70 kg = 490 = 500 mg (approx.)
$t_{1/2}$ = 3 × $S_{cr}$ = 3 × 4 = 12
Interval = 3 × $t_{1/2}$ = 3 × 12 = 36 hours
Schedule = 500 mg every 36 hours

Dosing on the basis of replacing half the loading dose every $t_{1/2}$ would result in this patient receiving 250 mg every 12 hours. This latter approach to dosing in renal impairment and that of the nomogram would result in less serum level fluctuation than the formula of Cutler and Orme.

Kanamycin is bound very little, if any, to serum proteins. Hemodialysis reduces kanamycin serum levels by about 50%, and giving half the loading dose, 3.5 mg/kg, after every dialysis should provide adequate serum levels. Peritoneal dialysis of kanamycin decreases the uremic serum $t_{1/2}$ significantly but not to a normal level.[120] To prevent decreases in serum levels during peritoneal dialysis, kanamycin should be added to the dialysis solutions in adequate amounts to equal desired serum levels of about 20 $\mu$g/ml.

*Tobramycin.* Tobramycin is an investigational amino-

### References

1. Kunin, C. M.: A Guide to Use of Antibiotics in Patients with Renal Disease, *Ann. Internal Med. 67*:151 (July) 1967.
2. Bennett, W. M. et al.: A Practical Guide to Drug Usage in Adult Patients with Impaired Renal Functions, *JAMA 214*:1468 (Nov. 23) 1970.
3. Kunin, C. M.: Antibiotic Usage in Patients with Renal Impairment, *Hosp. Pract. 7*:141 (Jan.) 1972.
4. Dettli, L. et al.: Multiple Dose Kinetics and Drug Dosage in Patients with Kidney Disease, *Acta Pharmacol. Toxicol. 29*:211 Supp. 3, 1971.
5. Bulger, R. J. and Petersdorf, R. G.: Antimicrobial Therapy in Patients with Renal Impairment, *Postgrad. Med. 47*:160–165 (Jan.) 1970.
6. Anon: Criteria for the Evaluation of the Severity of Established Renal Disease, *Arch. Internal Med. 128*:304 (Aug.) 1971.
7. Jelliffe, R. W.: New Developments in Drug Dosage Regimens, *J. Mond. Pharm. 15*:53 (Mar.) 1972.
8. Jelliffe, R. W.: Bedside Estimate of Creatinine Clearance, *Ann. Internal Med. 79*:604 (Oct.) 1973.
9. Siersback-Nielson, K. et al.: Rapid Evaluation of Creatinine Clearance, *Lancet*:1133 (May 29) 1971.
10. Oldstone, M. B. A. and Nelson, E.: Central Nervous System Manifestitations of Penicillin Toxicity in Man, *Neurology 16*:693–700 (July) 1966.
11. Smith, H. et al.: Neurotoxicity and Massive Intravenous Therapy with Penicillin, *Arch. Internal Med. 120*: 47–53 (July) 1967.
12. Raichle, M. E. et al.: Neurotoxicity of Intrave-

nously Administrered Penicillin G, *Arch. Neurol. 25*:232–239 (Sept.) 1971.

13. Kunin, C. M. and Maxwell, F. J.: Persistence of Antibiotics in Blood of Patients with Acute Renal Failure, III: Penicillin, Streptomycin, Erythromycin and Kanamycin, *J. Clin. Invest. 38*:1509–1519 (July-Dec.) 1959.

14. Plaut, M. E. et al.: Penicillin Handling in Normal and Azotemic Patients, *J. Lab. Clin. Med. 74*:12 (July) 1969.

15. Schreiner, G. E.: Dialysis of Poisons and Drugs, *Drug Intel. Clin. Pharm. 5*:322–334 (Oct.) 1971.

16. Hoffman, T. A., Cestera, R., and Bullock, W. E.: Carbenicillin in Hepatic and Renal Failure, *Ann. Internal Med. 73*:173–178 (Aug.) 1970.

17. Wallace, J. F. et al.: Evaluation of an Indanyl Ester of Carbenicillin, *Antimicrob. Agents Chemother.*: 223–226, 1970.

18. *Med. Letter 15*:29 (Mar. 30) 1973.

19. Whelton, A. et al.: Carbenicillin Concentrations in Normal and Diseased Kidneys, *Ann. Internal Med. 78*:659 (May) 1973.

20. Waisbren, B. A. et al.: Carbenicillin and Bleeding (Letter), *JAMA 217*:1243 (Aug. 30) 1971.

21. Ruedy, J.: The Effects of Peritoneal Dialysis on the Physiological Disposition of Oxacillin, Ampicillin and Tetracycline in Patients with Renal Disease, *Can. Med. Ass. J. 94*:257–261 (Feb. 5) 1966.

22. Lee, H. A. and Hill, L. F.: The Use of Ampicillin in Severe Renal Disease, *Brit. J. Clin. Prac. 22*:354–357 (Aug.) 1968.

23. Jusko, W. J. et al.: Ampicillin and Hetacillin Pharmacokinetics in Normal and Anephric Subjects, *Clin. Pharmacol. Ther. 14*:90 (Jan.-Feb.) 1973.

24. Jensen, H. A. et al.: Permanent Impairment of Renal Function After Methicillin Nephropathy, *Brit. Med. J. 4*:406 (Nov. 13) 1971.

25. Brauninger, E. G. and Remington, J. S.: Nephropathy Associated with Methicillin Therapy, *JAMA 203*: 103 (Jan. 8) 1968.

26. Baldwin, D. S. et al.: Renal Failure and Interstitial Nephritis Due to Penicillin and Methicillin, *N. Engl. J. Med. 279*:1245 (Nov. 28) 1968.

27. Kunin, C. M.: Clinical Significance of Protein Binding of the Penicillins, *Ann. N. Y. Acad. Sci. 145*:282 (Sept.) 1967.

28. Bulger, R. J. et al.: Effects of Uremia on Methicillin and Oxacillin Blood Levels, *JAMA 187*:319–322 (Feb. 1) 1964.

29. Rosenblatt, J. E. et al.: Mechanisms Responsible for the Blood Level Differences of Isoxazolyl Penicillins, *Arch. Internal Med. 121*:345–348 (Apr.) 1968.

30. Gravenkemper, C. F. et al.: Dicloxacillin Compared with Oxacillin and Cloxacillin, *Arch. Internal Med. 116*:340 (Sept.) 1965.

31. Williams, T. W. et al.: Effect of Hemodialysis on Dicloxacillin Concentration in Plasma, *Antimicrob. Agents Chemother.*:767, 1967.

32. McCloskey, R. V. and Hayes, C. P., Jr.: Plasma Levels of Dicloxacillin in Oliguric Patients and the Effect of Hemodialysis, *Antimicrob. Agents Chemother.*:770, 1967.

33. Klein, J. O. and Finland, M.: Antibacterial Action In Vitro and Absorption and Excretion of Nafcillin in Normal Young Men, *Amer. J. Med. Sci. 246*:44 (July) 1963.

34. Kunin, C. M. and Atuk, N.: Excretion of Cephaloridine and Cephalothin in Patients with Renal Impairment, *N. Engl. J. Med. 274*:654–656 (Mar. 24) 1966.

35. Tuano, S. B. et al.: Relation of the Kidney to Blood Level Differences After Parenteral Administration of Cephaloridine and Cephalothin, *Antimicrob. Agents Chemother.*:101, 1966.

36. Perkins, R. L. et al.: Cephalothin and Cephalori-

dine-Comparative Pharmacodynamics in Chronic Uremia, *Amer. J. Med. Sci. 257*:116 (Feb.) 1969.

37. Yamasaku, F. et al.: A Study of the Kinetics of Cephalosporins in Renal Impairment, *Postgrad. Med. J. 46*:57 (Oct. Supp.) 1970.

38. Kirby, W. M. M. et al.: Pharmacokinetics of the Cephalosporins in Healthy Volunteers and Uremic Patients, *Postgrad. Med. J. 47*:41–46 (Feb. Supp.) 1971.

39. Kabins, S. A. and Cohen, S.: Cephalothin Serum Levels in the Azotemic Patient, *Antimicrob. Agents Chemother.*:207–214, 1964.

40. Hansten, P. D.: Cephalothin, Gentamicin, Colistin Hazard, *JAMA 223*:1158 (Mar. 5) 1973.

41. Venuto, R. C. and Plaut, M. E.: Cephalothin Handling in Patients Undergoing Hemodialysis, *Antimicrob. Agents Chemother.*:50–52, 1970.

42. Linsell, W. D. et al.: Abnormal Urinary Deposits in Cephaloridine Therapy, *Postgrad. Med. J. 43*:90 (Aug. Supp.) 1967.

43. Foord, R. D.: Progress in Antimicrobial and Anticancer Chemotherapy, Proceedings Sixth International Congress on Chemotherapy, Tokyo, 1969, p. 597.

44. Dodds, M. G. and Foord, R. W.: Enhancement by Potent Diuretics of Renal Tubular Necrosis Induced by Cephaloridine, *Brit. J. Pharmacol. 40*:227–236 (Oct.) 1970.

45. Lawson, D. H. et al.: The Nephrotoxicity of Cephaloridine, *Postgrad. Med. J. 46*:36 (Oct. Supp.) 1970.

46. Fleming, P. C. and Jaffe, W.: The Nephrotoxic Effect of Cephaloridine, *Postgrad. Med. J. 43*:89–90 (Aug. Supp.) 1967.

47. Gabriel, R., Foord, R. W., and Joekes, A. M.: Reversible Encephalopathy and Acute Renal Failure after Cephaloridine, *Brit. Med. J. 4*:283–284 (Oct. 31) 1970.

48. McAllister, T. A.: Cephaloridine Nephrotoxicity (Letter) *Lancet 2*:710 (Sept. 30) 1972.

49. Winchester, J. F. and Kennedy, A. C.: Absence of Nephrotoxicity During Cephaloridine Therapy, *Lancet 2*: 514 (Sept. 9) 1972.

50. Kabins, S. A. and Cohen, S.: Cephaloridine Therapy as Related to Renal Function, *Antimicrob. Agents Chemother.*:922–932, 1965.

51. Kunin, C. M. and Finkelberg, Z.: Oral Cephalexin and Ampicillin-Antimicrobial Activity, Recovery in Urine and Persistence in Uremic Patients, *Ann. Internal Med. 72*:349 (Mar.) 1970.

52. Lindquist, J. A. et al.: Cephalexin in Patients with Renal Disease, *N. Engl. J. Med. 283*:720 (Oct. 1) 1970.

53. Bailey, R. R. et al.: The Effect of Impaired Renal Function and Hemodialysis on Urine Levels of Cephalexin, *Postgrad. Med. J. 46*:60 (Oct. Supp.) 1970.

54. Kabins, S. A. et al.: Cephalexin Therapy as Related to Renal Function, *Amer. J. Med. Sci. 257*:133 (Feb.) 1970.

55. Kunin, C. M. and Brandt, D.: Comparative Studies of Ampicillin, Cephalothin and Cephaloglycin, *Amer. J. Med. Sci. 255*:196 (Mar.) 1968.

56. Braun, P. et al.: Cephalexin and Cepaloglycin Activity in Vitro and Absorption and Urinary Excretion of Single Oral Doses in Normal Young Adults, *Appl. Microbiol. 16*:1684–1694 (Nov.) 1968.

57. Lowentritt, L. et al.: Cephaloglycin as a Urinary Antimicrobial in Patients with Reduced Renal Function, *J. Urol. 106*:615 (Nov.) 1971.

58. Nissenson, A. R. et al.: Effect of Renal Failure and Hemodialysis on Cephacetrile Pharmacokinetics, *Clin. Pharmacol. Ther. 13*:887 (Nov.-Dec.) 1972.

59. Kirby, W. M. and Regamey, C.: Pharmacokinetics of Cephazolin Compared with Four Other Cephalosporins, *J. Infect. Dis. 128*:Supp. 5341 (Oct.) 1973.

60. Craig, W. A. et al.: Pharmacology of Cephazolin and Other Cephalosporins in Renal Insufficiency, *J. Infect. Dis. 128*:Supp. 5347 (Oct.) 1973.

61. Levinson, M. E. et al.: Pharmacology of Cepha-

zolin in Patients with Normal and Abnormal Renal Function, *J. Infect. Dis. 128*:Supp. 5354 (Oct.) 1973.

62. McCloskey, R. V. et al.: Hemodialysis of Cephazolin, *J. Infect. Dis. 128*:Supp. 5358 (Oct.) 1973.

63. Rein, M. F.: Pharmacodynamics of Cephazolin in the Presence of Normal and Impaired Renal Function, *Antimicrob. Agents Chemother. 4*:366 (Sept.) 1973.

64. Whalley, P. J. et al.: Tetracycline Toxicity in Pregnancy, *JAMA 189*:337 (Aug. 3) 1964.

65. Horowitz, S. T. and Marymont, J. H., Jr.: Fatal Liver Disease During Pregnancy Associated with Tetracycline Therapy, *Obstet. Gynecol. 23*:826 (June) 1964.

66. Frimpter, G. W. et al.: Reversible Fanconi Syndrome Caused by Degraded Tetracycline, *JAMA 184*:111 (Apr. 13) 1963.

67. Albers, D. D. et al.: Renal Failure Following Methoxyfluorane Anesthesia and Tetracycline, *J. Urol. 106*:348 (Sept.) 1971.

68. Shils, M. E.: Renal Disease and The Effects of Tetracycline, *Ann. Internal Med. 58*:389 (Mar.) 1963.

69. Lew, H. T. and French, S. W.: Tetracycline Nephrotoxicity and Nonoliguric Acute Renal Failure, *Arch. Internal Med. 118*:125 (Aug.) 1966.

70. George C. R. and Evans, R. A.: Tetracycline Toxicity in Renal Failure, *Med. J. Austral. 1*:1271 (June 12) 1971.

71. Kunin, C. M. et al.: Persistence of Antibiotics in Blood of Patients with Acute Renal Failure–Tetracycline and Chlortetracycline, *J. Clin. Invest. 38*:1487 (Sept.) 1959.

72. Bateman, J. E. et al.: Fatal Complications of Intensive Antibiotic Therapy in Patients with Neoplastic Disease, *Arch. Internal Med. 90*:763 (Dec.) 1952.

73. Dimmling, T. et al.: Resorption und Ausscheidung von Oxytetracyline in Abhangigkeit von der Nieronfunktion, *Arzneim. Forsch. 7*:681, 1957.

74. Little, P. J. and Bailey, R. R.: Tetracyclines and Renal Failure, *N. Z. Med. J. 72*:183 (Sept.) 1970.

75. Fabre, J. et al.: The Kinetics of Tetracyclines in Man, *Schweiz. Med. Wochenschr. 101*:625, 1971.

76. Merier, G. et al.: Le Comportement de l'Oxytetracycline en Cas d'Insuffisance Renale, *Schweiz. Med. Wochenschr. 100*:1442, 1970.

77. Fabre, J. et al.: Influence of Renal Insufficiency on the Excretion of Chloroquine, Phenobarbital, Phenothiazines and Methacycline, *Helv. Med. Acta. 33*:307, 1966.

78. Bernard, B. et al.: Clinical Pharmacologic Studies with Minocycline, *J. Clin. Pharmacol. 11*:332 (Sept.-Oct.) 1971.

79. Lang, W.: Pharmacokinetics of Minocycline, Proceedings Minocycline Symposium, Bad Reichenhall, Germany, July 1971 (translation copy available from Lederle Laboratories).

80. McHenry, M. C. et al.: Minocycline in Renal Impairment (Abstract), *Clin. Pharmacol. Ther. 13*:146 (Jan.-Feb.) 1972.

81. George, C. R. et al.: Minocycline Toxicity in Renal Failure, *Med. J. Aust. 1*:640 (Mar. 31) 1973.

82. Reubi, F. and Munger, C.: Renale und Extrarenale Ausscheidung von Rolitetracycline bei patienten mit Normaler und Eingeschrankter Nierenfunktion, *Pharmacologia Clinica 1*:8–18, 1968.

83. Kunin, C. M. et al.: Distribution and Excretion of Four Tetracycline Analogues in Normal Young Men, *J. Clin. Invest. 38*:1950–63, 1959.

84. Leevy, C. M. et al.: Observations on the Distribution of C14 Oxytetracycline in Man, *Antibiot. Ann.*:258, 1958-59.

85. Shils, M. E.: Chlortetracycline Therapy with Renal Disease, *N. Engl. J. Med. 275*:113 (July 14) 1966.

86. Fabre, J. et al.: Absorption, Distribution and Excretion of Doxycycline in Man, *Schweiz. Med. Wochenschr. 97*:915 (May 17) 1967.

87. Mannhart, M. et al.: The Elimination of Doxycycline and its Reaction to Hemodialysis in Anuric Patients, *Schweiz. Med. Wochenschr. 101*:123 (Jan. 30) 1971.

88. Stein, W. et al.: Doxycycline Serum Levels in Patients with Renal Insufficiency, *Arzneim. Forsch. 19*:827 (May) 1969.

89. Cox, C. E. (Bowman Gray School of Medicine, Winston Salem, N.C.), data on file, Medical Department, Pfizer Labs.

90. Mahon, W. A. et al.: Studies on the Absorption and Distribution of Doxycycline in Normal Patients and in Severe Renal Impairment, *Can. Med. Ass. J. 103*:1031 (Nov. 7) 1970.

91. Merier, G. et al.: Behavior of Doxycycline in Renal Impairment, *Helv. Med. Acta. 35*:124 (Nov.) 1969.

92. Ritzerfeld, W. et al.: Doxycycline in Serum, Dialysate and Urine of Patients with Kidney Damage, *Int. J. Clin. Pharmacol. 3*:325 (Oct.) 1970.

93. Doluisio, J. T. and Dittert, L. W.: Influence of Repetitive Dosing of Tetracycline on Biologic T½ in Serum, *Clin. Pharmacol. Ther. 10*:690 (Sept.-Oct.) 1969.

94. Burgess, J. L. and Brichall, R.: Nephrotoxicity of Amphotericin B with Emphasis on Changes in Renal Tubular Function, *Amer. J. Med. 53*:77 (July) 1972.

95. Butler, W. R. et al.: Nephrotoxicity of Amphotericin B—Early and Late Effects in 81 Patients, *Ann. Internal Med. 61*:175 (Aug.) 1964.

96. McCurdy, D. K. and Elkinton, F. M., Jr.: Renal Tubular Acidosis Due to Amphotericin B, *N. Engl. J. Med. 278*:124 (June 18) 1968.

97. Bindschadler, D. D. and Bennett, J. E.: A Pharmacologic Guide to the Clinical Use of Amphotericin B, *J. Infect. Dis. 120*:427 (Oct.) 1969.

98. Vogel, R. A. and Crutcher, J. C.: Studies on the Bioassay and Excretion of Amphotericin B in Patients with Systemic Mycoses, *Antibiot. Med. 5*:501, 1958.

99. Morris, R. C., Jr.: Renal Tubular Acidosis Mechanisms, *N. Engl. J. Med. 281*:1405 (Dec. 18) 1969.

100. Koechlin, B. A. et al.: The Metabolism of 5-Fluorocytosine in the Rat and Its Disposition in Man, *Biochem. Pharmacol. 15*:435 (Apr.) 1966.

101. Schönebeck, J.: Studies on 5-Fluorocytosine and Its Relation to Candida Albicans, *Scand. J. Urol. Nephrol.*: Supp. 11 (Chapter 10) 1972, p. 35-44.

102. McLeod, D. C.: Error in Flucytosine Dosage, *Ann. Internal Med. 78*:978 (June.) 1973.

103. The Pharmacologic Basis of Therapeutics, 4th ed., The MacMillan Co., New York, New York.

104. Janetz, E.: Polymyxin, Colistin and Bacitracin, *Ped. Clin. N. Amer. 8*:1057 (Nov.) 1961.

105. MacKay, D. N. and Kay, D.: Serum Concentrations of Colistin in Patients with Normal and Impaired Renal Function, *N. Engl. J. Med. 274*:394–397 (Feb. 20) 1964.

106. Curtis, J. F. and Eastwood, J. B.: Colistin Sulphomethate Sodium Administration in the Presence of Severe Renal Failure and During Hemodialysis and Peritoneal Dialysis, *Brit. Med. J. 1*:484–485 (Feb. 28) 1968.

107. Goodwin, N. J. and Friedman, E. A.: The Effects of Renal Impairment, Peritoneal Dialysis and Hemodialysis on Serum Sodium Colistimethate Levels, *Ann. Internal Med. 68*:984–994 (May) 1968.

108. Wolinsky, E. and Hines, J. D.: Neurotoxic and Nephrotoxic Effects of Colistin in Patients with Renal Disease, *N. Engl. J. Med. 266*:759–762 (Apr. 12) 1962.

109. Cawthorne, T. and Ranger, D.: Toxic Effects of Streptomycin upon Balance and Hearing, *Brit. Med. J. 1*: 1444 (June 22) 1957.

110. Edwards, K. D. G. and Whyte, H. M.: Streptomycin Poisoning in Renal Failure, *Brit. Med. J. 1*:752 (Mar. 21) 1959.

111. Gordon, R. C. et al.: Serum Protein Binding of the Aminoglycoside Antibiotics, *Antimicrob. Agents Chemother. 2*:214 (Sept.) 1972.

112. Rodrigues, V. et al.: Gentamicin Sulfate Distribution in Body Fluids, *Clin. Pharmacol. Ther. 11*:257–281 (Jan.-Feb.) 1970.

113. McHenry, M. C. et al.: Gentamicin Dosage for Renal Insufficiency, *Ann. Internal Med. 74*:192 (Feb.) 1971.

114. Cutler, R. E. et al.: Correlation of Serum Creatinine Concentration and Gentamicin Half-Life, *JAMA 219*: 1037–1041 (Feb. 2) 1972.

115. Chan, R. A. et al.: Gentamicin Therapy in Renal Failure: A Nomogram For Dosage, *Ann. Internal Med. 76*:773-778 (May) 1972.

116. McCloskey, R. V. and Becker, G. G.: Evaluation of the Cutler-Orme Method for Administration of Kanamycin During Renal Failure, *Antimicrob. Agents Chemother.*: 161–164, 1970.

117. Cutler, R. E. and Orme, B. M.: Correlation of Serum Creatinine Concentration and Kanamycin Half-Life, *JAMA 209*:539–542 (July 28) 1969.

118. Kunin, C. M. et al.: Absorption of Orally Administered Neomycin and Kanamycin, *N. Engl. J. Med. 262*: 380–385 (Feb. 25) 1960.

119. Mawer, G. E. et al.: Nomogram for Kanamycin Dosage, *Lancet 2*:45 (July) 1972.

120. Greenberg, P. A. and Sanford, J. P.: Removal and Absorption of Antibiotics in Patients with Renal Failure Undergoing Peritoneal Dialysis, *Ann. Internal Med. 66*: 465–479 (Mar.) 1967.

121. Regamey, C. et al.: Comparative Pharmacokinetics of Tobramycin and Gentamicin, *Clin. Pharmacol. Ther. 14*:396 (May-June) 1973.

122. Lockwood, W. R. and Bower, J. D.: Tobramycin Serum of Normal and Anephric Patients, *Antimicrob. Agents Chemother. 3*:125 (Jan.) 1973.

# 49 Pharmacokinetics and Dosing of Antimicrobial Agents in Renal Impairment, Part II

Eric A. Jackson and Don C. McLeod

This chapter discusses the dosing consideration of antimicrobial agents when used in patients with renal impairment.

The drugs covered are the antituberculars, bacitracin, chloramphenicol, chloroquine, clindamycin, dapsone, erythromycin, lincomycin, neomycin, vancomycin, the urinary antiinfectives, sulfonamides, and trimethoprim. The data from this chapter and the preceding one are summarized in a table which uses the principle of keeping a constant dose and varying the dosing interval based on the degree of renal impairment.

## Antituberculars

*Isoniazid.* Isoniazid is rapidly and almost completely absorbed from the gut with peak serum levels occurring at one hour, and the serum being completely cleared of isoniazid by 12 hours. Most of the isoniazid dose is metabolized to inactive metabolites, namely acetyl-isoniazid and various isoniazid hydrazones. Several studies have established that there are two genetic phenotypes for isoniazid inactivation, so-called "rapid" and "slow" acetylators. Patients who are rapid acetylators have lower serum levels of active drug and excrete less than 5% of the dose in the urine as isoniazid. Slow acetylators have higher serum levels and excrete about 20–25% of the dose in the urine as isoniazid. Peripheral neuritis, the principle toxicity, occurs more frequently in slow than rapid inactivators and appears related to the higher serum levels ($>30$ $\mu$g/ml) of unchanged isoniazid.[1] Bowersox et al.[2] have studied the serum $t_{1/2}$ of isoniazid in renal failure. They did not classify patients as rapid or slow acetylators, but found a serum $t_{1/2}$ of 0.5–4.4 hours (mean 2.3 hours) in 11 normal persons. In 9 patients with serum creatinine ranging from 7.6–20.7 mg/100 ml, the serum $t_{1/2}$ varied from 0.75–7.6 hours (mean 3.7 hours). Although the serum $t_{1/2}$ of isoniazid increased in uremia, they found no progressive accumulation or toxicity with isoniazid given 300 mg daily. Bennett et al.[3] have recommended a dose of only 100 mg daily in the anuric patient, but Kunin[3] recommends the usual 300 mg dose in renal impairment. It appears that no dosage adjustment for isoniazid is required in renal impairment, except possibly for a slow acetylator who is practically anuric. If the chief toxicity of peripheral neuritis does occur, it is easily reversed with oral pyridoxine. In the case of a large isoniazid overdose, Glogner et al.[5] have shown that peritoneal dialysis is effective in lowering serum levels in renal impairment, but that it is of no benefit with normal renal function. Durr and Missmahl successfully hemodialyzed a woman attempting suicide with isoniazid.[6]

*Aminosalicyclic Acid (PAS).* This drug is metabolized principally by acetylation and to a minor degree by glycine conjugation. An oral dose of 4 g produces peak serum levels of 7.5 $\mu$g/ml within two hours, and blood levels are negligible within five hours after a single dose. Jenne et al.[7] have studied the serum $t_{1/2}$ of PAS in rapid and slow isoniazid acetylators. Rapid acetylators had a mean PAS serum $t_{1/2}$ of 43 minutes while slow acetylators had a mean $t_{1/2}$ of 48 minutes. This difference is insignificant. Serum protein binding was determined to range from 58–73% with a mean of 68%. Jenne et al. calculated the PAS clearance from serum to be 140 ml/min, and assuming protein binding to be 68%, deduced that about 66% of PAS urinary removal is due to tubular secretion. These figures represent a composite of unchanged PAS and its glycine conjugate. About 80% of a PAS dose is recovered in the urine, and half of this is the acetylated metabolite. The sodium salt of PAS largely eliminates the hazard of crystalluria due to the relatively insoluble excretion products. Studies on the pharmacokinetics of PAS in renal impairment have not been located, but Bennett et al.[3] report that it can cause acidosis and an increase in uremic symptoms. The increase in serum $t_{1/2}$ of free PAS would be insignificant therapeutically, but the metabolites could greatly accumulate.

*Ethambutol.* Ethambutol is an antitubercular with a rather low order of toxicity. The primary toxicity is a retrobulbar neuritis with a reduction of visual acuity, central scotoma and a green/red color blindness. This toxicity has proven to be reversible upon dosage reduction or discontinuance. The usual dose is 25 mg/kg in a single daily dose for 6–8 weeks and then 15 mg/kg daily. Toxicity may occur without this dosage reduction. A dose of 25 mg/kg produces a peak blood level of 5 $\mu$g/ml at 2 hours which declines to 0.5 $\mu$g/ml at 24 hours. The therapeutic level is generally 3 $\mu$g/ml or more. About 80% of the oral dose is absorbed with 20% appearing in the feces. About 70% of the oral dose is excreted in the urine unchanged, and 10% is excreted as metabolites. Uptake of ethambutol into erythrocytes results in levels about two to three times that of the serum. Using the above data of Peets et al.,[8] the normal serum $t_{1/2}$ of ethambutol is calculated to be about 6.6 hours.

Ethambutol accumulates greatly in renal impairment, and the dose must be appropriately lowered based on the degree of impairment. Pyle et al.[9] reported in 1966 a case of very high ethambutol serum levels in an azotemic patient with a blood urea nitrogen (BUN) level of 105–112 mg/100 ml. The serum level reached 14.5 $\mu$g/ml six hours after a dose of 18 mg/kg. Strauss and Erhardt[10] have found increased serum levels of ethambutol in patients with decreased glomerular filtration rate (GFR) due to renal tuberculosis. Using the data of Peets et al.,[8] the anuric serum $t_{1/2}$ can be estimated to be 32 hours. Table 1 gives general dosage guidelines for the use of ethambutol in renal impairment.

Wilson[11] has written that there is no correlation between ethambutol serum levels and visual toxicity, and this claim has been incorporated into some ethambutol reviews. The author presents no data or cites no reference to substantiate this, and all evidence seems to be to the contrary. The serum $t_{1/2}$ of any drug which is predominantly excreted in the urine unchanged should be expected to increase in renal impairment.

*Rifampin.* This is an antitubercular agent which also has activity against many gram-positive and gram-negative organisms. Serum levels of 0.2 $\mu$g/ml or less are effective against most strains of the tubercle bacillus.[12] Unchanged drug is concentrated in the bile but is reabsorbed in the gut. Rifampin is deacetylated by the liver, and during 24 hours only 9–15% of a dose is excreted unchanged in the urine.[13] Inactive metabolites are excreted primarily in the bile and are found in the feces. The serum $t_{1/2}$ of rifampin is about three hours but can range from 1.5–5 hours depending primarily on the liver function.[14] Spring and Dettli[15] have reported that the serum $t_{1/2}$ of rifampin is unchanged even in severe renal impairment, thus the drug may be dosed normally in renal impairment. Liver dysfunction may increase the serum $t_{1/2}$ with a resulting increase in adverse effects.[16] A rifampin-induced interstitial nephritis resulting in acute renal failure has been reported.[17] The oliguria may be present for several days, but has been reversible thus far.

*Cycloserine.* Cycloserine is a broad-spectrum antibiotic which in concentrations of 5–20 $\mu$g/ml inhibits tubercle bacilli. Adverse effects are common when the serum level is 30 $\mu$g/ml or more, and they consist primarily of CNS symptoms such as tremor, twitching, muscle spasms and convulsions. Doses of pyridoxine up to 100 mg will reverse the CNS effects of cycloserine.[18] Conzelman[19] has found that as much as 64% of a dose of cycloserine is recovered unchanged in the urine, and thus cycloserine should require considerable dosage adjustment in renal impairment. Studies reporting the use of cycloserine in uremia have not been located.

*Viomycin.* This drug is an antitubercular which is used as a reserve agent when other primary drugs are ineffective or contraindicated. Its toxicities are similar to those of streptomycin and include albuminuria, renal impairment, ototoxicity, hypokalemia and allergic reactions. Renal function usually recovers quite rapidly when treatment is stopped. Vestibular dysfunction is more common than with streptomycin. Since its toxicities are additive with those of streptomycin, the two drugs should not be used concomitantly. As with streptomycin, hearing loss may not be apparent until several days or weeks after therapy. Viomycin should be avoided whenever possible in a patient with renal impairment. No blood level and pharmacokinetic studies have been located in the renally-impaired patient, and although the dosage should be reduced, the exact proper adjustment is not known.[12]

*Pyrazinamide.* Pyrazinamide is an antitubercular which is occasionally used in combination with other drugs. Its chief toxicity is to the liver; and when a dose of 3 g daily is given orally, hepatotoxicity appears in about 15% of the patients and jaundice in 2–3%. Death due to hepatic necrosis is a rare occurrence. Because of its toxicity, pyrazinamide should be used only in hospitalized patients. Caccia[20] has reported serum levels of 45 $\mu$g/ml two hours after administration of 1 g of pyrazinamide, while Stottmeier[21] found peak serum levels to be 65 $\mu$g/ml after a dose of 20 mg/kg. Urine levels of 60–100 $\mu$g/ml were detected by Stottmeier 12 hours after oral administration, and serum accumulation should be expected in renal impairment. This action would tend to increase the incidence of hepatotoxicity. Serum levels as high as 300 $\mu$g/ml have been observed in icteric tuberculosis patients.[22]

## Bacitracin

Bacitracin has a gram-positive spectrum and is frequently used topically or for local instillation within the cranium during brain surgery. It is not nearly as sensitizing topically as many other antibiotics, and it is relatively nontoxic when applied to the surface of the brain. Eagle et al.[23] have reported that bacitracin is cleared by the kidneys at a rate similar to the GFR, and that after an i.m. injection, 87% of the dose is excreted in the urine within six hours. Zintel et al.[24] report, on the other hand, that no more than 30% of an i.m. dose is recovered in the urine within 24 hours. They concluded that considerable bacitracin is either retained or destroyed in the body. This same study reported that five patients receiving 200,000 units of bacitracin i.m. daily showed slight to very severe diminution in GFR, renal plasma flow and maximal tubular excretion of para-aminohippurate. Bacitracin is seldom used i.m. today, and the drug is particularly dangerous with preexisting renal impairment. Bacitracin accumulates in renal impairment and this could lead to further uremia.[25]

## Chloramphenicol

The primary toxicity of chloramphenicol is erythropoietic depression, and studies using $Fe^{59}$ indicate that this depression is more frequent than generally realized.[26] About 5–15% of a dose of chloramphenicol is excreted as active drug in the urine, the rest being excreted as inactive metabolites. The active drug is cleared by glomerular filtration, about 22–24 ml/min of blood being cleared in the patient with normal renal function. Kunin et al.[27] have studied the elimination rate of chloramphenicol in normal and anuric patients. The usual serum $t_{1/2}$ of the active drug was found to be 1.5–3.5 hours while the serum $t_{1/2}$ in the anuric patient was 3.2–4.3 hours. The kidney is thus of only minor importance in the elimination of the active drug, but Kunin found that the metabolites of chloramphenicol do accumulate and persist for many days after a dose in the anuric patient.

Suhrland and Weisberger[28] studied the incidence of erythropoietic depression in 16 patients with hepatic dysfunction, 19 patients with renal ipairment and 16 patients with normal hepatic and renal status. They found evidence of erythropoietic depression in 50% of the patients with hepatic dysfunction and 32% of the patients with renal impairment. None of the normal patients experienced toxic effects. Patients with both jaundice and ascites were particularly prone to toxicity. In every instance erythropoietic depression was correlated with a high free chloramphenicol serum level. The authors suggest that those patients developing toxic effects were either unable to conjugate at a normal rate or unable to excrete the free active drug.

Lindberg et al.[29] have studied the concentration of chloramphenicol in the urine in relation to renal function. After a 1-g dose, the maximum concentration of active drug in the urine was 150–180 $\mu$g/ml. The maximum urine levels decrease in a linear correlation to a decrease in the GFR. When the GFR, as measured by the creatinine clearance, falls below 20 ml/min, inadequate concentrations of active drug exist for most gram-negative urinary infections. Peak urine levels may be adequate but the level is not sustained long enough for a bacteriostatic drug such as chloramphenicol to be effective. Due to decreased effectiveness in urinary infections and increased toxicity, chloramphenicol is not a desirable drug for use in patients with renal impairment. If used in patients with renal insufficiency, however, the dose is the same as that for normal individuals. Kunin et al.[27] found that hemodialysis removed only small amounts of active antibiotic and some nitro compounds. Greenberg and Sanford[30] found that peritoneal dialysis does not alter the serum $t_{1/2}$ of active chloramphenicol. Therefore, no dosage adjustments are necessitated by either type of dialysis. Its occasional usefulness in pyelonephritis is not compromised with renal impairment.

## Chloroquine

Chloroquine is slowly excreted unchanged in the urine, 20% or more of a dose being recovered in 96 hours. The normal biological $t_{1/2}$ is 150–200 hours and this is increased somewhat in renal impairment. Fabre et al.[31] have shown that chloroquine does accumulate in renal impairment and the following dosing guidelines are suggested: (1) for short-term care of malaria, the classical dose of 1 g, then 300 mg twice daily for 10 days, can be maintained, even in renal impairment; and (2) in prolonged cases demanding treatment, an initial daily dose of 150 mg should be used with a $C_{cr}$ of 30–60 ml/min, or 100 mg daily for a $C_{cr} < 30$ ml/min; after two weeks these doses should be halved. Chloroquine toxicity upon long-term therapy may consist of lichenoid skin eruption and inverted T waves in the electroencephalogram, both reversible, and retinopathy which is not reversible. The use of chloroquine in rheumatoid arthritis and systemic lupus erythematosus should be closely monitored due to the kidney manifestations of these illnesses.

## Clindamycin

Clindamycin is a semi-synthetic derivative of lincomycin. It has a spectrum identical to lincomycin and exhibits cross resistance with lincomycin. Clindamycin is active against many gram-positive organisms and against most isolates of bacteroides, important organisms in anaerobic infections of the abdominal cavity.[32] Sensitive strains of streptococci and pneumococci are inhibited by serum levels less than 0.3 $\mu$g/ml. The minimum inhibitory concentration (MIC) for staphylococci ranges from 1–3 $\mu$g/ml. Ninety percent of an oral dose is absorbed in 24 minutes in fasting patients as compared with 2–4 hours for lincomycin.[33] It is also well absorbed when taken with food. Clindamycin seems to have a lower incidence of gastrointestinal irritation than lincomycin. Transient elevations of alkaline phosphatase and serum transaminases have been observed during clindamycin therapy.[34] Nine percent of the active drug is excreted in the urine, and 3.5% in the feces. The majority is excreted as inactive metabolites. Adequate serum levels are maintained by giving 150 mg every six hours. The normal $t_{1/2}$ is 2.4 hours and is only slightly increased (4–5 hours) in markedly reduced renal function. Consequently, dosing modifications are not necessary in any degree of renal impairment. Peritoneal and hemodialysis do not appreciably affect serum levels of the drug.[35] Although specific information is lacking in the literature, dosing modifications would seem necessary if renal and hepatic failure were both present.

## Dapsone

Dapsone is widely used in the treatment of leprosy and is regarded by many as the drug of choice. Dapsone is well absorbed in man with 80% or more of a dose being excreted as dapsone or its metabolites. About 15% of a dose is excreted in the urine as unchanged dapsone.[36] The serum $t_{1/2}$ in man is several days, and dapsone and its metabolites can be found in the urine for many days after an oral dose.[37] Dapsone has not been reported to be nephrotoxic. The most common toxicities encountered are hemolysis, methemoglobinemia, vomiting, neurological symptoms, skin rashes and an occasional infectious mononucleosis-like syndrome which may be fatal. Reports on the use of dapsone in renal impairment have not been located. Since only 15% of a dose is excreted unchanged in the urine, renal impairment would not be expected to greatly alter the serum $t_{1/2}$ or toxicity of dapsone. Dapsone has been reported as causing a case of nephrotic syndrome,[38] but this is probably a rare allergic reaction.

## Erythromycin

Erythromycin base and its esters are relatively nontoxic even in unusually high serum concentrations. An early study[39] on the use of i.v. erythromycin reported a prolonged blood level in one patient with renal impairment. This study showed that about 15% of a dose of erythromycin is excreted unchanged in the urine during the first 24 hours, most occurring in the first four hours. The average serum level at four minutes after i.v. infusion of 300 mg of erythromycin gluceptate was 41 $\mu$g/ml (20–82 $\mu$g/ml range) and at two hours was 2.6 $\mu$g/ml. In one uremic patient the two-hour serum level was in the normal range, but the six-hour serum level was the same as the two-hour level. Less than 1% of the dose was recovered in the urine. Kunin and Finland[13] found that the erythromycin serum $t_{1/2}$ of about 1.5 hours in normal patients is prolonged to as much as 5.8 hours in uremia. Nonrenal mechanisms are of primary importance in erythromycin elimination, and the usual dose and dosing interval may be safely used in renal impairment. Kunin and Finland also observed in one patient that liver disease did not appear to prolong the serum $t_{1/2}$ of erythromycin. With normal renal and hepatic function, choles-

tatic jaundice and elevated liver enzymes are occasionally associated with the estolate ester of erythromycin and this product is best avoided altogether.

## Lincomycin

Lincomycin is effective against many gram-positive pathogens, although it is not the drug of first choice for any organism. The MIC range is generally 0.5–2 $\mu$g/ml. The major side effect is severe and persistent diarrhea. This diarrhea has been occasionally associated with blood and mucus in the stool and has at times resulted in an acute colitis. The incidence of diarrhea is geater with oral dosage than with parenteral dosage. Changes in liver function tests (particularly elevations of serum transaminase) and jaundice have occasionally been observed following lincomycin therapy. Effective serum levels may be maintained by giving the drug orally every 6–8 hours and parenterally every 12 hours. Oral administration with food causes a significant decrease in absorption. Urinary excretion is small and variable. About 5% of an oral dose and about 15% of a parenteral dose are recovered in the urine. Tissue level studies indicate that biliary excretion is important. The normal serum $t_{1/2}$ is 4–5 hours. Peak concentrations and serum $t_{1/2}$ of lincomycin are threefold greater in patients with severe renal insufficiency than in normal individuals, according to a study by Reinarz and McIntosh.[40] Blood levels are not significantly altered by peritoneal dialysis or hemodialysis. The dosing interval only needs to be slightly altered in severe renal impairment (see Table 1). In patients with hepatic insufficiency, the serum $t_{1/2}$ is almost doubled even when renal function is normal (see Figure 1.)[41] Therefore, severe renal impairment accom-

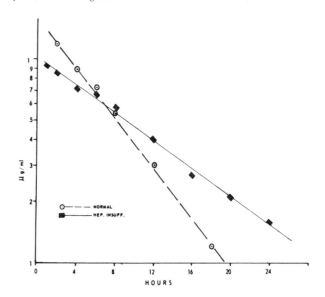

Figure 1. Comparison of lincomycin concentration in patients with normal hepatic function and in patients with hepatic functional impairment, plotted on a semilog scale[41]

panied by liver dysfunction necessitates further dosage adjustments, but specific guidelines have not been found.

## Neomycin

Neomycin is a very toxic drug when given systemically, and many cases of ototoxicity and nephrotoxocity have been reported. Profound hearing loss after the i.v. or i.m. use of neomycin was reported after the initial clinical introduction of the drug.[37] Oral neomycin gained popularity for the preparation of the bowel prior to surgery and in the treatment and prophylaxis of hepatic coma, and soon there were reports of its ototoxicity by this route.[42,43] There have also been reports of its ototoxicity after irrigation of granulated wounds,[44,45] rectal and colonic irrigations[46] and aerosol application for pulmonary infection.[47] Ototoxicity after use of a topical ointment augmented by DMSO has also been reported.[48] Permanent perception deafness and occasionally vestibular damage may result. With parenteral use there also has been nephrotoxicity (severe tubular necrosis) resulting in death.[49]

Kunin et al.[50] studied the absorption of neomycin when given orally. A 4-g dose resulted in peak serum levels of 4 $\mu$g/ml at one hour. About 1% of the oral dose was recovered from the urine and the authors observed that the drug accumulated in azotemic patients. Half of a parenteral dose is recovered unchanged in the urine of humans. Detection of toxicity is made more difficult since ototoxicity may not be noticeable until many days after cessation of therapy. Renal impairment greatly increases the likelihood of toxicity, and the drug must be used with great care in the renally-impaired patient. Krumlovsky et al.[51] have demonstrated that hemodialysis clears the blood of neomycin at the rapid rate of about 38 ml/min.

## Vancomycin

Vancomycin is a reserve antibioic that may be used in the treatment of staphylococcal infections resistant to pencillin G, methicillin, the isoxazolyl penicillins and other drugs more commonly used for staphylococcal infections. Vancomycin is excreted about 80% unchanged in the urine; extrarenal mechanisms are not an important factor in removal of the drug.[52] The most serious toxicity of vancomycin is a perceptive type of deafness which occurs almost exclusively in patients with renal impairment.[53] A single 500-mg injection produces serum levels of 5–10 $\mu$g/ml at 1–2 hours; prolonged levels of 80–100 $\mu$g/ml may produce deafness. In the normal patient the serum $t_{1/2}$ is about six hours, whereas in the oliguric patient the $t_{1/2}$ may be up to 240 hours (see Figure 2).[54] The pharmacokinetics of vancomycin in rela-

tion to renal function thus approaches that of inulin. In mild renal impairment a 1-g dose every 2–3 days is sufficient. In moderate impairment one dose every 3–10 days is adequate, while in severe impairment one dose is sufficient for at least 10 days. In this latter case one dose should suffice for an entire treatment. Vancomycin is dialyzable, but so slowly that the dosage schedule need not be modified for persons undergoing hemodialysis.[54]

## Urinary Antiinfectives

Urinary tract infections in the renally-impaired patient pose not only the problem of preventing toxic serum accumulation of the antiinfective agent, but also the problem of achieving an effective concentration of drug in the urine. The ideal urinary tract antiinfective should be rapidly cleared by the kidney in an active form, bactericidal in low concentrations, freely soluble in the urine and of a low order of toxicity to the kidney and other organs. In addition, the rate of metabolism or other extrarenal removal should be low so that in renal impairment adequate concentrations can be achieved in the urine. The drugs that best meet these criteria are the penicillins and cephalosporins, notably ampicillin and cephalexin for oral use. These drugs have been discussed in the preceeding chapter and special attention will be given in this section to those drugs used primarily or exclusively as urinary antiinfectives.

*Nitrofurantoin.* Nitrofurantoin is used exclusively as a urinary antiinfective. It is bactericidal in the urine to most gram-positive and gram-negative organisms. A urine concentration of 3–4 $\mu$g/ml will inhibit most strains of *E. coli* while 10 $\mu$g/ml inhibits some strains of *Proteus* and *Aerobacter*.[55] Concentrations much higher than these are needed for many gram-negative organisms encountered today. About 30–40% of a dose of nitrofurantoin is excreted unchanged in the urine,[56] and the remainder is rapidly inactivated.[57] The normal serum $t_{1/2}$ of nitrofurantoin is 20 minutes.[56] If dosed normally in azotemia, serum levels may reach 5–6 $\mu$g/ml, but the extrarenal inactivation still removes nitrofurantoin very rapidly. Three studies[55,58,59] have shown that urine concentrations of nitrofurantoin are a function of glomerular filtration, and in the azotemic patient inadequate urinary concentrations result. Increasing the dose is not an effective means of increasing urine levels due to the rapid extrarenal inactivation and the toxicity of relatively low serum levels. Loughridge[60] has described peripheral neuropathy due to nitrofurantoin, and Roelsen[61] has reported hypersensitivity reactions and severe polyneuropathy with accompanying muscle atrophy. Clearly, nitrofurantoin may be ineffective in moderate to severe renal impairment and should not be used in this circumstance.

*Nalidixic Acid.* This drug is a urinary antiinfective

**Table 1. Summary Information on Dosing Antimicrobial Agents in Renal Impairment**

| DRUG | SERUM $t_{1/2}$ (hr) NORMAL | OLIGURIC | ELIMINATION CONSTANT ($K_e$) NORMAL | OLIGURIC | % RECOVERED UNCHANGED IN URINE (NORMAL $C_{cr}$) | % BOUND TO SERUM PROTEINS | TOXICITY LIABILITY IN RENAL IMPAIRMENT | USUAL ADULT MAINTENANCE DOSE AND DOSING INTERVAL | MILD | MODERATE | SEVERE |
|---|---|---|---|---|---|---|---|---|---|---|---|
| **Penicillins** | | | | | | | | | | | |
| Penicillin G | 0.5 | 10 | 1.39 | 0.069 | 58–85% i.v. | 50% | Convulsions, hyperkalemia | 2–5 million U/8 hr | 8 | 8 | 12 |
| Carbenicillin | 1.0 | 15 | 0.69 | 0.046 | 40% p.o., 80–90% i.v. | 50% | Convulsions | 4–5 g/4 hr | 6 | 6–12 | 12 |
| Ampicillin | 1.3 | 20 | 0.53 | 0.035 | 20–65% p.o., 92% i.v. | 20% | Rashes | 250 mg/6 hr | 6 | (2–4 g) 6–12 | (2 g) 12 |
| Hetacillin | 1.3 | 20 | 0.53 | 0.035 | Similar to ampicillin | 20% | Rashes | 225 mg/6 hr | 6 | 6–12 | 12 |
| Methicillin | 0.5 | 4 | 1.39 | 0.17 | 70% i.m. | 39% | Interstitial nephritis | 1 g/4 hr | 4 | 4–8 | 8–12 |
| Dicloxacillin | 0.7 | 1.0 | 0.99 | 0.69 | 36% p.o., 39% i.m. | 96% | None | 500 mg/6 hr | (Avoid) | (Avoid) | (Avoid) |
| Cloxacillin | 0.5 | 0.8 | 1.39 | 0.87 | 30% p.o. | 94% | None | 500 mg/6 hr | 6 | 6 | 6 |
| Oxacillin | 0.4 | 0.5–1 | 1.73 | 0.69 | 21% p.o., 40% i.m. | 95% | None | 500 mg/6 hr | 6 | 6 | 6 |
| Nafcillin | 1.0 | ? | 0.69 | ? | 17% p.o., 36% i.m. | 89% | None | 500 mg/6 hr | 6 | 6 | ? |
| **Cephalosporins** | | | | | | | | | | | |
| Cephalothin | 0.5 | 18 | 1.39 | 0.039 | 60–90% i.v. | 56% | None | 1 g/4 hr | 4 | 4–8 | 8–12 |
| Cephaloridine | 1.5 | 20 | 0.46 | 0.035 | 70% i.m. | Low | Nephrotoxic | 500 mg–1 g/6–12 hr | 8–12 | 12–24 | 24–48 |
| Cephalexin | 0.9 | 30 | 0.77 | 0.023 | 90% p.o. | 12% | None | 250 mg/6 hr | (Avoid) 8–12 | (Avoid) 12–24 | (Avoid) 24–48 |
| Cefazolin | 1.9 | 56 | 0.36 | 0.012 | >90% | 86% | None | 500 mg/8 hr | 8–12 | 12–24 | 24–48 |
| **Tetracyclines** | | | | | | | | | | | |
| Tetracycline | 10 | 100 | 0.069 | 0.007 | 60% | 65% | Azotemia, acidosis, hepatoxicity, hyperphosphatemia | 250 mg/6 hr | 6–8 | 24–48 | 48–96 |
| Oxytetracycline | 8 | 66 | 0.087 | 0.011 | 70% | 35% | Same as tetracycline | 250 mg/6 hr | 8 | 8–21 | 21–36 |
| Chlortetracycline | (9) | (9) | 0.077 | 0.077 | 18% | 45% | Same as tetracycline | 250 mg/6 hr | (Avoid) | (Avoid) | (Avoid) |
| Demeclocycline | 14 | ↑ | 0.050 | — | 40% | 90% | Same as tetracycline | 300 mg/12 hr | (Inadequate information) | (Inadequate information) | (Inadequate information) |
| Methacycline | 14 | ↑ | 0.050 | — | 50% | 90% | Same as tetracycline | 300 mg/12 hr | (Inadequate information) | (Inadequate information) | (Inadequate information) |
| Rolitetracycline | 12 | 35 | 0.058 | 0.02 | 60% | 50% | Same as tetracycline | 350 mg/12 hr | 12 | 24–72 | 72–96 |
| Minocycline | 13 | ? | 0.053 | ? | 6% | 75% | Same as tetracycline (?) | 100 mg/12 hr | 18 | 18–24 | 24–36 |
| Doxycycline | 17 | 17 | 0.041 | 0.041 | 33% | 90% | None | 100 mg/24 hr | 24 | 24 | 24 |
| **Antifungals** | | | | | | | | | | | |
| Amphotericin B | 24 | 24 | 0.029 | 0.029 | 2–5% | ? | Nephrotoxicity, 80% of patients | 1 mg/kg/24 hr | 24 | 24 | (Avoid) |
| Flucytosine | 3 | 70 | 0.23 | 0.01 | 90% | 48% | None | 38 mg/kg/6 hr | 6–12 | 12–48 | 48–144 |
| Griseofulvin | 20 | 20 | 0.035 | 0.035 | 1% | ? | None | 500 mg/6 hr | 6 | 6 | 6 |

| DRUG | SERUM t½ (hr) NORMAL | SERUM t½ (hr) OLIGURIC | ELIMINATION CONSTANT (Ke) NORMAL | ELIMINATION CONSTANT (Ke) OLIGURIC | % RECOVERED UNCHANGED IN URINE (NORMAL Ccr) | % BOUND TO SERUM PROTEINS | TOXICITY LIABILITY IN RENAL IMPAIRMENT | USUAL ADULT MAINTENANCE DOSE AND DOSING INTERVAL | MAINTENANCE DOSE INTERVALS IN RENAL IMPAIRMENT (hr) MILD | MODERATE | SEVERE |
|---|---|---|---|---|---|---|---|---|---|---|---|
| *Polymyxins* | | | | | | | | | | | |
| Polymyxin B | 4.4 | 35 | 0.16 | 0.02 | 60% | Low | Azotemia, GFR, nephrotoxicity, neurotoxicity | 500 µg/kg/6 hr | | (See text) | |
| Colistin (Colistimethate) | 2.4 | 10 | 0.29 | 0.069 | 60–75% | Low | Nephrotoxicity, neurotoxicity | 1.5–2.5 mg/kg/12 hr | 24–36 | 36–72 | 72–90 |
| *Aminoglycosides* | | | | | | | | | | | |
| Streptomycin | 2.5 | 100 | 0.28 | 0.007 | 30–80% | 34% | Ototoxicity, nephrotoxicity | 1 g/12 hr | 24 | 24–72 | 72–96 |
| Gentamicin | 2 | 67 | 0.35 | 0.01 | 86–100% | 2% | Ototoxicity, nephrotoxicity | 1 mg/kg/8 hr | 8–12 | 12–36 | 48–96 |
| Kanamycin | 4 | 84 | 0.17 | 0.008 | 52–90% | 3% | Ototoxicity, nephrotoxicity | 7 mg/kg/12 hr | 18–24 | 24–72 | 72–96 |
| *Antituberculars* | | | | | | | | | | | |
| Isoniazid | 1.1 (rapid) 3.6 (slow) | 8 avg. | 0.63 (rapid) 0.19 (slow) | 0.087 | 5% (rapid) 25% (slow) | None | Peripheral neuritis | 100 mg/8 hr | 8 | 8 | 8 |
| Aminosalicylic acid | 0.7 | ↑ | 0.99 | — | 40% | 68% | Uremic distress, acidosis | 3 g/6 hr | 6 | (Avoid) | (Avoid) |
| Ethambutol | 6.5 | 32 | 0.11 | 0.022 | 70% | ? | Ocular toxicity | 25 mg/kg/day first 60 days | 24–48 | 48–96 | 96–120 |
| Rifampin | 2.75 | 2.75 | 0.25 | 0.25 | 9–15% | 75% | None | 600 mg/24 hr | 24 | 24 | 24 |
| Bacitracin | 1.5 | ↑ | 0.46 | — | 30% | ? | Nephrotoxicity | Systemic use rare, 50,000 U/6 hr | (Avoid) | (Avoid) | (Avoid) |
| Chloramphenicol | 2.5 | 4 | 0.28 | 0.17 | 5–15% | 60% | Erythropoietic depression | 250 mg/6 hr | 6 | 6 | 6 |
| Chloroquine | 150 | ↑ | 0.004 | — | ? | 50% | Retinopathy | 200 mg/12 hr | 6 | (See text) | |
| Clindamycin | 2.4 | 5 | 0.29 | 0.14 | 12% | 90% | None | 150 mg/6 hr | 6 | 6 | 6 |
| Erythromycin | 1.5 | 5.8 | 0.46 | 0.12 | 15% | 18% | None | 250 mg/6 hr | 6 | 6 | 6 |
| Lincomycin | 5 | 13 | 0.14 | 0.053 | 5–15% | ? | None | 250 mg/6 hr | 6 | 6–8 | 8–12 |
| Neomycin | 6 | ↑ | 0.12 | — | 50% | ? | Ototoxicity, nephrotoxicity | 4 g p.o. Single dose | | (See text) | |
| Vancomycin | 5 | 240 | 0.14 | 0.003 | 90% | 10% | Ototoxicity | 1 g/12 hr | 24–72 | 72–240 | 240 |
| *Urinary Antiinfectives* | | | | | | | | | | | |
| Nitrofurantoin | 0.33 | Slight | 2.10 | — | 30–40% | 25–60% | Polyneuropathy, hypersensitivity | 50–100 mg/6 hr | 6 | (Avoid) | (Avoid) |
| Nalidixic acid | 1.6 | 21 | 0.43 | 0.033 | (See text) | 93% | None | 500 mg/6 hr | 6 | 6 | (Avoid) |
| Methenamine | 2 | ↑ | 0.35 | — | 80% | ? | None | 500 mg–1 g/6 hr | 6 | 6 | (Avoid) |
| Trimethoprim | 10.6 | (See text) | 0.065 | — | 53% | 70% | (See text) | 160 mg/12 hr | | (See text) | |
| *Sulfonamides* | | | | | | | | | | | |
| Sulfisoxazole | 6 | 12 | 0.12 | 0.058 | 70% | 25% | Crystalluria | 1 g/6 hr | 6 | (Avoid) | (Avoid) |
| Sulfamethizole | ? | 58 | — | 0.012 | 90% | 90% | Crystalluria | 1 g/6 hr | | (See text) | |
| Sulfamethoxazole | 9.3 | (See text) | 0.074 | — | 30–50% | 50% | Crystalluria | 500 mg/12 hr | | (See text) | |

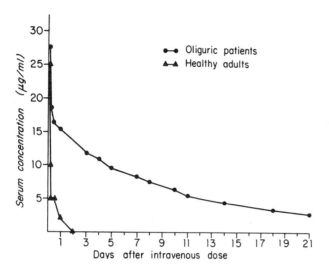

Figure 2. Average serum concentrations of vancomycin after single 1-g doses given i.v. to oliguric patients as compared to healthy patients[54]

useful against most gram-negative bacilli, a notable exception being *Pseudomonas aeruginosa*. It is probably most effective against Proteus species, but many sensitive gram-negative bacilli become resistant within a few days of therapy. Four metabolites of nalidixic acid have been identified; one of these, hydroxynalidixic acid, has an in vitro spectrum similar to nalidixic acid. The other metabolites are inactive. McChesney et al.[62] found a serum $t_{1/2}$ of 1.4–1.7 hours for nalidixic acid, and they also found that administration of sodium bicarbonate increased the amount of active drug excreted in the urine. About 80% of a dose is recovered in the urine, 20% being in an active form and 60% in a conjugated inactive form. The extent of conjugation may vary considerably, however, between individuals. Total concentration of nalidixic acid and its metabolites reach about 1000 $\mu$g/ml after a single 1-g dose in adults. Goff, Schlegal and O'Dell[58,59] studied the urinary excretion of nalidixic acid in uremic patients and found the same concentration in uremia as in patients with normal kidney function. The authors suggest that if nalidixic acid is used in renal impairment, a high initial dose be followed by the usual maintenance dose. Lowentritt and Schlegal[63] found the serum $t_{1/2}$ of nalidixic acid in the anuric patient to be about 21 hours. Skin rashes, photosensitivities, visual disturbances and convulsions occur occasionally with nalidixic acid therapy, and more rarely, cholestatic jaundice and blood dyscrasias may occur. It is not known if renal impairment increases the incidence of toxicity.

*Methenamine.* Methenamine mandelate and hippurate are used exclusively as urinary germicides, and their action is dependent upon the degradation of methenamine to formaldehyde in an acidic urine. The optimal acidity for this degradation is $pH$ 5.5 or less. No articles have been located on the use of methenamine in renal impairment. The American Hospital Formulary Service[64] states that since the efficacy of methenamine is dependent upon an adequate concentration of formalde-

hyde in the urine; and, since a therapeutic concentration is unlikely to be obtained in the presence of renal impairment, the drug is not likely to be therapeutically effective when renal function is significantly impaired.

**Sulfonamides**

The sulfonamides are bacteriostatic drugs active against a number of gram-negative and gram-positive organisms. Today their use is most commonly for urinary tract infections. The clinically useful sulfonamides are all absorbed rapidly from the gastrointestinal tract, and effective blood and urine levels are maintained by the oral route.

All of the sulfonamides are excreted in the urine either as the free drug or as the acetyl or glucuronide conjugate. Glomerular filtration is the primary mechanism of renal excretion, although active tubular secretion occurs with some of these drugs. Also, tubular reabsorption of varying degrees occurs with most sulfonamides. The long-acting sulfonamides, sulfamethoxypyridazine and sulfadimethoxine, remain in the body for extended periods of time because of a high degree of tubular reabsorption.

The $N^4$-acetyl derivative, the major metabolite for nearly all of the sulfonamides, does not possess antibacterial activity but does contribute to toxicity. Also, the acetylated metabolite crystallizes in the urine more readily than the free drug.[12] Because the acetylated fraction of most sulfonamides increases considerably as the serum $t_{1/2}$ increases, they are not recommended in moderate to severe renal impairment. All sulfonamides are bound loosely to plasma protein in varying degrees. Generally, the acetylated form is bound to a greater extent than the free drug, and the long-acting sulfonamides are more highly bound than the shorter-acting compounds.

These drugs may cause serious, sometimes fatal, adverse effects. The incidence of adverse effects is greater with the long-acting sulfonamides, and their use is not generally recommended. Many of the adverse effects are sensitivity reactions, i.e., various rashes, photosensitivities and erythema multiforme (Stevens-Johnson syndrome). Although Stevens-Johnson syndrome is most often associated with the long-acting drugs, other sulfonamides have caused this reaction. Sulfonamides are oxidants and may induce hemolytic anemia in persons with glucose 6-phosphate dehydrogenase deficiency. Agranulocytosis, aplastic anemia and thrombocytopenia have been associated with sulfonamide therapy, and liver damage may occur. The relationship of these reactions to renal impairment is not known. Crystalluria due to precipitation of the free drug and/or its $N^4$-acetyl metabolite in the urinary tract may cause renal damage. The incidence of crystalluria may be kept to a minimum by using a more soluble sulfonamide such as sulfisoxazole, by using the trisulfapyrimidine combination, by keeping the patient well hydrated or by alkalinizing the urine.

*Sulfisoxazole.* One of the most soluble sulfonamides, sulfisoxazole, is distributed only in extracellular body water. Weinstein et al.[65] have reported that 95% of a single dose is excreted by the kidneys in 24 hours. From 30–35% of the drug is acetylated and about 70% reaches the urine in the free form. Sulfisoxazole is bound about 25% to proteins.

Svec et al.[66] have shown that sulfisoxazole is much more soluble in the urine at *p*H values of 5–6 than is sulfadiazine. Nevertheless, precaution should be taken to insure an adequate output of urine—1,200–1,500 ml/day —in order to prevent crystalluria. Reidenberg et al.[67] studied the metabolism of sulfisoxazole in normal obese patients and in azotemic patients. From the elimination constants reported in this study a normal serum $t_{1/2}$ of 5.6 hours and an azotemic (BUN values ranging from 31–78 mg/100 ml) $t_{1/2}$ of 11.1 hours can be calculated. Goossens and van Oudtshoorn[68] report a normal $t_{1/2}$ of 6.3 hours for sulfisoxazole. They also found that by alkalinizing the urine the serum $t_{1/2}$ is reduced to 4.4 hours and the average percent acetylated is reduced from 35% to 26%.

In moderate to severe renal impairment, the fraction of acetylated (inactive) sulfisoxazole would increase in both the serum and urine. Due to the poor solubility of the acetyl metabolite, crystalluria is more likely to occur and effective free drug urine levels would be more difficult to obtain. Sulfisoxazole is thus not recommended for use in patients with moderate to severe renal impairment.

*Sulfamethoxazole.* This drug is very similar to sulfisoxazole; however, its rates of absorption and excretion are slower. Also, sulfamethoxazole is less soluble and more likely to precipitate in the urine than sulfisoxazole. About 60% of the total drug is excreted in 48 hours, and it is approximately 50% bound to plasma proteins. Only 30–50% of the drug reaches the urine in the free (active) form with 50–70% being acetylated.[64] This high degree of acetylation makes sulfamethoxazole less effective than sulfisoxazole against urinary tract infections. Craig and Kunin[69] have studied the kinetics of sulfamethoxazole when given in combination with trimethoprim. The serum $t_{1/2}$ of the nonacetylated drug in normal subjects was 9.3 hours. In severely uremic patients the serum $t_{1/2}$ ranged from 22–50 hours. Nonacetylated sulfamethoxazole was found to be normally bound about 62% to plasma proteins, but the binding is consistently reduced in uremic patients. Uremic patients with low serum albumin bound only 15% of the drug.

*Sulfadiazine.* Sulfadiazine is excreted rather slowly by the kidneys with only 60–85% of an oral dose being excreted in 48–72 hours. It is approximately 55% bound to plasma proteins. Due to its low solubility, crystalluria is a constant concern. From 15–40% of sulfadiazine in the urine is acetylated.[12] Adam and Dawborn[70] studied the effects of renal impairment on urinary excretion and plasma levels of two sulfonamides. They noted an accumulation in the plasma of free and conjugated sulfadiaz-

ine associated with toxic side effects and a significant reduction in urine concentration of free drug in renally-impaired patients. They suggest that sulfonamides are contraindicated in patients with serum creatinine levels greater than 5 mg/100 ml.

*Sulfamethizole.* This drug is absorbed and excreted very rapidly with 84–97% of the total drug being excreted in 10 hours. This rapid rate of excretion makes maintenance of effective blood levels very difficult, and the drug is useful only for urinary tract infections. Sulfamethizole is highly soluble and crystalluria rarely occurs. About 90% of the drug is bound to plasma proteins.[64] Lowentritt and Schlegel[63] reported an anuric $t_{1/2}$ of 58 hours. Significantly, only 2–9% of the drug in the urine is acetylated with about 90% reaching the urine in the free, active form. There is conflicting data regarding the excretion of free sulfamethizole in patients with impaired renal function. Schlegal et al.[58] and Goff et al.[59] found that patients with a creatinine clearance as low as 8 ml/min can excrete sulfamethizole in the urine to the same extent as normal individuals, provided the serum concentration is correspondingly elevated. They suggest initiating therapy with higher than normal doses (2 g every six hours for four doses) to provide serum levels great enough to produce effective urine concentrations in the first 24 hours, thereafter lowering the dose to the normal maintenance dose (1 g every six hours). These authors were measuring only free (active) sulfonamide using the modified Bratton-Marshall technique,[1] indicating that sulfamethizole's degree of acetylation remains low even in severe renal impairment. No toxic effects due to elevated serum levels were noted by these authors. Adam and Dawborn[70] noted, however, a reduction in urine concentration of free sulfamethizole in patients with renal impairment. They found increased serum levels of free and conjugated drug and an increased incidence of side effects. The findings of Adam and Dawborn are similar to those of Lippman and Marti[72] on sulfisomidine. One would expect the degree of acetylation of any sulfonamide to increase if the drug remains in the body for extended periods of time.

*Sulfisomidine (Sulfadimetine).* This drug has less antibacterial activity than sulfisoxazole but is acetylated to only a small degree (5–10%). About 80% of a single oral dose is excreted by the kidney in 24 hours and only 10% of this is acetylated.[12] Lippman and Marti[72] investigated the effect of renal function on the excretion of sulfisomidine. They found that the drug accumulated in the serum of renally-impaired patients with small amounts reaching the urine. Also, acetylation was found to be significantly increased when renal function was impaired, reducing the effective free drug concentration. Lippman and Marti were using low doses of sulfisomidine (125 mg four times daily), and this, along with the renal impairment, probably contributed to the ineffective urine concentrations.

*Sulfadimethoxine and Sulfamethoxypyridazine.* As mentioned earlier, the long-acting sulfonamides, sulfadimethoxine and sulfamethoxypyridazine, produce lower urine concentrations and are more likely to accumulate and cause toxic reactions than the other sulfonamides. A study by Madsen[73] on the excretion of long-acting sulfonamides in renal failure and hepatitis provides information that might be applicable to other sulfonamides. As would be expected, in renal insufficiency the total amount of long-acting sulfonamide excreted is low. In hepatitis the excretory rates of total drug did not differ significantly from normal. There was a greater percentage of free (active) drug excreted in the urine of patients with hepatitis, reflecting a decreased rate of metabolism. Madsen's results regarding acetylation rates differ markedly from those of Reidenberg et al.[67] who found the rate of acetylation of sulfisoxazole in one cirrhotic patient to be the same as for normal individuals.

### Trimethoprim

Trimethoprim is effective against a wide variety of bacterial species because of its antifolic acid activity. It inhibits the enzyme dihydrofolate reductase. Sulfonamides potentiate the antibacterial effect of trimethoprim. The drug is used clinically in combination with sulfamethoxazole because of its similar biological $t_{1/2}$. Craig and Kunin[69] have studied the serum $t_{1/2}$ of trimethoprim and sulfamethoxazole in both normal and uremic patients. The normal serum $t_{1/2}$ for trimethoprim was found to be 10.6 hours. In the severely uremic patients, the serum $t_{1/2}$ varied from 14–46 hours. One uremic patient with a persistently alkaline urine had a trimethoprim $t_{1/2}$ of 46 hours and a sulfamethoxazole $t_{1/2}$ of 22 hours. Another severely uremic patient with a persistently acidic urine had a trimethoprim $t_{1/2}$ of 14 hours and a sulfamethoxazole $t_{1/2}$ of 50 hours. In patients with a $C_{cr}$ of <10 ml/min, the serum $t_{1/2}$ of trimethoprim was generally less than that of sulfamethoxazole (Figure 3). Trimethoprim is normally bound 70% to plasma proteins, and this does not significantly change in renally-impaired patients, according to the data of Craig and Kunin.[69] The drug is removed by both glomerular filtration and tubular secretion. Normally about 53% of the trimethoprim dose is recovered unchanged in the urine. This decreases to 1–4% in patients requiring hemodialysis. Hemodialysis effectively removes trimethoprim and sulfamethoxazole.

A modified dosage schedule for trimethoprim-sulfamethoxazole seems to be indicated in moderate-severe renal impairment. Craig and Kunin recommend that with a $C_{cr}$ < 10 ml/min a full loading dose be followed by half the loading dose once or twice daily. In patients undergoing hemodialysis, a dose should be given at the beginning and end of the procedure. Urine levels in uremic patients were generally adequate to treat infections due to *E. coli* and *Proteus* species.

Kalowski et al.[74] have reported 16 cases of deteriora-

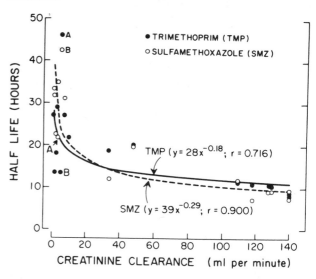

Figure 3. Relation between renal function (expressed by creatinine clearance) and half-life of nonacetylated sulfamethoxazole and trimethoprim in serum after a single oral dose of combined drugs (800 mg SMZ, 160 mg TMP); one uremic patient who received only trimethoprim (160 mg) is also included[69]

tion of renal function while receiving trimethoprim-sulfamethoxazole. The damage reversed in 13, but was permanent in three. Most of the patients had associated renal lesions and were receiving other drugs, although these were not recognized to be nephrotoxic. The authors postulate that the mechanism may have been acute tubular necrosis due to the time course, reversibility of damage in 13 of 16 patients, and renal biopsy results in two patients. Five of the patients received reduced doses as recommended in the literature. The acetylated sulfonamide metabolites accumulate in renal impairment and may have contributed to the deterioration. If trimethoprim-sulfamethoxazole is used with a reduced $C_{cr}$, the patient should be closely monitored for renal changes.

### Commentary

From the data discussed above it is possible to dose safely many antimicrobial agents in renal impairment. The data on certain drugs are incomplete and often not precise, and pharmacists and physicians trying to calculate exact doses must realize the limitations imposed. Even well studied drugs such as gentamicin are surrounded by controversy. The various gentamicin dosage recommendations vary greatly, particularly the resulting time with subtherapeutic serum levels present. Anyone recommending dosage adjustments in the clinical setting must understand the various theories and dosing guidelines and be able to justify his recommendations. The relative importance of dosage adjustments must also be well understood for the various drugs. It is pointless to attempt to calculate exact doses for a drug such as penicillin G which has such a wide margin of safety. It should be sufficient to empirically adjust the dose only when severe renal impairment exists. Due to the elimination kinetics and the margin between effective and toxic serum levels, the aminoglycosides require dosage adjustment even in mild renal impairment. Summary tables are helpful in alerting the clinician to needed dosage changes, but alone they are clearly insufficient.

In dosing in renal impairment, most authors recommend that the first dose of a drug be given in the usual manner. That is, the normal loading or maintenance dose is given, and then subsequent doses or the dosing intervals are adjusted according to the severity of renal impairment. This approach has apparently been generally satisfactory. A study by Gibaldi and Perrier[75] casts some doubt on this general principle. They have found that the apparent volume of distribution decreases in severe renal impairment, and the usual dose of a drug with a low margin of safety could perhaps be toxic. Their calculations of the volume of distribution were done from published articles on cephalexin, colistimethate, lincomycin, methicillin and insulin. The volume of distribution decreased by 20-50% with the drugs studied. Prospective studies are needed to assess the significance of this change in volume of distribution since it is an important factor in determining serum levels and possible toxicity. It is probably of little significance except in severe renal impairment where dosing adjustments are critical.

The clinician wishing to be able to accurately calculate doses of drugs to fit a variety of circumstances surrounding patients with renal impairment must have a working knowledge of basic pharmacokinetics. The texts of Wagner[76] and Goldstein et al.[77] provide considerable background on the derivation of kinetic formulas, but the formulas may prove difficult to apply easily in the clinical setting. Dettli et al.[78,79] have described a rather simple method of bedside calculation using the elimination constant of the drug in normal and anuric patients as the basis. Hirschman and Borgsdorf[80] have derived a formula to calculate the serum $t_{1/2}$ in various degrees of renal impairment when the normal serum $t_{1/2}$ and the percentage urinary excretion are known. From the new serum $t_{1/2}$, the proper dose to give at a specified interval can be easily determined. All of these formulas have limitations, and these should be understood well when calculating doses. Additional reviews include those by Schumacher,[81] Giusti and Hayton[82] and Kruger-Thiemer.[83]

Table 1 uses the principle of keeping a constant dose and varying the dosing interval based on the degree of renal impairment. This allows a concise table and is adequate for many drugs, but may not be appropriate for drugs with a low margin of safety when used in severe renal impairment. When this principle is followed, some critical drugs are dosed every several days. It is difficult for those administering drugs to adhere to such schedules, and subtherapeutic levels may be present for ex-

tended periods of time. A specific dose to be given at least once daily should offer several advantages. The above-mentioned articles discuss this type of dosage calculation, and they should be used for more accurate dosing.

## References

1. Harris, H. N.: Current Concepts on the Metabolism of Antituberculous Agents, *Ann. N.Y. Acad. Sci. 106*:43 (Feb.) 1963.

2. Bowersox, D. W. et al.: Isoniazid Dosage in Patients with Renal Failure (Abstract), *Amer. Rev. Resp. Dis. 105*:1020 (June) 1972.

3. Bennett, W. M. et al.: A Practical Guide to Drug Usage in Adult Patients with Impaired Renal Function, *JAMA 214*:1468 (Nov. 23) 1970.

4. Kunin, C. M.: Antibiotic Usage in Patients with Renal Impairment, *Hosp. Pract. 7*:141 (Jan.) 1972.

5. Glogner, P. et al.: Dialysis in Isoniazid Intoxication, *Deut. Med. Wochenschr. 96*:1307 (Aug. 6) 1971.

6. Durr, F. and Missmahl, H. P.: Extracorporal Hemodialysis of Isoniazid, *Deut. Med. Wochenschr. 90*:1174 (June 25) 1965.

7. Jenne, J. W. et al.: A Study of the Clearances, Metabolic Inactivation Rates and Serum Fall-Off Interaction of Isoniazid and PAS in Man, *Amer. Rev. Resp. Dis. 84*:371 (Sept.) 1961.

8. Peets, E. A. et al.: The Absorption, Excretion and Metabolic Fate of Ethambutol in Man, *Amer. Rev. Resp. Dis. 91*:51 (Jan.) 1965.

9. Pyle, M. M. et al.: A 4-Year Clinical Investigation of Ethambutol, *Amer. Rev. Resp. Dis. 93*:428 (Mar.) 1966.

10. Strauss, I. and Erhardt, F.: Ethambutol Absorption, Excretion and Dosage in Patients with Renal Tuberculosis, *Chemotherapy 15*:148, 1970.

11. Wilson, T. M.: Current Therapeutics—Capreomycin and Ethambutol, *Practitioner 199*:817 (Dec.) 1967.

12. Goodman, L. S. and Gilman, A.: The Pharmacologic Basis of Therapeutics, 4th ed., The MacMillan Co., New York, New York.

13. Cohn, H. D.: Clinical Studies with a New Rifamycin Derivative, *J. Clin. Pharmacol. 9*:19 (Mar.–Apr.) 1969.

14. Furesz, S. et al.: Absorption, Distribution and Elimination of Rifampin in Man, *Arzneim. Forsch. 17*:534, 1967.

15. Spring, P. and Dettli, L.: Pharmacokinetics of Rifampin in Normal and Pathologically Altered Elimination, Fifth International Congress of Chemotherapy, Vienna, 1967, p. 137.

16. Bergamini, N. et al.: A Clinical Survey of Rifampin, *Arzneim. Forsch. 20*:1546 (Oct.) 1970.

17. Ramgopal, V. et al.: Acute Renal Failure Associated with Rifampin, *Lancet 1*:1195 (May 26) 1973.

18. Epstein, I. G.: Pyridoxine and Its Relation to Cycloserine Neurotoxicity, *Antibiot. Ann.*:472, 1958–1959.

19. Conzelman, G. M.: The Physiologic Disposition of Cycloserine in the Human Subject, *Amer. Rev. Tuberc. 74*:739 (Nov.) 1956.

20. Caccia, P. A.: Spectrophotometric Determination of Pyrazinamide Blood Concentrations and Excretion Through the Kidneys, *Amer. Rev. Resp. Dis. 75*:105, 1957.

21. Stottmeier, K. D. et al.: The Absorption and Excretion of Pyrazinamide, *Amer. Rev. Resp. Dis. 98*:70 (July) 1968.

22. Kruger-Thiemer, E.: Theorie de Wirkung Bakteriostatischer Chemotherapeutika, *Jahresbericht Borstel. 5*:316, 1961.

23. Eagle, H. et al.: The Blood Levels and Renal Clearance of Bacitracin in Rabbits and Man, *J. Clin. Invest. 26*:919 (Sept.) 1947.

24. Zintel, H. A. et al.: The Absorption, Distribution, Excretion and Toxicity of Bacitracin in Man, *Amer. J. Med. Sci. 218*:439 (Oct.) 1949.

25. Jawetz, E.: Polymyxin, Colistin and Bacitracin, *Ped. Clin. N. Amer. 8*:1057 (Nov.) 1961.

26. Rubin, D. et al.: Early Detection of Drug Induced Erythropoietic Depression, *J. Lab. Clin. Med. 56*:453 (Sept.) 1960.

27. Kunin, C. M. et al.: Persistence of Chloramphenicol and Its Metabolites in the Blood of Patients and Renal Disease and Hepatic Cirrhosis, *J. Clin. Invest.* 38:1498, 1959.

28. Suhrland, L. G. and Weisberger, A. S.: Chloramphenicol Toxicity in Renal and Hepatic Disease, *Arch. Internal Med.* 112:747 (Nov.) 1963.

29. Lindberg, A. A. et al.: Concentration of Chloramphenicol in the Urine and Blood in Relation to Renal Function, *Brit. Med. J.* 2:724 (Sept. 24) 1966.

30. Greenberg, P. A. and Sanford, J. P.: Removal and Absorption of Antibiotics in Patients with Renal Failure Undergoing Peritoneal Dialysis, *Ann. Internal Med.* 66:465-479 (Mar.) 1967.

31. Faber, J. et al.: Influence of Renal Insufficiency on the Excretion of Chloroquine, Phenobarbital, Phenothiazines and Methacycline, *Helv. Med. Acta* 33:307, 1966.

32. *Med. Letter Drug Ther.* 12: (Oct. 16) 1970.

33. Wagner, J. G. et al.: Absorption, Excretion and Half-Life of Clinimycin in Normal Adult Males, *Amer. J. Med. Sci.* 256:25–37 (July) 1968.

34. McGeher, R. F. et al.: Comparative Studies of Antibacterial Activity in Vitro and Absorption and Excretion of Lincomycin and Clindamycin, *Amer. J. Med. Sci.* 256:279 (Nov.) 1968.

35. Cemino, J. E. and Tierno, P. M., Jr.: Hemodialysis Properties of Clindamycin, *Appl. Microbiol.* 17:446–448 (Mar.) 1969.

36. Ellard, G. A.: Absorption, Metabolism and Excretion of Dapsone in Man, *Brit. J. Pharmacol. Chemother.* 26:212 (Jan.) 1966.

37. Dharmendra et al.: Dapsone in the Treatment of Leprosy, *Leprosy in India* 22:174, 1950.

38. Belmont, A.: Dapsone-Induced Nephrotic Syndrome, *JAMA* 200:262 (Apr. 17) 1967.

39. Griffith, R. S. et al.: The Distribution and Excretion of Erythromycin Following IV Injection, *Antibiot. Ann.*:496, 1953–1954.

40. Reinarz, T. A. and McIntosh, D. A.: Lincomycin Excretion in Patients with Normal Renal Function, Severe Azotemia and with Hemodialysis and Peritoneal Dialysis, *Antimicrob. Agents Chemother.*:232-243, 1965.

41. Bellamy, H. M., Jr. et al.: Lincomycin Metabolism in Patients with Hepatic Insufficiency: Effect of Liver Disease on Lincomycin Serum Concentrations, *Antimicrob. Agents Chemother.*:36-41, 1966.

42. Last, P. M. and Sherlock, S.: Systemic Absorption of Orally Administered Neomycin in Liver Disease, *N. Engl. J. Med.* 262:385 (Feb. 25) 1960.

43. Halpern, E. B. and Heller, M. F.: Ototoxicity of Orally Administered Neomycin, *Arch. Otolaryng.* 73:675 (June) 1961.

44. Kelly, D. R. et al.: Deafness After Topical Neomycin Wound Irrigation, *N. Engl. J. Med.* 288:1338 (June 12) 1969.

45. Campanelli, P. A. et al.: Hearing Loss in a Child Following Neomycin Irrigation, *Med. Ann. D.C.* 35:541 (Oct.) 1966.

46. Fields, R. L.: Neomycin Ototoxicity Due to Rectal and Colonic Irrigation, *Arch. Otolaryng.* 79:67 (Jan.) 1964.

47. Fuller, A.: Ototoxicity Due to Long Term Use of Neomycin Aerosol, *Lancet* 1:1026 (May 7) 1960.

48. Herd et al.: Ototoxicity of Topical Neomycin Augmented by DMSO, *Pediatrics* 40:906 (Nov.) 1967.

49. Waisbren, B. A. and Spink, W. W.: Clinical Appraisal of Neomycin, *Ann. Internal Med.* 33:1099 (Nov.) 1950.

50. Kunin, C. M. et al.: Absorption of Orally Administered Neomycin and Kanamycin, *N. Engl. J. Med.* 262:380–385 (Feb. 25) 1960.

51. Krumlovsky, F. A. et al.: Dialysis in Treatment of Neomycin Overdose, *Ann Internal Med.* 76:443 (Mar.) 1972.

52. Lee, C. C. et al.: Distribution, Excretion and Renal Clearance of Vancomycin, *Antibiot. Ann.*:82, 1957.

53. Leach, W.: Ototoxicity of Neomycin and Other Antibiotics, *J. Laryng. Otol.* 76:774, 1962.

54. Lindholm, D. C. and Murray, J. S.: Persistence of Vancomycin in the Blood During Renal Failure and its Treatment by Hemodialysis, *N. Engl. J. Med.* 274:1047 (May 12) 1966.

55. Sachs, J. et al.: Effect of Renal Function on Urinary Recovery of Orally Administered Nitrofurantoin, *N. Engl. J. Med.* 278:1032 (May 9) 1968.

56. Reckendorf, H. K. et al.: Comparative Pharmacodynamics, Urinary Excretion and Half-Life Determinations of Nitrofurantoin, *Antimicrob. Agents Chemother.*:531, 1962.

57. Buzard, J. A. et al.: Studies on the Absorption, Distribution and Elimination of Nitrofurantoin in the Rat. *J. Pharmacol. Exp. Ther* 131:38 (Jan.) 1961.

58. Schlegal, J. N. et al.: Bacteriuria and Chronic Renal Disease, *Trans. Amer. Ass. Genito. Urin. Surg.* 59:32, 1967.

59. Goff, J. B. et al.: Urinary Excretion of Nalidixic Acid, Sulfamethizole and Nitrofurantoin in Patients with Reduced Renal Function, *J. Urol.* 99:371 (Apr.) 1968.

60. Loughridge, L. W.: Peripheral Neuropathy Due to Nitrofurantoin, *Lancet* 2:1133 (Dec. 1) 1962.

61. Roelsen, E.: Polyneuritis After Nitrofurantoin Therapy, *Acta. Med. Scand.* 175:145 (Feb.) 1964.

62. McChesney, E. W. et al.: Absorption, Excretion and Metabolism of Nalidixic Acid, *Toxicol. Appl. Pharmacol.* 6:292 (May) 1964.

63. Lowentritt, L. I. and Schlegal, J. N.: Treatment of Bacteriuria in Patients with Impaired Renal Function, *J. Urol.* 102:473 (Oct.) 1969.

64. American Hospital Formulary Service, American Society of Hospital Pharmacists, Washington, D.C.

65. Weinstein, L. et al.: The Sulfonamides, *N. Engl. J. Med.* 263:793-800 (Oct. 20) 1960.

66. Svec, F. A. et al.: New Sulfonamide (Gantrisin): Studies on Solubility, Absorption, and Excretion, *Arch. Internal Med.* 85:88-90 (Jan.) 1950.

67. Reidenberg, M. M. et al.: Rate of Drug Metabolism in Obese Volunteers Before and During Starvation and in Azotemic Patients, *Metabolism* 18:209–214 (Mar.) 1969.

68. Goossens, A. P. and van Oudtshoorn, M. C. B.: Determination of Pharmacokinetic Parameters for Urinary Excretion of Sulfafurazole Under Normal and Controlled Alkaline Urine Conditions, *J. Pharm. Pharmacol.* 22:224–226 (Mar.) 1970.

69. Craig, W. A. and Kunin, C. M.: Pharmacodynamic Effects of Urinary pH and Renal Impairment on Trimethoprim-Sulfamethoxazole, *Ann. Internal Med.* 78:491 (Apr.) 1973.

70. Adam, W. R. and Dawborn, J. K.: Urinary Excretion and Plasma Levels of Sulfonamides in Patients with Renal Impairment, *Aust. Ann. Med.* 19:250–254 (Aug.) 1970.

71. Bratton, A. C. and Marshall, E. K., Jr.: A New Coupling Component for Sulfanilamide Determination, *J. Biol. Chem.* 128:537–550 (May) 1939.

72. Lippman, R. W. and Marti, H. U.: Effect of Renal Function on Excretion of Sulfadimetine Given in Small Doses for Urinary Infection; *J. Urol.* 70:541 (Sept.) 1953.

73. Madsen, S. T.: A Comparative Study of the Excretion of Sulfonamide-Metabolites in Cases of Renal Failure and Hepatitis, *Chemotherapia* 1:1–9, 1966.

74. Kalowski, S. et al.: Deterioration in Renal Function in Association with Co-Trimoxazole Therapy, *Lancet* 1:394 (Feb. 24) 1973.

75. Gibaldi, M. and Perrier, D.: Drug Distribution in Renal Failure, *J. Clin Pharmacol.* 12:201 (May–June) 1972.

76. Wagner, J. G.: Biopharmaceutics and Relevant Pharmacokinetics, 1st ed., Drug Intelligence Publications, Hamilton, Illinois.

77. Goldstein, A. et al.: Principles of Drug Action, Hoeber Medical Division, Harper and Row, New York, New York.

78. Dettli, L. et al.: Multiple Dose Kinetics and Drug Dosage in Patients with Kidney Disease, *Acta Pharmacol. Toxicol.* 29:211 (Supp. 3) 1971.

79. Dettli, L. et al.: Drug Dosage in Patients with Impaired Renal Function, *Postgrad. Med. J.* 46:32 (Supp.) 1970.

80. Hirschman, J. and Borgsdorf, L.: DIAS Rounds, *Drug Intel. Clin. Pharm.* 5:251 (Aug.) 1971.

81. Schumacher, G. E.: Practical Pharmacokinetic Techniques for Drug Consultation and Evaluation. II: A Perspective on the Renal-impaired Patient, In *Clinical Pharmacy Sourcebook*, pp. 237-243.

82. Giusti, D. L. and Hayton, W. L.: Dosage Regimen Adjustments in Renal Impairment, *Drug Intel. Clin. Pharm.* 7:382 (Sept.) 1973.

83. Kruger-Thiemer, E.: Dosage Schedules and Pharmacokinetics in Chemotherapy, *J. Amer. Pharm. Ass. (Sci. Ed.)* 49:311, 1960.

# 50 Dosage Regimens of Antiarrhythmics, Part I: Pharmacokinetic Properties

René H. Levy and Gary H. Smith

A method is presented to develop individualized dosage regimens for cardiac antiarrhythmic drugs by applying steady-state kinetics (plateau principle) to pharmacokinetic parameters obtained from single dose studies.

The first step is to determine four fundamental drug parameters—the range of effective plasma levels, the volume of distribution, the biological half-life, and the fraction of drug absorbed. The significant data available in the literature on these four parameters for four drugs—lidocaine, procainamide, propranolol, and diphenylhydantoin—are presented. The ranges of effective levels, the volumes of distribution, and the biological half-lives for each agent are presented in tabular form. In several cases the data presently available are incomplete.

The application of these concepts to the calculation of maintenance dose and dosing intervals and to the handling of specific situations will be presented in the following chapter.

Cardiac arrhythmias, especially ventricular arrythmias, often constitute life-threatening situations, and their management remains a serious challenge to the clinician. In spite of the introduction of newer approaches such as electrical countershock and cardiac pacemakers, the requirement for maintenance and prophylactic therapy makes the continued study of antiarrhythmic agents important. The seriousness of most ventricular arrhythmias and the relatively narrow therapeutic range of most agents render drug administration complex and fraught with potential dangers. Consequently, it has become necessary for the clinician to increase his knowledge of the drug disposition (absorption, distribution, metabolism and excretion) of each agent utilized, ideally in each patient. However, the translation of drug disposition data into dosing guidelines useful in various clinical situations is yet unachieved not only in the case of antiarrhythmics, but for the majority of drugs. It is a major objective of clinical pharmacokinetics to narrow the gap between theory and practice. In a previous chapter, Schumacher[1] showed the applications of dosage regimen calculations in the evaluation of the tetracycline and penicillin antibiotics, and efforts of that type are critically needed.

The purpose of this chapter is to present a review of the significant pharmacokinetic properties of lidocaine, procainamide, propranolol, quinidine, and diphenylhy-dantoin. In the following chapter it will be shown how individualized dosage regimens can be developed when a few basic pharmacokinetic principles are utilized in conjunction with the appropriate pharmacokinetic parameters. Furthermore, these dosage regimen calculations will be reviewed with respect to the actual clinical picture including the appropriate use of serum concentrations as therapeutic guides.

## The Need for Dosage Regimen Calculations

For every agent approved for a given therapeutic use, one can find a standard dosage regimen from one of several reference sources, such as manufacturer's recommendations, and clinical pharmacology and medical textbooks. For many drugs, clinical experience has shown, however, that a significant fraction of patients do not respond adequately with those standard regimens. This is especially true for the antiarrhythmics. Recent investigations of the relationship between dosage and clinical response have shown that intersubject variability in drug absorption, distribution, metabolism and excretion are such that individualized dosage regimens are often necessary.[2-7] However, it should be emphasized at this point that in order to develop individual patient regimens, it is first necessary to dissociate the "standard" dosage regimen into its various components and then to understand how each component can vary and/or be adjusted under a specific clinical situation. This can be achieved best by analyzing a fundamental pharmacokinetic concept, the plateau principle.

The background for the pharmacokinetic considerations and equations presented in the next section can be found in one of several reference textbooks[8-11] and has, therefore, been omitted. Consequently, the following section contains only those concepts and definitions which are essential to the understanding of later applications.

### The Plateau Principle

The plateau principle is a general kinetic principle which applies to a wide variety of systems, from biochemical reactions to drug administration. Stated generally: If the rate of input into a system is constant and the rate of output from the system is exponential, the content of the system will accumulate until a steady state is reached. In terms of pharmacotherapeutics, this principle can be restated as follows: If a drug is administered at a constant rate (orally or parenterally) and its elimination from the body is exponential, the amount of drug in the body will accumulate until a steady state (or plateau) is reached.

A drug is administered at a constant average rate when it is given on a fixed-dose and fixed-time schedule such as once, twice or thrice daily (1 g/day is equivalent to 42.5 mg/hour or 0.70 mg/min) or when it is infused at a set flow rate. For most drugs (especially at low doses), elimination is an exponential process, i.e., the rate of elimination is not constant but increases proportionately as the amount of drug in the body increases. When the amount of drug present in the body is at a steady state, its rate of change is zero because the output rate has increased to a value equal to the constant input rate.

Under conditions of a constant rate of administration, the rate at which drug levels rise to the steady state is determined solely by the drug's biological half-life, $t_{1/2}$, which characterizes the exponential elimination process [$t_{1/2}$ is the time required for drug body levels to decrease by 50% (in the post distribution phase after intravenous administration or in the post absorption phase after oral or intramuscular administration); it is a biological constant of a given drug for a given individual at a given state of health]. At the end of the first half-life, the amount of drug in the body is equal to half the amount ultimately achieved at steady-state. At the end of the second, third and fourth half-lives, the amount of drug in the body represents 75%, 87.5% and 93.75%, respectively, of the steady-state amount. Thus, although theoretically steady-state is only achieved at infinite time, for practical purposes it is achieved (97%) within five half-lives.

### Continuous Mode of Administration: Intravenous Infusion

When a drug is infused at a constant rate, $R_0$, and is eliminated in a first-order fashion with a rate constant for elimination $K_e$, the steady state *amount* ultimately achieved in the body, $A_b^*$, is given by

$$A_b^* = \frac{R_0}{K_e} \tag{1}$$

From a practical standpoint, it is not possible to measure $A_b^*$. Fortunately, however, there exists a relationship between the amount of drug in the body at any time $A_b$ (including steady-state) and the corresponding drug *concentration* in blood, plasma ($C_p$) and tissues, as given by the definition of the apparent volume of distribution, $V_d$.

$$V_d = \frac{A_b}{C_p} \tag{2}$$

Thus, the plasma level at steady state $C_p^*$ is given by

$$C_p^* = \frac{R_0}{V_d K_e} \tag{3}$$

The product $V_d \times K_e$ is called total body clearance. Equation 3 can be written in terms of the biological half-life, $t_{1/2}$, which is related to the elimination rate constant $K_e$ by the following relationship.

$$t_{1/2} = \frac{0.693}{K_e} \tag{4}$$

$$C_p^* = \left[\frac{1.44 \, t_{1/2}}{V_d}\right] R_0 \tag{5}$$

### Intermittent Mode of Administration

When intermittent doses, D, of a drug are given at fixed, equally spaced dosing intervals, $\tau$, for a period of time of at least five half-lives, the amount of drug in the body will not reach a steady state, per se, in that it will continuously vary during the dosing interval. However, it will oscillate in a reproducible fashion between a maximum $(C_{pmax}^\infty)^a$ and a minimum $(C_{pmin}^\infty)^a$ during the dosing interval, and one speaks then of an *average* steady-state amount in the body $\bar{A}_b$ or plasma level $\bar{C}_p{}^b$ (Figure 1). In this case, $C_p$ is given by

---

[a] Since antiarrhythmics have a relatively narrow therapeutic range, it is pertinent to consider the magnitude of plasma level oscillations at steady state. In the case of intravenous administration, $(C_{pmax}^\infty - C_{pmin}^\infty) = D/V_d$, which is equal to the concentration achieved after administration of a single dose D. In the case of oral or intramuscular administration, the more rapid the rate of absorption, the greater the oscillation of plasma levels about $C_p$ during a dosing interval.

[b] The exact definition of $\bar{C}_p$ is $C_p = 1/\tau \int C_p dt$ where $\tau = t_2 - t_1$ and $C_p$ is the plasma level $t_1$ at anytime during the dosing interval.

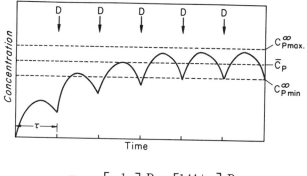

*Figure 1. Plasma concentration reaches a steady-state when multiple oral doses, D, of a drug are administered at fixed dosing intervals, τ.*

$$\overline{C}_p = \left[\frac{1}{V_d K_e}\right]\frac{D}{\tau} = \left[\frac{1.44\ t_{1/2}}{V_d}\right]\frac{D}{\tau} \qquad (6)$$

In the case of oral administration, only a fraction, f, of the administered dose, D, is ultimately available systemically $(0 < f < 1)$, and Equation 6 should therefore read

$$\overline{C}_p = \left[\frac{1.44\ t_{1/2}}{V_d}\right]\frac{fD}{\tau} \qquad (7)$$

Equations 5 and 7 can become very useful since they allow a calculation of steady-state or plateau plasma levels achieved for any given dosage regimen, if three basic pharmacokinetic drug parameters, $t_{1/2}$, $V_d$ and f are known. However, even when that is the case, Equations 5 and 7 are useful only if there exists a well-defined relationship between plasma levels and clinical effects. In the application section of this and the following chapter, it will be shown that in fact, four fundamental drug parameters—effective drug levels, biological half-life, volume of distribution, and fraction of a dose absorbed—are essential for adequate dosage regimen calculations. The following section will present a review of the pertinent information presently available on these basic pharmacokinetic parameters.

### Relationship Between Drug Plasma Levels and Clinical Effects

Table 1 contains the important information pertaining to effective and toxic plasma (or blood) levels for lidocaine, procainamide, propranolol and diphenylhydantoin, where each set of data is appropriately referenced. The importance of serum drug concentrations as therapeutic guides has been well discussed by Koch-Weser[5] in a recent review. For the purpose of this discussion it is necessary to note the following about antiarrhythmics: (1) they are reversibly acting drugs, i.e., their duration of action directly reflects their presence at the site of action; and (2) the concentration of unbound drug in plasma is in a constant dynamic equilibrium with its concentration at the site of action. Consequently, concentration of free drug in plasma should correlate well with pharmacological effect. In order for these relationships to be useful, however, they must have predictive capabilities, and consequently, they should result from well-controlled clinical studies of sufficiently large numbers of patients. Such an example is the study of Koch-Weser and Klein[3] where more than 1500 observations were made in 142 patients receiving procainamide. Seven plasma concentration ranges were studied with respect to four categories of clinical responses (ineffective, effective, minor toxicity and serious toxicity). These data illustrate two important points. A relatively narrow range of plasma levels (4–8 µg/ml) is considered optimal and is found to be effective in approximately 95% of the cases with less than 2% minor toxicity and no instance of serious toxicity. There is no clear and abrupt plasma level separating the categories of clinical responses mainly be-

**Table 1. Relationship Between Plasma Level and Clinical Effects**

| DRUG | NUMBER OF SUBJECTS | EFFECTIVE LEVELS (µg/ml) | TOXIC (µg/ml) | BLOOD OR PLASMA | REFERENCE |
|---|---|---|---|---|---|
| Lidocaine | 21 | 2–5 | 7–10 | plasma | 12 |
| | 10 | 1.2–6 | >10 | plasma | 13 |
| Procainamide | 142 | 4–8 | 8–16[a]; 16[b] | plasma | 3 |
| Propranolol | 12 | .04–.085 | | plasma | 14 |
| | 14 | >.03 | | blood | 15 |
| Diphenylhydantoin | 51 | 10–15 | | serum | 16, 17 |
| | 40 | 15–25 | | serum | 18 |
| | | | >25 | serum | 19 |
| | 174 | | 10–29 | serum | 17 |
| | 110 | | >30 | plasma | 20 |
| | 93 | 10–18 | >20 | plasma | 21 |

[a] Potentially toxic (minor toxicity).
[b] Serious toxicity.

cause of intersubject variability in efficacy and toxicity. (In fact, one observes the familiar bell-shaped distribution and dose-response curves.) However, in the case of procainamide at least, a fairly accurate *prediction* of clinical response can be made from plasma level measurements.

Table 1 shows that for the other antiarrhythmics, the pharmacokinetic information presently available is far from complete. Interestingly however, the values reported by various laboratories tend to converge toward certain plasma level ranges which can probably be utilized with a reasonable degree of prediction. These ranges may appear to be fairly wide, but in fact they are relatively narrow when compared to other groups of drugs such as some antibiotics.

A last comment refers to making the distinction between blood and plasma levels as they are reported in the literature (Table 1). The blood and plasma levels will be equal only in one instance—when the drug partitions equally between plasma and the cellular components of blood. More often than not, however, this partition ratio is not equal to one, and consequently, a given range of plasma levels will correspond to a different range of blood levels. It should be noted, however, that in several instances reports deal with plasma values because for many drugs plasma assays present less technical problems than the corresponding measurements in whole blood. Such is the case, for example, for gas chromatographic methods which are routinely used in the determination of lidocaine and diphenylhydantoin.

## Biological Half-Lives

Table 2 presents the pertinent information on biological half-lives for these same drugs. Again, the usefulness of these data is related to their predictive capability which in turn is directly dependent on the design of the studies from which they originate. Thus, it is important to ascertain the number of subjects utilized and to assess how the reported half-lives were determined, e.g., from intravenous or oral data. In the case of intravenous data the measured half-life could be shorter than the true post distribution half-life if blood samples are not drawn over a long enough period of time. With oral administration, the measured half-life would appear longer than the true elimination half-life in the case of absorption-rate-limited kinetics. It is also critical to recognize whether the subjects are normals or patients. In addition to obvious instances where disease state (renal or hepatic failure) can affect a drug's biological half-life rather drastically, it is likely that other factors, such as regional blood flow alterations in various disease conditions, can also affect the biological half-life.[22,23]

When all these parameters have been considered, it is necessary to analyze the level of agreement (or discrepancy) between the biological half-life values reported by the various laboratories. It can be seen, for example, that for lidocaine, procainamide and propranolol, the degree of consistency among the various sources is quite satisfactory, whereas in the case of diphenylhydantoin, the variability is somewhat disconcerting. In the case of

### Table 2. Biological Half-Lives of Antiarrhythmics

| DRUG | ROUTE | NUMBER OF SUBJECTS | RANGE (hours) | MEAN (hours) | REFERENCE |
|------|-------|--------------------|---------------|--------------|-----------|
| Lidocaine | i.v. | 10 | 1.2–2.2 | 1.8 | 31 |
| | i.v. | 5 | 1.4–1.9 | 1.5 | 31 |
| | i.v. | 5 | 1.3–1.8 | 1.5 | 32 |
| | i.v. | 5 | 1.2–1.7 | 1.4 | 33 |
| Procainamide | i.v. | 14 | 2.5–4.7 | 3.5 | 1 |
| | i.v. | 6 | 2.85 ± 0.25[a] | 2.85 | 34 |
| Propranolol | i.v. | 5 | 2.0–2.6 | 2.3 | 6 |
| | oral + i.v. | 9 | 2.3–5 | 2.5 | 35 |
| | oral | 9 | 2.2–4.0 | 3.1 | 6 |
| | oral | 10 | 2–3 | | 15 |
| Diphenylhydantoin | i.v. | 6 | 10.5–28.7 | 15.4 | 24 |
| | i.v. | 3 | 9.8–16.3 | 12.7 | 26 |
| | i.v. | 4 | 8–15 | 10.1 | 27 |
| | i.v. | 3 | 7.3–9.8 | | 29 |
| | i.v. | 2 | 9.1–11.2 | | 30 |
| | oral | 5 | 22–34 | 27 | 28 |
| | oral | 68 | 7–42 | 22 ± 9[b] | 25 |

[a] Mean ± standard error of the mean.
[b] Mean ± standard deviation.

the latter, it should be noted that intravenous studies appear to yield shorter half-lives which is consistent with the well-documented variable absorption of this drug.[7] Also, several reports have shown that diphenylhydantoin exhibits dose-dependent kinetics which explains the scatter of values reported by various authors.[24-30]

## Volume of Distribution and Total Body Clearance

Table 3 summarizes the values for volume of distribution and total body clearance. The caution required for the interpretation of literature data presented in Tables 1 and 2 is equally appropriate here. It should be recalled that the definition of volume of distribution is a poorly understood one because it is dependent on the pharmacokinetic model chosen to fit the experimental data. Consequently, one finds various volume terms in the same report and it becomes important to be able to select the terms useful for a given purpose. In the report of Rowland et al.,[31] there are three different volume terms which obviously have different values. The values presented in Table 3 are all $V_d$ terms as discussed by Riegelman et al.[35] for the one-compartment open model which assumes instantaneous distribution. This term has been selected because it refers to an equilibrium situation probably similar to that achieved after multiple doses of a drug. In general, information on volumes of distribution of drugs is quite scarce and antiarrhythmics are no exception. Lidocaine is the only drug for which there is more than one report available and the values obtained are in fair agreement. The values reported for total body clearance are even in better agreement which is not surprising in view of the fact that its calculation (from dose-area relationships) is model independent. It is our opinion that whenever possible one should report clearance as well as volume terms for the reason mentioned above, and also because the reciprocal of the clearance term is the proportionality constant between steady-state plasma level and infusion rate (Equations 3 and 6).

## Fraction of a Dose Systemically Available

Tables 1, 2, and 3 present the pertinent information presently available on three primary pharmacokinetic parameters. However, Equation 7 shows that a fourth parameter, the fraction of a dose ultimately available to the systemic circulation after oral administration, is required to calculate the average steady-state plasma level $\bar{C}_p$. A careful review of the literature on this subject shows that reliable data are scarce. There may be two reasons for this. First, f is a parameter which is dependent not only on the physical and chemical properties of the drug but also on dosage form factors and physiological variables, such as gastrointestinal motility and splanchnic blood flow. Although the influence of dosage form on biological availability is well documented, there are very few studies which attempt to evaluate this parameter under conditions relevant to clinical use. Thus, f should be defined for each dosage form commercially available (i.e., for each generic brand) in the various types of patients for whom it is intended, e.g., bedridden vs. ambulatory patients. A second reason why information is scarce is that a determination of f also requires that the drug be administered intravenously which renders the protocol of such a study somewhat demanding.

The studies of Koch-Weser et al.,[3,4] show that, except for patients with serious cardiovascular disturbances, f ranges between 0.75 and 0.95 for oral administration of procainamide. Lidocaine and propranolol are both metabolized to a very large extent and their metabolic clearance approaches to liver blood flow. Thus, they are both subject to the "first-pass effect"[6,36] whereby a significant fraction of a dose administered orally is metabolized at the first passage of portal blood through the liver before reaching the systemic circulation. In five subjects given 250 and 500 mg of lidocaine orally, f ranged between 0.21 and 0.46 with a mean of 0.35.[36] In a similar study where five subjects were given propranolol intravenously and in tablets, f varied between 0.16 and 0.60 with a mean of 0.32.[6] Accordingly, it was found that plasma propranolol levels varied sevenfold after oral

### Table 3. Volumes of Distribution of Antiarrhythmics

| DRUG | NUMBER OF SUBJECTS | $V_d$ (liters/kg) | $V_dK_e$ | REFERENCE |
|---|---|---|---|---|
| Lidocaine | 10 | 1.7 ± 0.7 | 9.16 ± 2.38 | 31 |
| | 5 | 1.6 ± 0.3 | 9.94 ± 1.98 | 31 |
| | 5 | 2.1 | 10.58 | 32 |
| Procainamide | 8 | 1.74–2.22 | 2.01 | 3 |
| Propranolol | 5 | 2.10 | | 6 |
| Diphenylhydantoin | 1 | 0.58 | | 30 |
| | 6 | 0.61[a] | | 24 |

[a] Calculated from the data of Glazko et al.[24]

dosage while the corresponding variation after an intravenous dose was only twofold.

### Quinidine

In the case of quinidine, there are no reliable values in the literature for the four parameters required for dosage regimen calculations. One major reason lies with the questionable specificity of the method of determination of this drug in plasma. Resnekov et al.[37] measured plasma levels in 20 patients following oral doses of a commercial sustained-release quinidine formulation. Each plasma level was determined by two commonly used methods, Hamfeldt and Malers[38] and Cramer and Isaakson.[39] The former method yields consistently higher values because it measures quinidine as well as some of its metabolites. It is based on the precipitation method of Brodie and Udenfriend[40] where quinidine extraction is effected simultaneously with plasma protein precipitation utilizing an alcohol-acetone mixture. The method of Cramer and Isaakson on the other hand is based on the extraction method of Brodie et al.[41] Cramer and Isaakson have shown that their method is more specific than the precipitation method of Brodie and Udenfriend[40] and that of Edgar and Sokolow.[42] Although the plasma concentration-time curve obtained by Resnekov et al. supports this fact, there is still some doubt as to the specificity of the method of Cramer and Isaakson since there is no absolutely specific method presently available to which it could be compared. The practical implications of these analytical considerations should now become evident. For example, it is difficult to define an effective range of plasma concentrations for quinidine unless the method of determination is specified. Thus, Resnekov et al. reported that the effective therapeutic range of plasma levels is 1–4 $\mu$g/ml for the method of Cramer and Isaakson, and 3–7 $\mu$g/ml for the method of Hamfeldt and Malers. Consequently, it would appear that, depending on its degree of specificity, a given method would yield a correspondingly different range of effective levels. An estimation of quinidine's half-life is also dependent on the species measured by a particular assay since it cannot be assumed that the drug and its metabolites have identical pharmacokinetics. Furthermore, in view of the extreme dependence of quinidine excretion on urinary $p$H,[43] one can expect an appreciable inter- and intrasubject variability in biological half-life. To our knowledge, any reliable determinations of the volume of distribution of this drug are not available. This is not surprising since quinidine is given in a single rapid intravenous bolus only very rarely, if at all, because of its toxicity (hypotension) by that route.[23]

### Summary and Conclusions

This chapter has presented the plateau principle approach to the evaluation of dosage regimens of anti-

arrhythmics. It was shown that four drug disposition parameters must be known in order to predict effective steady-state drug levels from a knowledge of maintenance dose and dosing interval.

A review of the significant data presently available in the literature on these four drug parameters (effective plasma levels, biological half-life, volume of distribution and fraction of a dose systemically absorbed) was presented. It was shown that an evaluation of literature data requires not only a knowledge of pharmacokinetics but also of the reliability of analytical methods. It was thus found that in several instances the data presently available are incomplete. The application of these concepts to the calculation of maintenance doses, dosing intervals and to the handling of specific clinical situations, will be presented in the following chapter.

### References

1. Schumacher, G. E.: Practical Pharmacokinetic Techniques for Drug Consultation and Evaluation, I: Use of Dosage Regimen Calculations, In *Clinical Pharmacy Sourcebook*, pp. 226-236.

2. Koch-Weser, J. et al.: Antiarrhythmic Prophylaxis with Procainamide in Acute Myocardial Infarction, *N. Engl. J. Med. 281*:1454-1460 (Dec. 4) 1969.

3. Koch-Weser, J. and Klein, S. W.: Procainamide Dosage Schedules, Plasma Concentrations and Clinical Effects, *JAMA 215*:1454-1460 (Mar. 1) 1971.

4. Koch-Weser, J.: Pharmacokinetics of Procainamide in Man, *Ann. N. Y. Acad. Sci. 179*:370-382 (July 6) 1971.

5. Koch-Weser, J.: Drug Therapy: Serum Drug Concentrations as Therapeutic Guides, *N. Engl. J. Med. 287*:227-231 (Aug. 3) 1972.

6. Shand, D. G. et al.: Plasma Propranolol Levels in Adults, *Clin. Pharmacol. Ther. 11*:112-120 (Jan.-Feb.) 1970.

7. Tyrer, J. H. et al.: Outbreak of Anticonvulsant Intoxication in an Australian City, *Brit. Med. J. 4*:271-273 (Oct. 31) 1970.

8. Swarbrick, J.: Current Concepts in the Pharmaceutical Sciences: Biopharmaceutics, Lea & Febiger, Philadelphia, Pennsylvania, 1970.

9. Wagner, J.: Biopharmaceutics and Relevant Pharmacokinetics, Drug Intelligence Publications, Hamilton, Illinois, 1971.

10. Gibaldi, M.: Introduction to Biopharmaceutics, Lea & Febiger, Philadelphia, Pennsylvania, 1971.

11. Notari, R.: Biopharmaceutics and Pharmacokinetics: An Introduction, Marcel Dekker, New York, New York, 1971.

12. Gianelly, R. J. et al.: Effect of Lidocaine on Ventricular Arrhythmias in Patients With Coronary Heart Disease, *N. Engl. J. Med. 277*:1215-1219 (Dec. 7), 1967.

13. Harrison, D. C. and Aldernon, E. L.: Relationship of Blood Levels to Clinical Effectiveness of Lidocaine, *In* Scott, D. B. and Julian, D. G. (ed.): The Treatment of Ventricular Arrhythmias, Williams and Wilkens, Baltimore, Maryland, 1971, pp. 178-189.

14. Coltart, D. J. et al.: Plasma Propranolol Levels Associated with Suppression of Ventricular Ectopic Beats, *Brit. Med. J. 1*:490-491 (Feb. 27) 1971.

15. McLean, C. E. and Deane, B. C.: Propranolol Dose Determinants Including Blood Levels Studies, *Angiology 21*:536-545 (Sept.) 1970.

16. Buchthal, F. and Svensmark, O.: Aspects of the Pharmacology of Phenytoin (Dilantin) and Phenobarbital Relevant to Their Dosage in the Treatment of Epilepsy, *Epilepsia 1*:373-384 (June) 1960.

17. Buchthal, F. et al.: Clinical and Electrocardiographic Correlation with Serum Levels of Diphenylhydantoin, *Arch. Neurol. 2*:624-630 (June) 1960.

18. Viukari, N. M. A.: Diphenylhydantoin as an Anticonvulsant: Evaluation of Treatment in Forty Mentally Subnormal Epileptics, *J. Ment. Defic. Res. 13*:212-218 (Sept.) 1969.

19. Stensrud, P. A. and Palmer, H.: Serum Phenytoin Determinations in Epileptics, *Epilepsia* 5:364–370 (Dec.) 1964.

20. Triedman, H. M. et al: Determination of Plasma and Cerebrospinal Fluid Levels of Dilantin in the Human, *Trans. Am. Neurol. Ass.* 85:166–170, 1960.

21. Bigger, J. T. et al.: Relationship Between the Plasma Level of Diphenylhydantoin Sodium and its Cardiac Antiarrhythmic Effects, *Circulation* 38:363–374 (Aug.) 1968.

22. Thompson, P. D. et al.: The Influence of Heart Failure, Liver Disease, and Renal Failure on the Disposition of Lidocaine in Man, *Amer. Heart J.* 82:417–421 (Sept.) 1971.

23. Bellet, S. et al.: Relation Between Serum Quinidine Levels and Renal Function, *Amer. J. Cardiol.* 27:368–371 (Apr.) 1971.

24. Glazko, A. J. et al.: Metabolic Disposition of Diphenylhydantoin in Normal Human Subjects Following Intravenous Administrations, *Clin. Pharmacol. Ther.* 10:498–504 (July-Aug.) 1969.

25. Arnold, K. and Gerber, N.: The Rate of Decline of Diphenylhydantoin in Human Plasma, *Clin. Pharmacol. Ther.* 11:121–134 (Jan.-Feb.) 1970.

26. Christensen, L. K. and Skoustad, L.: Inhibitions of Drug Metabolism by Chloramphenicol, *Lancet* 2:1397–1399 (Dec. 27) 1969.

27. Hansen, J. M. et al: Sulthiame (Ospolot) as Inhibitor of Diphenylhydantoin Metabolisms, *Epilepsia* 9:17–21 (Mar.) 1968.

28. Solomon, H. M. and Schrogie, J. J.: The Effect of Phenyramidol on the Metabolisms of Diphenylhydantoin, *Clin. Pharmacol. Ther.* 8:554 (July-Aug.) 1966.

29. Hansen, J. M. et al.: Dicoumarol Induced Diphenylhydantoin Intoxication, *Lancet* 2:265–266 (July 30) 1966.

30. Suzuki, T. et al.: Kinetics of and Diphenylhydantoin Disposition in Man, *Chem. Pharm. Bull.* 18:405–411 (Jan.) 1970.

31. Rowland, M. et al.: Disposition Kinetics of Lidocaine in Normal Subjects, *Ann. N. Y. Acad. Sci.* 179:383–398 (July 6) 1971.

32. Tucker, G. T. and Boas, R. A.: Pharmacokinetic Aspects of Intravenous Regional Anesthesia, *Anesthesia* 34:538–549 (June) 1971.

33. Boyes, R. N. et al.: Pharmacokinetics of Lidocaine in Man, *Clin. Pharmcol. Ther.* 12:105–116 (Jan.-Feb.) 1970.

34. Wiley, H. and Genton, E.: Pharmacokinetics of Procainamide, *Arch. Internal Med.* 130:366-369 (Sept.) 1972.

35. Riegelman, S. et al.: Concept of a Volume of Distribution and Possible Errors in Evaluation of This Parameter, *J. Pharm. Sci.* 57:128–133 (Jan.) 1968.

36. Boyes, R. N. and Keenaghan, J. B.: Some Aspects of the Metabolism and Distribution of Lidocaine in Rats, Dogs, and Man, *In* Scott, D. B. and Julian, D. G. (ed.): Lidocaine in the Treatment of Ventricular Arrhythmias, Williams and Wilkins, Baltimore, Maryland, 1971, pp. 140-153.

37. Resnekov, L. et al.: Sustained Release Quinidine (Kinidin Durules) in Maintaining Sinus Rhythm After Electroversion of Atrial Arrhythmias, *Brit. Heart J.* 33:220–225 (Mar.) 1971.

38. Hamfeldt, A. and Malers, E.: Determination of Quinidine Concentration in Serum in the Control of Quinidine Therapy, *Acta Societatis Medicorum Upsaliensis* 68:181–191, 1963.

39. Cramer, G. and Isaaksson, B.: Quantitative Determination of Quinidine in Plasma, *Scand. J. Clin. Lab. Invest.* 15:553–556, 1963.

40. Brodie, B. B. and Udenfriend, S.: The Estimations of Quinine in the Human Plasma with a Note on the Estimation of Quinidine, *J. Pharm. and Exper. Ther.* 78:154–158 (June) 1943.

41. Brodie, B. B. et al.: The Estimation of Basic Organic Compounds in Biological Material. II. Estimations of Fluorescent Compounds, *J. Biol. Chem.* 168:311–318, 1947.

42. Edgar, A. L. and Sokolow, M.: Experiences with the Photofluorometric Determination of Quinidine in Blood, *J. Lab. Clin. Med.* 36:478–484 (Sept.) 1950.

43. Gerhardt, R. F. et al.: Quinidine Excretion in Aciduria and Alkaluria, *Ann. Internal Med.* 71:927–933 (Nov.) 1969.

# 51 Dosage Regimens of Antiarrhythmics, Part II: Applications

René H. Levy and Gary H. Smith

Pharmacokinetic data presented in the preceding chapter are used to show How dosage regimens may be developed for antiarrhythmic drugs.

Dosage regimen calculations are presented for intravenous infusion of lidocaine and for oral administration of procainamide and propranolol. Dosing flow charts are presented for lidocaine and procainamide. While dosage regimens could be calculated for diphenylhydantoin, there are no reliable data on the fraction of administered dose available systemically and the volume of distribution of the drug. Clinical conditions where average doses of antiarrhythmics will lead to toxic effects are discussed.

The method of calculating dosage regimens is applicable to individual patient data and can serve as a useful guideline in managing patients.

In the preceding chapter,[1] a review of the plateau principle involving intravenous infusion and multiple oral dosing administration was presented. This led to the identification of four basic pharmacokinetic properties (therapeutically effective drug levels, biological half-life, volume of distribution, and fraction of a dose absorbed) which were reviewed for lidocaine, procainamide, propranolol, quinidine, and diphenylhydantoin. The data presented in the last chapter will be utilized here to show how dosage regimens can be developed. Furthermore, these dosage regimen calculations will be presented and discussed within the context of actual clinical situations in the form of dosing flow charts. The appropriate use of plasma level determination as therapeutic guides is also included.

## Continuous Mode of Administration: Intravenous Infusion

*Lidocaine.*

Problem: Knowing that the range of effective levels for lidocaine is 1-5 $\mu g/ml$, calculate a corresponding range of infusion rates.

Solution: Equation 3 of the previous chapter allows a direct calculation after rearrangement to the following form:

Infusion Rate = (Effective Level) x (Total Body Clearance)

$$R_o = C_p^*(V_d K_e)$$

If the desired level is 2 $\mu g/ml$:

$$R_o = \frac{2\mu g}{ml} \times 10 \frac{ml}{min\text{-}kg} = 20 \mu g/min/kg$$

(value for $V_d K_E$ taken from reference 1, Table 3) or for a 70-kg adult, $R_o = 1.4$ mg/min
If the desired level is 4 $\mu g/ml$, $R_0$ is also doubled and becomes 2.8 mg/min.

Comments:
1. It should be noted that these calculated infusion rates are quite consistent with those found in standard references; 1-4 mg/min reported in *Manual of Medical Therapeutics*[2] and *American Hospital Formulary Service,*[3] and 1-2 mg/min reported in the *Pharmacological Basis of Therapeutics.*[4]
2. These calculations show that commonly used infusion rates of 1 to 3 mg/min should yield plasma levels between 1.5 and 4 $\mu g/ml$ in an average patient without heart or liver failure.
3. Also important is the fact that these infusion rates will yield the corresponding plasma levels only after 5-8 hours (3-5 half-lives). Thus, to achieve a rapid response, there is a need for intravenous bolus doses to immediately achieve these levels.
4. The average intravenous bolus dose required to achieve a plasma level of 2 $\mu g/ml$ can be calculated from the equation $V_d = A_B/C_p$. However, if the calculation is made utilizing the $V_d$ term reported in Table 3 of reference 1, a value of 3.4 mg/kg is obtained which is severalfold larger than any of the recommended bolus doses. This example illustrates the importance of selecting the distribution volume term appropriate for a given purpose. Immediately following an intravenous bolus dose of lidocaine, the drug does not distribute into a volume $(V_d)$ of 1.7 liters/kg but in a much smaller volume, the so-called central compartment $(V_p)$ as discussed by Riegleman et al.[5] This central compartment comprises the plasma volume as well as those well perfused tissues which appear to instantaneously equilibrate with plasma. Rowland et al.[6] reported $V_p$ values of 0.44 liter/kg (10 subjects) and 0.48 liter/kg (5 subjects), whereas Boyes et al.[7] found a mean $V_p$ of 0.77 liter/kg (5 subjects). If 0.50 liter/kg is taken as a representative value, the above equation yields a dose of 1.0 mg/kg which would be necessary to achieve a plasma level of 2 $\mu g/ml$ immediately after an intravenous bolus injection. The initial level after the intravenous bolus injection

decreases rapidly due to distribution into peripheral, less well perfused compartments and would drop to approximately 0.5 μg/ml in one hour if no infusion was started simultaneously. Thus, the combination of a 1.0 mg/kg bolus and an infusion of 20 μg/min/kg administered simultaneously should immediately establish and maintain a plasma level of 2 μg/ml. This calculated 1.0 mg/kg bolus dose is quite consistent with the values found in standard reference sources.[2-4]

*Lidocaine Dosing Flow Chart.* When a patient presents with a diagnosis of an acute myocardial infarction with multiple ventricular arrhythmias, lidocaine will commonly be administered. The application of the kinetic rationale just discussed in the above comments to this clinical situation is illustrated in the dosing flow chart in Figures 1 and 2.

*Rationale for Lidocaine Flow Charts.* Toxicities and/or therapeutic failures from the use of lidocaine can often arise from mishandling of the infusion rate and lack of understanding of the plateau principle. One underlying constant in both lidocaine flow charts is that an additional bolus dose is always accompanied by a *proportional* increase in the infusion rate in order to maintain the transient increase in plasma level caused by the bolus. When this is not the case, i.e., the bolus is not accompanied by infusion, it is likely that arrhythmias will only be controlled in the few minutes following the bolus injection, thus leading to additional boluses. Ultimately the peripheral compartment which causes the initial rapid disappearance of lidocaine (after an intravenous bolus) becomes saturated and further bolus injections can lead to serious toxicity. Conversely, when the infusion rate is increased without a concomitant bolus injection, the desired clinical response may not be seen for several hours.

Patients A, $A_1$, $A_2$, B and $B_1$ represent the usual response to lidocaine therapy, i.e., patients who require plasma levels of 2–3 μg/ml.

Patients $B_2$, $B_4$, $B_5$ and $B_6$ represent the less usual and more difficult cases of lidocaine therapy. Cases similar to patient $B_2$ will rarely occur. Patient $B_4$ requires at least 4 μg/ml to respond whereas $B_5$ is refractory (in his case the clinician should consider another agent such as intravenous procainamide). The purpose of the

*Figure 1. Lidocaine dosing flow chart, part 1*

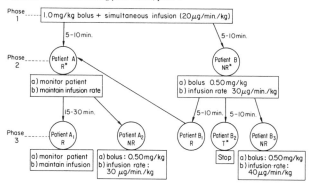

R* = Responding (arrhythmia controlled)
NR* = Not responding (arrhythmia not controlled)
T* = Toxic

*Figure 2. Lidocaine dosing flow chart, part 2*

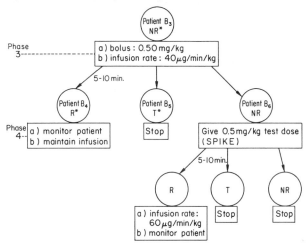

R* = Responding (arrhythmia controlled)
NR* = Not responding (arrhythmia not controlled)
T* = Toxic

"spike" dose for patient $B_6$ is to test whether he will respond at all to higher lidocaine levels. The "spike" dose constitutes a relatively safer approach than the other alternative of continuously increasing the infusion rate. Any toxicities caused by the "spike" dose will generally be of fast onset and fast disappearance, whereas those caused by elevated infusing rates are more insidious and of longer duration.

When toxicity occurs at any phase, after any dose, it is safer to stop all drug input and treat the symptoms if necessary.

## Discontinuous Mode of Administration: Oral Dosing

*Procainamide.*

Problem: Knowing the range of effective plasma levels of procainamide to be 4–8 μg/ml determine:

1. What dose should be given every six hours to maintain effective plasma levels.
2. How often should a 500-mg capsule be given to a 70-kg adult.

Solution: Part 1. Equation 7 in the previous chapter can be rearranged to give the oral dose (D) necessary to achieve an average level of 4 μg/ml:

$$D = \frac{C_p V_d \tau}{1.44\ t_{1/2} f} =$$

$$\frac{4\ (mg/liter) \times 2.0\ (liters/kg) \times 6\ (hr)}{1.44 \times 3.5\ (hr) \times 0.85} = 11.2\ mg/kg$$

(values for $V_d$, $T_{1/2}$ and f taken from reference 1.
For a 70-kg adult, D would be equal to 0.78 g every six hours, total daily dose 3.10 g. To achieve an average level of 6 μg/ml, D becomes 16.8 mg/kg.

Part 2. Equation 7 can also be rearranged to yield $\tau$:

$$\tau = \frac{1.44 t_{1/2} fD}{V_d C_p}$$

$$\frac{1.44 \times 3.5\ (hr) \times 0.85 \times 500\ mg}{140\ (liters) \times 4\ (mg/liter)} = 3.83\ hrs$$

Comments:
1. The values obtained above are in agreement with standard regimens found in various references.[2-4]
2. From plateau principle considerations, it becomes obvious that these regimens will achieve effective levels only after several doses (12–24 hours). When it is necessary to rapidly obtain effective levels, a priming dose is necessary. Procainamide is a good example where the useful "priming dose = 2X maintenance dose, when $\tau = t_{1/2}$" rule applies. This is based on the simple fact that following the administration of a priming dose, the amount of drug eliminated at the end of a dosing interval $\tau$ (when $\tau = t_{1/2}$) is equal to half of the priming dose. Consequently, if a maintenance dose equal to half of the priming dose is administered at the end of the dosing interval, it will exactly replace the amount of drug eliminated during the same time, and reestablish an amount of drug in the body equal to the priming dose. Thus, if a maintenance dose of 500 mg is given every four hours a priming dose of 1 g should be adequate.

*Procainamide Dosing Flow Chart.* Once a patient with ventricular arrhythmias has been well controlled with lidocaine, it is advantageous to convert the patient to oral medication when possible. Oral procainamide is often selected for this purpose. The dosing flow chart in Figure 3 is an example of how this can be accomplished.

*Rationale.* The patient is started on an i.m. dose firstly because it avoids the long wait of three to five half-lives for the achievement of steady-state, and secondly because it constitutes a reliable route of administration (i.e., the clinician can be certain that in most instances a significant fraction of the dose will rapidly reach the systemic circulation). Patient A represents the usual response since levels of 4 $\mu$g/ml will in general be achieved in one hour and maintained for at least another hour. Three hours later, patient A is started on a maintenance

dose equal to half the priming dose every half-life. Patients $A_1$ and $A_2$ represent usual cases. Patient $A_2$ is probably a "poor absorber" and his maintenance dose is increased because he previously responded (patient A) when effective levels were achieved (by i.m. administration). Patients B and C represent fairly unusual cases. Patient C could have a low procainamide clearance which would produce toxic levels or he might just be refractory to the drug and respond by toxicity. The purpose of the "spike" dose here is also to test whether patient B will respond at all to higher levels. Patient $B_1$ is an example of those patients who require levels above 8 $\mu$g/ml to respond, or it could be that the original i.m. dose did not achieve effective levels because of a large drug clearance or lack of absorption from the injection site. Since the "spike" dose has established that he requires higher doses, his oral maintenance dose is 9 mg/kg. Patients $B_4$ and $B_5$ are cases very similar to $A_1$ and $A_2$ where $B_5$ is probably a "poor absorber" and requires a higher oral dose. Patients $B_2$ and $B_3$ are examples of refractory patients in which case the clinician should consider switching to another oral agent such as quinidine.

*Blood Levels.* The dosing flow chart includes blood level measurements for patients $A_2$, $B_1$ and $B_5$, all of whom were not responding at some point which illustrates the fact that blood levels are not required in all instances but only in unusual cases. Their usefulness at this early stage (onset of therapy) is limited primarily by the fact that therapeutic decisions must often be made before having the results back from the laboratory. Nevertheless, when this information is available (hopefully 24 hours later while the patient is still in the hospital), it is possible to establish with certainty one of the several suppositions made previously. For example, if patient $A_2$ or $B_5$ exhibited a plasma level of 2-3 $\mu$g/ml, it could be concluded in all probability that he is a "poor absorber" and that his oral doses should be increased until he responds favorably. This information is of significant value in further management of these patients.

Blood level data is even more useful in prophylactic antiarrhythmic therapy where it is possible to wait one to two days to obtain the laboratory results.

*Propranolol.*

Problem:

1. Calculate the four hourly maintenance doses required to maintain plasma levels of 0.05 $\mu$g/ml.
2. Determine how often 40-mg tablets should be given to maintain those levels in a 70-kg adult.

Solution:

1. As in the case of procainamide, D is given by:

$$D = \frac{C_p V_d \tau}{1.44 t_{1/2} f} =$$
$$\frac{0.05 \ (\text{mg/liter}) \times 2.1 \ (\text{liter/kg}) \times 4 \ (\text{hr})}{1.44 \times 2.5 \ (\text{hr}) \times 0.30} = 0.39 \ \text{mg/kg}$$

Figure 3. *Procainamide dosing flow chart*

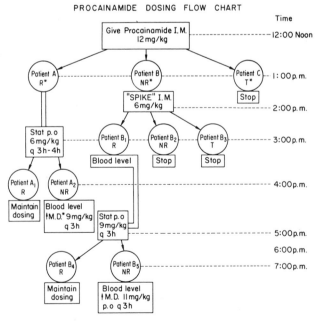

PROCAINAMIDE DOSING FLOW CHART

R* = Responding (arrythmia controlled)
NR* = Not responding (arrythmia not controlled)
T* = Toxic
M.D.* = Maintenance dose

(values for $V_d$, $t_{1/2}$ and f are taken from reference 1) or 27 mg for a 70-kg adult (163 mg total daily dose).

$$2. \quad \tau = \frac{1.44t_{1/2}fD}{V_dC_p} =$$

$$\frac{1.44 \times 2.5 \ (hr) \times 0.3 \times 40 \ (mg)}{147 \ (liter) \times 0.05 \ (mg/liter)} = 5.88 \ hours$$

(6 hours for practical purposes)

(total daily dose = 160 mg)

Comments: The above regimens were calculated assuming a value of 0.3 for f, the fraction of a dose systemically absorbed. As mentioned in the previous chapter, however, because of the "first-pass effect," there is a large intersubject variability in f. If the maintenance dose, D, and total daily dose are recalculated for the extreme values of reported by Shand et al[8] it is found that for an average 70-kg adult, the total daily dose ranges between 80 mg (f = 0.15) and 320 mg (f = 0.60). Interestingly, it is found in clinical practice that total daily doses required to control recurrent paroxysms of supraventricular tachychardia in different patients actually vary between 60 and 320 mg with mean doses of 120 to 160 mg. Thus, it seems probable that for propranolol the unpredictable effect of a given total daily dose is due at least in part to the intersubject variability in plasma level/dose ratio.

*Diphenylhydantoin.* In theory, dosage regimens could be calculated for diphenylhydantoin just as they were determined above for procainamide and propranolol. This is not possible, however, because of the lack of reliable data on f and $V_d$, which is quite surprising in view of the extensive use of this drug as a primary anticonvulsant. Also, it is quite possible that this drug exhibits dose-dependent kinetics, which would make the use of equation 7 (see preceding chapter) invalid at the higher dose levels.

*Dosage Regimens in Heart, Renal and Liver Failure.* The dosage regimen calculations presented so far were based on pharmacokinetic parameters obtained from normal volunteers and/or "normal" patients. There are certain clinical conditions where these average doses will lead to toxic effects because of altered pharmacokinetics. These changes are well documented in the case of antiarrhythmics and are summarized in Table 1. In the case of lidocaine, for example, the decrease in total body clearance found in heart failure and liver disease has been well quantified, and consequently, specific dosage adjustments can be performed. This is not the case with quinidine in renal and congestive heart failure where no distribution or elimination parameter was measured per se. Thus, even though it was found that plasma levels are increased in renal failure, it is not possible to determine accurately the fractional decrease in maintenance dose for a patient with a creatinine clearance of 50, 20 or 5 ml/min.

As long as it can be assumed that the ranges of effective and toxic levels are not changed in renal or liver failure, for example, it becomes apparent that equations 3 and 7 in the preceding chapter are also useful in disease conditions if the appropriate pharmacokinetic parameter is utilized. It should be remembered also that the effects of these disease conditions on the pharmacokinetic properties of a drug can fluctuate and tend to disappear as the patient's condition improves.

*Dosing Rationale and Clinical Management of Arrhythmias.* In this chapter, much emphasis has been put on the understanding and application of pharmacokinetic principles to the rational dosing of patients with arrhythmias. These equations can establish useful guidelines for managing an individual patient. They can lead to a better understanding of how to correctly employ these drugs in therapy. One additional important concept needs to be stressed at this point. The pharmacokinetic parameters used in these calculations are the average values for a patient population. They are all subject

**Table 1. Altered Pharmacokinetics of Antiarrhythmics in Heart, Liver, and Renal Failure**

| DRUG | DISEASE STATE | PARAMETER ALTERED | TYPE OF CHANGE | DOSING IMPLICATION | REFERENCE |
|---|---|---|---|---|---|
| Lidocaine | Heart failure | Total body plasma clearance | Decreased by 45% | ↓ $R_0$ proportionately | 9 |
| Lidocaine | Liver disease | Total body plasma clearance | Decreased by 45% | ↓ $R_0$ proportionately | 9 |
| Procainamide | Primary and secondary renal disease | Biological half-life | Increased by 100% | ↓ D or ↑ $\tau$ proportionately | 10 |
| Procainamide | Cardiac failure | Volume of distribution | Decreased by 25% | ↓ D or ↑ $\tau$ proportionately | 11 |
| Procainamide | Renal failure | Steady state plasma level | Increased | ↓ D or ↑ $\tau$ proportionately | 11 |
| Procainamide | Renal failure | Steady state plasma level | Increased | ↓ D or ↑ $\tau$ proportionately | 12 |
| Quinidine | Renal failure | Plasma levels after single dose | Increased | ↓ D or ↑ $\tau$ | 12 |
| Quinidine | Congestive heart failure | Plasma levels after single dose | Increased | ↓ D or ↑ $\tau$ | 12 |

to individual variation. Thus, unless he possesses the exact values of the parameters for his particular patient, the clinician cannot rely solely on pharmacokinetics or plasma levels when dosing patients. Good clinical judgment is still extremely important in assessing the overall therapy of each patient. "Do not treat a laboratory slip, treat the patient" remains an essential for good therapy.

## Summary and Conclusions

Formal theory of dosage regimens has been available for several years but has been "underutilized." The translation into useful therapeutic guidelines is by no means obvious, and several steps are required. These two chapters have presented a general approach involving an attempt to apply the well-known plateau principle. It was shown that three barriers must be crossed: (1) obtaining reliable pharmacokinetic parameters, (2) generating a dosing regimen, and (3) evaluating the "fit." The method proposed here utilizes mean literature data, but the theory is even more applicable to the individual patient's data.

We believe that the approach presented is quite general and can be applied to many other groups of drugs.

## References

1 Levy, R. H. and Smith, G. H.: Dosage Regimens of Antiarrhythmics, Part I: Pharmacokinetic Properties, In *Clinical Pharmacy Sourcebook,* pp. 291–297.

2. Rosenfeld, M. G. (ed): Manual of Medical Therapeutics, 20th ed., Little Brown and Co., Boston, Massachusetts, 1971, p. 147.

3. American Hospital Formulary Service, American Society of Hospital Pharmacists, Washington, D.C., 1972.

4. Goodman, G. and Gilman, A. (ed): The Pharmacological Basis of Therapeutics, 4th ed., Macmillan Co., New York, New York, 1971, p. 722.

5. Riegleman, S. et al: Concept of a Volume of Distribution and Possible Errors in Evaluation of this Parameter, *J. Pharm. Sci. 57*:128–133 (Jan.) 1968.

6. Rowland, M. et al.: Disposition Kinetics of Lidocaine in Normal Subjects, *Ann. N. Y. Acad. Sci. 179*:383–398 (July 6) 1971.

7. Boyes, R. N. and Keenaghan, J. B.: Some Aspects of the Metabolism and Distribution of Lidocaine in Rats, Dogs, and Man, *In* Scott, D. B. and Julian, D. G. (ed): Lidocaine in the Treatment of Ventricular Arrhythmias, Williams and Wilkins, Baltimore, Maryland, 1971, pp. 140-153.

8. Shand, D. G. et al.: Plasma Propranolol Levels in Adults, *Clin. Pharmacol. Ther. 11*:112–120 (Jan.-Feb.) 1970.

9. Thompson, P. D. et al.: The Influence of Heart Failure, Liver Disease, and Renal Failure on the Disposition of Lidocaine in Man, *Amer. Heart J. 82*: 417–421 (Sept.) 1971.

10. Wiley, H. and Genton, E.: Pharmacokinetics of Procainamide, *Arch. Internal Med. 130*:366-369 (Sept.) 1972.

11. Koch-Weser, J.: Pharmacokinetics of Procainamide in Man, *Ann. N. Y. Acad. Sci. 179*:370–382 (July 6) 1971.

12. Bellet, S. et al.: Relation Between Serum Quinidine Levels and Renal Function, *Amer. J. Cardiol 27*:368–371 (Apr.) 1971.

# 52 Keeping Bioavailability in Perspective

G. E. Schumacher

Some limitations of bioavailability analysis and the applicability of bioavailability considerations in clinical practice are discussed.

In estimating bioavailability, the potential biases associated with (1) using cumulative urinary excretion data, (2) using blood level data, and (3) estimating absorption when using intravenous administration as a reference are discussed. Also covered are bioavailability in relation to therapeutic effectiveness and single dose studies in relation to multiple dose regimens.

The subject of bioavailability as a scientific and professional consideration has generated a spate of literature in recent years. For the pharmaceutical scientist the subject represents an important area of research and evaluation in the development and production of dosage forms. The educator recognizes the subject as the logical culmination, demonstration and consequence of the various biopharmaceutic factors that he has been using for instruction. For the practitioner the topic is critical in the selection of reliable brands of dosage forms.

As a guide to the literature, papers delivered at two symposia are in print.[1,2] One textbook treats the topic in depth.[3] Ritschel has written perhaps the most lucid presentation of the subject for the practitioner.[4] Another paper aptly describes the various pharmacokinetic parameters employed in quantifying bioavailability.[5] A number of good papers have demonstrated the application of various methodologies in the evaluation of the bioavailability of numerous dosage forms.[6-14] Wagner has summarized the current status of bioavailability studies.[15]

This chapter will describe some of the practical pitfalls and limitations in bioavailability analysis that may have eluded the practitioner in his perusal of the literature and will attempt to place some perspective on the applicability of bioavailability considerations in clinical practice. The following topics will be discussed:

1. Some Factors That Bias the Estimation of Bioavailability
   a. Potential Bias in Using Cumulative Urinary Excretion Data
   b. Potential Bias in Using Blood Level Data
   c. Potential Bias in Estimating Absorption When Using Intravenous Administration as a Reference

2. Relationship of Bioavailability to Pharmacologic or Chemotherapeutic Response
   a. Bioavailability in Relation to Therapeutic Effectiveness
   b. Single Dose Studies in Relation to Multiple Dose Regimens

## Some Factors That Bias the Estimation of Bioavailability

Bioavailability is defined as the ratio of the amount of drug reaching the systemic circulation after administration of a sample dosage form as compared to a reference dosage form:

$$\%BA = \frac{(\text{Amount absorbed})_x}{(\text{Amount absorbed})_r} \times 100 \qquad (1)$$

$$\text{where } \%BA = \text{percent bioavailability}$$
$$x = \text{sample dosage form}$$
$$r = \text{reference dosage form}$$

In this context, bioavailability applies to (1) the relative absorption from *various dosage forms* of the *same drug*—capsule, tablet, injection forms, etc.—usually designating the intravenous injection form as the reference and (2) the relative absorption from a *single dosage form* of the *same drug* as supplied by various manufacturers—capsule brand A, capsule brand B, etc.—citing one of the brands as the reference. Bioavailability does not apply to the comparison of absorption from the dosage forms of drug A and drug B. The same drug must be used when employing bioavailability analysis.

### Potential Bias in Using Cumulative Urinary Excretion Data

One method of estimating bioavailability utilizes the measurement of the cumulative amount of unmetabolized drug excreted in the urine after administration of a single dose of drug. In order to assure the accurate assessment of the relative amount of drug absorbed from the various dosage forms it is necessary to collect urine samples until no more drug is excreted. The cumulative amount of drug excreted during this time interval is designated $Ae^{\infty}$. In terms of this parameter:

$$\%BA = \frac{Ae_x^{\infty}}{Ae_r^{\infty}} \times 100 \qquad (2)$$

where $Ae_x^{\infty}$ and $Ae_r^{\infty}$ = amount of unmetabolized drug excreted in infinite time after a single dose of the sample and reference dosage forms, respectively

To insure that more than 98% of the unmetabolized drug to be eventually excreted has indeed been excreted it is necessary to collect urine samples over an interval representing at least six biological half-lives of the drug. Collecting urine samples for less than this interval will not adequately describe the relative absorption from the various dosage forms; rather it will bias the results in favor of the more rapidly absorbed dosage forms.

An example of this type of bias is observed in a paper on the bioavailability of various tetracycline capsules presented at a 1969 symposium.[16] Bioavailability was calculated on the basis of an eight-hour urine collection. Since the biological half-life of tetracycline is 8–10 hours, it is apparent that urinary excretion was followed for no more than one half-life. In this case the ranking of the various capsules does not reflect the relative amount of drug absorbed, which is what bioavailability actually measures, but reflects the relative absorption rates from the capsules. The latter consideration is also an important parameter for single dose administration, but as will be mentioned later, it is a relatively unimportant consideration for drugs administered on a multiple dosing regimen. The reader is referred to the work of Barr et al.[7] for the proper application of cumulative urinary excretion in the estimation of tetracycline bioavailability as well as a demonstration of this technique in general.

### Potential Bias in Using Blood Level Data

Another method of estimating bioavailability utilizes the measurement of the area under the blood level vs. time curve for a single dose of drug, commonly denoted as AUC, as shown in Figure 1. In terms of this parameter:

$$\%BA = \frac{AUC_x}{AUC_r} \times 100 \qquad (3)$$

where $AUC_x$ and $AUC_r$ = area under the blood level vs. time curves for a single dose of the sample and reference dosage forms, respectively

A common method of assessing bioavailability which may reflect a bias in the calculations results from ranking dosage forms on the basis of peak blood levels achieved after a single dose, $C_{max}$, as shown in Figure 1. An example of this technique is noted in a well-publicized paper describing the bioavailability of various digoxin preparations.[17] Some background is necessary before discussing the potential bias in the digoxin paper.

Five factors influence the value of $C_{max}$: (1) dose administered, (2) fraction of dose absorbed, (3) absorption rate constant of the drug, $K_a$, (4) elimination rate constant of the drug, $K_e$, and (5) volume of distribution of drug in the body. For most drugs the absorption rate constant is much greater than the elimination rate constant ($K_a \gg K_e$). When this condition is true,

$$C_{max} \propto \frac{(AUC)(K_e)}{(e^{k_e t_{max}})} \qquad (4)$$

where $t_{max}$ = time at which $C_{max}$ is achieved

If a large enough number of patients is used in the study, the average volume of distribution and the average elimination rate constant ($K_e$) will usually remain constant when comparing the data obtained for the sample and reference dosage forms study groups. Thus, as shown in Equation 4 and the preceding discussion, $C_{max}$ values can usually be employed as a relative index of AUC, and therefore bioavailability, only when (1) $t_{max}$ values are approximately equal for the various dosage forms examined, (2) $K_a \gg K_e$, and (3) average $K_e$ and volume of distribution values remain constant for the sample and reference study groups. On the other hand, an increase in $t_{max}$ values usually suggests a decrease in the absorption rate constant ($K_a$) but it does not necessarily reflect a decrease in AUC values. So in the absence of equal $t_{max}$ values for the various dosage forms studied, the ranking of bioavailability on the basis of $C_{max}$ values can only be assumed to be presumptive but not conclusive evidence of the relative absorption of drug from the dosage forms.

Unfortunately, in the digoxin paper cited above,[17] the authors rank the relative bioavailability of the various dosage forms on the basis of relative $C_{max}$ values but the $t_{max}$ values for the dosage forms appear unequal from

*Figure 1. Blood level vs. time curve for single dose administration of oral dosage form*

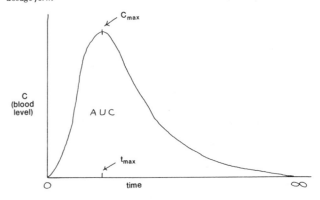

their data. Thus the conditions of Equation 4 are not achieved. Before the validity of this study can be assured it would be necessary to compare blood levels achieved upon multiple dosing, as will be discussed later.

Another method which introduces potential bias into the determination of bioavailability is not to measure AUC values over the full interval of the blood level vs. time curve (0 to ∞ in Figure 1) but to assess AUC for only a finite period of time (0 to t). If there is a difference in the absorption rate constants ($K_a$) for the various dosage forms and if the time interval used to assess the AUC is not longer than the interval required for absorption of the drug, then this technique of partial AUC measurement will bias the bioavailability results in favor of the more rapidly absorbed dosage forms. This technique does not provide an accurate assessment of relative bioavailability. A paper on the bioavailability of various phenylbutazone preparations[11] has been criticized[18] for using this technique. On the other hand, if $t_{max}$ values are approximately equal for the various dosage forms examined then the absorption rate constants are probably equal. In this case the method of partial assessment of AUC will provide a reasonable estimate of relative bioavailability because the variations in AUC are probably due to differences in the amount of drug absorbed. The justification for the latter technique is similar to the discussion associated with Equation 4.

### Potential Bias in Estimating Absorption When Using Intravenous Administration as a Reference

When the subject of relative absorption is not the comparative absorption from a single type of dosage form supplied from a variety of manufacturers (brands A, B, C, etc.) but concerns the comparative absorption of a drug from orally and intravenously administered dosage forms, then another type of potential bias results. Bias of this type is not of great clinical importance but it should be mentioned.

According to Equation 5 below, bioavailability also represents the ratio of absorption resulting from the administration of single doses of drug in oral and intravenous dosage forms:

$$\%BA = \frac{AUC_o}{AUC_{iv}} \times 100 \cong \frac{Ae_o^\infty}{Ae_{iv}^\infty} \times 100 \quad (5)$$

where subscripts o and iv = oral and intravenous dosage forms, respectively

Assuming complete absorption from the intravenous dosage form as a reference, then administering a drug in an oral dosage form which is known to be *completely* absorbed should result in 100% bioavailability. A number of studies suggest, however, that less than 100% bioavailability is achieved.[19-21] This is probably due to the (1) difference in the number of molecules passing through the liver (a primary metabolic site) on the first circulatory pass for oral as compared to intravenously administered drugs and/or (2) metabolism of drug in the gut wall prior to reaching the systemic circulation after oral administration. In other words, orally administered drug molecules must pass through the gastrointestinal membrane and then move *via* the hepatic portal system through the liver prior to reaching the central blood pool. For intravenously administered drugs, the gut wall is not a factor and only a small fraction of molecules pass through the liver on the first circulatory pass. Since absorption is often measured by analyzing blood or urine for unmetabolized drug, those drugs which are extensively metabolized by the liver and/or the gut wall may demonstrate an underestimate in comparative absorption from oral and intravenous dosage forms when employing Equation 5.

### Relationship of Bioavailability to Pharmacologic or Chemotherapeutic Response

For most drugs there is a relationship between the blood level and the pharmacologic or chemotherapeutic response.[22,23] Unfortunately, reliability on bioavailability estimates alone can often confound the significance of blood level determinations as a guide to therapeutic performance.

### Bioavailability in Relation to Therapeutic Effectiveness

Figure 2 is modified from the presentation of Withey et al.[12] and provides a basis for expanding this topic. Assume that these simplified geometric expressions of blood level vs. time profiles represent the oral administration of a single dose of a drug supplied by four different manufacturers. The AUC values for all of these forms are identical (2xy if x and y denote C and t, respectively). But in defining $C_{min}$ and $C_{max}$ as values representing the minimum level for response and the maximum "safe" level, respectively, it is apparent that the therapeutic responses resulting from the administra-

*Figure 2. Blood level vs. time curves for four different brands of the same oral dosage form*

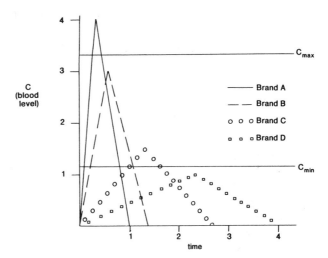

tion of a single dose of these four different brands with equal bioavailability will be quite different. Brand A is absorbed so rapidly that it reaches toxic levels, brand D is absorbed so slowly that it never achieves a therapeutic level, while brands B and C achieve effective and safe levels. Yet brand B provides a longer duration of effective concentration than does brand C.

### Single Dose Studies in Relation to Multiple Dose Regimens

Important as the above example is in depicting the fallibility of bioavailability analysis if not related to blood levels, the example suffers from a lack of clinical relevance for many drugs. Most drugs are administered on a multiple dosing regimen. It is well known that the administration of equal doses of a drug at equal dosage intervals results in the accumulation of drug in the body if the dosage interval is less than the time required for elimination of a single dose from the system. Since, as mentioned previously, the time required to eliminate a drug is at least six-fold greater than its biological half-life, blood levels increase with successive doses until a plateau state is reached in which the maximum, average and minimum blood levels are constant during successive dosing intervals.[24] This process is depicted in Figure 3. For example, if a drug is given at intervals corresponding with its biological half-life, the blood level will increase to plateau levels in about four half-lives, after which the level fluctuates between the $C_{max}$ produced by the first dose and twice that concentration. Using tetracycline capsules q8h with a half-life of eight hours as the example in Figure 3, a $C_{max}$ of 1 $\mu g/ml$ achieved by the first dose would result in a plateau state in about 30–35 hours after which the blood level would oscillate between 1–2 $\mu g/ml$. Administering the drug q6h or q12h would increase or decrease the plateau levels, respectively.

Now assume that 0.7 $\mu g/ml$ of tetracycline represents the $C_{min}$ value desired and that capsule brands A and B achieve $C_{max}$ values of 1.0 $\mu g/ml$ and 0.7 $\mu g/ml$, respectively, at similar $t_{max}$ values after the first dose. According to Equation 4 above, brand B may be considered only 70% as bioavailable as brand A, as a rough esti-

mate. Yet, upon reaching the plateau state during multiple dosing q8h, brands A and B will fluctuate between blood levels of 1.0–2.0 $\mu g/ml$ and 0.7–1.4 $\mu g/ml$, respectively. The concern over the use of brand B based on a single dose bioavailability estimate becomes unimportant during the clinically significant, multiple dosing situation. Brand A surely demonstrates greater bioavailability but the significance of this observation must often be judged in relation to the blood levels achieved and desired upon multiple dosing.

### Conclusion

When the practitioner encounters bioavailability data or is asked to render a judgment on the comparative evaluation of various brands of a drug he should discriminate between clinically significant and insignificant variations in bioavailability. Furthermore, he should be prepared to assess potential bias resulting from poor methodology that may invalidate some conclusions drawn from the data.

### References

1. Symposium on Formulation Factors Affecting Therapeutic Performance of Drug Products, *Drug Inform. Bull.* 3:1, 1969.
2. The Physiological Equivalence of Drug Dosage Forms, papers from the Symposium presented by the Food and Drug Directorate, Ottawa, Canada, June, 1969.
3. Wagner, J.: Biopharmaceutics and Relevant Pharmacokinetics, Drug Intelligence Publications, Hamilton, Illinois, 1971, ch. 24, 25, 39.
4. Ritschel, W.: Bioavailability in the Clinical Evaluation of Drugs, *Drug Intel. Clin. Pharm.* 6:246, 1972.
5. Barr, W.: Factors Involved in the Assessment of Systemic or Biologic Availability of Drug Products, *Drug Inform. Bull.* 3:27, 1969.
6. MacLeod, C. et al.: Comparative Bioavailability of Three Brands of Ampicillin, *Can. Med. Ass. J.* 107:203, 1972.
7. Barr, W. et al.: Assessment of the Biologic Availability of Tetracycline Products in Man. *Clin. Pharmacol. Ther.* 13:97, 1972.
8. Smolen, V.: The Determination of Drug Bioavailability Characteristics from Pharmacological Data, *Can. J. Pharm. Sci.* 7:1, 1972.
9. Smolen, V.: Applications of a Pharmacological Method of Drug Absorption Analysis to the Study of the Bioavailability Characteristics of Mydriatic Drugs, *Can. J. Pharm. Sci.* 7:7, 1972.
10. Wagner, J. et al.: In Vivo and In Vitro Availability of Commercial Warfarin Tablets, *J. Pharm. Sci.* 60:666, 1971.
11. Van Petten, G. et al.: The Physiologic Availability of Solid Dosage Forms of Phenylbutazone. Part I. In Vivo Physiologic Availability and Pharmacological Considerations, *J. Clin. Pharmacol.* 11:177, 1971.
12. Withey, R. et al.: The Physiologic Availability of Solid Dosage Forms of Phenylbutazone. Part II. Correlation of In Vivo Physiologic Availability and In Vitro Dissolution Parameters, *J. Clin. Pharmacol.* 11:187, 1971.
13. Mattok, G. et al.: Acetaminophen I. A Protocol for the Comparison of Physiological Availabilities of Ten Different Dosage Forms, *Can J. Pharm. Sci.* 6:35, 1971.
14. McGilveray, I. et al.: Acetaminophen II. A Comparison of the Physiological Availabilities of Different Commercial Dosage Forms, *Can. J. Pharm. Sci.* 6:38, 1971.
15. Wagner, J.: Generic Equivalence and Inequivalence of Oral Products, *Drug Intel. Clin. Pharm.* 5:115, 1971.

*Figure 3. Approach to plateau state upon multiple dose administration of an intravenous dosage form*

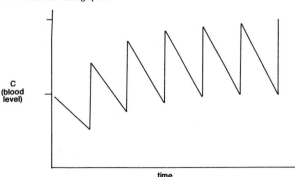

C (blood level)

time

16. Macdonald, H. et al.: Physiological Availability of Various Tetracyclines, *Drug Inform. Bull. 3*:76, 1969.

17. Lindenbaum, J. et al.: Variation in Biologic Availability of Digoxin from Four Preparations, *N. Engl. J. Med. 285*:1344, 1971.

18. Chiou, W.: Determination of Physiologic Availability of Commercial Phenylbutazone Preparations, *J. Clin. Pharmacol. 12*:296, 1972.

19. Rowland, M.: Influence of Route of Administration on Drug Availability, *J. Pharm. Sci. 61*:70, 1972.

20. Gibaldi, M. et al.: Influence of First-Pass Effect on Availability of Drugs on Oral Administration, *J. Pharm. Sci. 60*:1338, 1971.

21. Harris, P. and Riegelman, S.: Influence of the Route of Administration on the Area Under the Plasma Concentration-Time Curve, *J. Pharm. Sci. 58*:71, 1969.

22. Koch-Weser, J.: Serum Drug Concentrations as Therapeutic Guides, *N. Engl. J. Med. 287*:227, 1972.

23. Vesell, E. and Passananti, G.: Utility of Clinical Chemical Determinations of Drug Concentrations in Biological Fluids, *Clin. Chem. 17*:851, 1971.

24. Schumacher, G.: Practical Pharmacokinetic Techniques for Drug Consultation and Evaluation. I. Use of Dosage Regimen Calculations, In *Clinical Pharmacy Sourcebook*, pp. 226-236.

# 53 Potential Dangers of Common Drug Dosing Regimens

Paul J. Niebergall, Edwin T. Sugita, and Roger L. Schnaare

Various plasma level versus time profiles for procainamide and theophylline, based on different dosage regimens, were generated and compared using a digital computer program.

The usual 12-hour dosing period was compared to a 24-hour dosing period. A normal dose of procainamide given according to the usual q.i.d. regimen over a 12-hour period resulted in plasma levels that were below the therapeutic range for 12 hours out of each day. The same amount of drug given every four hours around the clock resulted in plasma levels that were always within the therapeutic range for this drug. The usual dose of theophylline given t.i.d., according to the usual definition of this term, resulted in plasma levels that were out of the therapeutic range for 14 hours out of each day. The same amount of drug given every six hours around the clock resulted in steady state plasma levels that were always within the therapeutic range for theophylline.

The results indicated that despite the time and effort devoted to the choice of drug and the amount of drug to be used for a given patient, the entire clinical effect observed for that patient might be markedly impaired by improper timing of the doses of the drug. This is primarily true for drugs with narrow therapeutic ranges, including diphenylhydantoin, lidocaine, lithium and quinidine, in addition to procainamide and theophylline.

Most drugs are given in multiple doses over a period of time. During the interval of treatment, the clinical effectiveness generally correlates reasonably well with plasma levels of drug[1-3] which should be kept within a certain therapeutic range. Plasma levels below this range will be inadequate in most patients, while concentrations above this range will result in an increase in the number and severity of side effects. Maintaining plasma levels within the therapeutic range for a particular drug can be achieved by proper selection of both dose and dosing regimen.

Upon the start of a multiple dosing regimen, the minimum and maximum plasma levels observed during any particular dosing interval tend to increase with succeeding doses until an equilibrium state has been achieved. During this equilibrium or steady state condition the minimum and maximum plasma levels are essentially the same from dose to dose. This drug accumulation and final equilibrium are shown in Figure 1.[a] The accumulation can be avoided and the equilibrium pattern established more rapidly if the drug is given at uniform dosing intervals equal to its biological half-life ($t_{1/2}$), with an initial dose equal to twice the maintenance dose as

shown in Figure 2. Thus, a drug with a $t_{1/2}$ of approximately eight hours should be given three times daily (t.i.d.) at eight-hour intervals, and a drug with $t_{1/2}$ of approximately six hours should be given four times daily (q.i.d.) at six-hour intervals.

Unfortunately, the term t.i.d. and q.i.d. are defined in many different ways. Earlier in this volume, Hermann[4] reported on a study in which 161 outpatients were given prescriptions with instructions for the drug to be taken twice daily (b.i.d.), t.i.d., or q.i.d. The large variety of ways in which these terms were interpreted by the outpatients (q.i.d. for one person meant every hour for four doses) led Hermann to suggest that these dosage regimens be defined for each situation taking into account both medication and patient criteria. Traditionally, this has been done by considering the daily dosing period to consist of either eight or twelve hours. In outpatient therapy, this generally means before, during, or after meals (t.i.d.) and another dose at bed time if needed (q.i.d.). Lewbart and Davis[5] found that in 56% of 457 hospitals responding to a questionnaire, drugs given on a t.i.d. schedule were given at 10-2-6 (10 a.m., 2 p.m., and 6 p.m.), 9-1-5, or 8-12-4, which are equivalent, and another 44% used t.i.d. schedules which were but a minor variation of these. This study also indicated that 95% of these hospitals used a q.i.d. dosing regimen of 10-2-6-10 or equivalent patterns such as 9-1-5-9 and 8-12-4-8. In many instances this is true regardless of the $t_{1/2}$ of the

---

[a] Since we were interested mainly in comparing the types of plasma level profiles obtained using various dosing schedules and not in the actual plasma levels at any given time, straight lines were used to connect the minimum and maximum plasma levels during each dosing interval. The lines would actually be slightly convex upward and concave downward.

Figure 1. Accumulation and steady state plasma level profile for a drug given every six hours

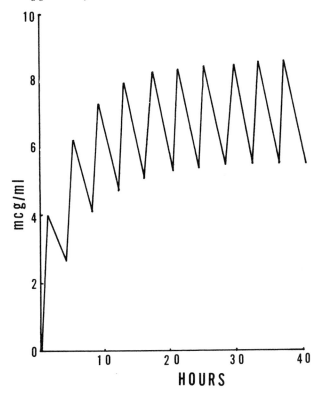

drug. The authors have found hospitals in which both potassium penicillin G ($t_{1/2}$ approximately one-half hour), and tetracycline ($t_{1/2}$ approximately ten hours) are both given according to the usual 10-2-6-10 type dosing schedule. Thus, for many drugs, it appears that for both inpatients and outpatients, doses are given at approximately four-hour intervals with a lapse of either 12 or 16 hours overnight during which time drug is being constantly eliminated from the patient's body. The validity of clustering the daily dosage into a short period, with a large no-dose period, as opposed to dosing during a 24-hour period at constant intervals apparently has not been questioned.

We derived the necessary questions and wrote a unique digital computer program[6] which would generate simulated plasma level versus time profiles for drugs in which both the dose and the dosing interval can be varied at will. This program was used to examine the 12-hour and the 24-hour dosing periods for theophylline with a therapeutic range of 10–20 $\mu$g/ml,[7-9] and procainamide with a therapeutic range of 4–8 $\mu$g/ml.[10] Both drugs are used in relatively severe conditions, have a narrow therapeutic range, elicit a high incidence of serious side effects, and are in many instances directed to be given t.i.d. or q.i.d. during a 12-hour dosing period.

Figure 2. Elimination of accumulation when the initial dose is double the maintenance dose and the dosing interval is equal to the biological half-life of the drug

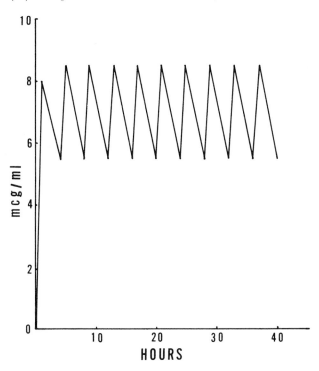

## Major Factors Influencing Plasma Levels

It would be helpful, before the 12-hour and the 24-hour dosing periods are compared, to quickly review those factors which contribute most to the observed plasma levels of a drug administered orally. These will be illustrated with procainamide using the following average values obtained or estimated from the work of Koch-Weser and Klein[10] which involved over 200 patients: the absorption rate constant, $k_a = 1.7$ hours$^{-1}$, and the elimination rate constant, $k_e = 0.198$ hours$^{-1}$. Figure 3 illustrates the effect of changing dose, in which the uppermost plasma level profile was obtained with a 0.75-g dose, the middle profile with a 0.5-g dose, and the lowest profile with a 0.25-g dose, each given every three hours around the clock. In this figure, and all those which follow, the dashed lines indicate the therapeutic range for the drug. As anticipated, the larger the dose, the higher the steady state plasma levels. Not as obvious is the fact that the larger the dose the greater the fluctuation between the minimum and maximum plasma levels during each dosing interval.

Figure 4 illustrates the effect of constant doses (0.5 g) given at various dosing intervals, $\lambda$. The uppermost plasma level profile was obtained with $\lambda = 2$ hours, the middle profile with $\lambda = 3$ hours, and the lowest profile with $\lambda = 6$ hours. Dosing at intervals less than the $t_{1/2}$ of the drug results in a greater degree of accumulation, but with less fluctuation of plasma levels within a dosing interval. Dosing at intervals greater than the $t_{1/2}$ results in lower plasma levels with much greater fluctuations.

*Figure 3. Effect of changing dose on the plasma level profile for procaina-mide given every three hours; A, dose = 0.75 g; B, dose = 0.50 g; C, dose = 0.25 g; dashed lines indicate therapeutic range*

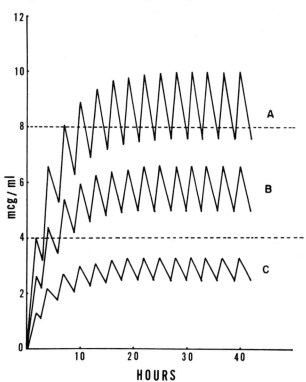

Thus it can be seen from Figures 3 and 4 that both the steady state plasma levels and the degree of fluctuation can be markedly altered by changing either the dose, the dosing interval, or both. For example, if plasma level fluctuations are an important consideration, as they should be for a drug with a narrow therapeutic range, it would be advisable to use smaller doses at more frequent dosing intervals, although this would be more bother-some for both the patient and the hospital staff.

While both the dose and the dosing interval can be varied by the individual designing the dosing regimen, one factor is generally beyond his control. That factor is the elimination rate constant of the drug which varies from patient to patient. In fact the elimination rate con-stant can change within a given patient as renal function decreases, if enzyme induction occurs, or with changes in urinary $pH$. The effect of increasing $t_{1/2}$ is illustrated in Figure 5, with procainamide given 0.5 g every three hours around the clock. The lowest profile represents the average $t_{1/2}$ of 3.5 hours, while the middle and upper-most profiles represent $t_{1/2}$ values of 5.0 and 7.0 hours, respectively.

Since elimination rate constants vary from patient to patient, all of the plasma level profiles simulated in this chapter represent those that would be obtained for the "average" patient and do not necessarily represent quan-titative levels for any given individual. The important issue here is not necessarily the exact levels reached for the drugs used, but rather the patterns of daily fluctuation of plasma levels, the potential dangers of

*Figure 4. Effect of changing the dosing interval on the plasma level of procainamide given in 0.50-g doses; A, $\tau$ = 2 hours; B, $\tau$ = 3 hours; C, $\tau$ = 6 hours; dashed lines indicate therapeutic range*

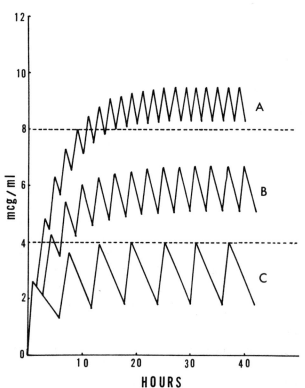

*Figure 5. Effect of changing the biological half-life on the plasma level profile for 0.50 g procainamide given every three hours; A, $t_{1/2}$ = 3.5 hours; B, $t_{1/2}$ = 5.0 hours; C, $t_{1/2}$ = 7.0 hours; dashed lines indicate therapeutic range*

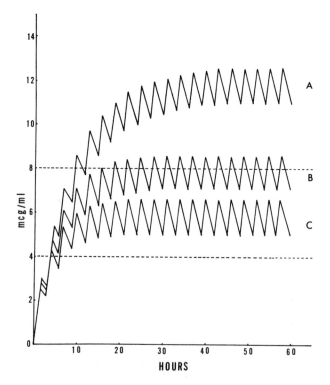

which would have to be assessed for each individual drug.

## Common Dosing Regimens

The package insert for a major brand of procainamide[b] suggests that for ventricular tachycardia, 1.0 g of procainamide should be given initially, followed by 0.5–1.0 g every four to six hours thereafter. Utilizing the data of Koch-Weser and Klein,[10] plasma levels were generated as a function of time for the situation in which 1.0 g of procainamide was given initially, followed by 0.5 g every four hours around the clock. The results, shown in Figure 6, illustrate the fact that the use of an initial dose equal to twice the maintenance dose eliminates the accumulation effect and results in therapeutic levels of procainamide within one hour. The plasma levels fluctuate within the therapeutic range and finally equilibrate with steady state levels between 4.3–6.8 $\mu$g/ml.

In many instances, however, the maintenance dose of this drug is given every four hours during a 12-hour period. One schedule the authors have seen frequently is the 10-2-6-10, q.i.d. pattern. If the instructions from the package insert were interpreted in this manner, 1.0 g of procainamide would be given for example at 10 a.m., followed by 0.5-g doses at 2 p.m., 6 p.m. and 10 p.m. during the first day of therapy, followed by 0.5 g at 10-2-6-10 thereafter. The plasma level versus time profile resulting from this interpretation of "every four hours" is shown in Figure 7. Although it is difficult to obtain from the figure, the computer printout showed that for the first day of therapy, therapeutic plasma levels could be maintained for only 17 out of 24 hours, and for the succeeding days the plasma levels would be below the therapeutic range for 12 out of every 24 hours.

The t.i.d. or 10-2-6 dose schedule is also used rather frequently for procainamide. The plasma level versus time profile for 1.0 g of procainamide given at 10 a.m., followed by 0.5 g at 2 p.m. and 6 p.m. the first day of therapy, and 0.5 g at 10-2-6 thereafter is shown in Figure 8. During the first day of therapy the plasma level of procainamide is below the therapeutic range for 12 hours. During the second and succeeding days, the plasma level is below the therapeutic range for 17 hours out of each full day.

Figures 6–8 demonstrate the fact that procainamide, with its narrow therapeutic range and short $t_{1/2}$ would be given only at constant dosing intervals around the clock. Even doubling the daily morning dose would not improve the plasma level pattern to any great extent if the common t.i.d. or q.i.d. schedules are used, since the long (12–16 hour) overnight no-dose period results in a marked decline in plasma levels during this period with the plasma level of procainamide being below the therapeutic range for an excessive amount of time.

The therapeutic range of theophylline is generally

*Figure 6. Plasma level profile for procainamide given 1.0 g initially then 0.50 g every four hours thereafter; dashed lines indicate the therapeutic range*

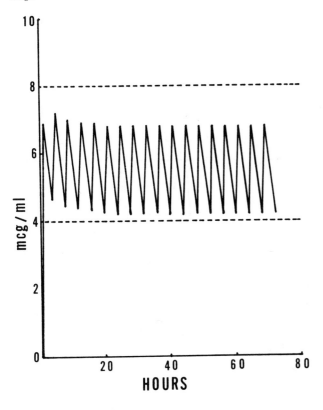

*Figure 7. Plasma level profile for procainamide given 1.0 g initially, then 0.5 g q.i.d. thereafter at 10-2-6-10; dashed lines indicate the therapeutic range*

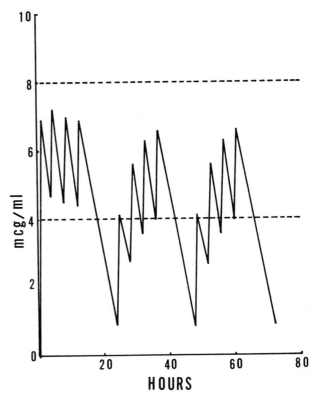

[b] Pronestyl, E. R. Squibb & Sons.

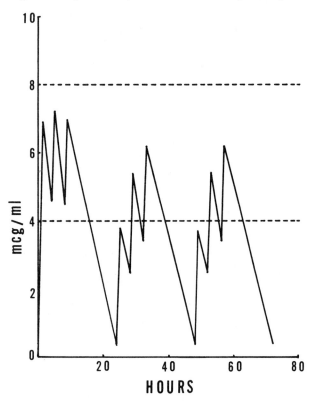

*Figure 8. Plasma level profile for procainamide given 1.0 g initially, then 0.5 g t.i.d. thereafter at 10-2-6; dashed lines indicate therapeutic range*

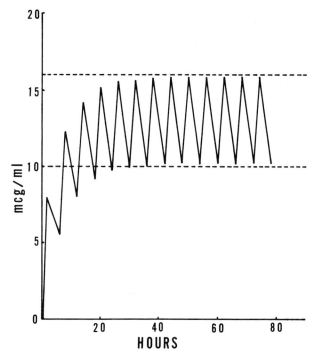

*Figure 9. Plasma level profile for 160 mg of theophylline given every six hours; dashed lines indicate therapeutic range*

given as being 10–20 μg/ml.[7-9] However, in one study Jenne et al.[7] found possible or definite toxicities in 12 out of 30 patients with plasma levels of theophylline greater than approximately 16 μg/ml, and only two toxicities in 53 patients with plasma levels below 15 μg/ml. Therefore, in this chapter we would prefer to use 10–16 μg/ml as a reasonable therapeutic range for theophylline. Plasma level profiles were simulated for theophylline using the data of Jenne et al.[7] and Schluger et al.[11] which gave the following estimated pharmacokinetic parameters: absorption rate constant, $k_a$ = 1.0 hours$^{-1}$; elimination rate constant, $k_e$ = 0.133 hours$^{-1}$. Since the average $t_{1/2}$ for theophylline is 5.2 hours,[7] it would be reasonable to give doses of this drug at six-hour intervals around the clock, resulting in four doses daily. The plasma level profile for 160 mg of theophylline given every six hours around the clock is shown in Figure 9. The steady state minimum and maximum plasma levels in each dosing interval are 10.2 and 15.8 μg/ml respectively. In many hospitals theophylline is given according to the usual t.i.d. or q.i.d. schedules. The plasma level profile for 160 mg of theophylline given t.i.d. at 10-2-6 is shown in Figure 10. This dosing schedule results in the plasma level of theophylline being above the therapeutic range for two hours, and below the range for 12 hours out of each day. The plasma level profile for 160 mg of theophylline given q.i.d. at 10-2-6-10 is shown in Figure 11. In this instance the plasma level of theophylline is above the therapeutic range for six hours and below the range for five out of every 24 hours. Thus, as was observed for

procainamide, due to the narrow therapeutic range and the relatively short $t_{1/2}$, theophylline should be given in four equal dosing intervals around the clock.

## Summary

The results of this study would tend to indicate that despite the time and effort devoted to the proper choice

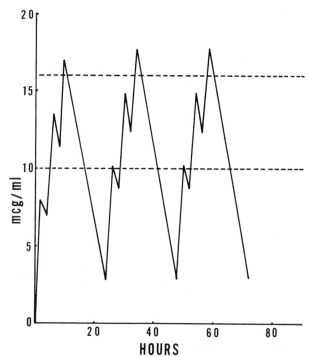

*Figure 10. Plasma level profile for 160 mg of theophylline given t.i.d. at 10-2-6; dashed lines indicate therapeutic range*

*Figure 11. Plasma level profile for 160 mg of theophylline given q.i.d. at 10-2-6-10; dashed lines indicate therapeutic range*

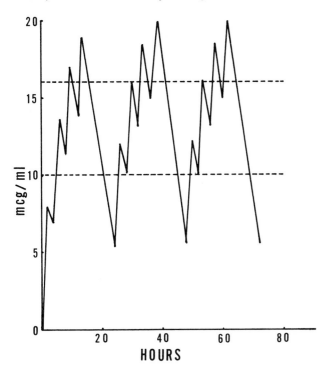

The computer program used to generate the data in this study is short, simple to use, and is available from us upon request. Since more and more hospitals are gaining access to time sharing computer services, it is hoped that the typical dosing regimens used in hospitals will be investigated via the simulation of average plasma level versus time profiles.

### References

1. Brodie, B. B.: Physicochemical and Biochemical Aspects of Pharmacology, *JAMA 202*:600-609 (Nov. 13) 1967.

2. Brodie, B. B. and Reid, W. W.: The Value of Determining the Plasma Concentration of Drugs in Animals and Man, *In* LaDu, B. N., Mandel, H. G. and Way. E. L. (eds.): Fundamentals of Drug Metabolism and Drug Disposition, Williams and Wilkins Co., Baltimore, Maryland, 1971, pp. 328-339.

3. Vesell, E. S. and Passananti, G. T.: Utility of Clinical Chemical Determinations of Drug Concentrations in Biological Fluids, *Clin. Chem. 17*:851–866 (Sept.) 1971.

4. Hermann, F.: The Outpatient Prescription Label as a Source of Medication Errors, In *Clinical Pharmacy Sourcebook*, pp. 175-179.

5. Lewbart, R. S. and Davis, N. M.: Hospital Variation in Medication Administration Schedules, *Hosp. Pharm. 4*:16–22 (May) 1969.

6. Niebergall, P. J., Sugita, E. T. and Schnaare, R. L.: Calculation of Plasma Level Versus Time Profiles for Variable Dosing Regimens, *J. Pharm. Sci.*

7. Jenne, J. W., Wyze, E., Rood, F. S. and MacDonald, F. M.: Pharmacokinetics of Theophylline, *Clin. Pharmacol. Ther. 13*:349–360 (May–June) 1972.

8. Jackson, R. H., McHenry, J. I., Moreland, F. B., Raymer, W. J. and Etter, R. L.: Clinical Evaluation of Elixophylline with Correlation of Pulmonary Function Studies and Theophylline Serum Levels in Acute and Chronic Asthmatic Patients, *Dis. Chest 45*:75–85 (Jan.) 1964.

9. Turner-Warwick, M.: Study of Theophylline Plasma Levels after Oral Administration of New Theophylline Compounds, *Brit. Med. J. 2*:67–69 (July 13) 1957.

10. Koch-Weser, J. and Klein, S. W.: Procainamide Dosage Schedules, Plasma Concentrations, and Clinical Effects, *JAMA 215*:1454-1460 (Mar. 1) 1971.

11. Schluger, J., McGinn, J. T. and Hennesey, D. J.: Comparative Theophylline Blood Levels Following the Oral Administration of Three Different Theophylline Preparations, *Amer. J. Med. Sci. 233*:296–302 (Mar.) 1957.

12. Koch-Weser, J.: Serum Drug Concentrations as Therapeutic Guides, *N. Engl. J. Med. 287*:227–231 (Aug. 3) 1972.

of drug and the amount of drug to be used for a given patient, the entire clinical effect observed for that patient might be markedly impaired by improper timing of the doses of the drug. This would be true primarily for drugs with narrow therapeutic ranges. In addition to procainamide and theophylline, other important drugs with narrow therapeutic ranges are:[12] diphenylhydantoin (10–20 $\mu$g/ml), lidocaine (0.5–1.3 $\mu$g/ml), lithium (0.5–1.3 mEq/liter), and quinidine (2–5 $\mu$g/ml). In other instances the therapeutic range is wide enough such that plasma level fluctuations due to the usual t.i.d. or q.i.d. dosing schedules would probably remain within the therapeutic range. One example of this might be nortriptyline with a therapeutic range of 50–140 $\mu$g/liter.[12]

# 54 Computerized Dosage Regimens for Highly Toxic Drugs

Frank J. Goicoechea and Roger W. Jelliffe

A quantitative, mathematical approach to the development of individualized dosage regimens using computer programs is described.

Computer programs have been developed for calculating dosage regimens of cardiac glycosides, kanamycin, gentamicin, streptomycin, and procainamide in patients with normal and impaired renal function. The programs compute peak and end-of-interval serum drug levels from data on past doses, body weight and blood urea nitrogen, serum creatinine levels or creatinine clearance.

An example of program execution for calculating procainamide dosage for a patient is presented.

The literature abounds with reports of iatrogenic drug disorders. Some of these are due to patient idiosyncrasies; they cannot be predicted in advance and thus are difficult to prevent. Many others, however, appear to be related to the duration of therapy, excessive dosage, or to deterioration of renal function during the course of therapy, thus leading to an excessive accumulation of drug and metabolite levels above the therapeutic range into a toxic range.[1-3] Such events are especially serious with those highly toxic drugs characterized by a high degree of renal excretion and by a narrow therapeutic index.

The incidence of such toxicity might be reduced or prevented by:

1. Closer patient monitoring by the physician and pharmacist.
2. Ability to predict reasonably effective drug plasma levels in advance.
3. Selection of the appropriate loading and maintenance dose based on the patient's weight and cardiac and renal function to achieve and maintain selected drug levels with reasonable accuracy for clinical purposes.
4. Ability to adjust these dosage regimens to changing renal function when it occurs.

In the past, dosage regimens have been derived either through an educated "guess," simplified formulae or by the eventual appearance of toxicity. Despite the ideal concept of individualized dosage, little real effort has been made to consider each patient as a single entity and thus to plan in advance to adjust his dosage quantitatively to his therapeutic needs, weight and hepatic, renal or cardiac function.

In contrast to the above approach, the clinical staff pharmacists and pharmacy residents at the Los Angeles County/University of Southern California Medical Center and pharmacy students at the University of Southern California School of Pharmacy, in collaboration with work done at the University of Southern California School of Medicine, have taken an active role in providing a careful, quantitative, mathematical approach to the development of individualized dosage regimens of cardiac glycosides,[4] kanamycin,[5] gentamicin,[6] streptomycin[7] and oral and intravenous procainamide[8,9] for patients with normal or impaired renal function, using computer programs which are available on an internationally accessible time-shared computer system.[a] The dosage regimens developed are adjusted to the patient's renal function, body weight and computed serum levels or computed total concentrations of drug in the body. They are also adjusted for oral or parenteral administration when appropriate. In the case of the cardiac glycosides,[4] the computer program is capable of replacing any mixture of digitalis leaf, digitoxin, digoxin or deslanoside which may have been given in the past with the single glycoside the physician now wishes to use. It is intended for adult patients with normal thyroid and hepatic function, normal electrolyte balance and no clinical evidence of malabsorption. It is based upon an initial mathematical analysis of the digitalis kinetics in patients with normal and reduced renal function. The pro-

[a] The Network Software Service of the General Electric Mark III system in the United States (General Electric Information Services, 7735 Old Georgetown Rd., Bethesda, MD 20014) (301) 654-9360 and Honeywell-Bull Information Systems in Europe.

grams for the other drugs[5-9] use generally similar mathematical descriptions and are intended for use in adult patients.

The programs have four basic parts:

1. Serial entry of individual past doses (up to 50, if past therapy was given) to estimate past and present total body drug levels and/or serum levels.
2. A description of relevant past and present clinical data, and a statement of usual effective therapeutic serum levels.
3. A place for selection by the physician, in consultation with the pharmacist, of the therapeutic goals or serum levels to be achieved in that patient, plus entry of his present renal function.
4. Computation and printout of dosage regimens to achieve and maintain the stated clinical goals, with the option to rerun the program with selection of different therapeutic goals if desired.

**Operation of the Programs**

Communication with the computer for the execution of the programs is through a remote terminal connected to the main computer via an ordinary telephone line, using an acoustic coupler.

As shown in Figure 1, the programs begin by asking whether or not the patient has had any previous therapy. If the answer is No, then the computer will skip to step 10, as shown, and ask for the patient's cardiac rhythm, the desired peak plasma level that the pharmacist and physician together think will be most useful, the patient's blood urea nitrogen, the desired dose interval and the

chosen route of administration. The computer (step 13) then computes and prints the loading dose to consider to achieve the chosen peak serum level with reasonable accuracy, given this patient's weight and renal function. It also prints the maintenance dose designed to maintain the peak serum concentration at the desired level, using the selected dosage interval.

On the other hand, if the patient had received previous therapy and a complete dosage regimen was desired, as shown in steps 3 and 4, Figure 1, the computer asks the operator for the total number of past doses. For each past dose, it asks for the dose, the renal function and the length of the dose interval which are entered as shown. Serial computation of past total body drug levels or serum levels is then performed, followed by a printout of the appropriate computed maximum and end-of-interval body concentrations of drug (or serum levels) during each dose interval.

If the patient had been on the drug for at least five drug half-lives, with stable renal function, the assumption can reasonably be made that the patient has closely approached a steady state situation, and one may enter into the computer only the data of doses received during the past five half-lives to produce a reasonable approach to a computed steady state in such a patient.

Next, the operator will be asked if the patient has had any possible toxicity. If so, he enters the manifestation of toxicity by typing the code, as instructed by the computer, and the date and serum level at which the toxicity occurred. The computer then asks for the patient's present cardiac rhythm and the other clinical data as described earlier. This is followed by a general statement of the range of therapeutic serum levels of the drug, and a request to enter the desired peak serum level, the patient's present renal function, the chosen dose interval and selected route of administration. If at the time the dosage regimen is to begin there is more drug present in the patient than the peak level selected, an appropriate waiting period is computed and printed. If the regimen developed is not satisfying to the pharmacist-physician team, or if it would be difficult for the patient to adhere to it as an outpatient, the operator may rerun the program, as shown in step 14, Figure 1, and enter different therapeutic goals. A different dosage interval might be chosen, for example. The programs will not accept selection of levels that are associated with a very high risk of serious toxicity.

Any member of the health team—physician, pharmacist, nurse or medical student—can be trained to use these programs. No previous computer experience is required. Nevertheless, the pharmacist, because of his training and background in pharmacology and pharmacokinetics, is in a unique position to utilize the reasoning behind the programs,[5-10] to take the greatest advantage of their use, and thus to perform a useful consultative service to the physician. Through daily drug monitoring, the pharmacist is able to evaluate changes

Figure 1. Flow sheet for procainamide program organization

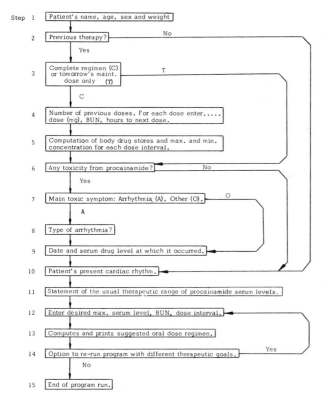

in those parameters such as renal function or electrolyte balance which may affect the biological half-life and sensitivity to a drug. If such changes occur, the pharmacist may use the computer programs to evaluate the effect of such changes upon the patient's present therapy and clinical response. If necessary, he may calculate a new maintenance dose adjusted to the patient's new renal function and may then initiate a change in the patient's therapy by presenting these findings and discussing them with the physician in charge of the case.

## Discussion

It is not within the scope of this chapter to discuss the mathematical models and development of these programs, which has already been done elsewhere.[4-10] It is, however, the intent of this report to describe ways in which these programs have been used by pharmacists to improve the quality of patient care. The pharmacy staff, pharmacy residents and pharmacy students at the LAC/USC Medical Center make use of programs such as the one described above for providing physicians with quantitative, individualized approaches to the development of dosage regimens of cardiac glycosides, kanamycin, gentamicin, streptomycin and procainamide. The role of the pharmacist, in a consulting capacity with the physician, has been to help to provide patients with dosage regimens individually tailored not only to the physician's desired clinical and therapeutic goals but also to the patient's body weight and renal function. These programs have also been a useful tool to monitor the computed levels of drugs in patients and to adjust dosages in those patients with unstable renal function, thus helping to keep serum levels of these drugs reasonably constant throughout such changes. If needed, dose regimens can be provided on a daily basis to compensate for such rapidly changing renal function.

The utility of such programs has already been shown for the cardiac glycosides[10] in a comparative study between a sample of patients who first received intuitive dosage regimens of digitalis and then received dosage according to a schedule provided by the computer programs. The study showed a reduction from a 35% incidence of digitalis toxicity at first, falling to 12% with computer assistance, a significant decrease ($p < 0.001$). Similarly, toxicity was only 4% for a comparable prospectively studied computer-assisted group.[10] Although no such comparative studies are yet available for the other drugs, the other programs have been very useful to the pharmacist and physician in predicting plasma drug levels with reasonable accuracy for clinical purposes.[4-9] Computed and measured serum levels thus are highly correlated.

It should be emphasized that such computer-assisted dosage regimens are only a therapeutic guideline. They should always be checked for errors, such as printing errors and errors due to static on the telephone lines, and should always be evaluated against the patient's overall clinical status, performance and apparent clinical requirements.

Figures 2A, 2B and 2C show the appearance of a representative computer program for procainamide dosage during execution. The program begins by considering a patient who was hospitalized with pulmonary edema and multiple ventricular extrasystoles. On admission, the patient's weight was 186 lbs, his height was 5 feet 8 inches, and his blood urea nitrogen was 20 mg/100 ml. In order to suppress the extrasystoles, the attending physician elected to treat the patient with 250 mg of oral procainamide every four hours after an initial dose of 500 mg. As the patient was reviewed on medical rounds, the pharmacist pointed out that for a patient of this weight and renal function, the above dosage regimen might not produce a therapeutic plasma level. The physician, however, elected to continue with the initial therapy. On the third day of therapy the patient still had multiple ventricular extrasystoles. The physician ordered a single dose of 750 mg of oral procainamide to be given immediately in an effort to control the arrhythmia. The pharmacist then evaluated the previous therapy by using the computer program. As shown in Figure 2A, he entered the patient's name, chart number, physician's name, weight, height and the number of previous doses of procainamide. Then a serial entry of each dose, the blood urea nitrogen level at that time and the length of each

*Figure 2A. Appearance of the representative program of procainamide as it is executed; this includes the calculation and printout of maximum and minimum serum levels of the drug based on the patient's past history of procainamide therapy*

```
PROGRAM TO RUN? PRON

RUNNING THE PRON PROGRAM ON G , E , CHART NUMBER 1483377
AGE= 56. YRS, SEX= M , HEIGHT= 5.FT  8. IN, WT= 186. LBS
WARD 6036, PHYSICIAN G , R

IS ALL THE ABOVE DATA CORRECT? (YES OR NO)
? YES

ARE YOU AN EXPERT IN THE USE OF THIS PRONESTYL PROGRAM?
? YES

PREVIOUS PRONESTYL RX?
? YES

COMPLETE REGIMEN OR JUST TOMORROW'S MAINT DOSE? (C, T, OR HELP)
? C
NUMBER OF PREVIOUS DOSES?
? 12

FOR EACH PREV DOSE, ENTER...
DOSE(MG),BUN(MG%),HRS TO NEXT DOSE

            DOSE,BUN,HRS
FOR DOSE # 1 ? 500,20,3
FOR DOSE # 2 ? 250,20,4
FOR DOSE # 3 ? 250,20,4
FOR DOSE # 4 ? 250,20,4
FOR DOSE # 5 ? 250,20,4
FOR DOSE # 6 ? 250,20,4
FOR DOSE # 7 ? 250,20,4
FOR DOSE # 8 ? 250,20,4
FOR DOSE # 9 ? 250,20,4
FOR DOSE # 10 ? 250,20,4
FOR DOSE # 11 ? 250,20,6
FOR DOSE # 12 ? 750,23,6
```

| DOSE | STORES (MG) | | CONC (MG/KG) | | PEAK | SERUM (MCG/ML) | |
|------|------|------|------|------|------|------|------|
| NUMBER | MAX | MIN | MAX | MIN | (HOURS) | MAX | MIN |
| 1 | 379.00 | 267.15 | 4.492 | 3.166 | 1.12 | 2.91 | 2.05 |
| 2 | 402.29 | 203.94 | 4.768 | 2.417 | .78 | 3.09 | 1.57 |
| 3 | 350.08 | 180.22 | 4.149 | 2.136 | .84 | 2.69 | 1.38 |
| 4 | 330.87 | 171.41 | 3.922 | 2.032 | .87 | 2.54 | 1.32 |
| 5 | 323.77 | 168.14 | 3.838 | 1.993 | .87 | 2.49 | 1.29 |
| 6 | 321.14 | 166.93 | 3.806 | 1.979 | .88 | 2.47 | 1.28 |
| 7 | 320.17 | 166.48 | 3.795 | 1.973 | .88 | 2.46 | 1.28 |
| 8 | 319.81 | 166.31 | 3.791 | 1.971 | .88 | 2.46 | 1.28 |
| 9 | 319.67 | 166.25 | 3.789 | 1.971 | .88 | 2.46 | 1.28 |
| 10 | 319.62 | 166.23 | 3.788 | 1.970 | .88 | 2.45 | 1.28 |
| 11 | 319.60 | 101.29 | 3.788 | 1.201 | .88 | 2.45 | .78 |
| 12 | 663.02 | 258.67 | 7.859 | 3.066 | 1.12 | 5.09 | 1.99 |

```
SERUM PRONESTYL LEVELS AT YOUR NEXT DOSE SHOULD BE   2.0 MCG/ML
```

*Figure 2B. Continuation of the execution of the procainamide program; this allows for a description of relevant past and present clinical data*

```
ANY POSSIBLE TOXICITY FROM PRONESTYL?
? NO
PATIENT'S PRESENT CARDIAC RHYTHM?
1=RSR, 2=AUR FIB, 3=PAC'S, 4=PNC'S, 5=PVC'S, 6=PAT, 7=AUR FLUTTER,
8=NODAL TACH, 9=V TACH, 10=1ST, 11=2ND,12=3RD DEGREE AV BLOCK,
13=SOME OTHER RHYTHM.
? 13
DESCRIBE THIS OTHER RHYTHM......USE UP TO 18 LETTERS.
? 1 AND 4
1 AND 4? IS THIS CORRECT? TYPE YES OR NO.
? YES

WHAT TYPE OF HEART DISEASE DOES THE PATIENT HAVE?
TYPE 1 FOR RHD,2 FOR ASHD,3 FOR HCVD,4 FOR LUETIC HD,
5 FOR CONGEN HD,6 FOR COR PULM,7 FOR SBE,8 FOR OTHER OR SEVERAL
? 2

WHICH OF THESE PROBLEMS DOES THE PATIENT HAVE?
TYPE 1 FOR INFARCT WITHIN 2 WEEKS,2 FOR OLDER INFARCT,3 FOR ISCHEMIA NOW.

TYPE 4 FOR AORTIC STENOSIS,5 FOR AI,6 FOR MS,7 FOR M INSUFF,
TYPE 8 FOR SEVERAL,OTHER,OR TO COMMENT.
TYPE 0 FOR NONE.
? 3

PATIENT'S PRESENT NEW YORK HEART ASSN. CLASS? (ENTER LIKE 2,B)
? 3,C
ENTER PATIENTS PRESENT BLOOD PRESSURE (SYST,DIAST)
? 130,90
THE APEX BEAT: HOW MANY CM BEYOND THE MCL?(0,1,2,ETC)
? 2
SPEED OF VENTRICULAR EJECTION?
1=VERY SLOW,2=SLOW,3=NORMAL,4=RAPID,5=VERY RAPID
? 4
DID PT HAVE RECENT ARTERIAL BLOOD GAS RESULTS? (YES OR NO)
? NO
```

dosing interval was made. The computer printout then showed that the computed maximum plasma procainamide level prior to the last dose was 2.45 µg/ml, well below suggested therapeutic levels.[11] This low computed result correlated well with the poor clinical response of the patient at that time.

Next, as shown in Figure 2B, the computer requested data of any possible toxicity from procainamide. If toxicity had been present, the computer would have asked for the main manifestation of toxicity, which the operator would have entered in a coded manner as instructed by the computer. The computer also requested additional information about the patient's clinical state, as shown in Figure 2B.

*Figure 2C. Conclusion of the execution of the procainamide program; this allows for selection of therapeutic goals or serum levels to be achieved, followed by a computation and printout of dosage regimens to achieve and maintain the desired clinical goals*

```
MAX SERUM PRON LEVELS OF 4 TO 8 MCG/ML ARE OFTEN EFFECTIVE.

DESIRED MAX SERUM LEVEL? BUN? DOSE INTERVAL?
? 4,21,6
YOU ENTERED  4.0 MCG/ML,  21.0 MG%, AND   6.0HRS? (YES OR NO)
? YES

    CONSIDER THIS ORAL DOSE PROGRAM:
DOSE     DOSE     SERUM LEVEL   TIME FOR MAX
NUMBER   (MG)     BEFORE DOSE      HOURS
  1      417.7        2.0           .8
  2      505.6        1.4           .8
  3      501.3        1.4           .8

AND THEREAFTER  501.5,  CHECK IT  501.5, MG,---G  6.0 HOURS,
IF RENAL FUNCTION DOES NOT CHANGE.

RERUN PROGRAM WITH DIFFERENT THERAPEUTIC GOALS?
? NO
NEVER TRUST A COMPUTER! LIKE A LAB, ITS RESULTS MAY HAVE ERRORS!

AS STATED EARLIER, ONLY YOU, THE USER, CAN BE RESPONSIBLE FOR
ACTING UPON THE BASIS OF THE OUTPUT SHOWN ABOVE.

IN ADDITION, EVEN IF YOUR GOALS AND THIS REGIMEN SEEM REASONABLE,
THEY MAY NOT FIT THE PATIENT. YOU ARE STILL RESPONSIBLE
FOR EVALUATING HIS RESPONSE TO THE REGIMEN YOU GIVE.

ALL INPUT AND OUTPUT HAS BEEN EVALUATED, CHECKED FOR ERRORS, CHECKED
FOR BEING CONSISTENT WITH THE PATIENT'S TOTAL CLINICAL PICTURE,
AND HAS BEEN VALIDATED BY THE RESPONSIBLE PERSON BELOW:

                       ................M.D. OR PHARM.D
(OUTPUT NOT VALID UNLESS DECLARED SO BY BEING SIGNED ABOVE)  04/18/73

PLEASE PUT THIS RECORD IN THE PATIENT'S CHART.
G ,E , CHART NO 1483377, ROOM OR WARD 6036
DR. G ,F  DATE  4/18/73
G
```

Finally, as shown in Figure 2C, the usual effective therapeutic levels[11] for procainamide are printed. The operator can select the desired peak serum level he wishes to achieve and maintain. As shown in this figure, the pharmacist considered achieving a peak serum level of 4 µg/ml. In order to achieve this new therapeutic goal the pharmacist also entered into the computer the present blood urea nitrogen level (21 mg/100 ml) and the desired dose interval of six hours. This was followed by the computation and printout of the suggested oral dosage regimen of procainamide to achieve these goals (418 mg, followed by 500 mg every six hours) adjusted to the patient's weight and renal function to achieve and maintain the desired peak serum level.

This new information was presented to the physician and discussed with him. The physician then ordered a dosage regimen of 500 mg, p.o., every six hours. Over the next few days, the number of ventricular extrasystoles decreased, and the patient was discharged from the hospital on the same oral dosage schedule.

It should be noted that dosage regimen for the physician to consider is intended to be used only as long as the patient's renal function does not change. If renal function should change, however, it is easy to recompute a regimen adjusted to the new renal function in a manner similar to that already shown above.

Before the program is terminated, a reminder is given to the operator that all the above data should be checked for possible errors and for consistency with the patient's total clinical picture before the new therapy is actually instituted. Figure 3 illustrates graphically the events described in the above patient by showing the correlation between his measured and computed plasma levels.

## Conclusion

The high incidence of drug-induced iatrogenic disorders not only emphasizes the importance of close patient

*Figure 3. This illustrates the clinical application of the computer program for predicting serum levels with reasonable accuracy (see text for explanation); the solid line describes the computed maximum and minimum serum levels achieved with the given doses; the circular symbol represents measured serum levels*

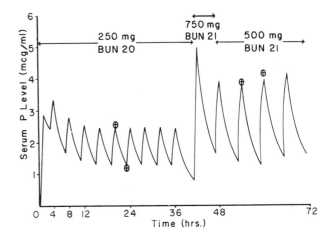

monitoring by the pharmacist and the physician but also shows the need for closer collaboration and understanding between the medical and pharmacy staff to help prevent adverse drug reactions by rational planning of dosage regimens of drugs such as cardiac glycosides, kanamycin, gentamicin, streptomycin and procainamide for patients with normal or impaired renal function.

## References

1. Ogilvie, R. I. and Ruedy, J.: Adverse Reactions During Hospitalizations, *Can. Med. Ass. J. 97*:1445–1457 (Dec.) 1967.

2. Ogilvie, R. I. and Ruedy, J.: An Educational Program in Digitalis Therapy, *JAMA 222*:50–55 (Oct.) 1972.

3. Jick, H. J.: Drug Surveillance Program, *Med. Sci. 18*:41–46 (July) 1967.

4. Jelliffe, R. W., Buell, J., Kalaba, R., Sridhar, R. and Rockwell, R.: A Computer Program for Digitalis Dosage Regimens, *Math. Biosci. 9*:179–193, 1970.

5. Jelliffe, R. W., Buell, J., Kalaba, R., Rockwell, R. and Knight, R.: Computer-Assisted Kanamycin Dose Programs, *Clin. Research 18*:137 (Jan.) 1970.

6. Jelliffe, R. W., Knight, R., Buell, J., Kalaba, R. and Rockwell, R.: Computer Assistance for Gentamicin Therapy, *Clin. Research 18*:441 (Apr.) 1970.

7. Jelliffe, R. W., Buell, J., Kalaba, R., Nagel, G., Bernstein, M. and Ivler, D.: A Computer Program for Streptomycin (S) Dosage with Separate Serum and Ear Compartment, submitted for consideration for Presentation at the Twelfth Interscience Conference on Antimicrobial Agents and Chemotherapy in Atlantic City, September 26–29, 1972.

8. Goicoechea, F. J., Wagers, R. W., Jelliffe, R. W.: A Computer Program for Oral Procainamide Dosage, *Circulation 46 Supp. II*:II-157 (Oct.) 1972.

9. Jelliffe, R. W., Goicoechea, F. J. and Wyman, M. G.: A Computer Program for Intervenous Procainamide Dosage, *Circulation 48 Supp. IV:* IV-169 (Oct.) 1973.

10. Jelliffe, R. W., Buell, J. and Kalaba, R.: Reduction of Digitalis Toxicity by Computer-Assisted Glycoside Dosage Regimens, *Ann. Internal Med. 77*:891-907 (Dec.) 1972.

11. Koch-Weser, J. and Klein, S. W.: Procainamide Dosage Schedules, Plasma Concentrations, and Clinical Effects, *JAMA 215*:1454, 1971.

# 55 Cost/Impact Analysis of Selected Clinical Pharmacy Functions in Three Hospitals

Paul J. Munzenberger, Larry N. Swanson, Robert E. Smith, Frances H. Zalewski, Jules I. Schwartz, and Len A. Billingsley

A preliminary study was conducted at three hospitals—two private hospitals and one public teaching institution—to collect data on the time and cost involved with the provision of inpatient clinical pharmacy services.

Pharmacists were assigned to medical units within each hospital, representing a total of 116 beds. The pharmacist participated on each assigned medical unit seven days a week at varying times during the day. The data were collected during 62-, 40-, and 44-day study periods at the three hospitals.

Results revealed that a patient could receive all four clinical pharmacy services—admission drug history, monitoring patient drug therapy, drug information, and discharge consultation—for $5.50, $9.10 and $5.54 at the three hospitals respectively. The results were based on an average hospital stay of ten days.

In September 1971, the *Journal of the American Pharmaceutical Association* published the Report of Task Force on the Pharmacist's Clinical Role.[1] Included in this report as areas for clinical involvement by the pharmacist were the following: (1) admission drug histories, (2) discharge drug consultations, (3) drug therapy monitoring and (4) drug information. Prior to and following this report, a number of studies have appeared in the literature investigating these roles. For example, Wilson and Kabat[2] and others[3,4] have discussed the positive effects of pharmacist initiated drug histories. Cooper has reported on the techniques for selection and monitoring of patients[5] while Cole and Sister Emmanuel,[6] Liberman,[7] Greiner[8] and Grissinger et al.[9] have considered the pharmacist's role in discharge drug consultations. While these articles have been concerned primarily with the effectiveness of pharmacists in these activities and the procedures for their implementation, we are aware of only two publications that attempt to attach a cost to clinical pharmacy services.[10,11] The purpose of this study was to collect time and cost data for the provision of the above inpatient clinical pharmacy services in a variety of hospital settings.

## Methodology

The study was conducted in three separate general medical and surgical hospitals within the city of Detroit.

Hospital A is a private institution with a bed capacity of 504 and is located in the northeast section of the city in a middle class neighborhood. Hospital B is the city-funded general hospital for Detroit and is located in the inner city area. It has a bed capacity of approximately 500 and its facilities are utilized by Wayne State University in the education and training of health care professionals. Hospital C is a private hospital with a bed capacity of 120 located in close proximity to hospital B. Prior to the initiation of this study, neither hospital A nor C provided the clinical pharmacy services under investigation, whereas these services have been provided for some time on many of the medical units of hospital B. The pharmacists providing the clinical services and data collection for this study were all Pharm.D. candidates who had completed the didactic and clinical clerkship portions of the doctoral program.

*Method of Data Collection at Hospital A.* The pharmacist assigned to this hospital was stationed on an internal medicine unit consisting of 42 beds for a total of 62 days during the summer of 1973. The pharmacist participated on the unit seven days a week at varying times during the day.

During the study period, the pharmacist attempted an admission drug history on all patients admitted to the unit. Unfortunately, some patients were unconscious or unable to communicate for other reasons and a reliable history was impossible for these patients. The taking of each drug history was timed with a stopwatch. The actual time spent with each patient was recorded as well as the time necessary for preparation and performance of such miscellaneous activities as locating the patient and the chart. The pharmacist-acquired drug history included known allergies and prescription and nonprescription medications taken by the patient prior to admission. At the completion of this study, a comparison was made, in a manner similar to that of Covington and Pfeiffer described elsewhere in this volume,[3] between the drug related information obtained by the pharmacist and that recorded by the physician in his history of the patient.

The pharmacist monitored each patient's chart daily, checking for possible drug interactions and appropriateness of therapy. Considered in this review were the patients' renal and hepatic status and the pharmacology and pharmacokinetics of the drugs involved. Drug related problems detected by the pharmacist were reported to the physician responsible for the care of the patient either verbally or via a written note left on the patient's chart. The pharmacist recorded the time required to monitor each patient's chart and the total time required each day for the monitoring function. The total time included the actual monitoring time and any necessary activity related to monitoring. Data were also tabulated on the number and type of problems detected and the outcome of each consultation.

The pharmacist responded to requests for drug information from the medical and nursing staffs of the assigned unit. Requests were initiated while the pharmacist was on rounds, at other times when she was available on the study unit or as a result of her consultations initiated by chart monitoring. The time required to research and answer these requests was recorded along with the specific request and the pharmacist's response.

The pharmacist attempted to provide a drug consultation to all patients discharged from the study unit. If the patient was discharged to a nursing home or if the pharmacist was not available on the unit at the time of discharge, a consultation was not provided. The instructions given to the patient included the name of the medication, when and how to use the medication, how to store the medication at home, what drugs or foods to avoid while taking the medication, any possible side effects, a review of the patient's condition where appropriate and any additional information required by the patient to assure maximum compliance and effect. In those cases where the patient did not receive any medications at discharge, the pharmacist reviewed the patient's disease state and the drugs and foods which should be avoided.

In cases where the pharmacist thought the patient might have compliance problems (e.g., the patient was given multiple drugs), a written instruction sheet was provided to supplement her oral consultation. With the aid of a stopwatch, each consultation was timed and the data recorded. Only that time actually spent with the patient was recorded.

*Method of Data Collection at Hospital B.* The study pharmacist at this hospital was assigned to two internal medicine units of 16 and 22 beds, respectively (total 38 beds), for a total of 40 days during the summer of 1973. Those clinical pharmacy services provided at hospital A were also provided at this hospital with only minor differences in methodology. Admission drug histories were timed with the exclusion of any preparation time. In addition, at patient discharge, the pharmacist did not provide written instruction sheets and only those patients discharged with medications received a consultation.

*Method of Data Collection at Hospital · C.* The pharmacist assigned to this hospital was stationed on a 36-bed internal medicine unit for a total of 44 days during the fall of 1973. The method of data collection at this hospital was identical to that of hospital B, with the exception that no pharmacist-acquired vs. physician-acquired drug history comparison was made.

**Results**

*Admission Drug Histories.* During the 62-day study period at hospital A, 28 admission drug histories were completed and 27 of these histories were timed. The average time required per history was 17 minutes. This figure represents the total time required for each history including any preparation or follow-up. If only the actual time spent with patients is considered, each history required an average of 13 minutes with a range of 5–22 minutes. The average number of histories completed per day was 0.45 and the average time required per day for the completion of admission drug histories by the pharmacist was 5.9 minutes. During the 40-day period a pharmacist was assigned to hospital B, 46 admission drug histories were completed and 37 of these were timed. The average time required per history was 11 minutes with a range of 7–25 minutes. These figures represent only the time actually spent with the patient and do not include any preparation or follow-up. At hospital B, the average number of admission drug histories completed per day was 1.1 while the average time required per day for the provision of this service was 12 minutes. During the 44-day study period at hospital C, 203 admission drug histories were completed and 188 of these were timed. The average time required per history was 5.2 minutes with a range of 1–17 minutes. Preparation and follow-up time were not included in these figures. At hospital C, the average number of admission drug histories completed per day was 4.6, while the average time required per day for the provision of this service was 23.9 minutes. Table 1 compares the admission drug history data collected at hospitals A, B and C.

Table 2 compares the pharmacist-acquired drug history at hospitals A and B with that portion of the physician's history concerned with drugs and allergies. No comparison was attempted at hospital C.

Analysis of the data presented in Table 2 reveals that:

## Table 1. Admission Drug Histories

| TYPE OF DATA | HOS-PITAL A | HOS-PITAL B | HOS-PITAL C |
|---|---|---|---|
| Total no. of histories completed | 28 | 46 | 203 |
| Total no. of histories timed | 27 | 37 | 188 |
| Average time required per history | 13 min. | 11 min. | 5.2 min. |
| Range of time required per history | 5–22 min. | 7–25 min. | 1–17 min. |
| Average no. of histories completed per day | 0.45 | 1.1 | 4.6 |
| Average total time required for histories per day | 5.9 min. | 12 min. | 23.9 min. |

(1) the pharmacist at hospital A recorded a higher incidence than the physician for all parameters and (2) the pharmacist at hospital B recorded a higher incidence than the physician for all parameters except the number of patients with allergies or hypersensitivities to foods and miscellaneous allergies or hypersensitivities. It must be noted that the pharmacists participating in this study were aware of the plan for this eventual comparison prior to the start of the study, whereas the physicians had no such knowledge. This prior knowledge may have influenced the intensity of the pharmacist-acquired histories and consequently biased the results.

*Monitoring Patient Drug Therapy.* The pharmacist assigned to hospital A was involved in 2176 chart monitoring events over the 62-day study period. An average of 35 patient charts were monitored per day requiring an average time of 83 minutes daily. The monitoring of each chart required an average of 2.4 minutes with a range of 0.25–3.8 minutes. The average monitoring time per patient chart represents the total time required per day for this clinical pharmacy function divided by the average daily number of charts monitored. During the study period, the pharmacist at hospital A detected 24 drug related problems as a result of this monitoring activity.

The pharmacist assigned to hospital B was involved in 1001 chart monitoring events over the 40-day study period. An average of 34.5 charts were monitored per day requiring an average time of 152 minutes daily. The monitoring of each chart required an average of 4.4 minutes with a range of 2.5–6.5 minutes. The pharmacist at hospital B detected 120 drug related problems as a result of this monitoring activity.

The pharmacist assigned to hospital C was involved in 1064 chart monitoring events over the 44-day study period.

## Table 2. Comparison of Physician-Acquired and Pharmacist-Acquired Drug Histories for Hospitals A and B[a,b]

| TYPE OF DATA | HOSPITAL A | | HOSPITAL B | |
|---|---|---|---|---|
| | PHYSICIAN-ACQUIRED INFORMATION | PHARMACIST-ACQUIRED INFORMATION | PHYSICIAN-ACQUIRED INFORMATION | PHARMACIST-ACQUIRED INFORMATION |
| Number of patients with allergies or hypersensitivities to drugs (includes serums and vaccines) | 9 | 12 | 2 | 5 |
| Number of patients with allergies or hypersensitivities to foods | 1 | 6 | 0 | 0 |
| Miscellaneous allergies or hypersensitivities (ragweed, insect bites, dust, etc.) | 3 | 9 | 1 | 1 |
| Number of legend drugs consumed immediately prior to admission | 44 | 73 | 33 | 88 |
| Number of patients with a history of missing doses at home | 0 | 6 | 0 | 13 |
| Number of patients with a history of consuming someone else's medication | 0 | 2 | 0 | 5 |
| Number of nonprescription medications consumed regularly during past year by patients sampled | 7 | 40 | 3 | 60 |

[a] Data from hospital A represent 28 drug histories while the data from hospital B represent 35 drug histories.

[b] Adapted from Covington and Pfeiffer: The Pharmacist-Acquired Medication History, In *Clinical Pharmacy Sourcebook,* pp. 351-354.

## Table 3. Drug Therapy Monitoring

| TYPE OF DATA | HOSPITAL A | HOSPITAL B | HOSPITAL C |
|---|---|---|---|
| Total no. of days drug therapy monitoring provided | 62 | 29 | 44 |
| Total no. of chart encounters | 2176 | 1001 | 1064 |
| Average no. of charts monitored/day | 35 | 34.5 | 24.2 |
| Average time for chart monitoring/day[a] | 83 min. | 152 min. | 80.8 min. |
| Average monitoring time/ patient chart | 2.4 min. | 4.4 min. | 2.9 min. |
| Range of monitoring time/ patient chart | 0.25–3.8 min. | 2.5–6.5 min. | 0.5–12.5 min. |
| No. of drug related problems detected | 24 | 120 | 51 |

[a] These figures represent the total time required to monitor patient charts/day.

An average of 24.2 charts were monitored per day requiring a total of 80.8 minutes per day. The monitoring of each chart required an average of 2.9 minutes with a range of 0.5–12.5 minutes. The pharmacist at hospital C detected 51 drug related problems. Table 3 compares the monitoring data collected from hospitals A, B and C.

*Drug Information.* A summary of the data collected concerning drug information requests appears in Table 4. As shown in this table, there were 20 drug information consultations at hospital A. The type of personnel requesting drug information from the pharmacist included physician interns (3), physician residents (6), staff physicians (3), nurses (3), and other pharmacists (5). This total of 20 consultations does not include those points of drug information initiated by the pharmacist as a result of chart monitoring. The average number of consultations per day was 0.32 and the average time required per consultation was 8.5 minutes. The average time required per day for drug information consultations was 2.7 minutes.

At hospital B, the pharmacist provided 143 drug information consultations. Unlike hospital A, this total includes those consultations initiated by the pharmacist as a result of drug therapy monitoring. The average number of consultations completed per day was 3.6. The average time required per consultation was 9.1 minutes and the average time required per day for this clinical pharmacy function was 32.7 minutes.

At hospital C, the pharmacist provided 51 drug information consultations. This total also included those consultations initiated by the pharmacist as a result of drug

therapy monitoring. The average number of consultations completed per day was 1.2. The average time required per consultation was 3.0 minutes and the average time required per day for this activity was 4.6 minutes.

Table 5 represents a summary of the total number of drug related suggestions made by the pharmacists at hospitals A and B. The data from hospital C were not collected in this form and are therefore excluded from this tabulation. A tabulation was made of the number of times a suggestion by the pharmacist to the physician yielded a change in drug therapy. For the purpose of analysis, suggestions were divided into three groups: (1) "continuity of therapy" included the improper duration of a medication regimen (too long or too short) or failure to continue chronic medication within the hospital that was prescribed prior to admission; (2) "drug therapy problems" included allergies, specific contraindications, inappropriate doses or dosage schedules, drug interactions, nursing drug problems or possible side effects encountered during the course of monitoring; and (3) "rational drug therapy" included the pharmacist's suggestions for drug changes when the drug of choice was not being used in a specific situation. As shown in Table 5, 40% of the pharmacist's suggestions concerned with continuity of therapy were followed by the physician at hospital A while 53.6% were followed at hospital B. Seventy-five percent of the suggestions concerned with drug therapy problems were followed at hospital A while

## Table 4. Drug Information Consultations

| TYPE OF DATA | HOSPITAL A[a] | HOSPITAL B | HOSPITAL C |
|---|---|---|---|
| Total no. of consultations | 20 | 143 | 51 |
| Average no. of consultations per day | 0.32 | 3.6 | 1.2 |
| Average time required per consultation | 8.5 min. | 9.1 min. | 3.0 min. |
| Average time required per day for consultations | 2.7 min. | 32.7 min. | 4.6 min. |

[a] Does not include drug information consults initiated as a result of drug therapy monitoring.

## Table 5. Pharmacist-Initiated Suggestions for Drug Therapy Change

| TYPE OF SUGGESTION | TOTAL NO. OF SUGGESTIONS | | NO. OF DRUG THERAPY CHANGES | | % OF CHANGE | |
|---|---|---|---|---|---|---|
| | HOSPITAL | | HOSPITAL | | HOSPITAL | |
| | A | B | A | B | A | B |
| Continuity of therapy | 5 | 28 | 2 | 15 | 40 | 53.6 |
| Drug therapy problems | 12 | 85 | 9 | 70 | 75 | 82.4 |
| Rational drug therapy | 5 | 14 | 1 | 9 | 20 | 64.3 |
| Total | 22 | 127 | 12 | 94 | 54.5 | 74 |

82.4% were followed at hospital B. Twenty percent of the suggestions concerned with rational drug therapy were followed at hospital A while 64.3% were followed at hospital B. Overall, 54.5% of the suggestions made by the pharmacist at hospital A resulted in a change in drug therapy while 74% of the suggestions made at hospital B resulted in a change in drug therapy.

*Discharge Consultations.* Thirty-one discharge consultations were completed at hospital A and 19 were timed by the pharmacist assigned to this facility. The average time required per patient consultation was 3.3 minutes with a range of 0.5–12.25 minutes. The average number of consultations completed per day for the 62-day study period was 0.5 while the average time required per day for discharge consultations was 1.7 minutes. At hospital B, during the 40-day study period, 40 discharge consultations were completed; 32 of which were timed. The average time required per patient consultation was 4.4 minutes with a range of 2–12 minutes. The average number of consultations completed per day during the study period was 1.0; therefore, the average time required per day for discharge consultations was also 4.4 minutes. At hospital C, 22 discharge consultations were completed and all were timed. The average time required per consultation was 5.8 minutes with a range of 1.0–15.5 minutes. The average number of consultations completed per day was 0.5 and the average time required per day for discharge consultations was 2.6 minutes. Table 6 compares the discharge consultation data obtained from hospitals A, B and C.

**Time and Cost Analysis**

*Hospital A.* As shown in Table 7, the average total time required per day to provide all four clinical pharmacy services was 93.3 minutes. Based on a pharmacist hourly rate of $8.00, the average cost to the hospital per day to provide all four services to the 42-bed unit would be $12.48. Admission drug histories required 6.0% of the total daily time. Again, based on a hourly rate of $8.00, the average cost to the hospital per day to provide this service would be $0.80 and the average cost for each admission drug history would be $1.76. The drug therapy monitoring function required the largest percentage of the total daily time (89.0%). This service would cost $11.06 per day if all patients were monitored and the average cost per patient chart would be $0.32. Drug information services required 3.0% of the total daily time.

The drug information consultation service would cost the hospital $0.36 per day and the average cost for each consultation would be $1.14. Discharge consultations required 2.0% of the pharmacist's total daily time. The average daily cost to the hospital for this service would be $0.22 and each consultation would cost $0.44. Based on a hospital stay of ten days, a patient could receive all four clinical pharmacy services during his hospitalization at a cost of $5.50.

*Hospital B.* As shown in Table 7, the average total time required per day to provide all four services was 201.1 minutes. Again based on a pharmacist hourly rate of $8.00, the average cost to the hospital per day to provide all four services to the 38 beds would be $26.82. Admission drug histories required 6.0% of the total daily time and this translated to an average daily cost to the hospital of $1.60. The average cost for each admission drug history would be $1.46. Drug therapy monitoring of patient charts required 75.6% of the total daily time. This service would cost $20.26 per day if all patients were monitored and the average cost per patient chart would be $0.58. Drug information services required 16.3% of the total daily time. This service would cost $4.36 per day and the average cost for each consultation would be $1.22. Discharge consultations required 2.1% of the total daily time and would cost the hospital $0.58, as would each consultation. Based on a hospital stay of ten days, a patient could receive all four pharmacy services during his hospitalization at a cost of $9.10.

*Hospital C.* Table 7 shows that the average total time required per day to provide all four services was 111.9 minutes. Again, based on a pharmacist hourly rate of $8.00, the average cost to the hospital per day to provide all four services would be $14.92. Admission drug histories required 21.4% of the total daily time and would thus cost the hospital an average of $3.18 per day. The average individual cost for each admission drug history would be $0.70. Drug therapy monitoring of patient charts required 72.2% of the pharmacist's total daily time, and this would translate to a cost of $10.78 per day

## Table 6. Discharge Consultations

| TYPE OF DATA | HOSPITAL A | HOSPITAL B | HOSPITAL C |
|---|---|---|---|
| Total no. of consultations completed | 31 | 40 | 22 |
| No. of consultations timed | 19 | 32 | 22 |
| No. of consultations completed/day | 0.5 | 1 | 0.5 |
| Average time required/ patient consultation[a] | 3.3 min. | 4.4 min. | 5.8 min. |
| Range of time for each consultation | 0.5–12.25 min. | 2–12 min. | 1.0–15.5 min. |
| Average time required/ day for discharge consultations | 1.7 min. | 4.4 min. | 2.6 min. |

[a] These figures represent only the time required for the actual consultation.

## Table 7. Time and Cost Analysis for Hospitals A, B and C[a]

| TYPE OF DATA | HOSPITAL A | HOSPITAL B | HOSPITAL C |
|---|---|---|---|
| Average total time/day for all four services | 93.3 min. | 201.1 min. | 111.9 min. |
| Average cost to hospital/day to provide all four services | $12.48 | $26.82 | $14.92 |
| Percent of total daily time required for admission drug histories | 6.0 | 6.0 | 21.4 |
| Average cost to hospital for each admission drug history | $1.76 | $1.46 | $0.70 |
| Average cost to hospital/day for admission drug histories | $0.80 | $1.60 | $3.18 |
| Percent of total daily time required for monitoring | 89.0 | 75.6 | 72.2 |
| Average cost to hospital for monitoring each patient chart | $0.32 | $0.58 | $0.38 |
| Average cost to hospital/day for monitoring patient charts | $11.06 | $20.26 | $10.78 |
| Percent of total daily time required for drug information | 3.0 | 16.3 | 4.1 |
| Average cost to hospital for each drug information consultation | $1.14 | $1.22 | $0.40 |
| Average cost to hospital/day for drug information consultations | $0.36 | $4.36 | $0.62 |
| Percent of total daily time required for discharge consultations | 2.0 | 2.1 | 2.3 |
| Average cost to hospital for each discharge consultation | $0.44 | $0.58 | $0.78 |
| Average cost to hospital/day for discharge consultations | $0.22 | $0.58 | $0.34 |
| Cost to hospital per average patient stay | $5.50 | $9.10 | $5.54 |

[a] Cost data are based on $8.00/hour pharmacist salary which does not include fringe benefits.

if all patients were monitored. The average cost per patient chart would be $0.38. Drug information services required 4.1% of the total time at a cost of $0.62 per day with an average cost for each consultation of $0.40. Discharge consultations required 2.3% of the total daily time; a daily cost of $0.34 and $0.78 for each consultation. Again, based on a hospital stay of ten days, a patient could receive all four services during his hospitalization at a cost of $5.54.

### Discussion and Conclusions

It seems apparent that the present scope of inpatient clinical pharmacy services has been reasonably well defined. Our primary objective was to attach some time and cost data to the provision of these services in at least three distinct types of hospital environments. Our ultimate goal was to provide some data which could hopefully be extrapolated to various other institutions interested in the establishment of clinical pharmacy programs.

As is apparent by much of the data, time, and hence cost figures, varied significantly among the three hospitals. These variances can most obviously be attributed to differences in the mode of operation of the individual hospital and the individual pharmacist and to the nature and severity of patient illness. For example, even though internal medicine units were chosen for all three hospitals, the patients at hospital B tended to have more serious illnesses and had a longer duration of hospitalization than those at hospital C. This was reflected in a lower turnover rate for hospital B and thus: fewer drug histories were performed, more time was required for each history and more time was needed to monitor each patient. Because of the teaching environment of hospital B where medical interns and residents play very active roles in patient management, a far greater number of drug information consultations was elicited by the pharmacist at this institution as opposed to either hospital A or C.

One could speculate on many other possibilities for differences in the time required to perform the various clinical services at each hospital. Of far greater importance is the recognition that time requirements differ among institutions and certainly between individual wards or units within the same institution. One must determine how to use the services of the clinical pharmacist in a given situation most efficiently. For example, it might be most beneficial to patient care at hospital C to use the pharmacist to take medication histories in lieu of other services. This type of an approach with appropriate time and cost data might also allow a director of a hospital pharmacy to establish part-time clinical programs when only limited funds are available.

All time and cost data were based on the actual time needed to perform each of the individual functions and did not include lag time between activities. The pharmacist at hospital B, for example, spent an average of 201.1 minutes (or 3.3 hours) per day engaged in the four specified clinical pharmacy services covering an average of 35 patients. However, he spent an average of 275 minutes (or 4.5 hours) per day on the unit. Therefore, approximately one hour and 15 minutes per day was not accountable to the four specified functions. With this data for this specific hospital and a comparable patient population, one might extrapolate that this pharmacist could provide all four clinical pharmacy services to 60–70 patients in an eight-hour day. One could further speculate that if the above variables remained reasonably constant, one would need approximately two pharmacists to provide the outlined clinical services (five days per week—one eight-hour shift/day) to the 118 internal medicine beds at hospital B. Extrapolation to the entire hospital would require time and cost data for the provision of these clinical pharmacy services to patients on other types of units besides internal medicine (e.g., surgical). Projections for hospitals A and C can be made in like manner.

We recognize the need for a large number of similar studies to fully assess the cost of clinical pharmacy services. However, it is hoped that this report will serve to provide some preliminary insight into costs of these newer areas of pharmacy participation.

## References

1. HSRD Briefs: Report of Task Force on the Pharmacist's Clinical Role: 1971, *J. Amer. Pharm. Ass.* NS11:482–485 (Sept.) 1971.

2. Wilson, R. S. and Kabat, H. F.: Pharmacist Initiated Patient Drug Histories, In *Clinical Pharmacy Sourcebook*, pp. 346-350.

3. Covington, T. R. and Pfeiffer, F. G.: The Pharmacist-Acquired Medication History, In *Clinical Pharmacy Sourcebook*, pp. 351-354.

4. Cradock, J. C., Whitfield, G. R., Menzie, J. W. and Fortner, C. L.: Postadmission Drug and Allergy Histories Recorded by a Pharmacist, *Amer. J. Hosp. Pharm.* 29:250-252 (Mar.) 1972.

5. Cooper, C. T.: Techniques for the Selection and Monitoring of Patients by Pharmacists, *Amer. J. Hosp. Pharm.* 29:334-337 (Apr.) 1972.

6. Cole, P. and Sister Emmanuel: Drug Consultation: Its Significance to the Discharged Hospital Patient and Its Relevance as a Role for the Pharmacist, In *Clinical Pharmacy Sourcebook*, pp. 168-176.

7. Liberman, P.: A Guide to Help Patients Keep Track of Their Drugs, *Amer. J. Hosp. Pharm.* 29:507–509 (June) 1972.

8. Greiner, G. E.: The Pharmacist's Role in Patient Discharge Planning, In *Clinical Pharmacy Sourcebook*, pp. 163-167.

9. Grissinger, S. E., Wolfe, L. W. and Cohen, M. R.: A Protocol for Consultation with Discharged Patients about Their Medications, *Hosp. Pharm.* 8:1175–1183 (No. 6) 1973.

10. Smith, W. E.: Clinical Pharmacy Services in a Community Hospital: DHEW Pub. No. HSM 72-3019 (Jan.) 1972.

11. Smith, W. E.: The Economic Feasibility of Clinical Pharmacy in the Hospital Setting, National Technical Information Service, U.S. Department of Commerce; Springfield, Virginia 22151.

# 56 Selection, Training, and Evaluation of Clinical Pharmacists

William A. Miller

Detailed procedures are reviewed for the selection, training, and evaluation of pharmacists involved in providing clinical pharmacy services.

Specific criteria are used in selecting pharmacists, in determining the type of training and staff development program required for the department, and in evaluating the performance of pharmacists for merit salary increases. Criteria are provided for evaluation of the following skills: (1) professional practice skills, (2) communication skills, (3) educational skills, (4) management skills, and (5) personal characteristics. A peer review system for the evaluation of pharmacists is outlined. Training and staff development programs designed to maintain the competence of the pharmacists are reviewed.

Probably the most important determinant of the quality of clinical pharmacy services in hospitals is the individual competence of the pharmacist involved in clinical practice. The standards of practice for hospital pharmacy have changed dramatically over the last 13 years since the American Society of Hospital Pharmacists prepared its Statement on the Abilities Required of Hospital Pharmacists. The skills required for comprehensive hospital pharmacy services are many and no longer can be possessed in total by one or more administrative pharmacists. The educational programs (B.S., M.S., Ph.D. and Pharm.D.) designed for training practitioners for clinical hospital pharmacy are diverse, and pharmacists graduate with varied backgrounds and levels of competence. Specialization in pharmacy practice is now being formally considered by the profession. The term "clinical pharmacy" is viewed by many as a broad or all encompassing term for a group of rapidly developing specialities in pharmacy practice. Postgraduate professional residency training is rapidly becoming much more prevalent and specialized, analogous to postgraduate medical training. Expertise is now being sought in highly specialized areas of pharmaceutical practice, education and institutional pharmacy administration. More students are now obtaining residency training and electing to pursue positions of clinical practice versus hospital pharmacy administration. Rosinski[1] has stated that the profession must (1) define the standards which practicing pharmacists should satisfy, (2) develop and make available to all practicing pharmacists a national examination embodying the standard, (3) develop continuing education courses that embody subject matter content related to the formulated standards and (4) establish a

mechanism through which continuing education programs can be accredited. These four steps must be carefully applied to clinical hospital pharmacy if a more uniform standard of practice is to be obtained. Specialization in hospital pharmacy must be defined. Postgraduate residency training must be better defined. Hopefully in the future students will be able to obtain a more uniform educational background with various options for professional practice. Then competence will be more easily determinable. Hospital pharmacy departments cannot wait for these changes to occur but must push ahead to provide clinical services as an integral component of hospital pharmacy service. Since the key determinant to the quality of clinical pharmacy services provided in hospitals is the individual competence of the pharmacist, a considerable amount of time must be devoted by hospital pharmacy directors to the selection, training and evaluation of pharmacists involved in providing clinical services. This chapter will present some practical procedures that directors of hospital pharmacy departments may modify and use in selecting, training and evaluating pharmacists providing clinical services.

## Professional Staffing Patterns

The current professional staff of the Department of Pharmacy, The Ohio State University Hospitals consists of 42 pharmacists, 12 residents, and 7 interns. Of these 42 pharmacists, 25 function primarily as clinical pharmacists on various medical and surgical units. The present annual turnover rate for pharmacists is 19%.

Each clinical pharmacist is assigned to a team of three

pharmacists and ten technicians. One of the three pharmacists is designated as a pharmacist coordinator and in this capacity is responsible for all direct patient care services provided for 90–150 inpatients. Each clinical pharmacist is rotated back to centralized areas of the department (i.e., intravenous admixtures, unit dose or ambulatory care dispensing) for approximately two months per year. This rotation is designed to keep the pharmacist abreast of centralized pharmacy services since clinical services are dependent upon them. This has also allowed minimum dichotomy to occur between pharmacists working in various areas of the department.

## Recruitment of Pharmacists

A number of methods are used to recruit pharmacists for clinical positions. These include:

1. Local recruitment of graduating pharmacy students from Ohio colleges of pharmacy
2. Promotion of pharmacy interns to staff pharmacist positions
3. Use of the American Society of Hospital Pharmacists Personnel Placement Service
4. Follow-up on individual letters of inquiry about clinical positions
5. Personal contacts with clinical faculty at other colleges training pharmacists for clinical practice.

## Selection of Pharmacists Involved in Providing Clinical Services

Pharmacists are selected based upon their ability to perform according to the job description for pharmacists (Appendix A). Skills required of clinical pharmacists have been categorized into five major groups: (1) professional practice skills, (2) communication skills, (3) educational skills, (4) management skills and (5) personal characteristics. For each of these skill categories specific criteria have been developed to further expand upon the job description responsibilities.

*Interview Procedure.* Each pharmacist applicant visits the department for a personal interview up to one and one-half days. Sometimes the applicant is interviewed twice; initially, to see if both parties are interested in intensively pursuing the possibility of employment of the individual, and secondly, to more formally interview the individual. The interview procedure includes the following:

1. Review of the completed application form and other biographical information (e.g., transcripts, letters of recommendation)
2. Personal interview with administrative members of the department
3. Personal interview with clinical practitioner members of the department
4. Tour of the department
5. Assignment of the applicant to one of the clinical practitioners working to allow direct observation of activities
6. Disease and drug screening examination
7. Clinical pharmacy conference presentation.

Throughout the interview an attempt is made to evaluate the applicant's abilities to perform in the five major skill categories.

*Pharmacist Entry Salary Levels.* Pharmacists enter the department at different salary levels based upon their educational background, experience and expected level of contribution to patient care. Three entrance levels have been designated and the following information is presented as a summary of the criteria that are used in establishing an appropriate entrance level for a clinical pharmacist.

*Entrance Level I*

1. Education
   a. Internship.
   b. Registered pharmacist.
   c. Bachelor of Science in pharmacy.
   d. Generally these individuals will have to self-educate themselves in areas of drug knowledge, communication skills, supervisory skills and educational skills that they have not had as a part of their formalized curriculum.
   e. Pharmacists entering at Level I will most often be rated on the Pharmacist Evaluation Form (Appendix B) at level (1–2) or (3–4) because they will lack education, experience and training in many of these areas.
   f. These individuals will generally score below average on the Department of Pharmacy "Disease and Drug Knowledge Screening Examination" given to pharmacist applicants.
2. Experience.
   These individuals will generally have had *minimal* experience in functioning as a pharmacist and will not be able to readily adapt to our positions without several months of on-the-job training and experience.
3. Level of Contribution.
   The level of contribution for these individuals will increase as they learn through experience more drug knowledge, how to supervise pharmacy technicians and coordinate their service responsibilities.

*Entrance Level II*

1. Education.
   a. Internship completed.
   b. Registered pharmacist.
   c. Bachelor of Science in pharmacy with considerable job experience or a Master of Science or Doctor of Pharmacy degree.
   d. These individuals will most often be rated on the Pharmacist Evaluation Form at level (3–4) or (5–6) because of their experience or additional educational training.
   e. Those individuals with a Master of Science or Doctor of Pharmacy degree will generally have had the following courses (or equivalents):
   —Clinical pharmacology
   —Biopharmaceutics
   —Pharmacokinetics
   —Statistics and experimental design
   —Scientific writing
   —Radiopharmaceuticals
   —Clinical pharmacy clerkship
   —Hospital pharmacy administration
   —Personnel management
   —Electronic data processing
   These are courses which the average Bachelor of Science student does not obtain in his curriculum.

f. These individuals will generally score above average on the Department of Pharmacy "Disease and Drug Knowledge Screening Examination" given to pharmacist applicants.

2. Experience.

These individuals will have more experience as a pharmacy practitioner than individuals entering at Level I. These individuals will have a greater drug knowledge and will initially be more effective communicators and supervisors. Little on-the-job experience and training will be required.

3. Level of Contribution.

These individuals should be able to effectively perform many of the functions listed on the Pharmacist Evaluation Form immediately. They should be able to help less knowledgeable pharmacists to understand drug therapy and to effectively communicate and supervise.

*Entrance Level III*

1. Education.
   a. Internship completed.
   b. Registered pharmacist.
   c. Master of Science in pharmacy or Doctor of Pharmacy degree.
   d. Residency in hospital or clinical pharmacy.
   e. Pharmacists entering at this level will most often be rated on the Pharmacist Evaluation Form at level (5–6) or (7) because of their educational background and residency experience.
   f. Additional course work as listed in 1-e under Entrance Level II.
   g. These individuals will generally score considerably above average on the Department of Pharmacy "Disease and Drug Knowledge Screening Examination."

2. Experience.

These individuals will have benefited from a hospital or clinical residency program designed to train them in various areas of clinical hospital pharmacy practice.

3. Level of Contribution.

These individuals should be able to provide leadership within the department in improving and developing pharmacy services. They should be able to contribute at a level much higher than pharmacists entering at Level I and II.

*Assessment of Professional Practice Skills.* The specific criteria developed to define the professional practice abilities of the pharmacist are shown in Appendix B, part A.

*(1) Previous Educational Background and Experience.* If the pharmacist has had previous clinical experience and qualifies at Entrance Level II or III, this can be assessed easily by asking him to describe the scope and depth of his practice. Often when a pharmacist states that he has had clinical experience, he means experience with intravenous admixtures, unit dose and floor liaison activities. Although these are essential activities they do not constitute indepth clinical experience.

*(2) Clinical Pharmacy Conferences.* Applicants applying for Entrance Level II or III may be asked to make a presentation to the staff to demonstrate their expertise and competence in an area of drug therapeutics. The question of the depth of knowledge that a pharmacist has in a given area of therapeutics is easily assessed through the presentation and the ensuing discussion. Every effort is made by the staff not to humiliate or embarrass the applicant by asking him questions that he is obviously not prepared to answer.

*(3) Disease and Drug Knowledge Screening Examination.* Each applicant is asked to take a disease and drug knowledge screening examination. The results of this examination are used to detect the applicant's current scope and depth of knowledge about important disease and drug therapy principles and concepts. This has allowed us to place less emphasis on how the individual has become competent (i.e., whether the individual has a B.S., M.S., Ph.D. or Pharm.D. degree or whether he has gained his knowledge through self-education and practice). The examination also helps the applicant understand what is expected in terms of disease and drug content knowledge.

The applicant is required to take the following sections of the examination which are considered basic to all areas of clinical practice:

1. General pathology
2. Major disease concepts and diagnosis
3. Drug interactions
4. Biopharmaceutics and pharmacokinetics
5. Adverse drug reactions.

In addition the applicant selects one of the following specialized areas of drug therapeutics with which he feels most familiar:

1. Infectious disease drug therapy
2. Cardiovascular disease drug therapy
3. Renal disease drug therapy
4. Hematological disease drug therapy
5. Neoplastic disease drug therapy
6. Gastrointestinal disease drug therapy
7. Respiratory disease drug therapy
8. Psychiatric disease drug therapy
9. Neurological disease drug therapy
10. Endocrine disease drug therapy
11. Dermatological disease drug therapy.

The results of this portion of the examination are used to evaluate the applicant's depth of knowledge in specific therapeutic areas. The examination is primarily multiple choice and is based upon material presented in the clinical teaching program for undergraduate and graduate pharmacy students (see Appendix C).

*(4) Peer Review.* Applicants are asked to accompany a clinical pharmacist for a two- to four-hour time interval. During this time the applicant has the opportunity to view first hand the functions of the pharmacist. An effort is made by the staff to realistically portray the pharmacist's activities so that applicants do not accept positions under false pretenses. During this time the pharmacist has an opportunity to find out more about the applicant's clinical experience through questions or comments which the applicant may make while reviewing patients or providing specific clinical services.

In the future, more specific techniques will be developed to perform a peer analysis of applicants and more emphasis will be placed on this interview method for pharmacists entering at Level II or III.

*Assessment of Communication Skills.* The specific criteria developed to define the communication skills needed by the pharmacist are shown in Appendix B, part B. Communication skills are assessed throughout the interview process by everyone participating. Attention is paid to whether the applicant is able to express himself and demonstrate confidence in his abilities. Formal oral communication skills are assessed during the applicant's presentation at the clinical pharmacy conference. No specific methods are used to assess written communication skills other than reviewing the letters sent to the department by the applicant.

*Assessment of Supervisory Skills.* The specific criteria developed to define the supervisory skills needed by the pharmacist are shown in Appendix B, part C. These skills are assessed by reviewing the applicant's previous supervisory and administrative training and experience. Since technicians participate in many important pharmacy functions such as intravenous admixture compounding, unit dose dispensing and drug administration, it is important that they be closely supervised in order to assure drug use control. The pharmacist must be able to delegate technical functions to technicians without losing control of these functions. By delegating technical functions the pharmacist is able to spend more time performing functions requiring professional judgment.

*Assessment of Educational Skills.* The specific criteria developed to define the educational skills needed by the pharmacist are shown in Appendix B, part D. Since the department of pharmacy is in a university hospital, one of our basic objectives is teaching. Approximately 40% of the pharmacists in the department have joint academic and service appointments in the college of pharmacy and the hospitals. In addition to our formalized teaching programs, the department conducts its own training program for technicians and provides inservice education to nurses and physicians. The applicant's educational skills are assessed by reviewing his previous teaching experience and interest. During the applicant's presentation of a clinical pharmacy conference, teaching skills are noted by determining how well the subject matter is presented.

*Assessment of Employee Characteristics.* The specific criteria developed to define the general employee characteristics of pharmacist applicants are shown in Appendix B, part E. These characteristics are very important in the overall analysis of whether a pharmacist is desirable for employment in the department. There is no place for mediocrity at the professional level in the department. Every pharmacist must be motivated toward the achievement of a high level of professional practice and esteem.

## Evaluation of Pharmacists Involved in Providing Clinical Pharmacy Services

Pharmacists are evaluated for professional performance on an annual basis. The results of the evaluation are used in recommending annual merit increases. The evaluation consists of the following procedure:

1. Each pharmacist self-evaluates himself with an evaluation form (Appendix B).
2. A group evaluates each pharmacist with the same evaluation form. This group is composed of peer pharmacists as well as members of the administrative staff.
3. The associate director of the department then reviews the evaluation results with the pharmacist.
4. The evaluation is used in order to make merit salary adjustments for the next fiscal year.

The evaluation form consists merely of a composite of the specific criteria that have been previously listed for the five basic skill areas. The pharmacist and his evaluators are asked to rate the pharmacist according to the scale described on the evaluation form.

After these evaluations are complete, the information is summarized and transferred onto a personnel department form (Figure 1). Each of the skill areas are weighted differently depending upon their overall importance in the performance of the pharmacist's job. Professional practice skills are considered the most important and are thus weighted more heavily (i.e., 35%).

Once the evaluation is complete, all of the specific comments are reviewed with the pharmacist involved. During this session, the associate director gives the pharmacist honest feedback on his performance to date. This feedback includes discussion of the pharmacist's special talents and his weaknesses. At the end of this conference, the pharmacist identifies some personal pro-

*Figure 1. The personnel department form used in the evaluation of pharmacists*

Form # 8806
(441517)

**THE OHIO STATE UNIVERSITY HOSPITALS**
**DEPARTMENT OF PERSONNEL**
**MERIT INCREASE PROGRAM**

GROUP 2

Name________ Title________ Cost Center________

☐ Present Rate Exceeds Maximum ☐ Present Rate Within 5% of Maximum

Needs Improvement — Meets Expectations — Exceeds Expectations — Superior

1 2 3 4 5 6 7

1. Professional Knowledge (Recommended Weight 25) Weight Used____ Score
Evaluator Comments:

2. Communications Skills (Recommended Weight 20) Weight Used____ Score
Evaluator Comments:

3. Management Skills (Recommended Weight 20) Weight Used____ Score
Evaluator Comments:

4. Educational Skills (Recommended Weight 20) Weight Used____ Score
Evaluator Comments:

5. Employee Characteristics (Recommended Weight 15) Weight Used____ Score
Evaluator Comments:

OVERALL EVALUATION— Use Whole Numbers Only Score
Evaluator Comments:

Employee Comments:

Increase: ____ % ____ Hour

New Hourly Rate: ____

Employee Date

Evaluator Date

Administrator Department Head Date

Questions regarding the Merit Increase Program should be refered to the Wage and Salary Administration Office 2-0854

fessional goals for the next year. This helps the pharmacist to constructively improve his performance.

*Peer Evaluation.* A considerable amount of emphasis is placed in the evaluation on the opinion of the pharmacist's peers. Peer evaluation consists of both objective and subjective statements of the pharmacist's skills in the five basic areas. More objective peer evaluation will be achievable in the future after more objective criteria are developed to measure the pharmacist's ability to perform in each of these skill areas. A pharmacist's work is also reviewed by analyzing the things he does while reviewing patient profiles, rounding with physicians, monitoring drug therapy for specific types of patients (e.g., congestive heart failure, hypertension, infectious, etc.) and counseling patients.

### Training of Pharmacists Involved in Providing Clinical Pharmacy Services

Because pharmacy practice is rapidly changing, there is a need for training and continuing education programs in pharmacy departments to help pharmacists learn new information and maintain their professional competence.

*Pharmacist Orientation and Training.* Pharmacists are oriented initially to the overall philosophy and organization of the pharmacy department. Subsequent to this initial orientation the pharmacist is rotated through all of the central service areas of the department which support the clinical pharmacist. This includes the following approximate orientation schedule:

1. Unit dose dispensing—two weeks
2. Intravenous admixture service—ten days
3. Ambulatory care dispensing—two days
4. Drug information center—two days
5. Clinical orientation—two weeks
6. Dodd Hall, Upham Hall and Means Hall pharmacy services—two days
7. Drug administration training—one week.

In addition, the pharmacist is trained to initiate cardiopulmonary resuscitation and to assist during emergencies. After the central orientation, the pharmacist is trained by other clinical pharmacists to provide specific clinical services.

*Disease and Drug Knowledge Training.* Based upon the results of the disease and drug knowledge screening examination, pharmacists may be encouraged to take an audio-tutorial basic pathology course to review or improve their disease knowledge. This pathology course, entitled "Modular Concepts in Human Disease," consists of 135 30-minute tapes with accompanying instructional books and is available from Harmon C. Bickley, Ph.D., Department of Pathology, College of Medicine, University of Iowa.

Drug knowledge is reviewed and updated through teaching conferences designed to review basic principles and concepts in the use of drugs. Teaching conferences are presented throughout the year for new pharmacists

and as review sessions for pharmacists already on the staff. A list of past clinical pharmacist teaching conferences is in Appendix D.

*Continuing Professional Competence of the Pharmacist.* A tremendous emphasis is placed throughout the department on the maintenance of professional competence. Departments of pharmacy must expect their professional staff to maintain competence through continuing education. The department supports the travel of pharmacists to various professional meetings for this purpose. Beyond this, the department expects each pharmacist to actively read the hospital and medical literature in order to keep abreast of new information. The pharmacists in the department have a conference each day from 3:00 p.m. to 4:00 p.m. This time was selected because the maximum number of pharmacists are available due to a one-hour overlap between day and evening shifts. Appendix E illustrates a typical weekly conference schedule.

The pharmacists all have areas of drug expertise for which they are personally responsible. Pharmacists are expected to:

1. Review current literature in their drug therapy areas and report significant findings at journal club.
2. Serve as drug consultants to other pharmacists less knowledgeable about a given drug therapy area.
3. Maintain a reference file of the best articles published in the area of therapeutics through use of the Med Line and Mechanized Information Center Services as well as our drug information center and university library facilities.

At the end of each conference, time is devoted to the exchange of information between pharmacists. Interesting drug therapy cases are reviewed at this time. Service and drug information questions are asked and are either resolved or referred by the use of a "Drug Therapy and Operational Problem Note" to an appropriate person (Figure 2). Members of the drug information and administrative staff are present at each conference to give immediate feedback to the pharmacists concerning any topic.

*Figure 2. The drug therapy and operational problem note*

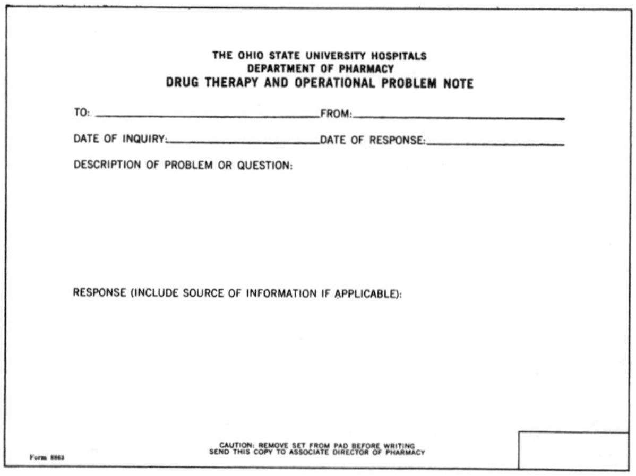

THE OHIO STATE UNIVERSITY HOSPITALS
DEPARTMENT OF PHARMACY
DRUG THERAPY AND OPERATIONAL PROBLEM NOTE

TO: _____ FROM: _____

DATE OF INQUIRY:_____ DATE OF RESPONSE:_____

DESCRIPTION OF PROBLEM OR QUESTION:

RESPONSE (INCLUDE SOURCE OF INFORMATION IF APPLICABLE):

CAUTION: REMOVE SET FROM PAD BEFORE WRITING
SEND THIS COPY TO ASSOCIATE DIRECTOR OF PHARMACY

Form 8663

## Conclusion

Directors of pharmacy departments must devote a substantial amount of their effort to the selection, evaluation and training of pharmacists involved in providing clinical pharmacy services. If these programs are successful the result will be competent clinical pharmacists providing quality clinical pharmacy services.

## Reference

1. Rosinski, G. F.: Strengthening Professional Competence, *J. Amer. Pharm. Ass. NS13*:403 (Aug.) 1973.

## Appendix A

### Clinical Pharmacists' Responsibilities

I. Clinical Services
   A. Obtains patient drug histories and communicates all pertinent information to the physician
   B. Identifies drugs brought into the hospital by patients
   C. Provides drug information
   D. Assists in drug product selection
   E. Monitors the patient's total drug therapy for:
      1. Effectiveness/ineffectiveness
      2. Side effects
      3. Adverse drug reactions
      4. Toxicities
      5. Drug interactions
      6. Incompatabilities (therapeutic, chemical, laboratory)
   F. Counsels patients on:
      1. Medications to be self-administered in the hospital
      2. Discharge medications
   G. Communicates with:
      1. Physicians on patient care rounds to provide drug information concerning therapeutics
      2. Nurses concerning medication problems or questions
   H. Participates actively in cardiopulmonary emergencies by:
      1. Procurement and preparation of needed drugs
      2. Charting all medications given
      3. Performing cardiopulmonary resusitation, if necessary
   I. Provides inservice education to:
      1. Pharmacists, pharmacy interns, residents and students
      2. Nurses and nursing students
      3. Physicians and medical students
II. Coordination and Supervision of Drug Administration Activities on Patient Care Units
   A. Reviews and interprets all medication orders
   B. Verifies the technicians work for accuracy and completeness by:
      1. Checking all medication orders and procedures necessary to add, delete, or change an order in the unit dose system
      2. Checking all record keeping functions
   C. Procures drugs from the central pharmacy, as needed
   D. Assists in training new pharmacy technicians
   E. Assists the technicians in dealing with new procedures or difficult patients
   F. Acts as a liaison between the technician and nurse, the pharmacy department and the nursing unit, and the pharmacy department and the floor coordination committee.

## Appendix B

### Pharmacist Evaluation Performance Criteria

Each performance criterion should be rated at one of four levels—(7) indicates that the individual has unusual strength or ability in this area. It would not be expected that any individual could be rated in this category on more than a few criteria, (5–6) indicates that the individual exceeds expectations or abilities in this area; (3–4) indicates that the individual performs satisfactorily in this area and it is expected that more criteria would normally be rated here than any other area; (1–2) indicates need for improvement in this area, and it is assumed that everyone would be rated in this category for some criteria. The N.A. designation may be used by the individual being rated to indicate that his assignments did not include responsibilities related to that criterion. The N.A. designation may be used by the rater or the reviewer when he is unable to judge that particular criterion.[a]

A. Professional Practice Skills
   1. Ability to innovate new concepts of clinical practice.
   2. Ability to have professional impact with physicians, nurses and others primarily concerned with patient care.
   3. Depth and breadth of practical technical and academic knowledge for being an effective clinical pharmacist.
   4. Growth and authority in specific assigned clinical areas.
   5. Skills in perceptive observation of the patient's response to drug therapy.
   6. Skills in making professional judgment based on scientific clinical knowledge and the unique characteristics of the individual patient situation.
   7. Skills in the performance of technical pharmaceutical functions (motor skills).
   8. Effectiveness in extemporaneously answering drug information requests.
   9. Effectiveness in utilizing the drug information center for answering drug information requests.
   10. Ability to obtain a useful, concise medication history.
   11. Effectiveness in discharge medication counseling.
   12. Effectiveness in self-medication counseling.
   13. Ability to perform outpatient medication counseling.
   14. Effectiveness in monitoring drug therapy for:
      a. Effectiveness/ineffectiveness.
      b. Drug interactions.
      c. Adverse drug reactions, side effects or allergic responses.
   15. Ability to influence the prescribing patterns of physicians (appropriate drug selection).
B. Communication Skills
   1. Effective communication and ability to establish rapport with nurses.
   2. Effective communication and ability to establish rapport with physicians.
   3. Effective communication and ability to establish rapport with patients.
      a. Compassioniate concern for the patient.
      b. Ability to communicate with relatives.
   4. Effectiveness in communications with pharmacy technicians.
      a. Technical aspects of the unit dose drug administration program.
      b. Individual patient's progress and response to drug therapy.
      c. Drug therapy plans for patients.
   5. Effective communications and liaison with other professional staff (dietary, social service, etc.).
   6. Ability to influence patterns of patients' care through effective, diplomatic communication and established rapport with staff (does this person turn off people with his approach?).
   7. Exhibits skill in using effective written communications.
C. Management Skills
   1. Ability to organize, operate and supervise the logistical aspects of his service responsibilities.
   2. Ability to effectively supervise and control technicians in assigned areas (achieve cooperation, motivate individual performance, reinforce responsibilities of technicians and prevent unauthorized expansion of these responsibilities).
   3. Effectiveness in coordinating his area of service responsibility with other areas of the department.
   4. Ability to work within an organization or structure according to the expectations of his superiors.
   5. Ability to follow policies and live within regulations. (Does he go against the grain or present objections and recommendations diplomatically?)
   6. Effectiveness in getting people to accomplish his objectives, follow his methods and accept his direction.

---

[a] Only the criteria are presented here; check blanks for the rating levels have been omitted.

7. Ability to apportion effort and time according to predetermined priorities.

8. Ability to adapt to and analyze changing situations and make good judgments and recommendations accordingly.

9. Ability to consistently withstand pressures and tensions inherent in the job without losing effective control; to remain calm and effective in dealing with crisis situations; to assist subordinates in maintaining constructive attitudes under all conditions.

10. He is unusually perceptive of problem areas and initiates direct actions to solve them, or when appropriate, suggests well thought out solutions or approaches to the solution through the proper channels.

11. He requires a minimum of supervision and motivation in assigned responsibilities.

12. Ability to prevent technicians from assuming responsibilities which are clearly pharmacist's responsibilities.

13. Ability to recognize personnel problems and to document them, and to follow through with appropriate disciplinary action.

14. Ability to maximally utilize technicians to perform technicial functions involved in the unit dose drug administration program.

15. Ability to evaluate technician performance and review the evaluation with the technician.

D. Educational Skills

1. Ability to assist instructors in the education and training of under graduate pharmacy students, interns and residents.

2. Ability to assist in instructing student nurses in drug administration procedures.

3. Ability to instruct pharmacy technician trainees.

4. Effectiveness in conducting inservice programs for nurses, physicians or pharmacists.

5. Participation in continuing education programs (seminars, inservice programs).

6. Effectiveness in maintaining his own professional competence.

E. Employee Characteristics

1. Character and life style which reflect favorably upon his position, his employer and his profession.

2. Satisfaction of assistant, associates and director of department with quality, quantity and nature of performance.

3. Ability to reflect a good image of the department.

4. Effectiveness in achieving recognition for the department through individual accomplishments or professional prestige.

5. Quality and quantity of published papers, verbal presentations and other evidence of creativity and scholarship.

6. The degree of respect he accords patients, subordinates, peers and supervisors.

7. Participation in civic, church, and other activities which reflect a balance of interests and activities.

8. The degree of respect that has been accorded to him by patients, subordinates, peers and supervisors.

9. Ability to demonstrate in his work the capacity and desire to broaden his perspectives, increase his own value, widen his horizons and integrate his actions into departmental objectives.

10. Appointments, honors and awards which distinguish the individual in the profession.

11. Participation in professional organizational activities.

12. Demonstrates promptness and has good attendance record.

13. Demonstrates willingness to serve the department beyond normal expectations in time of personnel shortages, vacations, etc.

## Appendix C

### Disease and Drug Knowledge Screening Examination Sample Questions

#### General Pathology

1. All of the following are functions of the humoral immunologic systems EXCEPT:
   a. neutralize virus, toxins and venoms
   b. protect against extracellular pyogenic pathogens
   c. fix and activate complement
   d. responsible for graft rejection
   e. cause lysis of foreign cells

2. Plasma cells are:
   a. thought to be closely related in origin to the basophil
   b. smaller than lymphocytes
   c. detected early in acute inflammation

   d. the primary source of immunoglobulins
   e. phagocytic

3. In the cellular type of immune response:
   a. no humoral antibody can be detected
   b. the reaction results in the "sensitizing" lymphocytes
   c. immunization can occur in a lymph node
   d. antigen is involved .
   e. all of the above

#### Antibiotics

(There may be more than one correct answer for each question)

1. Mrs. Johns is being placed on gentamicin 80 mg every eight hours. What tests would you use to monitor the side effects of this drug?
   a. SGOT, SGPT
   b. BUN
   c. Serum creatinine and/or creatinine clearance
   d. CBC with retics
   e. Hgb/Hct

2. Mr. K is to receive Loridine 1 g q 4 hours around the clock for his infection. This dose:
   a. may cause dizziness and reversible loss of hearing.
   b. is the maximum recommended daily dose.
   c. is probably an overdose since it is higher than the maximum daily recommended dose.
   d. is likely to precipitate transient deafness, eight cranial nerve damage, proteinuria and irreversible kidney damage.
   e. is likely to cause diarrhea if given for any length of time because of its action on the organisms of the gastrointestinal tract.

3. Ampicillin is the most allergenic of the presently available penicillin products. Patients taking ampicillin and one of the drugs listed below exhibit hypersensitivity reactions three to four times more than patients taking ampicillin alone.
   a. Diuril
   b. Benemid
   c. Estrogen
   d. Allopurinol
   e. Phenobarbital

## Appendix D

### Clinical Pharmacist Training Conferences

University, Hospital and Departmental Organization
Goals and Objectives for the Department, Short and Long-Term
Principles of Supervision
Personnel Policies and Procedures
Principles of Communication
Written Communications
Nonverbal Communications
Aseptic Techniques
Unit Dose Packaging
Radiopharmaceutical Component of Clinical Pharmacy Services
Investigational Drugs, Formulary System, Pharmacy and Therapeutics Committee
Drug Information Services
Principles in Drug Literature Evaluation
Emergency Care—Drugs
Emergency Care—Cart and Equipment
The Patient as an Individual
Rational Drug Prescribing
Medication History Determination
Monitoring Drug Therapy Effectiveness
Adverse Drug Reactions
Drug Interactions—Overview
Drug Interactions—Absorption and Distribution
Drug Interactions—Metabolism and Excretion
Thyroid Disorders
Diabetes Mellitus
Antiinfectives
Urinary Tract Infections
Pneumonia
Nosocomial Infections
Sepsis
Myocardial Infarction
Angina Pectoris
Arrhythmias

Congestive Heart Failure
Peripheral Vascular Diseases
Hematology—Introduction
Anemia
Leukemia
Hodgkin's Disease and Lymphomas
Solid Tumors
Hypertension
Acute Renal Failure
Chronic Renal Failure
Peptic Ulcer Disease
Alcoholic Cirrhosis and Hepatic Failure
Inflammatory Bowel Disease
Surgical Management of Gastrointestinal Diseases
Psychiatry
Physical Medicine
Chronic Obstructive Pulmonary Disease
Neurology
Opthalmology

## Appendix E

**Pharmacist Conference Schedule**
**3:00 p.m.–4:00 p.m.**
**Week of November 12–16**

MONDAY     JOURNAL CLUB
Current Literature on BCG Vaccine
New England Journal of Medicine Articles
Immunosuppressive Agents
American Journal of Medicine (October)

TUESDAY     TRAINING CONFERENCE
Rational Drug Prescribing

WEDNESDAY     CLINICAL CONFERENCE
Thyroid Disorders

THURSDAY     TRAINING CONFERENCE
The Patient As An Individual

FRIDAY     CASE PRESENTATION
Ampicillin Rash

# 57 Activity Analysis of Clinical Pharmacists

Thomas S. Thielke

The activity patterns of clinical pharmacists were studied.

Two groups of pharmacists in one hospital were studied: (1) general clinical pharmacists functioning in association with a decentralized unit dose system, and (2) clinical pharmacists who administered medications in addition to the duties performed by the other group. Activities were categorized as technical, consultative, and personal and miscellaneous. Technical activities consumed 44% of the first group's time and only 21% of the second group's time. The first group spent 29% of its time on consultative activities; the second group, 43%.

Over the last few years there have been many articles describing proposed or implemented pharmacy systems and emphasizing the terms "unit dose" and "clinical pharmacy." Most systems described in these papers were either in a trial stage or implemented on a fraction of the total beds with few systems functioning throughout the hospital. The mechanics of these systems have varied as much as the definitions of clinical pharmacy. It was always difficult to relate the description and function of the drug distribution system to the definition and function of the "clinical pharmacist." The goals of each never seemed to be headed in the same direction. In some cases where the pharmacists was directly tied to the distribution function, it was difficult to clearly trace his function through the many flow charts, checks and balances.

What types of activities does a clinical pharmacist perform when working under a unit dose drug distribution system? At University of Wisconsin Hospitals, a study was undertaken to demonstrate how a clinical pharmacist with two to three years of experience in the patient care area provides pharmacy service through consultative, technical and educational activities.

## Background

During the summer of 1965, University of Wisconsin Hospitals experimented with a completely decentralized unit dose drug distribution system for 90 beds. Although problems were encountered in several of the procedures and certain modifications were necessary, it was felt that decentralized pharmacy service was not only feasible but was definitely the procedure of choice for this hospital.

Following the study period, the experimental system was thoroughly reviewed and some major changes were made. As a result, a combined centralized-decentralized unit dose drug distribution system was implemented in July 1966 and expanded throughout the hospital by the spring of 1969. The centralized function includes the packaging and medication preparation functions, and the decentralized function includes the pharmacists' activities in the patient care area. Upon completion of expansion of the unit dose system to the entire hospital (750 beds), the role of the pharmacist in the patient care area was evaluated.

Several organizational and procedural changes resulted from the evaluation. These changes were made in order to streamline and standardize the unit dose drug distribution system. This eventually resulted in increased time spent by the pharmacist in professional and educational activities and a decrease in his technical duties.

In January 1970, the University of Wisconsin unit dose drug distribution system functioned as shown in the flow chart in Figure 1. Emphasis should be placed on the fact that the pharmacist and his profile are the center of activity with the input being the medication order by the physician and the output being the drug administration and charting by nurses who utilize the pharmacist's profile.

*Figure 1. Scheme of operation for the Wisconsin Information Service and Medication Distribution system*

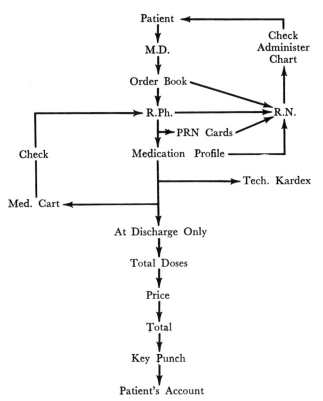

## The Study

Upon standardizing the mechanics of the unit dose system, we turned our efforts to study the activities of the decentralized clinical pharmacists (hereafter referred to as floor pharmacists). The floor pharmacist played a vital role in the unit dose drug distribution system, but we wanted to know what types of duties and functions they perform from 7 AM to 11:30 PM, seven days a week. To determine this, we acquired the services of two senior industrial engineering students who were looking for an independent study to fulfill requirements for graduation. They were aided by the hospital industrial engineer who counseled them throughout the study. Their purpose was to analyze and evaluate the "pharmaceutical function" at University of Wisconsin Hospitals, pharmaceutical function being defined as the activities of the floor pharmacists.

Initially, time was spent with the students in order to give them an insight into activities of the floor pharmacists. A slide presentation was shown and the theoretical activities of the system were discussed in detail. At the same time, procedures for function expansion, system development, information gathering and information reporting were established. Upon developing a list of restraints of the system, an activity sampling study was conducted for the purpose of gathering information and verifying the theoretical activities received from written procedures. From this initial sampling, an expanded list of activities was developed and some were combined to prevent overlap. After finalizing the list of activities, a 44-hour, two-minute interval work sampling study was conducted. This resulted in 1,320 two-minute interval samples which covered all seven days of the week and all the working hours of the day from 7 AM to 11:30 PM. These periods of time were randomly covered and confidence intervals were calculated from work sampling charts.

During the time the study was conducted, a trial system was being carried out on the fourth floor of the hospital which was made up of three nursing units totaling 110 beds. This system differed from the rest of the hospital in that the pharmacist was administering all medications in addition to his other activities. Because of these added duties, a pharmacist working with the trial system was responsible for 30 to 60 beds. This differs from the rest of the hospital where a pharmacist was responsible for approximately 120 beds.

The activities of the fourth floor pharmacists were also studied in order to make a comparison with the general floor pharmacists' activities. The activity list was expanded to include medication administration and certain other relevant activities; 1,050 two-minute samples were taken. The results of the general and fourth floor samplings are presented in Table 1.

## Discussion

The activities were categorized into three general types: technical, consultative, and personal and miscellaneous. The five technical duties represented 43.7% of the general floor pharmacist's time and the five consultative services represented 28.8% of his time. The remaining 27.5% of the time was made up of personal and miscellaneous duties. Therefore, in the spring of 1970, a pharmacist working on the general floors spent a little less than one-half of his time on technical activities. This was probably a result of designing the system around the service function and later expanding the consultative role. It is interesting to note that three general activities (transcribing orders, checking and correcting medication carts, and walking) took about 40% of the pharmacist's time. The floor pharmacist at University Hospitals is forced into these activities because of the lack of any electronic data processing or transportation systems and the physical design of the nursing units. These activities could be significantly reduced by utilizing an on-line EDP system, some type of mechanical transportation system and a more convenient physical plant structure.

Table 1. Percent Time Spent by General Floor Pharmacists and Fourth Floor Pharmacists in Daily Activities

| ACTIVITY | % TIME GENERAL FLOOR PHARMA-CISTS | % TIME FOURTH FLOOR PHARMA-CISTS |
|---|---|---|
| *Technical* | | |
| Transcribing orders | 14.72 | 5.77 |
| Writing out *prn* cards | 3.83 | 1.56 |
| Ordering iv's & calling central unit dose | 4.71 | 1.42 |
| Revising & updating medication profiles | 7.29 | 8.22 |
| Checking & correcting medication carts | 13.17 | 4.20 |
| *Consultative* | | |
| Consulting with medical personnel & attending conferences | 14.08 | 16.59 |
| Consulting with patients | 1.13 | 6.29 |
| Going to control area for supplies or information | 6.94 | 4.89 |
| Checking drug information & self-education | 4.91 | 11.01 |
| Teaching | 2.79 | 4.06 |
| *Personal and Miscellaneous* | | |
| Breaks and personal needs | 7.34 | 13.92 |
| Walking | 13.15 | 7.25 |
| Other | 5.89 | 5.78 |
| *Administering Medications* | | |
| Including taking blood pressure and apical pulse and communicating with patient while administering medication | — | 9.07 |

What happens when the function and staffing patterns of the floor pharmacist are changed? This question is answered by the results of the activity sampling on the fourth floor shown in Table 1.

Again the activities are broken down into technical, consultative, and personal activities with medication administration as a separate category. The technical activities made up 21.2% of the fourth floor pharmacist's time, a substantial reduction from the general floors. Consultative activities made up 42.9% of the pharmacist's time; a substantial increase over the general floors. The personal and miscellaneous category remained about the same (approximately 27%) although the walking time was reduced because the pharmacist was only covering 30 to 60 beds instead of 120.

The most significant reduction in technical activities for the fourth floor pharmacists occurred in the time spent transcribing orders and checking medications carts. This was partially caused by the reduction in the number of beds covered by the pharmacist. However, the time that was saved did not all go into medication administration which accounted for only 9% of the pharmacist's time. The fourth floor pharmacist was spending more time consulting with medical personnel and checking drug information for physicians. The time for teaching patients and other medical personnel

also was increased significantly. Therefore, the reduction in the amount of time spent performing technical activities resulted in an increase in consultative services.

Most of the pharmacists working on the nursing units during the study had been on the staff of University Hospitals during the first two years of implementation of the unit dose drug distribution system. During this time these pharmacists spent about 80-90% of their time performing technical and mechanical functions. These technical functions have been gradually reduced with more professional or consultative services taking their place. At the same time the service function provided by the pharmacy department was maintained and even increased to cover the entire central service area. This was done by redefining the responsibilities and work load of the pharmacy technicians and reorganizing the entire distribution function. This reorganization resulted in a more efficient service.

During this same time period, these floor pharmacists were also gaining valuable patient care experience which never could not be gained by any other form of learning. With the advent of clinical pharmacy education, the pharmacy staff was kept up to date by presenting to them all the information given to the undergraduate and graduate clinical pharmacy students. This was done through summer continuing education programs and inservice education by the medical staff of the hospital.

**Recent Changes**

Recently, changes have been made in the drug distribution system to allow the floor pharmacist to spend more time in consultative services such as patient histories, chart and work rounds, and patient teaching. Some of these changes are:

1. The number of times medication carts are delivered to the floor to be checked by the pharmacist has been reduced.
2. Clinical pharmacy team supervisors who are responsibile for four to nine nursing units have been introduced. The responsibilities of these supervisors include undergraduate student teaching in the patient care area, supervision of all pharmacists, interns, residents, and technicians assigned to their team, and overall responsibility for all central service functions on their nursing units. This structure has added a larger degree of flexibility for the floor pharmacist because the supervisor is available to screen questions, to relieve the floor pharmacist so he may attend conferences or rounds, and to aid the pharmacist in case of emergencies.
3. Medication technicians have been introduced to the floor where the pharmacist administers medications. This technician is supervised by the pharmacist, but performs the actual mechanics of administering medications to the majority of the patients on the fourth floor. This has lessened the amount of time the pharmacist spends on medication administration.

## Conclusion

It is a lot easier to begin with a service-oriented system and then slowly move to the consultative aspects of professional pharmacy practice. It should always be the pharmacist's responsibility to maintain tight control over distribution and administration of drugs in the hospital, and this function should never be sacrificed in order to provide a more rewarding professional atmosphere for a clinical pharmacist. This will satisfy the hospital administrators, service, fiscal and patient care needs, and at the same time, gradually introduce the pharmacist to the clinical aspects of hospital pharmacy practice where he can become an accepted and needed member of the health care team.

# 58 Evaluation of the Pharmacist as a Drug Therapy Advisor on Ward Rounds

J. Heyward Hull, III and Fred M. Eckel

The contribution of a pharmacist serving as a drug information source while actively participating as a member of a medicine team was studied.

The pharmacist attended work rounds for six months and provided drug information upon request. He actively followed the patients, critically reviewed their drug therapy, and offered unsolicited suggestions for changes in their regimen when drug-related problems were suspected.

The pharmacist received 197 drug information questions. Two-thirds of the requests were answered at the time requested. The most common categories of drug information questions were drug use or indications, ingredients or strengths of a drug, dosage, absorption, fate or excretion of a drug, toxicities or side effects of a drug, and equivalents or comparisons of drugs. Two-thirds of the requests were initiated by the physician with primary responsibility for the care of the patient. The pharmacist's ability to answer questions at the time of request increased from 56.7% during the first three months of the study to 69.2% the second three months. The pharmacist offered 68 unsolicited drug therapy suggestions. Over one-third of the suggestions related to observed or potential side effects from drugs. Greater than 50% of the suggestions were related to observed or potential adverse drug reactions. Two-thirds of all suggestions were accepted by the physicians as measured by a written drug order change within 24 hours. The percentage of suggestions accepted by physicians declined as the academic level of physicians increased.

It is concluded that the pharmacist can contribute to direct patient care and physician education through active participation on a medical team.

The potential value of a pharmacist assigned to a medicine team as a drug information source and drug therapy advisor is being discussed frequently by pharmacists. A number of articles either describe the pharmacist's participation in ward rounds or suggest the logic of this involvement.[1-23] However, despite the enthusiasm generated by authors, most of these articles have provided no documentation, or only anecdotal evidence, to support claims of patient care benefit resulting from pharmacist involvement with medicine teams. Only three studies have provided any insight into the nature of the contribution by a pharmacist.[4,24,25] If the pharmacist is to rightfully lay claim to usefulness as the drug expert on a medical team, then the value of this involvement must be documented.

In an attempt to evaluate this role, a study was conducted in the spring of 1971 with the following objectives:

1. To determine to what extent the physician would request drug information from a pharmacist if he were regularly available as a member of medical ward rounds.
2. To determine the nature of the requests, according to categories of information, and to simultaneously determine the pharmacist's ability to answer the requests in the various categories.
3. To determine the relative drug information needs of the various members of the medical team.
4. To determine the effect of having a pharmacist actively monitoring a patient's drug therapy on a medical service by identifying types of pharmacists' suggestions and the willingness of physicians to alter drug therapy on the recommendation of a pharmacist.

The study was conducted at North Carolina Memorial Hospital (NCMH), a university teaching hospital. At NCMH, medical care is handled by physician teams in medicine, surgery, pediatrics, obstetrics and other specialties. The members of a physician team vary with the service. A general medicine team is made up of an attending physician, one junior attending resident, three interns (which may include one acting intern, a fourth-year medical student) and three third-year medical students. There are four medicine teams in the hospital, each of which is responsible for 20 to 30 patients, depending on the census. All members of the medicine house staff rotate through each of these teams. Each team provides care for a broad range of diseases (diabetes, renal disease, congestive heart failure, etc.). Patients with these conditions require the greatest number and widest variety of drugs. It was felt that drug information needs of a medical service would therefore be greater than for those of the other services.

Since the pharmacist planned to participate actively with the medical team on a part-time basis, it was necessary to determine the most useful activities for the pharmacist. Two meetings of the team as a group were considered: morning work rounds and attending (teaching) rounds.

Morning work rounds are conducted primarily for reviewing changes in each patient's status over the past day and to plan the patient's care for the immediate future. Each patient is visited, his diagnostic or treatment program (including drug therapy) is reviewed, and appropriate adjustments are made for the coming day.

Attending rounds are held primarily for teaching purposes. Newly admitted patients are examined by one of the medical students who presents the patient's past and present medical history, chief complaint, diagnosis and care plan to the team. Results of his workup are compared with that of the admitting intern, and discussion regarding the diagnosis follows. Although treatment plans are included in these discussions, primary emphasis is upon diagnosis.

Of these two group meetings, morning work rounds seemed most suitable for the purposes of the study. The strong service orientation results in greater emphasis on the patient's treatment. It was decided that the pharmacist would attend the morning work rounds regularly and would participate in attending rounds if time permitted.

Members of a general medicine team rotate on a monthly basis. It was decided that the pharmacist would remain with the same medicine team throughout the study period to enable him to participate with the greatest possible number of different physicians. Approval for the addition of the pharmacist to the medical team was obtained from the pharmacy and therapeutics committee.

The pharmacist who participated in rounds was enrolled in the second year of a combined Master of Science degree/residency program in hospital pharmacy. He had obtained his Bachelor of Science degree in pharmacy in 1963. For the five years prior to his return to graduate school he had practiced community pharmacy. He did not take any special courses in his graduate program to prepare him for this project.

## Methods

The pharmacist accompanied the team on medical work rounds each morning for 135 days over a period of six months (January 29, 1971 to July 29, 1971). Each session lasted from one to one and one-half hours. In addition, the pharmacist spent two to three hours each day in reviewing the charts of the patients on the service. The service maintained an average of about 20 patients during the study period (ranging from 11 to 33).

Since the pharmacist wanted to be knowledgeable about the patient as well as participate in ward rounds to answer questions, it was necessary to extract a significant amount of information from the chart. The pharmacist recorded pertinent patient information on 3″ by 8″ sheets kept in a looseleaf notebook. The information usually recorded was: patient's name and vital statistics, chief complaint, intern's working diagnosis, drug allergies, and most important, the chronologic record of the patient's hospital drug regimen. In addition, on the back of the sheet was recorded relevant admission laboratory data and progress notes recorded by either the physicians or nurses.

The pharmacist stated his purpose as "following the team to learn more about drug therapy as it relates to the disease condition." In addition he volunteered to "attempt to answer questions that might arise during rounds" and obtained permission to raise questions if he suspected unusual or inappropriate use of drugs. The pharmacist attended rounds five to six days per week. All requests for drug information or suggestions offered to the team were recorded discreetly on a 3″ by 5″ file card kept in the patient notebook and were later transferred to a logbook daily.

Drug information requests were classified using the Piecoro format.[4] By this method, the requests were first classified according to one of three major categories: pharmaceutical, pharmacological or therapeutic. Second, the requests were identified within that major category according to specific type (e.g., if the question was, "What is the mechanism of action of allopurinol?" the request was recorded first as pharmacological, then specifically for mechanism of action). In addition, the type of physician making the request and whether the request could be answered spontaneously were tabulated.

Suggestions were classified in a somewhat different manner, using a technique designed by the investigator. Each suggestion was classified according to the type of drug therapy problem. Each suggestion was also classified according to the recommended change offered as a solution to the problem. Again, the physician to whom the suggestion was offered and whether or not the suggestion was accepted were recorded. Acceptance of a suggestion was considered to be any order changed consistent with the nature of the suggestion. For example, if the physician ordered Cytoxan for a patient and the pharmacist suggested that uric acid levels be monitored, then the suggestion offered would be recorded under "side effects from drug" and under "recommended special patient monitoring." If an order was subsequently written for serum uric acid determinations, the suggestion would be considered as having been accepted.

**Table 1. Classification of Drug Information Requests According to Major Category**

| CATEGORY | NO. REQUESTS | % |
|---|---|---|
| Pharmaceutical | 61 | 31.0 |
| Pharmacological | 81 | 41.1 |
| Therapeutic | 55 | 27.9 |
| TOTAL | 197 | 100.0 |

**Table 2. Percentage of Requests Answered at the Time Requested According to Category**

| CATEGORY | NO. ANSWERED/TOTAL | % |
|---|---|---|
| Pharmaceutical | 43/61 | 70.5 |
| Pharmacological | 46/81 | 56.8 |
| Therapeutic | 36/55 | 65.5 |
| TOTAL | 125/197 | (63.5) |

## Results

While on rounds, the pharmacist communicated with the other members of the team 265 times regarding the drug therapy of patients on the service. Of this total, 197 (74.3%) were questions asked of the pharmacist by the team members (drug information requests), and 68 (25.7%) were unsolicited suggestions offered by the pharmacist to the team regarding suspected drug-related problems uncovered as a result of monitoring therapy. Collectively there were 1.96 physician-pharmacist interactions per ward round, with a range of zero to eleven.

*Drug Information Requests.* A summary of the drug information requests is shown in Table 1. Eighty-one (41.1%) of the 197 total requests were pharmacologic in nature, 61 (31%) were pharmaceutical requests, and 55 (27.9%) were therapeutic requests.

The pharmacist's ability to respond to the request im-

**Table 3. Classification of Drug Information Requests According to Category and Physician Type**

| CATEGORY | PHYSICIAN TYPE[a] | | | | | TOTAL |
|---|---|---|---|---|---|---|
| | A | R | I | AI | MS | |
| **PHARMACEUTICAL** | | | | | | |
| 1. Name of drug | | 1/1 | 1/2 | | | 2/3 |
| 2. Ingredients or strength | | 3/4 | 10/14 | 1/3 | | 14/21 |
| 3. Storage or stability | | | 0/1 | | | 0/1 |
| 4. Physical or chemical properties | | | 2/2 | | | 2/2 |
| 5. Incompatibilities or compatibilities | | | | 0/1 | | 0/1 |
| 6. Dosage forms or package size | | 1/1 | 6/7 | | | 7/8 |
| 7. Source of supply or availability | 1/1 | | 3/4 | 2/2 | | 6/7 |
| 8. Cost | | 2/2 | 0/2 | | | 2/4 |
| 9. Identification | 1/1 | 2/2 | 2/3 | | | 5/6 |
| 10. Characterization of a drug | | 1/3 | 3/3 | 0/1 | 1/1 | 5/8 |
| TOTAL | 2/2 | 10/13 | 27/38 | 3/7 | 1/1 | 43/61 |
| **PHARMACOLOGICAL** | | | | | | |
| 1. Dosage | 1/1 | 1/1 | 9/14 | 2/4 | | 13/20 |
| 2. Pharmacological actions or effects | | 0/1 | 1/4 | 1/1 | 2/2 | 4/8 |
| 3. Mechanism of action | 1/1 | 1/1 | 2/3 | | 2/2 | 6/7 |
| 4. Absorption, fate, or excretion | | 8/10 | 4/8 | 2/2 | | 14/20 |
| 5. Contraindications | | 0/1 | 2/4 | | | 2/5 |
| 6. Toxicities or side effects | 0/1 | 4/6 | 2/9 | 0/1 | 1/3 | 7/20 |
| 7. Antidote | | 0/1 | | | | 0/1 |
| TOTAL | 2/3 | 14/21 | 20/42 | 5/8 | 5/7 | 46/81 |
| **THERAPEUTIC** | | | | | | |
| 1. Use or indication | 0/1 | 6/7 | 9/10 | | 2/4 | 17/22 |
| 2. Equivalents or comparisons | | 2/3 | 7/13 | 2/2 | 0/1 | 11/19 |
| 3. Evaluation of a new drug | | | | 1/1 | | 1/1 |
| 4. Details of a clinical procedure | | | 0/3 | 0/1 | | 0/4 |
| 5. Method of administration | | 1/2 | 4/5 | 1/1 | 1/1 | 7/9 |
| TOTAL | 0/1 | 9/12 | 20/31 | 3/4 | 4/7 | 36/55 |
| CUMULATIVE TOTAL | 4/6 | 33/46 | 67/111 | 11/19 | 10/15 | 125/197 |

[a] A = attending; R = resident; I = intern; AI = acting intern; MS = medical student. Numerator value = number answered at time of request; denominator value = total number of requests.

341

## Table 4. Questions Answered at Time of Request According to Month of Study

| MONTH | NO. ANSWERED | TOTAL QUESTIONS | % |
|---|---|---|---|
| 1. February[a] | 20 | 34 | 58.8 |
| 2. March | 18 | 32 | 56.3 |
| 3. April | 13 | 24 | 54.2 |
| 4. May | 13 | 18 | 72.2 |
| 5. June | 17 | 24 | 70.8 |
| 6. July | 44 | 65 | 67.7 |
| TOTAL | 125 | 167 | (63.5) |

[a] Including three days in January

## Table 5. Drug Information Requests According to Physician Type

| PHYSICIAN TYPE | NO. REQUESTS | % |
|---|---|---|
| Attending | 6 | 3.1 |
| Resident | 46 | 23.4 |
| Intern | 111 | 56.3 |
| Acting intern | 19 | 9.6 |
| Medical student | 15 | 7.6 |
| TOTAL | 197 | 100.0 |

mediately was determined within each of the three major categories, as shown in Table 2. The highest percentage of questions answered at time of request was in the pharmaceutical category (70.5%). This was followed by the therapeutic category (65.5%), and finally, the pharmacological category (56.8%). For all categories, the pharmacist felt his knowledge was adequate to satisfactorily answer 63.5% of the questions at the time requested.

A more detailed classification within each category is seen in Table 3. The classification here is according to subclass within each category of request and according to the type of physician asking the question. For each request subclass, the total number of requests is recorded as a denominator value and the number of questions answered at the time requested is recorded as the numerator value.

The number of questions received as well as the pharmacist's ability to respond at the time of request was determined on a monthly basis as shown in Table 4. For the first three months the pharmacist averaged responding at the time of request 56.7% of the time. During the second three months, however, his ability to respond at the time of request increased to 69.2% of the time. The best percentage was recorded in the fourth month when 72.2% of the requests were answered at the time requested.

Table 5 shows the number of drug information requests according to the type of physician who asked them. The interns accounted for 111 (56.3%) of the 197 drug information requests. There were 46 (23.4%) requests asked by the residents, 19 (9.6%) requests asked by the acting intern, 15 (7.6%) requests by the medical students, and 6 (3.1%) requests by the attending physicians. If the values from the intern and acting intern are combined, 130 (66.0%) requests were initiated by physicians with primary responsibility for the care of the patient.

*Suggestions to Physicians.* As a result of regularly monitoring the patient's drug therapy by chart review, the pharmacist offered a total of 68 suggestions during the study period. Classification of the suggestions according to the type of drug therapy problem is seen in Table 6. A numerator-denominator arrangement has been used here also, with the numerator value representing the number of suggestions accepted by the physician and the denominator representing the number of suggestions offered by the pharmacist.

It may be seen that 26 (38.3%) of the 68 suggestions were related to either observed or potential side effects from one or more drugs in the patient's regimen. Fourteen of these suggestions were accepted. Twelve (17.6%) of the suggestions fell into the general category "to improve chances of effective therapy." Nine of the 12 (75%) were accepted.

Suggestions were next classified according to the recommended change as a solution to the problem as shown in Table 7. Using an alternative drug was the most commonly recommended change, accounting for 13 (19.1%) of the 68 total suggestions. This proposed change was acceptable to the physician contacted 85% of the time. Other commonly suggested changes were adding an additional drug and altering the route or method of administration. Although only occurring twice, recommendations not to use particular drugs were not accepted by the physicians.

The suggestions offered and the response elicited were determined according to the academic level or position of the physician on the team as shown in Table 8. Eight (88.9%) of nine suggestions were accepted by the acting intern; 30 (68.2%) of 44 suggestions were accepted by the intern; and 6 (42.9%) of 14 were accepted by the resident. The only suggestion offered to an attending physician was accepted. There were no suggestions offered to medical students since they did not function in a decision-making capacity. Overall, 45 (66.2%) of the 68 suggestions offered to the physicians on the medical team resulted in changes in therapy.

## Discussion

The results of this study indicate that a pharmacist participating as a member of a medicine team can serve

**Table 6. Suggestions Classified According to Type of Drug Therapy Problem and Physician Type**

| CATEGORY | PHYSICIAN TYPE[a] | | | | | TOTAL |
|---|---|---|---|---|---|---|
| | A | R | I | AI | MS | |
| 1. To provide more accurate dose | | | 2/5 | | | 2/5 |
| 2. Side effects from drug[b] | 1/1 | 2/6 | 9/17 | 2/2 | | 14/26 |
| 3. Allergic reaction[b] | | 1/1 | 1/1 | | | 2/2 |
| 4. Toxicity (dose-related)[b] | | 1/2 | 3/3 | 2/2 | | 6/7 |
| 5. Drug-drug interaction[b] | | 1/1 | 2/3 | 1/2 | | 4/6 |
| 6. Drug-laboratory test interaction[b] | | 0/2 | | | | 0/2 |
| 7. Ineffective dose | | | 1/1 | | | 1/1 |
| 8. Physical incompatibility (i.v.) | | | 1/1 | 1/1 | | 2/2 |
| 9. Improve chances of effective therapy | | 1/2 | 7/9 | 1/1 | | 9/12 |
| 10. Order inappropriately written or recorded | | | 4/4 | 1/1 | | 5/5 |
| TOTAL | 1/1 | 6/14 | 30/44 | 8/9 | | 45/68 |

[a] A = attending; R = resident; I = intern; AI = acting intern; MS = medical student. Numerator value = number accepted; denominator value = total number of suggestions.
[b] Observed or potential.

as a drug information source. That a physician is willing to use a pharmacist in an advisory role is indicated by the average of approximately two physician-pharmacist encounters concerning drugs per ward round session. Although a total of 265 communications over a six-month period is not a dramatic documentation of the potential value of the pharmacist, it must be recognized that this was the first experience in a direct contact relationship for both the pharmacist and the physicians on the teams. It seems reasonable to assume that if the phar-

macist is a useful addition to the medical team, the number of contributions by the pharmacist would increase.

Of the communications with members of the medicine team, 197 were initiated by physicians or medical students, and 68 were initiated by the pharmacist. Closer inspection of these interactions suggest the nature of the usefulness of the pharmacist on a medicine team.

*Drug Information Requests.* The pharmacist received requests from all members of the medicine team. The

**Table 7. Suggestions Classified According to Recommended Change and Physician Type**

| CATEGORY | PHYSICIAN TYPE[a] | | | | | TOTAL |
|---|---|---|---|---|---|---|
| | A | R | I | AI | MS | |
| 1. Use alternative drug | | | 8/10 | 3/3 | | 11/13 |
| 2. Add additional drug | | 0/2 | 3/7 | 2/2 | | 5/11 |
| 3. Increase dose of drug | | | 2/2 | | | 2/2 |
| 4. Decrease dose of drug | | 0/1 | 1/1 | | | 1/2 |
| 5. Discontinue drug | | 4/6 | 2/3 | | | 6/9 |
| 6. Change administration times | 1/1 | | 3/4 | 2/3 | | 6/8 |
| 7. Change drug dosage form | | | 1/2 | | | 1/2 |
| 8. Change route or method of administration | | | 7/10 | 1/1 | | 8/11 |
| 9. Special monitoring of patient | | 2/4 | 3/4 | | | 5/8 |
| 10. Do not use drug | | 0/1 | 0/1 | | | 0/2 |
| TOTAL | 1/1 | 6/14 | 30/44 | 8/9 | | 45/68 |

[a] A = attending; R = resident; I = intern; AI = acting intern; MS = medical student. Numerator value = number accepted; denominator value = total value of suggestions.

**Table 8. Acceptance of Suggestions According to Physician Type**

| PHYSICIAN | NO. ACCEPTED/TOTAL | % |
|---|---|---|
| Attending | 1/1 | 100.0 |
| Resident | 6/14 | 42.9 |
| Intern | 30/44 | 68.2 |
| Acting Intern | 8/9 | 88.9 |
| TOTAL | 45/68 | (66.2) |

greatest number of questions—81 (41.1%)—were of a pharmacologic nature. That greater than two-thirds of the questions were from categories other than pharmaceutical indicates that the pharmacist was accepted as a source of information beyond that associated merely with the drug product.

Although the number of drug information requests in the subcategories (e.g., dosage, antidotes, etc.) (Table 3) is too small to provide firm conclusions, it appears that the information needs of the team vary somewhat according to physician type. For example, it may be seen that the intern has the need for simple information, such as the dosage, ingredients and/or strength of a drug. The resident, however, generally appears to have mastered this knowledge and wants more subtle and sophisticated information. His needs more often fall into the areas of absorption percentages, metabolism or routes of excretion of drugs. While information needs for dosage or strength of a drug often represent convenience more than contribution by the pharmacist, these two classes combined made up only approximately one-fifth of the questions.

Of the 197 drug information requests, the pharmacist answered 125 (63.5%) at the time requested. As might have been expected, the pharmacist more consistently responded immediately to requests in the pharmaceutical category (70.5%). This was followed by requests in the therapeutic category (65.5%), and finally, the pharmacologic category (56.8%). That the pharmacist only answered slightly more than one-half of the requests in the pharmacologic category at the time requested has several implications. Either requests in this category were more sophisticated, requiring a review of the literature, or the educational background of the pharmacist in pharmacology was not well developed. It must be recognized, however, that this represents the ability or background of only one pharmacist and the results of this study cannot be extrapolated to all pharmacists.

To further appreciate the significance of the percentages of questions answered at the time the request was initiated, several things must be considered. At the beginning of the study, the pharmacist often was hesitant to provide answers to questions until a literature search was completed. This was due to a lack of confidence in both his answer and his ability to provide it. The major reason for hesitation was the pharmacist's lack of knowledge of the influence of disease on the patient or patient response to the drug. An exception to this was requests in the pharmaceutical category. Inquiries in this category related primarily to the drug product, and the pharmacist felt confident to respond immediately, perhaps because of traditional pharmacy experiences.

The lack of a simple answer to some of the questions made answering them without reviewing the literature somewhat foolhardy. For example, one question asked of the pharmacist was, "Could cholestyramine be used effectively in a patient who had ingested an overdose of Darvon, to bind it up in the gastrointestinal tract and prevent absorption?" Although it may seem logical that cholestyramine or another drug might work in this situation, the answer should be documented in the literature to determine the degree of effectiveness, the dosage required and other supportive care required in the management of the patient. Thus, while the percentages of questions answered at the time of request provide some insight into the ability of the pharmacist to respond from memory, this information has significance only when results are qualified by the degree of sophistication of the question group. The sophistication of the questions were not considered in this study. Piecoro[4] found that 72% of the drug information requests directed to a pharmacist on attending rounds could be answered at the time requested.

The number of questions answered at the time of request increased from 56.7% during the first three months to 69.2% during the second three months. Several things may have contributed to this increase. Often questions or potential problems could be anticipated by remarks recorded in the patient's progress notes in the chart. As the pharmacist improved his ability to use the chart, these comments provided clues to future questions. For example, one chart progress note stated: "At home, patient only takes Quadrinal (?)." Another stated: "Unexplained elevation in eosinophil count. Will R/O allergy to Aldomet." Remarks such as these allowed the pharmacist to prepare for the anticipated question which would probably be asked the following morning on rounds.

The knowledge learned from discussions with other team members during work rounds provided a great source of clinical drug use experiences for the pharmacist. A similar benefit from rounds was learning the therapeutic "idiosyncrasies" of the attending physicians. This allowed the pharmacist to prejudge, to a degree, the reception that might be given a suggestion or answer to a question offered later. Much of the knowledge obtained from these sources could be used by the pharmacist at a later time.

Another somewhat common occurrence which helped the pharmacist improve his performance was repetitive questions. During the study period, questions for commonly used drugs such as digoxin or gentamicin came up several times. If the pharmacist could not answer the question on the first request, he usually was able to provide the information when it was requested again.

Many questions were asked as the result of a leading question by the pharmacist. For example, during a discussion of the patient's diarrhea problem, the pharmacist might inquire if the patient were still being given a particular drug. This would usually lead the physician to ask if the drug often caused diarrhea. An approach such as this served two purposes. First, it assured the pharmacist that the patient was in fact still taking the drug; second, it allowed the physician to initiate the inquiry and take action to change therapy or not, depending upon his relative concern for the two problems of the patient. It was found that this approach, although somewhat conservative, worked very well as a mechanism to emphasize a point or idea without having to force an issue in what might have been a gray area in the pharmacist's knowledge.

*Suggestions to Physicians.* The 68 suggestions offered to a member of the medicine team during the study represents greater than 25% of the pharmacist's formal contributions regarding drug therapy. Approximately two-thirds (66.0%) of these suggestions were accepted as useful information. This acceptance rate implies that a pharmacist may be able to serve in a useful capacity as a drug therapy monitor. Two areas of potential contribution from a pharmacist appear to be (1) providing information that improves the likelihood that use of a drug will be both rational and effective, and (2) predicting or detecting undesired drug reactions (Table 6).

Although the individual classification of the observed or potential problems (Table 6) which stimulated the suggestions provide some insight into the needs of the various physician groups, the numbers in each category are much too small to allow any definite conclusions to be drawn. The greater number of suggestions directed to the intern is reflected by his relatively greater degree of responsibility for the patient. It also documents a general effort by the pharmacist not to "go over the head" of the intern to get therapy changed whenever possible.

The average percentage of suggestions accepted (66.2%) is of interest. At the beginning of the study it was felt that one benefit of a pharmacist associating with a medical team, rather than geographic location on a nursing unit, would be a better acceptance rate, perhaps due to the opportunity to make suggestions at the time decisions regarding therapy were being made. It was hoped that this would improve the likelihood that the suggestion would be accepted, since it would avoid the connotation of wrongness associated with the physician having to change orders written earlier. Smith,[24] in a recent two-month departmental study of the utilization of clinical pharmacy services in a 680-bed private community medical center, found physician acceptance of the pharmacist's information 86.5% of the time. Most of the pharmacists in the study were geographically located on the nursing units and shared responsibility for

the drug distribution system as well. It is unclear whether the difference in acceptance between Smith's study and the present study is due to differences in physician attitudes, differing needs in community versus university teaching hospitals, variations in measurement parameters, or some other factors.

There was a definite decline in the percentage of suggestions accepted with increasing level of experience or academic position of the physician. Although the acting intern accepted 88.9% of the suggestions offered to him, the resident accepted only 42.9%. It is difficult to determine if the lower rate of acceptance by the residents was primarily due to the quality of the suggestion offered or a general reluctance to accept information from a pharmacist. Surprisingly, Smith[24] found no significant difference in the acceptance of suggestions among private physicians in the community (85%), residents (87%) and interns (90%).

Unfortunately, measurement of the quality of the information provided in terms of its clinical appropriateness was not possible in this study, other than determining the physicians' reaction to the information. Nor was there any quantitative measure of the positive influence on the care of the patient when this information was used. Although it was felt by the pharmacist that the information offered represented a useful contribution, it is entirely possible that some of the suggestions which were accepted for use did not represent the best approach to the therapeutic management of the patient. Conversely, on several occasions, well documented information, which was felt useful by the pharmacist, was not accepted. Other studies should be undertaken to resolve these important questions. Included in these studies must be objective measurement of cost-to-benefit ratios for such services.

## Conclusion

The problems encountered in attempting to passively provide drug information from a central service in the hospital pharmacy have been aptly described by Bouchard:[26] "Physicians, in general, have little feel for what they do not know about drugs...(and therefore)...do not always recognize situations where questions should be asked." Since the pharmacist in any situation where he is not familiar with the patient or his problems must wait for the physician to recognize his own limitations, the quality of his potential contribution must of necessity be compromised. The pharmacist in this study chose to actively monitor patients by chart review and participate in medical ward rounds as a point of contact. This approach represents one method to increase the availability of drug information as well as increase the likelihood of its use. It is felt that many of the questions which were asked would not have been asked, let alone answered, had the pharmacist not been conveniently available.

Many suggestions offered to the team members related

to observed or potential adverse drug reactions. Melmon[27] has suggested that as many as 70 to 80% of the adverse drug reactions seen in hospitalized patients can be predicted from data available on either the drug or the patient in whom the drug is being used. He also suggests that "most of these are preventable without compromise of the therapeutic benefits of the drug." If this is a reasonably close estimate, then a major contribution of the pharmacist might be in reducing the number of these untoward reactions.

It is possible and perhaps likely that many of these observed or potential drug therapy problems would have eventually been recognized, regardless of the intervention by the pharmacist. However, it seems reasonable to assume that in a significant number of these patients, recognition of the problem might not have occurred until an adverse reaction to the drug signaled its existence. These reactions can have serious consequences. For example, studies have shown that 20 to 30% of patients on digitalis preparations experience an adverse reaction.[28-30] Also shown is that approximately 10% of these patients die as a result of this toxicity.[31] Obviously, waiting for the onset of toxicity of this drug to take appropriate measures to correct therapy is not an acceptable approach to dealing with the potential problem. Other drugs carry similar potential dangers.

Less well documented, but perhaps equally significant, are the problems associated with ineffective drug therapy resulting from various causes. Many of these might easily be prevented by a pharmacist if he were knowledgeable concerning the therapeutic goals of the physician. Information regarding the physician's intent has not always been conveniently accessible to pharmacists in the past. No meaningful clinical involvement can be established by the pharmacist unless he has access to this information. Direct physician contact overcomes this obstacle.

The pharmacist, as the person on the medicine team with a high index of suspicion for drug-related problems such as these, can provide a potentially valuable resource to complement the physician whose primary focus is upon diagnosing and treating the ill patient. Although additional studies are needed to document the value of a pharmacist as a member of a medical care team, this study indicates that the pharmacist does have a contribution to make to patient care and physician education.

### References

1. Goddard, J. L.: Drugs in the Hospital, *Hosp. Formul. Manage.* 2:35–37 (Feb.) 1967.
2. Smith, W. E.: The Future Role of the Hospital Pharmacist in the Patient Care Area, *Amer. J. Hosp. Pharm.* 24:228–231 (Apr.) 1967.
3. Smith, W. E.: Role of a Pharmacist in Improving Rational Drug Therapy as Part of the Patient Care Team, *Drug Intel.* 1:244–249 (Aug.) 1967.
4. Piecoro, J. J., Jr., Wolf, H. H. and Knapp, D. A.: A Pharmacist on Hospital Ward Rounds, *J. Amer. Pharm. Ass.* NS7:630–633 (Dec.) 1967.
5. Canada, A. T., Jr.: Clinical Pharmacy: A Course for the Future Pharmacist's Role, *Amer. J. Pharm. Educ.* 32:70–74 (Feb.) 1968.
6. Goddard, J. L.: Pharmacy's Future: Trials and Triumphs, *Hosp. Formul. Manage.* 3:31–33 (Feb.) 1968.
7. Hartshorn, E. A.: Pharmacy (Annual Administrative Reviews), *Hospitals* 42:127–130 (Apr. 1) 1968.
8. Canada, A. T., Jr.: The Role of the Clinical Pharmacist, *Amer. J. Pharm.* 140:152–156 (Sept.–Oct.) 1968.
9. Pratt, S., Beck, A. V. R. and Sperandio, G. J.: Experience in a New Clinical Pharmacy Training Program, *Amer. J. Hosp. Pharm.* 25:559–563 (Oct.) 1968.
10. Masaki, B. W.: Clinical Rounds Enable the Health Team to Appreciate the Rx Man's Knowledge, *Amer. Prof. Pharm.* 34:21–27 (Nov.) 1968.
11. Emmanuel, Sister: Experience with a Course in Clinical Pharmacy, Part Two: Lectures, Patient Rounds and Other Laboratory Experiences, *Amer. J. Hosp. Pharm.* 25:682–690 (Dec.) 1968.
12. Paxinos, J.: What Role can Pharmacists Play in the Clinical Environment, *Hosp. Topics,* 47:75–78 (May) 1969.
13. Bell, J. E., Grimes, B. J., Bouchard, V. E. and Duffy, Sister M. G.: A New Approach to Delivering Drug Information to the Physician Through a Pharmacy Consultation Program, *Amer. J. Hosp. Pharm.* 27:29–37 (Jan.) 1970.
14. Whitney, H. A. K., Jr., Blissitt, C. W. and Kinsella, R. A.: A Clinical Teaching Environment, *Hospitals* 44:132–137 (Feb. 1) 1970.
15. Hill, W. T., Jr., Blair, W. T. and Mitchell, N. M.: Satellite Service, *Hospitals* 44:96–102 (Mar. 16) 1970.
16. Thompson, C. O., Schwartau, N. W., Trites, D. K. and Lechwart, J. F.: Pharmaceutical Communications in the Clinical Environment, *Amer. J. Hosp. Pharm.* 27:277–293 (Apr.) 1970.
17. Smith, D. L.: Pharmacist on a Ward, *Can. J. Hosp. Pharm.* 23:108–112 (May–June) 1970.
18. Bailey, D. E. and Plein, E. M.: A Study of Clinical Pharmacy Practice in a Small Private Hospital, *Hosp. Pharm.* 5:5–14 (Aug.) 1970.
19. Nagata, R. E., Jr.: Implementation of Clinical Pharmacy Through Training, *Hosp. Pharm.* 5:4–9 (Dec.) 1970.
20. Thompson, M.: Clinical Pharmacy in the Small Hospital, *Amer. J. Hosp. Pharm.* 28:205–207 (Mar.) 1971.
21. Sandler, A. and Altbach, H.: Clinical Training for Veterans Administration Pharmacy Interns, *Amer. J. Hosp. Pharm.* 28:260–266 (Apr.) 1971.
22. Silverman, H. M. and Simon, G. I.: Physician Reaction to a Clinical Pharmacist, In *Clinical Pharmacy Sourcebook,* pp. 379-381.
23. Thielke, T. S.: Activity Analysis of Clinical Pharmacists, In *Clinical Pharmacy Sourcebook,* pp. 334-337.
24. Smith, W. E.: Clinical Pharmacy Services in a Community Hospital (Case Study Series), U.S. Department of Health, Education, and Welfare, Pub. No. HSM 72-3019, January 1972.
25. Bell, J. E., Bouchard, V. E., South, J. C. and Duffy, Sister M. Gonzales: A New Approach to Delivering Drug Information to the Physician through a Pharmacy Consultation Program-Evaluation Results, In *Clinical Pharmacy Sourcebook,* pp. 368-378.
26. Bouchard, V. E.: Toward a Clinical Practice of Pharmacy, *Drug Intel. Clin. Pharm.* 3:342–347 (Dec.) 1969.
27. Melmon, K. L.: Preventable Drug Reactions—Causes and Cures, *N. Engl. J. Med.* 284:1361–1368 (June 17) 1971.
28. Rodensky, P. L. and Wasserman, F.: Observation on Digitalis Intoxication, *Arch. Internal Med.* 108:61–78, 1961.
29. Billar, G. D., Smith, T. W., Abelmann, W. H., Haber, E. and Hood, W. B., Jr.: Digitalis Intoxication: A Prospective Clinical Study with Serum Level Correlations, *N. Engl. J. Med.* 284:989–997 (May 6) 1971.
30. Ogilvie, R. I. and Rudy, J.: An Educational Program in Digitalis Therapy, *JAMA* 222:50–55 (Oct. 2) 1972.
31. Jelliffe, R. W.: Reduction of Digitalis Toxicity by Computer-Assisted Digitalis Dosage Program. Quantitative Relationship to Serum Potassium, *Fed. Proc.* 30:284, 1971.

# 59 Pharmacist-initiated Patient Drug Histories

Roger S. Wilson and Hugh F. Kabat

This study examined the efficacy of pharmacists developing patient drug histories for newly admitted hospitalized patients.

One hundred patients were interviewed by a pharmacist on the day after admission to determine the medications they had taken during the six-month period prior to admission. Only 57 percent of the medications found by the pharmacist were recorded by the attending physician during the patients' admission interview. Although the physician recorded 70 percent of the patients' prescribed medications, he recorded only 37 percent of the nonprescription medications found by the pharmacist.

Over 90 percent of the patients were cooperative with the pharmacist interviewer. Almost one out of four patients had a particular drug problem which they discussed with the pharmacist. The pharmacist and physicians recorded essentially the same information on drug dependence, allergies, and previous reactions to drugs. Almost 40 percent of the patients interviewed revealed that they did not utilize their prescription drugs exactly as directed by their physician.

The primary problem involved in pharmacist initiated patient drug histories was the amount of time required.

In this study the pharmacist was able to obtain a more complete patient drug history than the physician. The economics of the situation suggest that patient drug histories should be taken by pharmacists practicing in the patient care setting or during a daily round to interview all new patients.

During the past several years there has been an increasing effort by hospital pharmacists to extend their services beyond those necessary to maintain the integrity of the drug distribution system. Several authors have suggested that the pharmacist, if based in the patient care setting, can make a valuable contribution to patient care through participation in the drug selection process, supervision of unit dose drug distribution, monitoring of patient drug therapy and taking and evaluating patient medication histories.[1]

Traditionally, a drug history has been taken along with the patient's admission history. At the beginning of this century, when the present system of history taking was firmly established, there was little drug therapy that was capable of altering the natural course of most diseases. Many prescribed medications were pharmacologically impotent and could not cause much benefit, harm or diagnostic interference. Accordingly, the physician, when taking a medical history, paid scant attention to ascertaining what previous treatment had been given. Since then, there has been a therapeutic revolution and numerous potent drugs are now available which can profoundly influence the outcome of many diseases. At the same time, they may produce clinical features closely resembling naturally occurring disorders and even obscure the correct diagnosis. Wilson noted the importance of a complete drug history when he stated, "It cannot be too strongly emphasized that no clinical history is complete without a list of drugs taken during the previous six months. Unfortunately, this is rarely achieved."[2]

While some hospitals for many years have been requiring their employees to interrogate newly admitted patients on the subject of allergies and/or drugs recently taken, it appears that the majority has initiated this procedure only in the last five years. The California Hospital Association surveyed its member hospitals to determine their policies and practices concerning soliciting information on allergies and drugs being taken by newly admitted patients. Sixty-nine percent of the 229 reporting hospitals required their employees to obtain information on allergies from newly admitted patients. However, only 39 percent had a similar policy for drugs recently taken. Of those hospitals reporting affirmatively (171) to either question, 18 percent required physician employees to conduct these interviews and seven percent reported that both physicians and nonphysician employees were designated for this activity. Nonphysician employees including registered nurses, clerks, licensed vocational nurses or aides (pharmacists were not mentioned) conducted these interviews in the remaining 75 percent of the hospitals.[3] Of course, solicitation of information on these topics by a nonphysician does not relieve the attending physician of his responsibility to check the answers and inquire further when indicated.

## Purpose of the Study

The purpose of this study was to compare pharmacist initiated patient drug histories with histories taken by physicians. The study was conducted in the 1085-bed Minneapolis Veterans Administration Hospital. Over a 30-day period, one pharmacist interviewed 100 male patients, ranging in age from 20 to 84, in order to obtain prescription and nonprescription drug histories during the six-month period prior to hospital admission. The pharmacist's individual findings were compared with the drugs recorded in the patient's chart by the physician during his interview of the patient at the time of admission.

The pharmacist's interviews were conducted on the day after admission because of other required patient procedures and interviews on the admission day. Because only one pharmacist was available for interviewing, only four medical units were selected for the study. Each day the pharmacist received a "Gains and Losses Report" from the medical records department listing all new admissions for the previous day. The pharmacist visited the four medical units once daily and interviewed, if possible, all new admissions. On some occasions an additional call back was necessary.

Figure 1 shows the questions asked by the pharmacist.

*Figure 1. Questions the pharmacist asked patients during the drug history interview*

1. Were you using any drugs prior to being admitted to the hospital? Did you bring them to the hospital with you?
2. Have you used any other drugs during the past six months, including shots administered at your doctor's office?
3. Have you used any drugs recently that are not prescription drugs, such as analgesics, antacids, effervescent salts, laxatives, antidiarrheals, vitamins or other patent medicines?
4. Have you used any external preparations, such as lotions or ointments?
5. Have you used any drugs for nerves, heart or sleep?
6. Do you have any known allergies or reactions to any drugs? Also, any dependence on any drugs? Does your physician know of these?
7. Did you take your prescription drugs regularly or as directed by your physician? If not, why?
8. Have you had any particular problems with your drugs with which I might help?

## Description of Patients Interviewed

Only certain patients were selected for the study. A preliminary discussion with physicians disclosed that they placed little reliance on drug history information obtained from senile or alcoholic patients, so these were excluded from the sample. Patients too ill to be interviewed and those transferred or away from the patient care unit for an extended period of time were similarly excluded from the sample. Patients admitted directly from other health care facilities where their drug ingestion was controlled and recorded in an accompanying chart were also excluded from the study.

Table 1 summarizes the spectrum of diagnoses represented by the patients in this study.

### Table 1. Primary Diagnosis of Patients Included in the Study

| DIAGNOSIS | NO. |
|---|---|
| Gastrointestinal disorder | 29 |
| Cardiovascular disorder | 29 |
| Arthritis or gout | 7 |
| Pulmonary disorder | 8 |
| Blood disorder | 6 |
| Diabetes | 6 |
| Renal disorder | 2 |
| Miscellaneous and unknown | 13 |
| | 100 |

## Patient Acceptance of Pharmacist

Almost all patients responded very favorably to the pharmacist interviewer. Those who did not were seriously ill or emotionally upset about some matter. Each patient interviewed was rated on a scale of one to three based on the following criteria:

1. Patient did not want to answer questions or was totally disinterested in talking to the pharmacist.
2. Patient responded with yes/no answers but was cooperative.
3. Patient answered questions well and appeared interested in talking about his drugs.

Table 2 shows the number of patients with each rating.

### Table 2. Patient Cooperation During Pharmacist Interview

| SCALE | NO. |
|---|---|
| 1 | 9 |
| 2 | 8 |
| 3 | 83 |
| | 100 |

After a drug history was taken by the pharmacist, the patient's chart was examined and the drugs recorded by the physician were compared with those recorded by the pharmacist. The base line for each patient was the total number of prescription and non-prescription drug products he said he had taken during the previous six months. Thus, all drug products recorded by either physicians or the pharmacist were included — if both the physicians and the pharmacist recorded the same drug product, it was counted only once.

## Study Findings

The total number of prescription and nonprescription drug products taken by the 100 patients in this study during the six-month period prior to admission was 261. This total included 156 prescription medications and 105 nonprescription items with an average of 2.6 different medications per patient (see Table 3).

Table 3. Prescription and Nonprescription Medications Recorded by Physicians and by the Pharmacist

| INTERVIEWER | NO. OF MEDICA-TIONS | NO. OF PRESCRIP-TION PRODUCTS | NO. OF NONPRE-SCRIPTION PRODUCTS |
|---|---|---|---|
| Physicians and pharmacist | 143 | 106 | 37 |
| Physicians only | 6 | 4 | 2 |
| Pharmacist only | 112 | 46 | 66 |
| | 261 | 156 | 105 |

Of the 261 prescription and nonprescription medications recorded, 55 percent were recorded by both the physicians and the pharmacist. However, 43 percent of the drug products noted in the study were not recorded by the physicians. Physicians did record a few drugs (six) which had been undetected by the pharmacist. Only about 57 percent of the prescription and nonprescription medications taken by the patients in the previous six months were included in their medical histories when physicians alone took the histories.

In this study, physicians recorded over 70 percent of the prescription medications in the patients' medical histories but only 37 percent of the nonprescription medications. The dramatic difference between the performance of the pharmacist and physicians in recording nonprescription medications may have been the result of a more complete interview on drug usage by the pharmacist. Or this difference may have been caused by the physicians' consideration of these medications as clinically unimportant, in which case an effort should be made to make physicians more aware of the effects of common nonprescription drug products. Interactions between prescribed and nonprescribed medications taken prior to hospitalization could greatly affect a patient's medical condition. For example, most common antacids will prevent or delay the absorption of tetracycline.[4] Salicylates, in large doses, such as those taken by arthritic patients, may intensify the action of oral anticoagulants or the oral antidiabetic agent, tolbutamide, and, in other instances, cause gastric irritation or hemorrhage in patients with a history of gastrointestinal disease.[5,6]

An important part of taking drug histories is not only disclosure of drug utilization but also specific identification of all drug products. Physicians were able to identify the specific drug product patients were taking only 77 percent of the time compared with an 86 percent identification rate for the pharmacist (see Table 4). No effort was made to validate these identifications.

Table 4. Prescription and Nonprescription Drug Products Specifically Identified During Patient Drug History Interviews

| INTER-VIEWER | PRESCRIP-TION MEDICATIONS RECORDED | PRESCRIP-TION PRODUCTS IDENTIFIED | NONPRE-SCRIPTION MEDICATIONS RECORDED | NONPRE-SCRIPTION PRODUCTS IDENTIFIED |
|---|---|---|---|---|
| Physicians | 110 | 91 | 39 | 24 |
| Pharmacist | 152 | 122 | 103 | 97 |

Moreover, physicians identified only 62 percent of the nonprescription drug products found during their patient interviews compared to 95 percent for the pharmacist. This difference in ability to identify specific brands of a drug product or the specific drug in a therapeutic class is probably due to the pharmacist's greater familiarity with drug products.

When the prescription drugs disclosed by interview were arranged according to the *American Hospital Formulary Service* therapeutic classifications, it was noted that the pharmacist recorded significantly more cough syrups, parasympatholytic, vasodilating, analgesic, tranquilizer, sedative-hypnotic and antidiarrheal drugs than the physicians did during their patient interviews. In all other therapeutic classifications, there were no significant differences in numbers of drugs recorded by physicians or the pharmacist. These differences may have been due to a more complete interview by the pharmacist and a special effort to find specific drugs such as those used for the heart, nerves and sleep. Or possibly physicians felt that these drugs were not important enough to include in the patients' medical histories. However, the use of these drugs may affect a patient's medical progress because of possible drug interactions with other commonly used drugs. Physicians recorded only two sedative-hypnotic drugs compared to eleven recorded by the pharmacist. This class of drugs may seem unimportant or easily forgotten but drugs such as chloral hydrate and the barbiturates may intensify the action of oral antidiabetic agents and may also antagonize the action of the oral anticoagulants and diphenylhydantoin.[7] These examples again illustrate the need for a complete drug history which includes both prescribed and nonprescribed medications taken by patients during the six months prior to admission.

In this study the pharmacist recorded 103 nonprescription items during patient interviews compared with only 39 of the physicians (see Table 5).

Table 5. Classification of Nonprescription Drugs Recorded by Physicians and the Pharmacist

| CLASSIFICATION | NO. RECORDED BY PHYSICIANS | NO. RECORDED BY THE PHARMACIST |
|---|---|---|
| Antacids | 18 | 33 |
| Analgesics | 8 | 29 |
| Laxatives | 4 | 13 |
| Effervescent salts | 1 | 5 |
| Vitamins | 0 | 8 |
| Cough syrups | 2 | 4 |
| External preparations | 1 | 3 |
| Others | 5 | 8 |

The pharmacist recorded many more analgesics, antacids, laxatives, effervescent salts, vitamins, external preparation and expectorants. Again, these differences may be the result of a more complete interview by the pharmacist and a special effort to record nonprescribed medications or possibly the physicians' feeling that these medications are not important enough to include in the patients' medical history.

In general, physicians appeared to be most concerned about drugs being used at the time of admission and less concerned about drugs discontinued prior to admission, despite the fact that a number of drugs have a latent activity period of up to several months after administration. An example might be a patient receiving gold injections from his private physician several months prior to admission. High concentrations are retained by the kidney for months after a single intramuscular injection. As another example, it is also important to know that a patient has been on long-term steroid therapy prior to admission if surgery is anticipated. Of the 110 prescription medications recorded by the physician, 92 percent were products which were being taken at the time of admission. In the case of the 152 prescription medications recorded by the pharmacist, 82 percent were being used by the patient at the time of admission. Thus, of the prescription medications recorded by physicians, only 8 percent had been discontinued in the six-month period prior to admission as compared with 18 percent of those recorded by the pharmacist (see Table 6).

This difference may be due to the fact that the pharmacist asked specifically about drugs used during the six-month period prior to admission and the physicians may not have done this.

Table 6. Time Period between Discontinuation of Medication and Hospital Admission

| INTERVAL | NO. OF DRUGS | % |
|---|---|---|
| Taking drugs on admission | 124 | 82 |
| Discontinued less than 2 weeks prior to admission | 4 | 3 |
| Discontinued 2-4 weeks prior to admission | 15 | 10 |
| Discontinued 1-3 months prior to admission | 5 | 3 |
| Discontinued 4-6 months prior to admission | 4 | 3 |
| | 152 | 100 |

No patients in this study admitted any drug dependence. Seventeen patients told the pharmacist that they had had drug reactions in the past. This was identical to the responses recorded in the charts by the physicians during their patient interviews.

Sixteen percent of the patients interviewed by the pharmacist spontaneously asked questions about their medications and another six percent expressed a desire to discuss problems regarding personal drug usage. These patients were primarily those with chronic illnesses such as arthritis or peptic ulcer who required long-term drug therapy. This illustrates the need for more patient contact by the pharmacist if the patient's needs for drug information are to be met.

Almost 40 percent of the patients interviewed by the pharmacist admitted that they do not utilize their prescription drugs as directed by their physician. Table 7 summarizes the reasons given for the deviations.

Table 7. Reasons Given by Patients for Deviation from Physician's Prescribed Directions

| RESPONSE | NO. |
|---|---|
| Take drugs only when necessary | 9 |
| Forget drugs occasionally | 7 |
| High cost | 5 |
| Dislike drugs unless very ill | 6 |
| Discontinued because of ineffectiveness | 5 |
| Discontinued because of side effects | 2 |
| Supply ran out | 2 |
| Can not take drugs to work | 1 |
| Not interested | 1 |
| Take more often due to declining effectiveness | 1 |
| | 39 |

**Problems Experienced**

The greatest obstacle to pharmacist initiated patient drug histories was the time required to engage in this activity. Although it required just over 9 minutes to conduct the average interview, an additional 24 minutes per patient were required to reach the patient care area, to locate a specific patient and to identify his drug products. The pharmacist recorded more medications than physicians, but a more efficient method must be found before the system can be economical. Perhaps the pharmacist could do the interviews as part of the admission procedure in concert with the admitting physician or perhaps this activity can be part of the responsibility of a clinical pharmacist based in the patient care area.

### References

1. Owyang, E., et al.: The Pharmacist's New Role in Institutional Patient Care, *Amer. J. Hosp. Pharm.* 25:624-630 (Nov.) 1968.

2. Wilson, G. M.: Ill Health Due to Drugs, *Brit. Med. J.* 1:1065-1069 (Apr. 30) 1966.

3. Mills, D. H.: Allergic Reactions to Drugs, *Calif. Med.* 101:4-8 (July) 1964.

4. Juul Christensen, E. K., et al.: Influence of Gastric Antacids on the Release *In Vitro* of Tetracycline Hydrochloride, *Pharm. Weekblad.* 102:463-473 (May 26) 1967.

5. Solomon, H. and Schrogie, J.: The Effect of Various Drugs on the Binding of Warfarin-C to Human Albumin, *Biochem. Pharmacol.* 16:1219-1226 (July) 1967.

6. Stowers, J. M. et al.: Clinical and Pharmacological Comparison of Chlorpropamide and other Sulfonureas, *Ann. N.Y. Acad. Sci.* 74:689-695, 1959.

7. Orrenius, S., et al.: Phenobarbital-Induced Synthesis of the Microsomal Drug Metabolizing Enzymes System and its Relationship to the Proliferation of Endoplasmic Membranes, *J. Cell. Biol.* 25:627-639 (June) 1939.

# 60 The Pharmacist-acquired Medication History

Tim R. Covington and Frederick G. Pfeiffer

In an effort to further demonstrate the pharmacist's clinical abilities and potential contribution to improving drug therapy, 58 pharmacist-acquired medication histories were compared with the medication histories obtained from the same inpatients by physicians.

Particular attention was directed toward determining the extent to which patients knew which drugs they were taking prior to admission, the reliability of these patients in taking scheduled doses as outpatients, frequency with which these patients consumed another patient's prescription drugs, frequency at which nonprescription drugs were consumed prior to admission, and the detection of allergies.

In comparing physician-acquired data with pharmacist-acquired data, several things were obvious. Physicians did not generally obtain a comprehensive medication history. The pharmacist was more proficient in acquiring comprehensive medication histories. Much of the information obtained in the pharmacist-acquired medication history revealed that a significant percentage of patients were poorly informed about many aspects of drug therapy.

The authors conclude that hospital pharmacists must take a more active role in counseling patients regarding their drug therapy.

The objective of this presentation is to further illustrate how the pharmacist may effectively contribute to patient care by fulfilling certain clinical responsibilities requiring direct patient-pharmacist communication. Although there are several opportunities for direct patient-pharmacist communication, this presentation deals specifically with the pharmacist's role in medication history acquisition and the subsequent need to counsel ambulatory outpatients and patients upon discharge from the hospital regarding proper drug usage.

## The Problem

Basic to effective patient interviewing and counseling is the ability to communicate. Effective communication depends largely upon the pharmacist's ability to communicate verbally and interpret nonverbal responses.[1] While it is not within the scope of this paper to enumerate specific communicative techniques, one should not minimize the importance of developing effective communication skills as is revealed in the following nursing service incident-accident report:[2]

> Mr. Smith, on April 14, 1966, was given some liquid pHisoHex soap and instructed to take a shower before going to surgery. Instead of taking a shower with pHisoHex he drank it. Because he didn't go to surgery on April 14 Mr. Smith was again given some liquid pHisoHex soap so he could take a shower. Instead, he drank it again. This morning the patient complained to the doctor that the "medicine" made him vomit.

The pharmacist's potential contribution in the acquisition of medication histories is great, but there has been little documentation of his expertise in this area. Physician-acquired medication histories are generally sketchy.[3] Often little effort is made to determine what drugs the patient may have been taking prior to admission. Failure to acquire this information has significant medicolegal implications in that many maintenance drugs should be continued during hospitalization while other drugs having residual effects after discontinuation, such as reserpine or monoamine oxidase inhibitors, may alter the normally predictable response to the treatment regimen. In addition, the physician-acquired medication history is often lacking in information concerning the patient's reliability in taking scheduled doses, frequency with which patients consume other patients' legend drugs, nonprescription drug usage patterns and alcohol consumption patterns. Finally, often the only entry in the physician-acquired medical history concerning medication is the response of the patient when questioned about drug allergies. Even this vital question is not always asked or appropriately documented as was revealed in a study conducted in a university teaching hospital. In this study a retrospective analysis of 270 patient charts revealed that 42 (16%) of the patients were apparently not asked if they had drug allergies, or if they were asked, the response was not recorded.[4] Questions concerning allergies should always be asked and documented lest the patient sustain an unnecessary, expensive and potentially life-threatening allergic reaction.[1]

## Methodology

In an effort to demonstrate the pharmacist's ability and expertise in acquiring patient medication histories, 58 inpatients on medicine and surgery units of a 500-bed, municipal, acute care, general hospital were selected at random and interviewed by a pharmacist. Information was recorded on a medication history data sheet. Physician-acquired facts relative to a patient's medication history were transcribed from the chart onto one of these forms and then compared with the data obtained from the same patient by the pharmacist.

## Results

*Allergies or Hypersensitivities.* Perhaps the most surprising finding in this study was the relative infrequency with which physicians documented the patient's history of allergies or hypersensitivities to drugs or other chemicals (see Table 1). In only 32 (55%) of the 58 charts was there an entry indicating the physician had asked the patient about prior allergies or hypersensitivities.

While physician-acquired histories noted 5 patients with prior drug allergies, pharmacist-acquired medication histories revealed 15 prior drug allergies including 6 to penicillin, 2 to sulfonamides, and 1 to aspirin. The interviewing pharmacist was careful in assuring that the patient understood the definition of "allergy." In addition, the pharmacist was cautious not to suggest specific allergies that might bias the response. The contrast of reported drug allergies (8.6% of patients according to the physicians and 25.8% of patients according to the pharmacist) speaks well for the pharmacist's communicative skill and ability to extract pertinent information from patients.

The pharmacist also revealed 12 food allergies, 3 allergies to pets, and 6 allergies to miscellaneous agents which contrasts sharply with physician-acquired data. Finally, in an effort to determine whether there was any familial genetic correlation of allergies or hypersensitivities, it was revealed that 11 of the 15 patients with a history of allergies had at least one member of their immediate family prone toward allergies or hypersensitivities.

*Prescription Drug Consumption.* Many of the questions asked by the pharmacist are not routine in a

Table 1. Comparison of Physician-Acquired and Pharmacist-Acquired Medication Histories for 58 Patients

| TYPE OF DATA | PHYSICIAN ACQUIRED INFORMATION | PHARMACIST ACQUIRED INFORMATION |
|---|---|---|
| **ALLERGY AND HYPERSENSITIVITY** | | |
| Number of times question was asked by physicians as evidenced by entry in chart | 32 | — |
| Number of patients with allergies or hypersensitivities to drugs (includes serums and vaccines) | 5 | 15 |
| Number of patients with allergies or hypersensitivities to foods | 2 | 12 |
| Number of patients with allergies or hypersensitivities to pets | 1 | 3 |
| Miscellaneous allergies or hypersensitivities (ragweed, insect bites, dust, etc.) | 1 | 6 |
| Number of individuals whose immediate family had history of allergies or hypersensitivities | 0 | 12 |
| **PRESCRIPTION DRUG CONSUMPTION** | | |
| Legend drugs consumed immediately prior to admission (number represents prescriptions) | 38 | 193 |
| Number of times above question was asked by physicians as evidenced by entry in the chart | 21 | — |
| **RELIABILITY OF PRESCRIPTION DRUG CONSUMPTION** | | |
| Number of patients with a history of missing doses at home | 0 | 23 |
| **CONSUMPTION OF ANOTHER INDIVIDUAL'S PRESCRIPTION DRUGS** | | |
| Number of patients with a history of consuming someone else's medication | 0 | 9 |
| **NONPRESCRIPTION MEDICATION CONSUMPTION** | | |
| Number of nonprescription medications consumed regularly during past year by patients sampled | 2 | 237 |

physician-acquired medication history but are, nevertheless, essential in maximizing patient safety and rational drug therapy. Regarding prescription drug consumption, the pharmacist documented that the 58 patients sampled were consuming 155 more prescription drugs immediately prior to admission than was revealed in their charts. Physicians documented that 38 prescription drugs were being consumed prior to admission, or 0.65 drugs per patient. The pharmacist determined that 193 prescription drugs were being consumed immediately prior to admission, or 3.2 drugs per patient (see Table 1).

Entries in the chart suggested that physicians inquired into prior prescription drug usage only 21 times, although the question may have been asked and not recorded in the chart. At any rate, prior drug usage should be recorded for the benefit of other physicians and health professionals who may become involved with the case.[5]

*Self-Medication Schedules.* When asked by the pharmacist if they ever failed to consume prescription drugs as prescribed, 23 patients reported a history of missing doses (see Table 1). Comments such as, "Sometimes I forget," "When I run out I usually get a refill in a day or two," "I stop taking them when I start to feel better" or "I cannot afford the medicine" were not uncommon. One female reported she failed to take her oral contraceptive for four days in the midst of the 20 tablet cycle. One study revealed an epileptic patient who did not take his Dilantin and phenobarbital until he "got bad."[5]

Many patients are much too casual about taking drugs. At one extreme are individuals who consume drugs in excess. An example of excessive ingestion was revealed by a 19-year-old, unmarried student nurse presenting with severe iron deficiency anemia, excessive menstrual flow and symptoms of endometrial adenocarcinoma. By chance the physician asked about medication she was consuming and discovered that she had been taking six oral contraceptive tablets per day for three of every four weeks over a period of 20 months. This was done to "guarantee" conception control![6] At the other extreme are patients who abandon their drug therapy regimen for a variety of reasons. Drug defaulting by the drug-consuming public is a tremendous public health problem that has not received the attention it warrants. It is most common for chronically ill patients such as those with rheumatic fever, tuberculosis, diabetes, ulcers, psychiatric disorders, and so forth, to default.[7] It has been estimated that only two-thirds of 6,000 patients on drug therapy and under the care of the Tuberculosis Control Section of the Philadelphia Department of Health take their medication properly.[8] In addition, reports of patients from lower socioeconomic levels selling their drugs or leaving them on buses are not uncommon.[1]

Clearly, there is a great need for some health professional, logically the pharmacist, to vigorously counsel patients on their particular drug therapy regimen, emphasizing the actions of the drugs, why and how the physician's instructions should be carefully followed, and the importance of acquiring refills as prescribed.[9]

*Consumption of Another Individual's Prescription Drugs.* In this study, nine (15.5%) of the patients interviewed by the pharmacist revealed a history of occasionally taking someone else's prescription drugs. This question was not asked of the patient by any physician as evidenced by no documentation in the charts. Through malinformed self-diagnosis based on symptoms that resembled those under treatment in other individuals, patients have reported the consumption of a friend's or relative's "nerve pills," sedatives, digitalis for lower back pain, pink pain pills for headache, green water pills for fluid, diet pills for stimulation, and amitriptyline HCl, 10 mg, to make the patient "feel better."[5] Obviously these patients were not aware of the specificity, toxicity and interaction potential of pharmaceuticals. The pharmacist, once again, is the individual best suited by education, training and practice locus to fulfill this public education function. Failure to fulfill this function is a default of professional responsibility.

*Nonprescription Medication Consumption.* While nonprescription medications are potential sources of drug-drug interactions, adverse drug reactions and iatrogenic disorders, it is significant that only two chart entries concerning prior nonprescription drug usage were recorded by physicians. In sharp contrast, the pharmacist determined that the 58 patients in this study regularly consumed 237 nonprescription drugs during the past year (see Table 1). This represents an average regular consumption of 4.1 drugs per patient. One patient consumed 14 nonlegend drugs at regular intervals. Many of these proprietary medications were flagrantly misused and abused, laxatives being the most commonly abused nonprescription drug, followed closely by aspirin. In many instances it was quite obvious that patients do not consider proprietary medications as drugs.

One particular patient, hospitalized with congestive heart failure, correlated his regular ingestion of Alka-seltzer with swelling in his ankles. The interview revealed that his genuine respect for the potency, specificity and toxicity of prescription drugs did not apply to nonprescription medication. As a result, he allowed Alka-seltzer, with a sodium content of 532 mg per tablet, to complicate his primary disease state.

Aspirin was seen to produce varying degrees of nephropathy, complicate a peptic ulcer and prolong bleeding time in patients consuming anticoagulants.

Also of great importance is the fact that many proprietary products are of questionable efficacy. At the least, they are expensive, but more importantly, their use may delay a person from seeking appropriate medical attention. The consumer is continuously victimized by Madison Avenue marketing practices which extol the virtues of a particular panacea, while never mentioning a word about contraindications or side effects.

The time is long overdue for the pharmacist to project himself into the role of a nonbiased health educator-at-large, informing and protecting drug conscience people from their own misinformation relative to nonprescription medications.[1]

*Alcohol Consumption.* Finally, the pharmacist should inquire into the patient's alcohol consumption pattern as alcohol ingestion and concurrent drug therapy may be the source of significant problems for the patient. Guidelines as to what degree of alcohol consumption constitutes a light, moderate or heavy drinker should be set since arbitrary assignment of these terms are of little use.

## Conclusion

Data such as those presented here point out quite vividly the need to acquire a comprehensive medication history and to properly counsel hospitalized patients at discharge and ambulatory outpatients regarding their drug therapy. If the physician does not have the time or inclination to acquire a thorough medication history, he certainly cannot be expected to thoroughly counsel patients regarding proper use of all drugs. The burden, then, is upon the pharmacist to educate and advise the public in drug therapy related matters.

In addition to monitoring drug therapy of inpatients and outpatients via the patient drug profile it is our contention that the pharmacist should generally make the patient aware of the following points upon dispensing a prescription:[10,11]

1. For whom the medication is intended
2. The intended therapeutic use of the medication
3. The name of the medication
4. How to use the medication
5. When to use the medication
6. How long to use the medication
7. Maximum daily dose
8. Side effects
9. What to avoid
10. Storage
11. Miscellaneous auxiliary instructions.

The entire efforts of the health care team become futile if the patient fails to take his medication correctly while at home. The pharmacist, through oral and written communication, can and must do more toward decreasing confusion and increasing the reliability of the self-medicating public. Increased clinical activity by the pharmacist in the acquisition of medication histories and the counseling of patients must occur in order to improve patient care and hasten the evolution of the pharmacist's appropriate professional identity.

## References

1. Covington, T. R.: Interviewing and Advising the Patient, *In* Francke, D. E. and Whitney, H. A. K. (ed.): Perspectives in Clinical Pharmacy, 1st ed., Hamilton Press, 1972.

2. Zinner, N. R.: Clean Inside and Out (Correspondence), *New Engl. J. Med. 281:*853, 1969.

3. Wilson, R. S. and Kabat, H. F.: Pharmacist Initiated Patient Drug Histories In *Clinical Pharmacy Sourcebook,* pp. 346-350.

4. Yim, M. K.: Drug Hypersensitivities of Hospitalized Patients, Thesis for Master of Science in hospital pharmacy at Jefferson Medical College Hospital (May) 1967.

5. Covington, T. R. and Whitney, H. A. K.: Patient Pharmacist Communication Techniques, *Drug Intel. Clin. Pharm. 5:*370-376 (Nov.) 1971.

6. Symmers, W. S.: Curiosa and Exotica—How Many Have You Been Taking?, *Brit. Med. J. 4:*767 (Dec. 26) 1970.

7. Roth, H. P. et al.: Measuring Intake of a Prescribed Medication, *Clin. Pharmacol. Ther. 11:*228-237 (Mar.-Apr.) 1970.

8. Anon.: Deja Vue (Editorial), *Arch. Envir. Health 20:*449 (Apr.) 1970.

9. Anon.: Keep on Taking the Tablets . . ., *Lancet 2:*195-196 (July 25) 1970.

10. Brands, A. J.: Complete Directions for Prescription Medication, *J. Amer. Pharm. Ass. NS 7:*634-635 (Dec.) 1967.

11. Vreugdenhil, P. P.: Patient, Pharmacist, Physician, Prescription, *Can. Pharm. J. 9:*18-21 (Jan.) 1970.

# 61 Pharmacist-physician Drug Consultations in a Community Hospital

Gerald G. Briggs and William E. Smith

Data on pharmacist-physician drug information consultations in a 680-bed community hospital were collected over a three-month period and analyzed.

Analysis included the number of consultations, the type of physician using the pharmacist for drug information, the type of consultation, the drug class involved in consultation, the number of consultations involving actual or potential drug therapy problems, and physician acceptance of pharmacist recommendations. Consultations averaged 32 per day, mostly with private physicians, and usually involved the dose or schedule of a drug. The greatest number of consultations involving a single drug class occurred for anti-infectives. More consultations were initiated by pharmacists for potential drug therapy problems than for actual problems, but the frequencies of physician-initiated consultations in the two categories were similar. Physicians usually accepted the pharmacist's recommendations on drug therapy.

The data provide a baseline for future comparisons and will aid in the design of studies to identify the patient benefits of the pharmacist's clinical practice.

Memorial Hospital Medical Center of Long Beach is a 680-bed community teaching medical center. Pharmacy services were decentralized in 1968 and now include six satellite pharmacy units serving the fifth, fourth, third and second floors, the minimal care unit and Children's Hospital. An outpatient pharmacy is located on the main floor of the hospital. Excluding pharmacists in administrative positions, 19 pharmacists provide 24-hour, seven-day-a-week pharmacy services. One pharmacist per shift is assigned to each pharmacy unit between the hours of 7:30 a.m. and 12 midnight. One pharmacist services the entire medical center from 12 midnight to 7:30 a.m. The medical staff is composed of 550 private physicians of whom approximately 240 actively practice at the Center. In addition, Memorial Hospital Medical Center has an intern and resident program of 40 physicians. Medical, nursing and pharmacy students also receive training at Memorial.

The clinical involvement of the pharmacist in patient care is a major departure from pharmacy's traditional and relatively passive role of drug distribution on the health care team. Pharmacists are often placed in patient care areas and given two major responsibilities: drug distribution and drug consultation. Of the two, his primary function has historically been drug distribution. However, as pharmacy technicians are trained to perform distribution tasks, the pharmacist should find an increasing amount of time available for drug consultation.

Drug consultation is defined in this report as the flow of drug information from the pharmacist to other members of the health care team or the patient. The purpose of this information flow is to minimize drug therapy problems and, thereby, to improve patient care. The pharmacist as an interpreter of the myriad of drug information available today for the physician, the nurse, and the patient may be depicted as shown in Figure 1.

Historically, the physician, and to a certain extent the nurse, have acted as their own interpreters in correlating the drug literature with their clinical experience (pathways A, A', B and B', Figure 1). This role was satisfactory in the past due to the relative lack of drug information. Today, the physician and the nurse still rely to a major degree on their clinical experience (pathways A' and B') in their respective roles of prescribing and administering drugs. However, the input into the systems, pathways A and B, becomes less desirable as the com-

Figure 1. *Flow of drug information, showing the pharmacist as an interpreter of drug literature for the physician, nurse and patient*

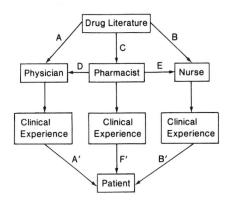

355

plexity of drug knowledge and drug utilization increases. Consequently, the pharmacist's input, pathways D, E and F′, resulting from his knowledge of the drug literature and his clinical experience, could be a significant factor in assuring that the patient receives the best possible drug therapy.

The past several years have seen a proliferation of information pertaining to drug-drug interactions, known or predicted adverse effects, drug-laboratory test interferences, drug-cost comparisons, drug metabolism-excretion-distribution and mechanism, posology, etc. There is apparently no convenient and effective method whereby a physician or a nurse may readily have access to these data. The need for someone such as a pharmacist in clinical practice to provide this information in a usable form for the physician's and nurse's evaluation is readily apparent.

A survey of the drug consultation activity of the clinical pharmacy services at Memorial Hospital Medical Center of Long Beach (MHMC) was conducted during 1971. All consultations between physicians and pharmacists occurring over a 93-day period were recorded and analyzed. Consultations occurring through the drug information service at the Center were excluded.

## Collection of Data

A data collection form was designed to enable the pharmacist to record relevant information on all consultations during the data collection period. The drug information consultation report form is shown in Figure 2. A description of the form is provided in Appendix A.

The objective of the survey was to clarify six different aspects of the pharmacist-physician drug consultation activity at Memorial Hospital Medical Center:

1. Number of consultations and the types of physicians using pharmacists for drug information
2. Types of consultation
3. Drug classes occurring in consultations
4. Number of consultations involving potential drug therapy problems
5. Number of consultations involving actual drug therapy problems
6. Number of recommendations made by pharmacists and accepted by physicians.

## Number of Consultations and Physician Types

Data on 2,933 consultations were collected over the 93-day study period, an average of 32 per day, 81% of which dealt with specific patients. Of the total number, private physicians were involved in 58% (1,701) and residents-interns in 42% (1,232), corresponding to daily averages of 18.3 and 13.2, respectively. Table 1 shows the mean number of consultations per day by physician-initiated and pharmacist-initiated classification.

The private physician total was further analyzed to determine the division of consultations by physician specialty. In Table 2, the specialties appearing most often

Figure 2. Drug information consultation report form

are shown. The surgery and medical disciplines accounted for 72% of the private physician-pharmacist drug consultations.

The actual composition of the active medical staff is not known since this group varies from time to time. About 550 private physicians have staff privileges at Memorial Hospital Medical Center, and of this number, approximately 200 are surgeons and 100 are internal medicine specialists. During the survey period, internal medicine specialists were involved in almost twice as many consultations per physician as were surgeons.

The ratio of active private physicians to residents and interns at Memorial Hospital Medical Center was on the order of 6 to 1 (240 to 40), but the ratio of drug consultations in which each group participated with pharmacists was 1.4 to 1 (1701 to 1232). The average number of consultations per private physician was seven (1701/240) and per resident-intern, 31 (1232/40). This suggests that house staff physicians with less experience and clinical knowledge need more drug information than private

## Table 1. Mean Number of Consultations Per Day According to Initiator of Consultation and Physician Type

| INITIATOR | PRIVATE PHYSICIANS | RESIDENTS AND IN-TERNS | ALL PHYSI-CIANS |
|---|---|---|---|
| Physician | 11.0 | 8.7 | 19.8 |
| Pharmacist | 7.3 | 4.5 | 11.8 |
| Mean Number/Day | 18.3 | 13.2 | 31.6 |

## Table 2. Percent of Consultations by Private Physician Specialty[a]

| SPECIALTY | % OF CONSULTATIONS |
|---|---|
| Surgeons | 38 |
| Medicine | 34 |
| General Practice | 12 |
| Ob/Gyn | 4 |
| Pediatrics | 4 |
| Miscellaneous[b] | 8 |

[a]Total number of consultations between private physicians and pharmacists: 1,701.
[b]Pathologists, radiologists, neurologists, psychiatrists and anesthesiologists.

physicians, and that they will utilize the pharmacist in clinical practice with greater frequency in respect to their absolute numbers than will their more experienced colleagues. However, house staff physicians also spend a substantially larger part of their time on duty at the Hospital and thus they are in contact with pharmacists much more than private physicians.

### Type of Consultation

Each consultation was classified according to the type of question or problem represented. Before beginning the survey, 24 categories were identified, 23 being separate and distinct types of drug information. The 24th, a "general" category, was utilized as a miscellaneous grouping. Upon completion of the survey, an attempt was made to breakdown the "general" category into additional distinct groupings, but so many types of different drug information were produced that the category was left as originally defined.

Eleven of the 23 distinct groupings produced 86% of the consultations (Table 3) with the "general" category accounting for an additional 10%. The 12 remaining types of drug information accounted for 4%. Definitions and examples of the 24 types of drug consultations are shown in Appendix B.

The most frequent type of drug information desired or offered during the survey concerned the dose or schedule of a drug. These types, plus information regarding the drug of choice for a particular disease state, occurred in almost one-half of the consultations for both private physicians and house staff members.

As shown in Table 4, physicians of both types initiated the consultations for these types of drug information an average of 60–66% of the time. The question posed by the data is whether physicians are lacking available reference sources for these particular information needs or whether they are utilizing the pharmacist because he is readily available to them. Based on an examination of the types of questions asked by physicians and the number of reference books available to them at each nursing core station, the answer seems most likely to be the pharmacist's availability.

Tables 3 and 4 provide other insights into drug information needs. Consultations involving drug-drug interactions, drug interference with laboratory tests and drug

## Table 3. Classification of Drug Consultations According to Physician Type

| CONSULTATION CLASSIFICATION | ALL PHYSICIANS NO. | ALL PHYSICIANS % | PRIVATE PHYSICIANS NO. | PRIVATE PHYSICIANS % | RESIDENTS AND INTERNS NO. | RESIDENTS AND INTERNS %[a] |
|---|---|---|---|---|---|---|
| (All types) | 2933 | 100 | 1701 | 100 | 1232 | 100 |
| Dose schedule | 819 | 28 | 421 | 25 | 398 | 32 |
| Drug of choice | 528 | 18 | 306 | 18 | 222 | 18 |
| Drug availability | 310 | 11 | 232 | 14 | 78 | 6 |
| Toxicity (adverse reaction) | 282 | 10 | 186 | 11 | 96 | 8 |
| Identification | 121 | 4 | 65 | 4 | 56 | 5 |
| Toxicity (overdose) | 119 | 4 | 62 | 4 | 57 | 5 |
| Method of administration | 85 | 3 | 50 | 3 | 35 | 3 |
| Drug-lab test interference | 76 | 2 | 50 | 3 | 26 | 2 |
| Comparison | 68 | 2 | 38 | 2 | 30 | 2 |
| Drug-drug interaction | 49 | 2 | 31 | 2 | 18 | 1 |
| Stability/ incompatibility | 48 | 2 | 35 | 2 | 13 | 1 |
| General | 306 | 10 | 159 | 9 | 147 | 12 |
| (Subtotal) | 2811 | 96[b] | 1635 | 96 | 1176 | 95 |

[a]Percent of total number of consultations for each physician group.
[b]Twelve other types of drug information accounted for the remaining 4% of total consultations.

stability or incompatibility were few in number, totaling only 49, 76 and 48, respectively. These low frequencies could imply lack of awareness by both physicians and pharmacists, but more likely, reflect both knowledgeable prescribing and immaturity of these aspects of pharmacological knowledge.

### Classification of Drugs Covered in Consultations

Most consultations collected during the survey dealt with a specific drug or drugs. However, 107 (4%) were concerned with laboratory tests, intravenous administra-

## Table 4. Percent of Drug Consultation Types Initiated by Physicians

| CONSULTATION CLASSIFICATION | PRIVATE PHYSICIAN TOTAL NO. | PRIVATE PHYSICIAN % PHYSICIAN INITIATED | RESIDENTS AND INTERNS TOTAL NO. | RESIDENTS AND INTERNS % PHYSICIAN INITIATED |
|---|---|---|---|---|
| (All Types) | 1701 | 60 | 1232 | 66 |
| Dose/schedule | 421 | 65 | 398 | 69 |
| Drug of choice | 306 | 60 | 222 | 69 |
| Drug availability | 232 | 69 | 78 | 68 |
| Toxicity (adverse reaction) | 186 | 51 | 96 | 60 |
| Identification | 65 | 98 | 56 | 98 |
| Toxicity (overdose) | 62 | 12 | 57 | 28 |
| Method of administration | 50 | 66 | 35 | 69 |
| Drug-lab test interference | 50 | 30 | 26 | 35 |
| Comparison | 38 | 91 | 30 | 100 |
| Drug-drug interaction | 31 | 37 | 18 | 44 |
| Stability/incompatibility | 35 | 77 | 13 | 92 |
| General | 159 | 72 | 147 | 81 |

**Table 5. Classes of Drugs Involved in Consultations According to Physician Type**

| DRUG CLASSIFICATION | ALL PHYSICIANS | | PRIVATE PHYSICIANS | | RESIDENTS AND INTERNS | |
|---|---|---|---|---|---|---|
| | NO. | % | NO. | % | NO. | % |
| (All drugs) | 2826 | 100 | 1639 | 100 | 1187 | 100 |
| Anti-infective | 726 | 26 | 469 | 29 | 257 | 22 |
| Central nervous system | 546 | 19 | 324 | 20 | 222 | 19 |
| Electrolytic, caloric, water balance | 385 | 14 | 198 | 12 | 187 | 16 |
| Blood formation and coagulation | 262 | 9 | 164 | 10 | 98 | 8 |
| Cardiovascular | 194 | 7 | 79 | 5 | 115 | 10 |
| Hormones and synthetic substitutes | 181 | 6 | 89 | 5 | 92 | 8 |
| Autonomic | 125 | 4 | 72 | 4 | 53 | 4 |
| Gastrointestinal | 106 | 4 | 55 | 3 | 51 | 4 |
| Vitamins | 85 | 3 | 65 | 4 | 20 | 2 |
| Antineoplastic | 45 | 2 | 32 | 2 | 13 | 1 |
| Expectorants and cough preparations | 44 | 2 | 19 | 1 | 25 | 2 |
| (Subtotal) | 2699 | 96[a] | 1566 | 96 | 1133 | 95 |

[a] Only the top eleven classifications are shown.

tion equipment or other items which could not be classified in this section. The drugs involved in consultations were classified according to the *American Hospital Formulary Service* of the American Society of Hospital Pharmacists.

Three drug categories account for 59% of the consultations as shown in Table 5: anti-infective, central nervous system, and electrolytic, caloric and water balance agents. In general, the relative frequencies of the classifications were similar for the two physician groups and reflected the usage of these agents at Memorial Hospital Medical Center as measured by doses administered.

**Drug Therapy Problems**

*Potential Problems.* In clinical pharmacy services, many drug information consultations should relate to potential drug therapy problems. The study criteria for the definition of a potential drug therapy problem required two things: (1) consultation for a specific patient and (2) a change in therapy to prevent a drug complication. Table 6 represents the application of these criteria to consultations between pharmacists and physicians.

*Actual Problems.* Although a basic function of the patient monitoring pharmacy service may be to minimize drug therapy problems, adverse drug reactions will and do occur. Consequently, criteria were established for consultations involving actual drug therapy problems:

The consultation had to be patient specific, and the individual initiating the consultation had to believe that a drug therapy problem existed and that an alteration of the drug regimen was necessary to eliminate the problem. In Table 7, data are presented which resulted from the application of this definition.

As shown by both sets of data, pharmacists were more inclined than physicians to initiate consultations over what they considered to be potential or actual drug therapy problems, 40% vs. 6% in one case, 16% vs. 6% in the other case. At least four explanations can be offered in interpretation of these data.

First, physicians do not always contact a pharmacist when a drug therapy problem exists or could exist. When the physician recognizes a problem, either potential or actual, and he has the knowledge to eliminate it, he will do so without consulting anyone. If he lacks the specific knowledge to remedy the situation, he will consult a reference source which may or may not be a pharmacist. On the other hand, the pharmacist upon recognition of a drug therapy problem must take this knowledge to the physician because there is no one else, excluding the nurse, to whom he can go. The instances which can be handled by pharmacist-nurse consultations, such as preventing drug-drug interactions by alteration of the dosing schedule, are relatively few (based on data collected during the study but not shown in this chapter). Further, our pharmacists are focusing their total clinical efforts on the elimination of drug therapy compli-

**Table 6. Consultations Involving Potential Drug Therapy Problems According to Initiator of Consultation and Physician Type[a]**

| INITIATOR | PRIVATE PHYSICIAN | | RESIDENTS AND INTERNS | | TOTAL | |
|---|---|---|---|---|---|---|
| | NO. | % | NO. | % | NO. | % |
| Physician | 56 | 5 | 52 | 6 | 108 | 6 |
| Pharmacist | 253 | 37 | 182 | 43 | 435 | 40 |
| Total | 309 | 18 | 234 | 19 | | |

[a]Total consultation for private physicians—1,701; for residents and interns—1,232.

**Table 7. Consultations Involving Actual Drug Therapy Problems According to Initiator of Consultation and Physician Type[a]**

| INITIATOR | PRIVATE PHYSICIAN | | RESIDENTS AND INTERNS | | TOTAL | |
|---|---|---|---|---|---|---|
| | NO. | % | NO. | % | NO. | % |
| Physician | 51 | 5 | 68 | 8 | 119 | 6 |
| Pharmacist | 118 | 17 | 56 | 13 | 174 | 16 |
| Total | 169 | 10 | 124 | 10 | | |

[a]Total consultation for private physicians—1701; for residents and interns—1,232.

cations, perhaps more so than physicians. A basic function of clinical pharmacy practice is to search out drug therapy problems, preferably before they occur, and bring this information to the attention of the physician for his evaluation and subsequent action. Finally, pharmacists and physicians may very well differ on what constitutes a drug therapy problem. What may be considered by the pharmacist as a problem requiring resolution may be dismissed by the physician as a necessary complication in reaching the ultimate therapeutic goal.

### Acceptance of Recommendations

About four of ten drug consultations involved a recommendation by the pharmacist. In some cases, the recommendation was to make no change when the physician was considering a change. In other cases, the advice was to alter the therapy then in existence or contemplated. The recommendations occurred for both physician-initiated and pharmacist-initiated consultations and involved most of the consultation types. Once a recommendation was made, it could be either accepted or rejected by the physician. The responsibility for deciding the status of a recommendation was left with the pharmacist recording the consultation. No attempt was made by the authors to verify affirmative replies by observing changes in the medical chart corresponding to the recommendation. However, all pharmacists participating in the survey were requested to verify the result of their recommendations by that method. Studies are planned in the future to identify the patient care results from drug consultation services.

Table 8 illustrates that recommendations made by pharmacists concerning a patient's drug therapy were usually accepted by physicians. Of the 1163 recommendations made, 1026 or 88%, were recorded as accepted. This high acceptance rate is an indication of the physician-pharmacist relationship that exists at Memorial Hospital Medical Center.

### Conclusion

The information collected in this survey provides a measure of the drug consultation efforts of pharmacists assigned to patient care areas at Memorial Hospital Medical Center. It demonstrates that our pharmacists in

clinical practice are utilized by private, resident and intern physicians with the degree of utilization weighted toward the latter two types of physicians. A physician training program is a definite asset for a pharmacy service encompassing drug consultations as one of its primary goals, but it is not a requirement for such a service.

The basic type of information exchanged between physicians and pharmacists concerned dosage and scheduling, or both, and the drug of choice for a particular disease state. Areas of recent major interest to health professionals such as adverse drug interactions and drug interference with laboratory tests were low in frequency. Assuming these subjects are as important as is generally considered, an opportunity exists for the pharmacy staff at Memorial Hospital Medical Center to improve patient care by expanding its efforts in these fields and communicating this knowledge to the physician.

Drug classifications corresponding to high prescribing habits of physicians at Memorial Hospital were also found to correspond to high consultation frequencies, particularly for anti-infectives, central nervous system drugs and electrolytic, caloric and water balance agents. This knowledge can be utilized for determining the direction which in-hospital training programs, pharmacy conferences and other educational programs should take.

Drug consultations related to drug therapy problems were especially emphasized by pharmacists in their contacts with physicians, accounting for over one-half of pharmacy-initiated consultations. Of all consultations between physicians and pharmacists, almost one-third could be assigned to the categories of either existing or potential drug therapy problems. The impact on patients involved in these consultations was not measured.

There seems little doubt that pharmacists are contributing to the drug therapy regimens of patients at Memorial Hospital Medical Center. This contribution in terms of frequency and type of information has been characterized. With the results of this study as a baseline, future surveys will help to establish how the drug consultation aspect of this pharmacy program is evolving. These surveys will also assist in the design of studies aimed at identifying patient benefits from pharmacists practicing in patient care areas.

### Appendix A
### Data Report Form

When a consultation was conducted, a completed drug information consultation report form contained the following data prior to analysis:

A. General
1. External—Consultations initiated by a physician and directed to the pharmacist.
2. Internal—Consultations initiated by a pharmacist, when he thought drug information was needed, and directed to a physician.
3. Rounds—Identified if consultation occurred on patient rounds.
4. Date and shift—Day and time of consultation.

**Table 8. Acceptance by Physicians of Pharmacist Recommendations to Change Drug Therapy**

| PHYSICIAN TYPE | TOTAL NO. CON-SULTA-TIONS | NO. RECOM-MENDA-TIONS | NO. AND % RECOM-MENDA-TIONS ACCEPTED | |
|---|---|---|---|---|
| Private Physician | 1701 | 695 | 600 | 86% |
| Residents and Interns | 1232 | 468 | 426 | 91% |

5. Telephone consult—Identified if consultation occurred via telephone.
6. Patient data—Identified if consultation related to a specific patient and if so, identified that patient by Memorial Hospital Medical Center number, sex, age and class of patient; abbreviations used for class of patient were:

| | |
|---|---|
| Med = Medical | Psy = Psychiatric |
| OB = Obstetrical | Sur = Surgical |
| Gyn = Gynecological | Ped = Pediatric |
| Isol = Isolation unit | ICU = Intensive medical care unit |
| ER = Emergency room/ outpatient | ISU = Intensive surgical care unit |

B. Professional Status
1. Private physician by specialty.
2. Resident physician by specialty.
3. Intern.
4. Other.
C. Information Provided
1. Verbal—Consultation by voice.
2. Written—Consultation by note or written article.
3. Information source—Source utilized if information provided was from other than personal experience.
D. Question/Problem
1. A brief resume of the question or problem with drug(s) involved but without specific patient data.
2. Actual problem—Identified if a drug therapy problem existed at the time of the consultation.
3. Potential problem—Identified if the consultation was made to prevent a drug therapy problem from occurring.
E. Answer/Recommendation
1. A brief resume of the answer or recommendation given in response to the question or problem.
2. Was change recommended?—Identified if the pharmacist suggested a change in the current or comtemplated drug therapy.
3. Accepted—Identified if the answer or recommendation was accepted.
4. Rejected—Identified if the answer or recommendation was not accepted.
F. Pharmacy—Identified the pharmacy unit to which the pharmacist was assigned at the time of consultation.

## Appendix B
## Types of Consultation

1. Dose schedule—The therapeutic dose and/or schedule of a drug.
   Examples: *External*—"What is the dose of ampicillin in this child?"
   *Internal*—"Every 8 hours for acetaminophen is inadequate for antipyresis."
2. Drug of choice—The best drug for the patient's condition under discussion.
   Examples: *External*—"Patient not responding to Arfonad, what can I use?"
   *Internal*—"Culture shows staph coag (+) which is resistant to antibiotic now being used."
3. Drug availability—The physical availability of the drug to the hospital.
   Examples: *External*—"Is Dalmane available?"
   *Internal*—"Phenergan injectable has been recalled."
4. General—A miscellaneous category.
   Examples: *External*—"Please supply me with information on procarbazine."
   *Internal*—"Would you like a review of our heparinization procedures?"

5. Toxicity (adverse reaction)—A side effect of the drug.
   Examples: *External*—"Can propylthiouracil cause agranulocytosis?"
   *Internal*—"Patient anorexic and nauseated after taking digoxin."
6. Identification question or problem relating to the identification of a drug.
   Examples: *External*—"What is the red capsule the patient was taking prior to admission?"
   *Internal*—Same as external example.
7. Toxicity (overdose)—An adverse reaction occurring from too high of a dose of the drug.
   Examples: *External*—"My patient took 150 mg Dalmane. Is that dose dangerous?"
   *Internal*—"650 mg aspirin is ten times the recommended dose for this child."
8. Method of administration—The various routes by which a drug may be given.
   Examples: *External*—"Can Keflin be given orally?"
   *Internal*—"I.M. ampicillin is not the route of choice in this patient."
9. Drug-lab test interference—A drug interfering with a laboratory test to provide misleading test results.
   Examples: *External*—No example.
   *Internal*—"Keflin will interfere with Clinitest glucose determination."
10. Comparison—Comparing two or more drugs in one or more aspects.
    Examples: *External*—"Are there any advantages of Terramycin over plain tetracycline?"
    *Internal*—"Do you think Vistaril is having similar effects for preoperative medication as Phenergan?"
11. Drug-drug interaction—Two or more drugs interacting in vivo to give a different effect from that expected if both were acting independently.
    Examples: *External*—"What is the interaction between tricyclics and sympatholytics?"
    *Internal*—"Iron and tetracycline given together will decrease the absorption of both."
12. Stability/incompatibility—A drug that is unstable or incompatible in vitro as ordered.
    Examples: *External*—"Can Aramine be mixed in D5W-LR?"
    *Internal*—"Ampicillin is not stable in intravenous solutions for 24 hours."
13. Order clarification—A physician's written order that required interpretation before implementation.
    Examples: *External*—No example.
    *Internal*—"No directions were given with your drug order."
14. Lab test—Utilized when a laboratory test was suggested or discussed (excludes "drug-lab test interference").
    Examples: *External*—"Will you explain the pharmacy study on saliva test for determining digitalis toxicity?"
    *Internal*—"Do you want daily ACT's taken?"
15. Intravenous therapy—Questions relating to intravenous therapy.
    Examples: *External*—"Will you explain the difference between the IVAC pump and the IVAC controller?"
    *Internal*—"Your patient's i.v. orders need renewal."
16. Hemogram—A patient's drug history submitted to the pathologist to aid in the interpretation of a series of blood tests.
    Examples: *External*—No example.
    *Internal*—"Written history for hemogram."
17. Drug contraindicated (disease)—Drug(s) contraindicated for use in a specific disease state.
    Examples: *External*—No example.
    *Internal*—"You ordered Darvon Compound for your patient with a bleeding gastric ulcer. The aspirin in the drug will aggravate the problem."
18. Drug contraindicated (allergy)—A drug contraindicted for a specific patient because of a previous allergic reaction.

Examples: *External*—No example.
   *Internal*—"Your patient is allergic to penicillin and ampicillin has been ordered."

19. Drug metabolism—The metabolism of a drug.
   Examples: *External*—"How are short-acting barbiturates metabolized?"
      *Internal*—No example.

20. Drug distribution—The distribution of a drug in the body.
   Examples: *External*—"Does nafcillin cross the blood-brain barrier?"
      *Internal*—No example.

21. Drug excretion—The excretion of a drug from the body.
   Examples: *External*—"Where is ampicillin excreted?"
      *Internal*—No example.

22. Drug mechanism of action—The method by which a drug exerts its effect in the body.
   Examples: *External*—"Where is site of action of Lasix?"
      *Internal*—No example.

23. Toxicity (allergic reaction)—A hypersensitivity reaction to a drug.
   Examples: *External*—"Does cross-hypersensitivity occur between Keflin and penicillin?"
      *Internal*—"Patient has rash over entire body. Gantanol most probable cause."

24. Drug cost—The cost of a drug.
   Examples: *External*—"What does our ampicillin cost?"
      *Internal*—"This antibiotic is expensive. Comparable agent which is less expensive is available."

# 62 A New Approach to Delivering Drug Information to the Physician Through a Pharmacy Consultation Program — Evaluation Methodology

J. Edward Bell, Vincent E. Bouchard, John C. South, and Sister M. Gonzales Duffy

The methodology used to evaluate a hospital clinical pharmacy program is discussed.

The primary objective of the study was to determine the extent to which the pharmacist provides drug information to the physician and to measure physician response to, and acceptance of, this information. Drug information provided by pharmacists to physicians caring for 123 surgical and 48 medical patients was studied. One set of data considered each drug information communication as an observation and included the physician's response to that communication. A second set of data considered each patient as an observation and categorized the patients with respect to the pharmacists' contribution to their care. The data for response-expected communications were analyzed statistically to determine if the physicians' responses could be related to any of the variables measured. Physicians were questioned to test the hypothesis that physician response was a direct result of information provided by the pharmacist.

The results of the study are presented in the following chapter.

During the past several years the profession of pharmacy has demonstrated increasing concern for the drug information needs of the physician. The development of pharmacy-based drug information centers represents a potential solution to the problem which the drug literature poses to the physician. Concurrently, the institutional practice of pharmacy has undergone a shift in emphasis toward clinical involvement.

The basic premise underlying the value of the drug information center concept is *not* that the pharmacist is an expert in all aspects of the clinical use of drugs. Rather, the pharmacist trained and experienced in the use of the drug literature can, when faced with a particular request, retrieve appropriate documents, interpret their contents, and apply the information to the situation which prompted the physician's question.[1]

For a drug information service to realize its maximum potential, appropriate and necessary information must be disseminated to the physician at its point of use—in the clinical areas of the hospital.[2,3] In order to call upon the resources of a drug information center the physician must first recognize his need for information. In a previous article,[4] we suggested that the need for informa-

tion is inversely proportional to the physician's awareness of that need. The pharmacist must therefore take the initiative in this regard.

The development of clinical pharmacy is predicated on the assumption that the pharmacist, in the patient care area, can disseminate drug information virtually at the patient's bedside. It is expected that the pharmacist, in addition to responsibility for drug control, will selectively communicate information to physicians when and where it is needed.[5-8] That the information be clinically relevant is a necessary corollary. In many institutions the pharmacist functions in the clinical areas of the hospital and makes a direct contribution to patient care. The provision of drug information to the professional staffs of the hospital has emerged as a major component of the pharmacist's patient-oriented services.

The pharmacy consultation program at Mercy Hospital of Pittsburgh, initiated in 1968, represents one such service and provides a formal mechanism for the communication of drug information to the physician.[4] Each patient included in the program is followed, with few exceptions, from admission to discharge. A medication history is obtained and the patient's condition evaluated with respect to drugs taken prior to admission. On a continuous basis (generally daily), the patient is monitored for drug interactions and laboratory test effects, adverse reactions (prospective and retrospective), contraindications, appropriateness of and response to therapy, and other drug-related considerations such as dosage, route of administration, and dosage schedule. The pharmacist, on an individual patient basis, provides unrequested drug information which he feels may be useful to the physician in that particular case. A form, the drug information communication sheet, is inserted in each patient's chart for this purpose. Appropriate utilization of the information is at the physician's discretion.

Verbal communications and discussion with the physician have obvious advantages and are utilized whenever possible. However, considering the nature of the patient chart and the communication function which it serves, written notes offer other advantages whether discussion has taken place or not. Consequently, the pharmacist attempts to record, if only briefly, the nature of any dialogue concerning the patient's therapy. Regardless, written notes provide a basis for independent, objective, prospective follow-up to determine utilization of the information provided. Therefore, only written communications were included in this study.

When the description of the consultation program was published[4] the service included two physicians' patients—an average census of eight to twelve. Since then the program has been expanded to several nursing units and three individual physicians with from 130 to 150 patients being actively monitored at any given time. During this expansion period a study was undertaken to characterize the pharmacists' activity. In this chapter the objectives and the methodology utilized for the study are presented and data collection and analysis are discussed. The results of the evaluation are presented in the following chapter.

## Objectives

This study was an attempt to determine the extent of the pharmacist's contribution to patient care resulting from his drug information-related activities within the context of the pharmacy consultation program at Mercy Hospital. The objectives were:

1. To determine the extent to which the pharmacist provides drug information to the physician and to measure physician response and acceptance of this information
2. To determine the scope of the information provided and to attempt to correlate various types of information with physician acceptance
3. To identify the sources of the information provided
4. To test the correlation of (1) above with certain patient physician and pharmacist variables
5. To compare acceptance of unsolicited information provided in the clinical areas with that requested by the physician from the drug information center.

The first objective was the major purpose of the study.

While the others were pursued insofar as the data allowed, they were essentially secondary to identifying pharmacist activity and physician response.

It is anticipated that information from this research will be useful in establishing the extent and value of the pharmacist's contribution to patient care as a result of his concern for the appropriate and rational use of drugs and his efforts to provide physicians with information in this regard. Additionally, identification of the necessary scope of informational resources would be useful to institutions anticipating such a service.

It is also hoped that the study will provide parameters which will define the circumstances in which the pharmacist has the greatest potential for service. These parameters might then be applied prospectively to identify patients more likely to benefit from such a program. This would provide guidelines for the implementation of similar services in institutions which may not have sufficient resources for a hospitalwide program.

Documented evidence of the pharmacist's direct contribution to patient care should encourage all hospitals and hospital pharmacists to develop clinically oriented drug information services insofar as their resources allow.

## Methodology

Barker suggested a method for evaluating the effectiveness of drug information services.[9] If a physician actually applies the information he has obtained from a drug information service to the care of his patient, some evidence of this should be documented in the patient's medical record. Depending upon the nature of the question and the reply, the physician might alter the patient's drug therapy, request laboratory tests, or make some comment or observation in the progress notes. An independent observer, with knowledge of the information provided, could then assess the value of the information to the physician. Drug information provided via a clinical pharmacy service should be amenable to analysis by the same technique.

Evaluation of unsolicited information provided by the pharmacist to the physician had several components in this study:

1. Objective prospective evaluation of information provided regarding a sample of surgical patients (surgical patient sample)
2. Objective prospective evaluation of information provided with respect to a sample of medical patients (medical patient sample)
3. Objective retrospective evaluation of the information provided from the drug information center as a result of formal consultation requests from physicians to the center
4. Subjective questionnaire assessment of the physicians' impressions of the value of the information provided via the pharmacy consultation program.

With the exception of the physician questionnnaire, the methodology proposed by Barker was utilized.

## Patient Selection

All patients admitted during a single month to the nursing units served by the program were included in the surgical patient sample. Subsequent to admission three of the 126 patients were discharged or transferred within 24 hours and were therefore disqualified. Patients transferred to these units from another patient care area were not included. For the purposes of the study a patient was considered discharged if transferred to a nursing area not served by the program although the pharmacist may have continued monitoring. Medical patients were chosen at random from two medical units in the hospital according to the same criteria applied to the surgical patients. Forty-nine medical patients were admitted to the study. One was subsequently disqualified under the 24-hour criterion.

The 123 surgical and 48 medical patients included in the study were followed and drug information was provided to their respective physicians by the assigned pharmacist.

Five pharmacists were involved in the study. It was not possible to use the same pharmacists for the surgical and medical samples. Differences exist among the pharmacists with respect to formal education and length of clinical experience (Table 1).

## Data Collection and Analysis

The drug information-related activities of the pharmacists were monitored by a pharmacist-observer. Each patient's chart was reviewed daily and two independent sets of data were collected: communication data and patient data.

## Communication Data

The first set of data considered each communication as an observation and included the physicians's response

to that communication. A communication was defined as a written note from the pharmacist to the physician which concerned one particular aspect of a patient's drug therapy. Thus, if a note consisted of two items (which may or may not have been related) to which the physician could respond independently, it was regarded as two communications.

Communications, based on the nature of the information conveyed, were classified *a priori* by the observer as to whether a response was expected on the part of the physician. The response took the form of some evidence in the patient's chart that the information had been read, accepted and utilized. For example, if salicylates were ordered for a patient who also had a history of ulcer disease, the pharmacist might suggest that a nonirritating drug be substituted or that antacids be administered concurrently. The observer would classify this as a "response-expected" communication, the expected response being either a change of analgesics or an order for an antacid. In another situation, however, a communication might convey information to the physician without suggesting that any action be taken. For example, a particular diagnostic test result may have been altered by the administration of a drug. The physician *might* respond to a communication of this nature by discontinuing the drug and repeating the test. However, this would be the exception rather than the rule. In most instances the particular result would be discounted and no further action taken. Such communications were classified as "no response-expected" and were not subsequently evaluated for physician reaction.

If a communication was recorded as response-expected, the patient's chart was reviewed for response until one of three possible results was apparent to the observer: evidence that the information was accepted and utilized by the physician *(positive response)*; evidence that the physician did not agree with the information or felt it was not applicable to the situation in question *(negative response)*; lack of any reference, explicit or implicit, to the information communicated *(no response)*. A successful communication was defined as one determined to be response-expected and to which a positive response occurred.

The following data were recorded for each communication:

1. Patient data
   a. Age
   b. Sex
   c. Number of diagnoses
   d. Length of stay to date of communication
   e. Type of hospitalization, as:
      short-term (12 days or less)
      long-term, convalescent
      long-term, intensive
   f. Number of different drugs administered in previous 24 hours
   g. Number of laboratory test results reported in previous 24 hours
2. Pharmacist (not necessarily pharmacist assigned to that patient)
3. Communication

### Table 1. Pharmacist Education and Clinical Experience

| PHARMACIST | SAMPLE | EDUCATION | CLINICAL EXPERIENCE |
|---|---|---|---|
| A | Surgical | B.S. (Pharm.) | 1.5 months |
| B | Surgical | Pharm. D. candidate | 5.5 months |
| C | Surgical | Pharm. D. | 7 months |
| D | Medical | Pharm. D. | 9 months |
| E | Medical | Pharm. D. candidate | 18 months |

a. Source of information:
  pharmacist personal knowledge, or specific reference
b. Type of information, as:
  product (e.g., dosage, route of administration)
  drug-laboratory test interference
  drug-drug interaction
  adverse reaction
  contraindication
  drug-of-choice (appropriateness of drug therapy)
c. Number of words and symbols in the communication
d. Time lapse between the event to which the information refers and the time of communication (in days)
e. Response-expected or no response-expected
f. Response, as: positive, negative, none
4. Physician data
a. Time lapse between communication and response (in days)
b. Clinical department
c. Staff level: intern, resident, attending
5. Study group: medical or surgical

The source used to obtain the information conveyed to the physician was noted by the pharmacist in each instance. Other data were collected by the observer.

A classification system was developed for the several types of information found in pharmacists' communications. For example, the patient's diuretic therapy, depending on the particular drug, may induce potassium loss. If the commnication suggested that another diuretic would therefore be more appropriate, the communication was recorded as "drug-of-choice." However, this could also be considered an adverse effect, implying corrective measures, or possibly a drug-induced laboratory test modification. Communications were therefore classified as to type with respect to the relevance of the information to the particular patient's situation.

## Patient Data

The second set of data collected considered each patient as an observation and categorized the patients with respect to the pharmacists' contribution to their care. The quantification of the effects of a service such as the pharmacy consultation program on patient care is perhaps possible under present day systems research methodology. However, such an undertaking was beyond the scope of this study. Therefore, an operational definition of "contribution to improved patient care" was employed. If at least one response-expected, positive response communication had transpired between the pharmacist and the physician, the patient was classified as "yes" with respect to improved care as a result of the information provided via the consultation program. Obviously, no potential for improved care existed if no communications were documented or if only response-expected, negative response communications occurred. If the information provided consisted of no response-expected and/or response-expected, no response communications only, the patient was recorded as "questionable."

At the time of discharge the following data were collected for each patient in the study:

1. Patient data
  a. Age
  b. Sex
  c. Number of discharge diagnoses
  d. Length of stay
  e. Type of hospitalization (as above for communication data)
  f. Total number of different drugs administered during stay
  g. Highest number of different drugs administered in a 24 hour period
  h. Total number of laboratory tests reported
  i. Number of different laboratory tests reported
2. Pharmacist assigned to that patient
3. Communications
  a. Number of independent communications
  b. Number from each source
  c. Number of each type
  d. Number response-expected
  e. Number positive response
  f. Number negative response
  g. Number no response
4. Physicians in attendance or in consultation
  a. Names
  b. Clinical department
5. Contribution to care, as: yes, no, questionable
6. Study group: medical or surgical

## Data Analysis

The data for response-expected communications were analyzed to determine if the physicians' responses could be related to any of the variables measured. Analysis of the patient data attempted to relate the variables considered to the ability of the pharmacists to directly contribute to patient care according to the operational definition. Various statistical procedures were used, each appropriate to respective portions of the analysis.

Chi square analysis was used for data presented in the form of $r \times k$ contingency tables[10] such as a table of response to communication by type of information provided. The null hypothesis was that the observed distribution did not differ significantly from a chance distribution. The $p$ value obtained indicates the probability of obtaining a value equal to or greater than Chi square ($\chi^2$) under the null hypothesis. The significance of the contingency coefficient, $C$, a measure of correlation,[11] is related to the significance of $\chi^2$.

A test of difference between arithmetic means[12] was employed when the data represented normally distributed continuous variables such as age or length of stay. The number of standard errors difference ($z$) was obtained. The value of $p$ represents the probability (two-tailed test) of obtaining a value as large or larger than the $z$ under a hypothesis of no difference between the populations from which the samples were drawn.

The Mann-Whitney U Test[13] was utilized for the analysis of continuous variables, such as numbers of drugs and tests, not assumed to be normally distributed. For large samples ($n > 20$), the sampling distribution of the statistic computed, $U$, approaches the normal distribution. A value for $z$ is therefore derived. The probability, $p$, associated with the observed value of $z$ is that for a two-tailed test under a hypothesis of no difference.

The number of standard errors difference ($z$) between two proportions[14] was computed to test for significance of difference between proportions, or percentages, such as the percentage of successful communications in the medical and surgical samples. The $p$ value derived corresponded to that derived in testing the difference between two arithmetic means.

Multiple correlation and regression analysis[15] of the patient data were undertaken in addition to employing tests of significant difference. All quantitative "patient" variables were included with the number of successful communications being the dependent variable. The unexplained residuals were analyzed with respect to qualitative variables such as assigned pharmacist and physician clinical department. Appropriate $p$ values are given for the correlation coefficient, $r$,[16] and the statistic which reflects the significance of the regression equation, $F$.[17]

## Consultations: Drug Information Center

During the study period 24 consultations were received in the Drug Information Center. Each represents a request from a physician to see a patient regarding a particular problem. After reviewing the patient's care the pharmacist, if indicated, offered written recommendations in the patient's chart.

The medical records of the 24 patients were obtained and the pharmacist's consultations reviewed. If response on the part of the physician was anticipated as a result of the consultation, the record was examined to determine if the physician had utilized the information provided or implemented the pharmacist's recommendations.

## Physician Questionnaire

While the data collected during the course of the surgical and medical patient studies might indicate an association between a communication by the pharmacist and some action by the physician, this would not necessarily demonstrate a causal relationship. A questionnaire was therefore designed to test the hypothesis that physician response was a direct result of information provided by the pharmacist (Figure 1).

The first three questions related to the physicians' impressions of the value of several types of information and his own and the pharmacists' competence to deal with various issues related to drug therapy. Questions four to eight related to the actual value of the information provided. The results of question seven (usefulness of the medication history) are not presented in this chapter.

*Figure 1. The physician questionnaire used to test the hypothesis that physician response was a direct result of information provided by the pharmacist (continued on page 367)*

*Figure 1. (continued)*

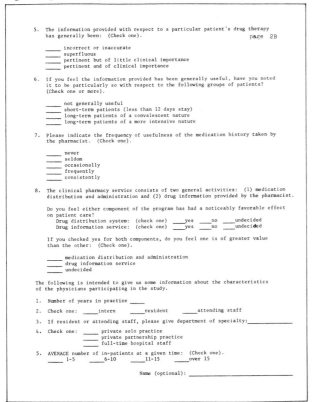

It was included to gather information for another study being conducted concurrently.[18] The last section of the questionnaire requested the physician to supply certain demographic variables.

The questionnaire was distributed to 50 physicians. The physicians selected were those involved in the care of the patients in the surgical and medical samples. Only physicians attending those patients on whom the pharmacist initiated communication were included. Table 2 shows the number of physicians in the questionnaire sample by patient group and staff level.

The patients in the surgical sample were served by a unit dose drug distribution system while the medical patients were not. Therefore two versions of question eight were used. Pages 1 and 2a were distributed to medical

sample physicians. Question eight on page 2b assured that the surgical sample physicians' attitude toward the drug information service would not be confused with their impression of the value of the distribution system. Only the results of the portion of the question related to the drug information service were included for evaluation.

A cover letter from the associate administrator of the hospital accompanied the questionnaire. Two weeks after the initial mailing a follow-up letter was sent.

Thirty-one questionnaires were returned. Five physicians explained that their experience with the clinical pharmacy service was not sufficient to allow them to answer some of the questions and returned incomplete questionnaires. Therefore, 26 replies were suitable for analysis.

The low number of negative responses to questions which could be considered the dependent variable precluded the use of regression analysis for the physician questionnaire. However, correlation coefficients were derived to attempt to associate responses among various questions.

### References

1. Anon.: The Hospital Pharmacist and Drug Information Services, *Amer. J. Hosp. Pharm.* 25: 381–382 (July) 1968.
2. Walton, C. A.: The Problem of Communicating Clinical Drug Information, *Amer. J. Hosp. Pharm.* 22: 458–463 (Aug.) 1965.
3. Canada, A. T.: Drug Information Service: Application to Immediate Patient Care, *Hosp. Pharm.* 1: 33–34, 1966.
4. Bell, J. E. et al.: A New Approach to Delivering Drug Information to the Physician Through a Pharmacy Consultation Program, *Amer. J. Hosp. Pharm.* 27: 28–37 (Jan.) 1970.
5. Canada, A. T.: The Role of the Clinical Pharmacist, *Amer. J. Pharm.* 140: 152–156 (Sept.-Oct.) 1968.
6. Rosenberg, J. M.: Mercy Hospital—St. John's Clinical Pharmacy Program, *Hosp. Pharm.* 3: 22–23 (Sept.) 1968.
7. Durant, W. J. and Zilz, D. A.: Wisconsin Information Service and Medication Distribution, *Amer. J. Hosp. Pharm.* 24: 625–631 (Nov.) 1967.
8. Smith, W. E.: The Future Role of the Hospital Pharmacist in the Patient Care Area, *Amer. J. Hosp. Pharm.* 24: 228–231 (Apr.) 1967.
9. Barker, K. N.: Role of Research in Evaluating Pharmaceutical Services in Hospitals, *Amer. J. Hosp. Pharm.* 26: 200–209 (Apr.) 1969.
10. Siegel, S.: Non-Parametric Statistics for the Behavioral Sciences, McGraw-Hill Co., New York, New York, 1956, pp. 104–111, 175–179.
11. Ibid.: pp. 196–202.
12. Spurr, W. A. and Bonini, C. P.: Statistical Analysis for Business Decisions, Richard D. Irwin, Inc., Homewood, Illinois, 1967, pp. 289–293.
13. Siegel, W.: op. cit., pp. 116–127.
14. Spurr, W. A. and Bonini, C. P.: op. cit., pp. 308–310.
15. Ibid.: pp. 589–612.
16. Edwards, A. L.: Experimental Design in Psychological Research, Holt, Rinehart and Winston, New York, New York, 1962, p. 79.
17. Ibid.: pp. 104–106.
18. La Verde, S., Doctor of Pharmacy Thesis, Duquesne University, 1970.

### Table 2. Staff Level and Patient Group of Physicians in the Questionnaire Sample

| | PATIENT GROUP | | |
|---|---|---|---|
| STAFF LEVEL | MEDICAL | SURGICAL | TOTAL |
| Attending | 12 | 14 | 26 |
| Resident | 2 | 10 | 12 |
| Intern | 6 | 6 | 12 |
| Total | 20 | 30 | 50 |

# 63 A New Approach to Delivering Drug Information to the Physician Through a Pharmacy Consultation Program — Evaluation Results

J. Edward Bell, Vincent E. Bouchard, John C. South, and Sister M. Gonzales Duffy

The results of a study which measured the frequency of pharmacists providing drug information in a clinical pharmacy service and the physicians' acceptance and utilization of the information are reported.

Other objectives of the study were to (1) characterize the type of information provided, (2) correlate patient, physician, and pharmacist variables with provision and acceptance of information, and (3) compare acceptance of unsolicited information with that of requested information.

Among the results, it was shown that, in general, physicians read, accepted, and utilized the information provided by pharmacists. The major portion of the information provided was without recourse to the literature. It appeared that a minimum period of experience may be necessary before a pharmacist can begin to function effectively in a consultation role.

One-fourth of the patients included in the study profited from the information provided by the pharmacist. The patients who benefited tended to be those who received more drugs, underwent a greater variety of laboratory tests and required longer periods of hospitalization. The physicians who found the information useful tended to be those who had been in practice longer and had a smaller inpatient service.

It is concluded that this clinical pharmacy service is an effective mechanism for the dissemination of drug information to physicians.

In two previous articles and in the preceding chapter[1,2] we have described our pharmacy consultation program and reviewed the objectives, methodology, and data collection and analysis of a study undertaken to evaluate it.

Briefly, the pharmacy consultation program is a clinical pharmacy service providing a "formal" mechanism for the dissemination of unsolicited drug information to the physician. Pharmacists, each responsible for a group of patients, monitor the patients' medication therapy and hospital course. The pharmacist provides information and offers suggestions, on an individual patient basis, via a communication sheet inserted in each patient's chart.

The primary objective of the study was to measure the frequency with which pharmacists provide information and the physicians' acceptance and utilization of this information. Additionally, we attempted to (1) characterize the type of information provided, (2) correlate pa-

tient, physician and pharmacist variables with provision and/or acceptance, and (3) compare acceptance of unsolicited information with that requested by the physician from the drug information center.

Communications were reviewed by an observer and categorized as to whether the pharmacist's note was such that some subsequent action should be taken by the physician (response-expected) or not (no response expected). If a response was anticipated (change of therapy, order laboratory test, etc.), the chart was reviewed daily until the result could be classified as positive, negative or no response. The observer also collected data concerning all communications, physicians, pharmacists and patients (whether notes were written or not) included in the study. Additionally, we sought the physicians' subjective assessment of the program and the information provided by the pharmacists via questionnaire.

This chapter presents and discusses the results of the evaluation of the pharmacy consultation program.

## Table 1. Summary of Communications, Response Classification and Physician Response

| SAMPLE | RESPONSE EXPECTED (A) | RESPONSE POSITIVE (B) | RESPONSE NEGATIVE (C) | NONE (D) | NO RE-SPONSE EXPECTED (E) | B/A × 100 | A + E N | B/N |
|---|---|---|---|---|---|---|---|---|
| Surgical (N = 123 patients) | 44 | 34 | 2 | 8 | 9 | 77% | 0.43 | 0.28 |
| Medical (N = 48) | 40 | 26 | 4 | 10 | 11 | 65% | 1.06 | 0.54 |
| Totals | 84 | 60 | 6 | 18 | 20 | | | |

### Communication Data

The communications recorded during the surgical and medical patient studies are summarized in Table 1. A total of 104 communications (A + E) were written: 84 response-expected and 20 no response-expected. The observed difference between the proportion of positive responses to response-expected communications (B/A) in the two samples was not significant ($p = 0.13$). However, the ratios of communications to patients [(A + E)/N] and response-expected, positive response communications to patients (B/N) differed considerably between the surgical and medical patient samples. This would indicate that, while there was no difference in physician acceptance in the two samples, there did appear to be variation in the amount of information provided. The increase in information, however, did not result in an increase in the number of patients classified "yes" with respect to pharmacist contribution (see below and Table 2).

The response-expected communications were divided into two groups: successful (positive response) and unsuccessful (negative and no response). The data collected regarding each communication were analyzed for significant difference between the two groups. Separate analyses were conducted for the medical sample, the surgical sample and the two groups combined, with corrections for missing data as necessary. The respective statistical tests used are shown in Table 2.

Tables 3 to 9 give the results of the analysis of each variable for the medical and surgical samples combined. No significant differences were found. Physician re-

## Table 2. Statistical Tests Utilized in the Analysis of Communication Data

| STATISTICAL TEST | VARIABLES |
|---|---|
| Difference between two arithmetic means | Age |
| Chi square[a] | Sex[b] |
| | Number of discharge diagnoses |
| | Type of hospitalization |
| | Assigned pharmacist |
| | Type of information |
| | Source of information |
| | Time lapse between event and communication[b] |
| | Time lapse between communication and response[b] |
| | Physician clinical department |
| Mann-Whitney U test | Duration of stay to date of communication |
| | Number of drugs administered in previous 24 hours |
| | Number of laboratory results reported in previous 24 hours |

[a] Application of chi square requires certain criteria regarding the expected frequencies or counts under a hypothesis of no difference. No cell may have an expected frequency less than one and not more than one-fifth of the cells less than five. In testing 2 × 2 tables only the former requirement applies. Adjacent categories may be combined in order to meet the criteria provided there is some rational basis for the combination (cf. the preceding chapter).

[b] Negative results obtained; data not presented in tables.

## Table 3. Relationship of Variables[a] to Physician Response

| VARIABLE | RESPONSE SUCCESSFUL | RESPONSE UNSUCCESSFUL | Z[b] | p[c] |
|---|---|---|---|---|
| Patient age | 58.6 | 58.1 | .15 | 0.88 |
| Length of stay to date of communication | 11.2 | 7.8 | 1.18 | 0.24 |
| Number of laboratory test results reported[d] | 3.8 | 4.1 | .50 | 0.62 |
| Number of words in the communication | 16.6 | 17.2 | .10 | 0.92 |

[a] Average value for each variable given.

[b] Number of standard errors difference.

[c] Probability of no difference.

[d] In the 24 hours previous to the communication.

**Table 4. Number of Discharge Diagnoses Related to Physician Response**

| SAMPLE | NUMBER OF DIAGNOSES | RESPONSE | | RESULTS |
|---|---|---|---|---|
| | | SUCCESSFUL | UNSUCCESSFUL | |
| Combined | 1-2 | 28 | 8 | $\chi^2 = 4.23$ |
| | 3-4 | 17 | 7 | $C = .22$ |
| | 5-6 | 7 | 7 | $.3 > p > .2$ |
| | 7-8 | 8 | 2 | |

**Table 5. Type of Hospitalization Related to Physician Response**

| TYPE OF HOSPITALIZATION | RESPONSE | | RESULTS |
|---|---|---|---|
| | SUCCESSFUL | UNSUCCESSFUL | |
| Short-term | 14 | 3 | $\chi^2 = 1.64$ |
| Long-term, convalescent | 12 | 7 | $C = .14$ |
| Long-term, intensive | 34 | 14 | $.5 > p > .3$ |

sponse was apparently not related to any of the measured variables.

Chi square analysis of communication response with respect to individual pharmacist was not possible. The data are shown in Table 6. The expected frequencies of the individual cells did not meet the criteria for chi square analysis and the only rational basis for combination of categories (pharmacists) was into medical and surgical. The resultant contingency table is a portion of Table 1 which was discussed previously.

The small expected frequencies in the contingency table relating type of information communicated to physician response did not meet the criteria for use of chi square (Table 7). As there was no rational basis for combining types of information to increase the expected frequencies, the last three categories were analyzed as a separate contingency table.

The absence of "successful" responses to drug-laboratory test interference data may be related to the greater clinical experience of the physician. A communication concerning a particular laboratory result, written by a pharmacist less experienced clinically than the physi-

**Table 6. Individual Pharmacist Communications Related to Physician Response**

| PHARMACIST | RESPONSE | |
|---|---|---|
| | SUCCESSFUL | UNSUCCESSFUL |
| A | 4 | 2 |
| B | 18 | 4 |
| C | 12 | 4 |
| D | 2 | 0 |
| E | 24 | 14 |

cian, may have anticipated a response and was therefore recorded as response-expected. However, the physician may have felt the result was "explained" by the drug and, in terms of relevance to the patient's diagnosis and condition, was not worth pursuing further as suggested by the pharmacist.

Concerning contraindications, the physician's greater experience may have taught him that many of the "contraindications" in the literature are in fact quite relative rather than absolute. Alternatively, he may have agreed

**Table 7. Type of Information Communicated Related to Physician Response**

| TYPE OF INFORMATION | RESPONSE | | RESULTS |
|---|---|---|---|
| | SUCCESSFUL | UNSUCCESSFUL | |
| Product, dosage, etc. | 5 | 1 | |
| Drug-laboratory test interference | 0 | 3 | |
| Drug interaction | 4 | 1 | |
| Adverse reaction | 29 | 10 | $\chi^2 = 4.61$ |
| Contraindication | 4 | 5 | $C = .25$ |
| Drug of choice | 18 | 4 | $p = .10$ |

**Table 8. Source of Information Communicated Related to Physician Response**

| SAMPLE | RESPONSE | SOURCE PHARMACIST KNOWLEDGE | REFERENCE MATERIAL | RESULTS |
|---|---|---|---|---|
| Combined | Successful | 43 | 17 | $\chi^2 = .04$ $C = .02$ $.9 > p > .8$ |
| | Unsuccessful | 17 | 7 | |

with the pharmacist but, in either case, concluded that the "contraindicated" drug still represented the best choice.

In order to test for difference in physician response related to the source of the pharmacists' information, the communications were grouped according to whether the pharmacist obtained the information from a specific reference or not. Those communications which were not the result of review of reference material represented communications containing information that was part of the respective pharmacist's knowledge. These represented almost three-fourths of the communications written during the two periods studied. The data and results of analysis are presented in Table 8 and indicate no difference in physician response.

Review of the individual communications revealed several "sets" each representing a group of communications containing essentially the same information. It therefore appears that once specific information has been obtained from a reference, in one situation, that knowledge becomes part of the pharmacist's "expertise" and he can successfully apply it to other situations as they develop. Essentially then, as the pharmacist gains experience, an increasing proportion of his communications would be written without recourse to reference material.

The references which were utilized by the pharmacists during the studies did not represent what could be considered an extensive collection. They consisted of *The Pharmacological Basis of Therapeutics*, the *American Hospital Formulary Service*, *Side Effects of Drugs*, the *Cecil-Loeb Textbook of Medicine*, the Iowa Drug Information Service (University of Iowa), and the drug interaction and drug-laboratory test interference tables available in the periodical literature.

Chi square analysis could not be utilized to test for difference with respect to physician clinical department. Combination of adjacent categories results in a "medical" and "surgical" grouping identical to that of Table 1. The data are presented in Table 9.

While it was not possible to associate any of the several variables with physician response, an attempt was also made to explain the difference in number of successful communications per patient (B/N, Table 1). Table 10 lists the pharmacists and the respective numbers of successful communications and assigned patients. If the number of successful communications is corrected for the number of assigned patients (40A/B) a weighted number of successful communications is obtained (column C).

Chi square analysis of column C gave $\chi^2 = 17.03$ ($p < .01$). Chi square analysis of column C for pharmacists B, C, and D showed no significant difference ($.3 > p > .2$). The observed difference in the quantity of information provided in the two samples might therefore be attributed to the activities of pharmacist A in the surgical sample and E in the medical sample. Reference to the

**Table 9. Clinical Departments Related to Physician Response**

| DEPARTMENT | RESPONSE SUCCESSFUL | UNSUCCESSFUL |
|---|---|---|
| Medicine | 27 | 14 |
| Orthopedics | 15 | 3 |
| Neurosurgery | 9 | 3 |
| General Surgery | 6 | 1 |
| Physical Medicine | 3 | 3 |

**Table 10. Pharmacists and Respective Numbers of Successful Communications Weighted to Number of Assigned Patients**

| PHARMACIST | SUCCESSFUL COMMUNICATIONS (A) | ASSIGNED PATIENTS (B) | WEIGHTED COMMUNICATIONS (C) |
|---|---|---|---|
| A | 4 | 37 | 4 |
| B | 18 | 40 | 18 |
| C | 12 | 40 | 12 |
| D | 2 | 8 | 10 |
| E | 24 | 40 | 24 |

### Table 11. Number of Patients by Clinical Sample and Pharmacist Contribution

| | CONTRIBUTION | | | | |
| SAMPLE | YES (A) | NO (B) | QUESTIONABLE (C) | TOTAL (N) | % YES[a] (A/N) |
|---|---|---|---|---|---|
| Medical | 12 | 30 | 6 | 48 | 25 |
| Surgical | 28 | 90 | 5 | 123 | 23 |
| Combined (total) | 40 | 120 | 11 | 171 | 23.4 |

[a] Data collected for subsequent studies[3] (in preparation) indicate this has risen to over 50%. We feel this has bearing on our comments regarding pharmacist experience.

pharmacists' educational and clinical experience characteristics given in the preceding chapter (Table 1) shows that A and E also represent the two extremes with respect to experience. Column C of Table 10 is not consistent with educational level.

It is reasonable to assume that the pharmacist's ability to recognize situations in which information should be provided would increase as he gained clinical experience. Pharmacist experience may therefore account for the observed difference in the numbers of successful communications in the two samples.

The effects of other variables, however, cannot be excluded. The medical and surgical samples were not matched, and in fact, showed significant differences ($p$'s all < .01) in age, number of discharge diagnoses, length of stay, number of different drugs administered, highest number of drugs in a 24-hour period, total number of laboratory tests and number of different laboratory tests. The effects of these variables are considered in the regression analysis of the patient data. Additionally, there may be differences in other factors not considered in this study or an inherent difference in the drug therapy between patients designated as "medical" and "surgical."

### Patient Data

Classification according to pharmacist contribution of the patients in the medical and surgical samples is shown in Table 11. The percentage of patients classified "yes" was approximately the same for both groups.

Analysis of the data collected for each patient showed several significant differences with respect to the "yes" and "no" groups. Patients classified as "questionable" were excluded. As with the communication data, surgical and medical groups were analyzed separately and as a combined sample. Again, the values given are for the combined sample. The various statistical tests used are given in Table 12.

### Age

The results of the analysis of the first variable, age, with respect to pharmacist contribution are shown in

Table 13. The results indicated a significant difference in patient age between the "yes" and "no" groups in the combined sample. The data revealed a tendency for pharmacist contribution to the care of older patients. While the differences in the medical and surgical samples separately were not significant at the 0.05 level, a consistently higher average age was obtained for the yes group.

### Number of Discharge Diagnoses

The surgical and medical samples could not be analyzed for difference with respect to number of diagnoses. The expected frequencies under the null hypothesis did not meet the criteria for use of chi square, and combining adjacent categories gave results not significant at the 0.05 level. The data and the results for the combined sample were significant and are given in Table 14. The patients in the study sample with higher numbers of diagnoses tended to be those for whom the pharmacist was able to make a contribution.

### Table 12. Statistical Tests Utilized in the Analysis of Patient Data

| STATISTICAL TEST | VARIABLES |
|---|---|
| Difference between two arithmetic means | Age<br>Length of Stay |
| Chi square | Sex[a]<br>Number of discharge diagnoses<br>Type of hospitalization<br>Assigned pharmacist[a]<br>Physician clinical department[a] |
| Mann-Whitney U test | Total number of different drugs administered<br>Highest number of drugs in a 24 hour period<br>Total number of laboratory test results reported<br>Total number of different laboratory test results reported |

[a] Negative results obtained; data not presented in tables.

## Table 13. Relationship of Variables[a] to Pharmacist Contribution

| VARIABLE | CONTRIBUTION | | $Z$[b] | $p$[c] |
|---|---|---|---|---|
| | YES | NO | | |
| Patient age | 56.1 | 49.1 | 2.44 | .015 |
| Length of stay | 21.7 | 9.8 | 4.63 | <.000006 |
| Total number of different drugs | 11.9 | 6.1 | 5.77 | <.000006 |
| Highest number of drugs in 24 hours | 5.9 | 4.2 | 4.36 | <.000006 |
| Total number of laboratory tests | 45.7 | 14.7 | 4.30 | <.000006 |
| Number of different laboratory tests | 16.1 | 9.5 | 4.33 | <.000006 |

[a] Average value for each variable given.
[b] Number of standard errors difference.
[c] Probability of no difference.

### Length of Stay

The data demonstrated a significant relationship between pharmacist contribution and length of hospitalization. As presented in Table 13, the average length of stay for the yes group was at least twice that of the no group. It might therefore be surmised that a longer hospital stay increases the probability that a patient will be included in the group for which the pharmacist makes a contribution.

### Type of Hospitalization

Classification of patients according to type of hospitalization serves, in this study, to separate patients with a longer than average stay into two groups: those of a convalescent nature and those requiring intensive management. Patients with average or less than average duration of stay were considered as a single class: short-term. Analysis of pharmacist contribution with respect to type of hospitalization is shown in Table 15.

Visual inspection of the data indicates the difference lies in a greater proportion of the long-term patients being included in the yes group than the short-term patients. Chi square analysis showed that the difference between the long-term convalescent and long-term intensive patients was not significant. This tends to support the relationship between length of stay and phar-

macist contribution. However, these results further indicate that the association is not dependent on the general intensity of care. Patients with a greater than average stay tended to be those for whom the pharmacist made a contribution, whether designated "convalescent" or "intensive."

### Numbers of Drugs and Laboratory Tests

Analysis of the patient data for total number of different drugs administered, highest number of different drugs administered in a 24-hour period, total number of laboratory test results reported and number of different laboratory test results reported gave highly significant differences with respect to the yes and no pharmacist contribution groups (Table 13). The averages given indicate that the patients in the yes group received more drugs and had a greater number and variety of laboratory analyses than patients in the no group.

Considering that the pharmacists' communications to the physicians related exclusively to the patients' drug therapy, the data would be expected to show the above results with respect to numbers of drugs. In order to successfully provide information to the physician the pharmacist must first recognize that some aspect of the patient's drug therapy warrants attention. The frequency of such situations would be expected to be a function of the number of drugs administered to the patient.

### Table 14. Number of Discharge Diagnoses Related to Pharmacist Contribution

| CONTRI-BUTION | NUMBER OF DIAGNOSES | | | | RESULTS |
|---|---|---|---|---|---|
| | 1 | 2 | 3 | 4 OR MORE | |
| Yes | 13 | 10 | 5 | 12 | $\chi^2 = 9.59$ |
| | | | | | $C = .24$ |
| No | 59 | 37 | 11 | 13 | $.05 > p > .02$ |

### Table 15. Type of Hospitalization Related to Pharmacist Contribution

| SAMPLE | TYPE OF HOSPITALIZATION | CONTRIBUTION | | RESULTS |
|---|---|---|---|---|
| | | YES | NO | |
| Combined | Short-term | 13 | 87 | $\chi^2 = 22.14$ |
| | Long-term, convalescent | 10 | 17 | $C = .35$ |
| | Long-term, intensive | 17 | 16 | $p < .001$ |

Another conclusion might be that successful communication by the pharmacist would often result in a change in drug therapy, inflating the numbers of different drugs administered to the patients in the yes group. However, the difference in the means shown in Table 13 does not support this argument. If every successful communication resulted in a change of drug the average increase in number of drugs for the yes group would be only 1.5 (60 ÷ 40).

The difference in numbers of tests cannot be conclusively interpreted. The pharmacist gleans the major portion of his knowledge of the patient from the chart, rather than the physician or the patient directly. An increased number and/or variety of laboratory results would therefore increase the pharmacist's knowledge of the patient's problems and current condition. It may be speculated that this results in a greater likelihood that the pharmacist will recognize situations in which drug information should be brought to the physician's attention. The pharmacist's interpretation of laboratory results, in lieu of or in addition to information in other sections of the chart, may lead him to recognition of adverse effects, awareness of the coexistence of contraindications, judgments regarding the appropriateness of drug therapy, or recognition of the need for additional therapy.

The observed differences in numbers of laboratory tests may also be related to some other variable such as number of diagnoses (variety of tests), length of stay (number of tests) or type of hospitalization (number and/or variety of tests); all of which are significant with respect to pharmacist contribution.

## Assigned Pharmacist; Clinical Department

Analysis of the patient data for pharmacist assigned and specialty of the attending physician against pharmacist contribution did not reveal any significant differences. Data for these are not presented.

It should be recognized, in relation to the communication data and the discussion of pharmacist experience, that circumstances often necessitated that a pharmacist initiate a communication concerning a patient assigned to another pharmacist. Therefore, the data obtained were not comparable to that given in Table 6 or 10.

## Regression Analysis of Patient Data

Multiple correlation and regression analysis of the continuous patient variables (type of hospitalization excluded) was undertaken with the number of response-expected, positive response communications as the dependent variable. Table 16 lists the variables included and the correlation coefficients among the several variables. Coefficients above 0.148 are significant at the 0.05 level and those above 0.193 at the 0.01 level. The table therefore demonstrates a high degree of intercorrelation among the variables. All the coefficients are significant at $p = 0.05$ and all but three at $p = 0.01$.

The independent variable which explains the greatest proportion of the variance of the dependent variable is the first to be included in the regression equation. In successive steps the next variables to be included are the ones which will account for the greatest proportion of the variance unexplained by the variables already included. The net effect is to consider and eliminate independent variables which appear to be significantly correlated with the dependent variable but whose effect on the dependent variable is explained by correlation with another independent variable.

For example, total number of laboratory test results may, hypothetically, be purely a function of length of stay. The two variables would be highly correlated with each other. The one more highly correlated with the dependent variable would be included first; thereby accounting for the effect of the other. The mathematical assumption is that both variables are measures of the same quality or attribute. In a practical sense, neither

### Table 16. Correlation Coefficients of the Continuous Patient Variables

| VARIABLE | | X1 | X2 | X3 | X4 | X5 | X6 | X7 |
|---|---|---|---|---|---|---|---|---|
| Age | X1 | | | | | | | |
| Number of diagnoses | X2 | .3463 | | | | | | |
| Length of stay | X3 | .3621 | .3511 | | | | | |
| Total number of different drugs administered | X4 | .1980 | .3779 | .6965 | | | | |
| Highest number of drugs in a 24 hour period | X5 | .1476 | .3287 | .4685 | .8037 | | | |
| Total number of laboratory tests | X6 | .1821 | .3714 | .4830 | .5950 | .4095 | | |
| Number of different laboratory tests | X7 | .2821 | .6080 | .5396 | .6280 | .4758 | .6760 | |
| Number of response-expected, positive response communications | X8 | .1916 | .3311 | .4209 | .4338 | .2794 | .3552 | .4137 |

may be the "true" variable in the patient. Continuing with the above example, length of stay and number of laboratory test results may be significant only insofar as they reflect seriousness of illness.

The patient variables found to be significant in the regression analysis are shown in Table 17. The appropriate statistics for each step of the stepwise regression are included. $R$ is the coefficient of multiple correlation, and $R^2$ indicates the proportion of the variance in the dependent variable explained by the independent variables included at that point in the stepwise regression.

The variables found to be significantly different between the yes and no groups in the previous section (Patient Data) might then be reconsidered. While seven variables showed significant difference only three entered the regression equation at a significant level. It appears that age, number of diagnoses, highest number of drugs in a 24-hour period, and total number of laboratory tests are important statistically only because they are related (correlated) with total number of different drugs, number of different laboratory tests and length of stay.

The results of the regression analysis suggested that the pharmacists in the study tended to initiate successful communications regarding those patients receiving more drugs, undergoing a greater variety of laboratory analyses, and requiring a longer period of hospitalization. Possible explanations of these results were discussed previously. However, the results also suggested, since number of diagnoses did not enter the regression equation at a significant level, that the more important relationship may be seriousness of the patient's illness rather than multiplicity of medical problems.

The residuals (unexplained variance in the dependent variable) of the final regression equation were grouped and averaged for each pharmacist and each physician clinical department. Such a procedure would indicate if the unexplained variance in the number of response-expected, positive response communications could be related to the assigned pharmacist or the physician's clinical department.

The results did not reveal a pattern consistent with either pharmacist experience or educational level. Regarding clinical department, the results for physical medicine indicated that the pharmacist's performance

### Table 17. Results of Regression Analysis of Patient Data with Number of Response-Expected, Positive Response Communications as the Dependent Variable

| VARIABLE | $R$ | $R^2$ | $F$ | $p$ |
|---|---|---|---|---|
| Total number of different drugs | .434 | .188 | 38.95 | <.01 |
| Number of different laboratory tests | .472 | .223 | 7.44 | <.01 |
| Length of stay | .491 | .241 | 3.91 | .01 |

### Table 18. Response to Question 5: "The Information Provided ··· Has Generally Been:"

| RESPONSE | FREQUENCY |
|---|---|
| Incorrect or inaccurate | 0 |
| Superfluous | 0 |
| Pertinent but of little clinical importance | 4 |
| Pertinent and of clinical importance | 22 |

was considerably better than that expected by the significant variables in the regression analysis.

### Drug Information Center Consultations

Of the 24 formal consultations received in the drug information center, 15 were classified as response-expected. Review of the patients' records demonstrated implementation of the pharmacists' recommendations by the physician in 13 instances. The percentage of successful consultations (87%) was not significantly different than that of the unsolicited information provided via the pharmacy consultation program (71%; $p = 0.13$).

It should be noted, however, that the 13 and 24 consultations, respectively, represented those associated with approximately 30,000 patient-days of hospitalization in Mercy Hospital. The 60 successful and 104 total communications recorded in the study of the pharmacy consultation program had a service base of 2,045 patient-days. This indicated that the pharmacist, on an unsolicited basis, can successfully bring considerably more drug information to the patient's bedside than the physician would otherwise request.

### Physician Questionnaire

Tabulation of the complete questionnaires revealed a favorable attitude toward the pharmacy consultation program on the part of the physicians who responded. The responses to questions 5 and 8 are summarized in Tables 18 and 19. Apparently the physician recognizes the information provided by the pharmacist as directly responsible for appropriate action on his part.

The responses to questions 1 to 4 are tabulated in Table 20 as frequencies of each response. Zeroes are omitted. The table is in the same format as the ques-

### Table 19. Response to Question 8: "···the Drug Information Service Has a Noticeably Favorable Effect on Patient Care"

| RESPONSE | FREQUENCY |
|---|---|
| Yes | 23 |
| No | 1 |
| Undecided | 2 |

**Table 20. Frequencies of Physician Responses to Questions 1 to 4**

| QUESTION | RESPONSES[a] | | | | |
|---|---|---|---|---|---|
| | NC | LC | SC | MC | GC |
| Question 1: Importance of: | | | | | |
| Drug effects on laboratory results | | 1 | 6 | 8 | 11 |
| Drug interactions | | | 2 | 5 | 19 |
| Adverse effects of drugs | | | 3 | 4 | 19 |
| Contraindications | | | 3 | 1 | 22 |
| Choice of most appropriate drug | | | 2 | 8 | 16 |
| Question 2: Physician competence: | | | | | |
| Drug effects on laboratory results | 1 | 8 | 11 | 4 | 2 |
| Drug interactions | | 6 | 10 | 9 | 1 |
| Adverse effects of drugs | | | 9 | 10 | 7 |
| Contraindications | | | 7 | 11 | 8 |
| Choice of most appropriate drug | | | 4 | 15 | 7 |
| Question 3: Pharmacist competence: | | | | | |
| Drug effects on laboratory results | 1 | | 5 | 7 | 13 |
| Drug interactions | | | | 8 | 18 |
| Adverse effects of drugs | | | 3 | 9 | 14 |
| Contraindications | | 2 | 5 | 10 | 9 |
| Choice of most appropriate drug | 3 | 5 | 8 | 7 | 3 |
| Question 4: Information provided: | | | | | |
| Drug effects on laboratory results | 4 | 3 | 9 | 5 | 5 |
| Drug interactions | 1 | 2 | 2 | 7 | 14 |
| Adverse effects of drugs | | 1 | 9 | 12 | 4 |
| Contraindications | | 2 | 10 | 7 | 7 |
| Choice of most appropriate drug | 1 | 3 | 13 | 6 | 3 |

[a] See Figure 1 for response code.

tionnaire and legends appropriate to each question may be found in Figure 1.

Because of the high percentage of favorable responses it was not possible to characterize physicians in terms of response to questions 5 and 8. Therefore an attempt was made to relate physicians' responses to question 4 to attitudes as demonstrated in answers to questions 1, 2, and 3 and to practice characteristics. Responses to questions 1 to 4 (20 responses) were given scores from 0 to 4 (left to right). The individual scores were totaled for each question to gain an index of each physician's response. The four totals for each questionnaire and the respective number of years in practice (raw number), staff level (scored: intern = 1; resident = 2; attending = 3) and average number of inpatients (scored 1 to 4) were correlated. Table 21 lists the responses and practice variables which showed significant correlation.

The results indicated that physicians who felt the five types of information were of concern in patient care (question 1) tended to be those who believed the pharmacist was competent to provide information regarding these (question 3) and that the information provided was of import (question 4). Additionally, these physicians tended to be those with a smaller average inpatient service. It also appeared that physicians who have been in practice longer tended to have confidence in the abilities of the pharmacist.

The individual responses to question 4 (scored 0 to 4)

*Figure 1. The physician questionnaire used to test the hypothesis that physician response was a direct result of information provided by the pharmacist (continued on p. 377)*

*Figure 1. (continued)*

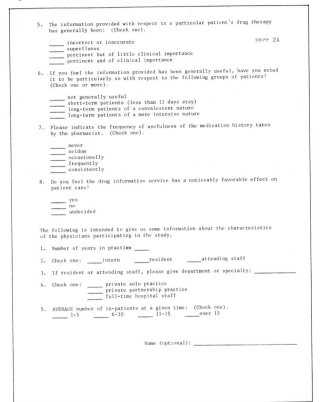

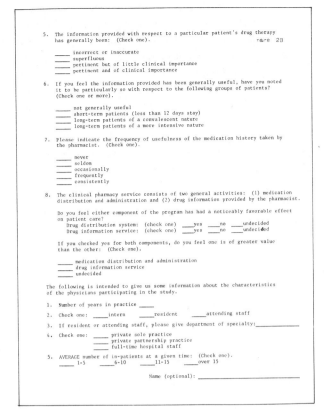

were also correlated with the individual responses to questions 1 to 3 and to the physicians' practice data. No meaningful correlations were obtained among the question responses and no significant correlations were found with the physician practice characteristics.

## Summary and Conclusions

The results of evaluation of the pharmacy consultation program indicate that the pharmacist, functioning in the clinical areas of the hospital, can successfully disseminate drug information at its point of use. In general, physicians read, accepted and utilized the information provided in the patients' charts by pharmacists and recognized the consultation program as having a favorable effect on patient care. Providing unsolicited information resulted in a considerable increase in the dissemination of clinically useful drug information and was not taken adversely by the physician.

The scope of reference material required to provide

such a service is not impressive. The references utilized by the pharmacists during the evaluation periods represented sources generally available in hospitals if not in the hospital pharmacy itself. Additionally, the major portion of the information was provided without recourse to the literature.

The ability of the pharmacist to function as a therapeutic advisor to the physician may be related to length of clinical experience. While the results are not conclusive, it appears that a minimum period of experience may be necessary before a pharmacist can begin to function effectively.

The patients most likely to benefit from continuous monitoring and provision of information when appropriate by a qualified pharmacist demonstrate certain characteristics. They tend to be those who receive a greater number of drugs, undergo a greater variety of laboratory tests and require longer periods of hospitalization than the average. Although multiplicity of diagnoses was also a significant characteristic, seriousness of illness may represent a stronger relationship.

**Table 21. Significant Correlations of Responses to Questions 1 to 4 and Practice Characteristics**

| CORRELATED VARIABLES | | CORRELATION COEFFICIENTS | p |
|---|---|---|---|
| Question 1 | Question 3 | +0.3955 | <.05 |
| Question 1 | Question 4 | +0.4477 | <.05 |
| Question 1 | Average number of inpatients | −0.3886 | <.05 |
| Question 3 | Years in practice | +0.4445 | <.05 |

One-fourth of the patients included in the study profited from information provided by the pharmacists. More communications were written per patient for medical patients. This may have been related to variation in the pharmacists involved in the respective studies.

The physicians who felt the information provided was of most practical importance tended to be those who had been in practice longer and had a smaller inpatient service. However, the preponderance of positive responses on the questionnaire indicated that physicians with opposite characteristics also regarded the service as contributing to patient care. The correlation appears to be one of degree.

Considering the quantity of communications recorded and the degree of physician acceptance, the pharmacy consultation program appears to be an effective mechanism for the dissemination of drug information to the physician.

### References

1. Bell, J. E. et al.: A New Approach to Delivering Drug Information to the Physician Through a Pharmacy Consultation Program. Part I: The Pharmacist; Part II: The Physician, *Amer. J. Hosp. Pharm. 27:* 28–37 (Jan.) 1970.

2. Bell, J. E. et al.: A New Approach to Delivering Drug Information to the Physician Through a Pharmacy Consultation Program-Evaluation Methodology, In *Clinical Pharmacy Sourcebook,* pp. 362-367.

3. Young, W. W., Doctor of Pharmacy Thesis, Duquesne University, Pittsburgh, 1972.

# 64 Physician Reaction to a Clinical Pharmacist

Harold M. Silverman and Gilbert I. Simon

After six months of a pilot program of clinical pharmacy activities, questionnaires were sent to all physicians with whom the clinical pharmacist had worked.

Of 27 house staff physicians surveyed, 17 replied. The majority of respondents indicated that the functions of the clinical pharmacist were desirable.

Over the past several years we have heard a great deal about the functions, responsibilities and training of the clinical pharmacist.[1-6] In September 1969, a clinical pharmacy program was instituted at Lenox Hill Hospital, a 576-bed, general, voluntary, community hospital serving mainly the upper east side of Manhattan, but also serving patients from throughout metropolitan New York City.

There are several groups of distinctly different individuals with whom the clinical pharmacist must interact if he is to be successful in his endeavors. As defined by the limits of our program, these groups are nurses, hospitalized patients and physicians. Our clinical pharmacist consults with the nursing staff on matters pertaining to the use and storage of drugs. Interaction between the clinical pharmacist and the patient comes at two primary points. First, at the time of admission, an interview is conducted if it is considered to be pertinent to the situation. Second, at time of discharge, the clinical pharmacist must be sure that the patient understands the directions for drugs he will be taking at home. Effective interaction between clinical pharmacist and physician is important for several reasons. First, the physician is, to date, the primary consumer of the services of our clinical pharmacist. Second, creation of a medical demand for clinical pharmacists will insure a need for these specialists within the other segments of the hospital's population. Third, most drug information provided by the clinical pharmacist is directed toward the physician.

Our clinical pharmacist performs several daily functions in satisfying the requirement for physician inter-action. He attends work rounds and teaching rounds on one of the nursing units he covers. During these rounds, cases are presented and he may either be asked questions or offer comments. He reviews all medication profiles for the patients on these floors two or three times a week. If incompatibilities are found, they are brought to the attention of the physician. At the same time, the reason behind the incompatibility is explained and alternate suggestions for therapy are made.

## Method of Study

Beginning in March 1969, questionnaires were sent to all house staff and attending staff physicians with whom the clinical pharmacist had worked. A different questionaire was sent to each type of physician (see Figures 1 and 2).

The questionnaire sent to attending staff physicians required a responding letter while the questionnaire sent to the house staff physicians merely required circling of a number under each question. The effectiveness of the two types is revealed by the returns received. Seventeen out of a possible 24 house staff physicians responded (70.8%) while only 6 out of a possible 27 of the attending staff physicians responded (22.2%).

## Results

The results obtained from house staff physicians are shown in Table 1. The rating system on the

*Figure 1. Questionnaire sent to house staff physicians*

**LENOX HILL HOSPITAL**

100 EAST 77TH STREET / NEW YORK, N. Y. 10021 / TRAFALGAR 9-8000

Dear Dr.

During the past several months, the Pharmacy Department has had an experimental program in operation in which you were involved.

Since July 1, 1969, Mr. Harold Silverman, our Clinical Pharmacist, has been making rounds on 4 East, 4 West, 5 West. He has attempted to be of service to physicians, nurses and, ultimately, the patient by providing informational services on drugs, drug products, pharmacology and toxicology.

Mr. Silverman's work is involved with an academic program offered by the College of Pharmaceutical Sciences of Columbia University leading to the Doctor of Pharmacy (Pharm.D.) degree. Within the next two years we expect that this program, and consequently the presence of Clinical Pharmacists in patient care areas, will expand to the point where we will have a large number of clinical-pharmacists-in-training at Lenox Hill.

We are interested in obtaining a written evaluation of Mr. Silverman's activities in the light of:

(a) The benefits offered by the presence of the clinical pharmacist on the nursing unit.

(b) Value of the information provided.

(c) If there were a clinical pharmacist available to you for every patient you had in the hospital, would you actively seek his services?

(d) In your opinion, does the value offered by the clinical pharmacist justify his presence?

Since this program is in the formative stages, I am vitally interested in your comments and suggestions. I hope you will take the time to reply in written form. However, should your schedule not permit this, you may dictate your answer to our pharmacy secretary.

Sincerely,

Gilbert I. Simon, Director
of Pharmacy Services

house-staff questionnaire covered a scale of 0 to 10, where 0 was the least favorable rating and 10 the most favorable. For ease of evaluation, these responses have been grouped into three larger categories. Values of 0 - 3 represent an essentially negative response. Values from 4 - 7 represent an essentially neutral to a moderately positive rating. Values from 8 - 10 represent a strongly positive or definitely favorable response.

We assumed that the pharmacist serving in the clinical capacity should have a large store of pharmaceutical knowledge, an adequate recall of therapeutic knowledge (indications, toxicities and interactions), the ability to comprehend medical terminology, and the ability to communicate verbally. Therefore, four questions specifically asking how well the clinical pharmacist rated in these areas were included. All of the responding house staff, except one, gave the clin-

*Figure 2. Questionnaire sent to attending staff physicians*

LENOX HILL HOSPITAL
PHARMACY DEPARTMENT

CLINICAL PHARMACY PROGRAM - EVALUATION SHEET

Please mark the numerical value corresponding to your opinion on each of the following questions. 10 is the highest evaluation and 0 is the lowest.

a. Ability of Clinical Pharmacist to comprehend medical terminology.

0 1 2 3 4 5 6 7 8 9 10

b. Ability of Clinical Pharmacist to communicate verbally.

0 1 2 3 4 5 6 7 8 9 10

c. Quality of pharmaceutical information provided.

0 1 2 3 4 5 6 7 8 9 10

d. Quality of therapeutic information provided.

0 1 2 3 4 5 6 7 8 9 10

e. Was the presence of the Clinical Pharmacist helpful in treating your patients?

0 1 2 3 4 5 6 7 8 9 10

f. If there was a clinical Pharmacy Service established at Lenox Hill Hospital, would you call for Clinical Pharmacy consultations?

0 1 2 3 4 5 6 7 8 9 10

g. Should there be a Clinical Pharmacist available for every hospitalized patient?

0 1 2 3 4 5 6 7 8 9 10

h. Do you feel the cost of maintaining such a service is justified by the advantages provided there in.

0 1 2 3 4 5 6 7 8 9 10

i. Should there be a similar program established in the Out Patient Department?

0 1 2 3 4 5 6 7 8 9 10

j. Should several Clinical Pharmacists be attached to the Home Care Program?

0 1 2 3 4 5 6 7 8 9 10

Signed_____ Date_____

Please list any additional comments you may have below.

ical pharmacist a strongly favorable rating on the questions referring to the abilities to comprehend the situation and verbalize his thoughts. The quality of information provided by our clinical pharmacist was rated in three questions; all responses to these questions, with the exception of five, characterized the clinical pharmacist's performance as excellent.

The next three questions were included to determine if the physical presence of the clinical pharmacist was of particular value or if the pharmacist's presence via telephone or requested consultation would suffice. We concluded from the combination of (1) a moderately favorable response to the question of how helpful the clinical pharmacist was in treating patients, (2) a

## Table 1. House Staff Physician Evaluation of the Clinical Pharmacist

| QUESTION | EVALUATION | | |
| --- | --- | --- | --- |
| | 0-3 | 4-7 | 8-10 |
| a. Comprehend medical terminology | 1 (5.9%) | — | 16 (94.1%) |
| b. Verbal communication | — | 1 (5.9%) | 16 (94.1%) |
| c. Quality of pharmaceutical information | 1 (5.9%) | 1 (5.9%) | 15 (88.2%) |
| d. Quality of therapeutic information | 1 (5.9%) | 2 (11.8%) | 14 (82.4%) |
| e. Helpful in treating patients | 1 (5.9%) | 3 (17.6%) | 13 (76.5%) |
| f. Would you request pharmacy consults | — | 4 (23.5%) | 13 (76.5%) |
| g. Should service be expanded to cover all patients | 4 (23.5%) | 5 (29.4%) | 8 (47.1%) |
| h. Is cost justified* | — | 7 (43.8%) | 9 (56.2%) |
| i. Should program be expanded to OPD | 4 (23.5%) | 5 (29.4%) | 8 (47.1%) |
| j. Should program be extended to home care services* | 7 (43.8%) | 7 (43.8%) | 2 (12.5%) |

*One medical resident replied "no opinion" to two questions.

highly favorable response to the suggestion of the establishment of a clinical consultation service and (3) a more negative response to the suggestion that the services of a clinical pharmacist be provided for all patients, that the physical presence of the clinical pharmacist was of no particular value.

It appears that in the eyes of the practitioner, the clinical pharmacist can make a definite contribution to patient care. However, his physical presence may not be required. Possibly, there should be a clinical pharmacy consultation service established in the hospital whose members would see patients only when called in by house staff to deal with a particular problem, or on their routine rounds.

The last three questions were used to see if we could define a future pathway for the extension of this service. Most respondents felt that if there was significant benefit to the patient, the cost of the clinical pharmacy program was immaterial. The questions about extension of the service to the Outpatient Department and Home Care Services revealed the following results: 47.1% felt the service should definitely be extended to the OPD, 29.4% felt the service had possibilities in the OPD and 23.5% felt the service has no place in the OPD. Only two persons felt that the services of the clinical pharmacist should be definitely extended to our Home Care program. The Home Care program is one in which professional services are provided to patients within their homes. This may involve visits by a nurse, dietician, physical therapist or social worker to follow up on problems which were treated acutely in the hospital but which also require long term, follow-up care by specifically trained professionals. The balance of responses were divided equally among the opinions that the pharmacist has no place on the Home Care Service or that he may be of some limited value to the Home Care program.

## Discussion and Conclusion

The functions of the clinical pharmacist were considered desirable by the majority of house staff physicians in our survey. If our results are compared to those of others who have attempted to provide clinical pharmacy services, we can see certain differences and similarities. Sister Emmanuel[7] reported physician reaction to the presence of senior pharmacy students in the clinical environment. The results are overwhelmingly in favor of the training of clinical pharmacy practitioners to provide improved patient services as well as more specialized services to the physician. Baily and Plein[1] reported that a clinical pharmacist was well accepted by the physicians with whom he had the opportunity to work. Smith[8] and Ginsberg and Birmingham[9] did not tabulate their results as to physician re-

sponse. However, both sources indicated a general acceptance in philosophy of the clinical pharmacists but some reluctance in their actual utilization by the physician. McLean[10] and Bosomworth and Miller[11] painted similar roles for the clinical pharmacist but ones which were molded to their particular situations.

The most important point to be kept in mind is that clinical pharmacy practice must be tailored to the individual hospital situation. The large, teaching institution may have a vastly different attitude towards the utilization of clinical pharmacists than the small, general, community hospital or the large long term care institution. In evaluating the clinical pharmacy service to be provided, one should consider the size and types of care offered by the institution in question, the size and present attitudes of medical, nursing and paramedical staffs, the availability of trained clinical pharmacists and the financial position of the institution.

We may assume that our training program, which is affiliated with the Doctor of Pharmacy Degree offered at the College of Pharmaceutical Sciences of Columbia University, provides our candidates with the proper background to do an effective job. Our results indicate that the best way for us to establish the clinical pharmacist in the hospital would be in a consulting capacity, to be called in on difficult cases and to make routine rounds with treating physicians.

## References

1. Baily, D. E. and Plein, E. M.: A Study of Clinical Pharmacy Practice in a Small Private Hospital, *Hosp. Pharm.* 5:5-14 (Aug.) 1970.
2. Kapnick, R. L. et al.: Physician's Assessments—Present and Future Pharmacy Practice, *J. Amer. Pharm. Ass.* NS10:460-465 (Aug.) 1970.
3. Ward, O., Hanan, Z. I. and Durgin, Sister J. M.: The Practice of Clinical Pharmacy in Pediatrics, *Hosp. Pharm.* 5:15, 18, 19, 22 (Aug.) 1970.
4. Hansten, P. D. and Owyang, E.: Role of the Pharmacist in Assessing the Effects of Drugs on Clinical Laboratory Results, *Amer. J. Hosp. Pharm.* 25:298 (June) 1968.
5. Provost, G. P.: A New Dimension in Pharmaceutical Education (Editorial), *Amer. J. Hosp. Pharm.* 24:349 (July) 1967.
6. Mehl, B. et al: An Experiment in Clinical Pharmacy in a Large Hospital, *Amer. J. Hosp. Pharm.* 25:631 (Nov.) 1968.
7. Sister Emmanuel: Experience With a Course in Clinical Pharmacy, Part Three: Evaluating the Course from Several Aspects, *Amer. J. Hosp. Pharm.* 26:100-113 (Feb.) 1969.
8. Smith, W. E. et al.: Clinical Pharmacy: General Hospital, *Hospitals* 44:86 (Nov. 1) 1970.
9. Ginsberg, M. P. and Birmingham, P. H.: Clinical Pharmacy: Long-term Care Institution, *Hospitals* 44:94 (Nov. 1) 1970.
10. McLean, W. M. et al.: A Trinity of Units—Patient Pharmacist and Doses, Part Two. The Patient-Unit Pharmacist, *Amer. J. Hosp. Pharm.* 26:398-403 (July) 1969.
11. Bosomworth, P. P. and Miller, W. A.: Current Trends in Medical Education and Their Impact on Pharmacy, *Amer. J. Hosp. Pharm.* 26:523-528 (Sept.) 1969.

# 65 Physicians' Attitudes Toward Clinical Pharmacy Services

J. Dennis Andrews and Anthony S. Manoguerra

Physicians' attitudes toward clinical pharmacy services were studied through questionnaires sent to 50 interns and residents who had worked with clinical pharmacists.

Sixty-six percent of the physicians responded to the 10-point questionnaire. They indicated a desire to have a pharmacist available, and they utilized him both when in the area serviced by the pharmacist and after leaving the area. The physicians also felt that pharmacists were not disadvantageous on ward rounds, provided the pharmacists gave accurate and clinically useful information (verbal answers preferred). They saw a potential role for the pharmacist in a private practice situation and said that they would utilize him in such a setting.

Clinical pharmacy services throughout the country have been established and expanded at a tremendous rate during the last several years. With the changes in pharmacy education that are occurring, we can expect that the future growth of clinical pharmacy services will be even more rapid than in the past. With these increases in new services, there is a greater need to evaluate their effect on patient care. This chapter reports the attitudes of physicians toward the clinical pharmacy services at the University of California Medical Center, San Francisco (UCSF) as determined by a survey.

Clinical pharmacy services at UCSF grew out of a satellite pharmacy established on the general surgery ward of H. C. Moffitt Hospital in 1966.[1] At that time the pharmacist was responsible for unit dose drug distribution to the ward, and attempts were made to begin clinical involvement.[2] In 1969, it was decided to centralize the unit dose drug distribution so that the pharmacist assigned to the ward would have more time for direct patient care activities. Since that time, the level of distribution responsibility has been decreased. Twenty-four-hour service is provided with this pharmacist responsible only for emergency distribution of medications. The majority of his time is now freed for clinical service and teaching and functioning as a member of the cardiopulmonary resuscitation team.

In 1970 the service was expanded to provide 16-hour coverage of one of the general medicine wards of the hospital. The pharmacy staff here does not have any drug distribution responsibility.

Clinical service to other areas of the hospital have developed on an unscheduled basis through extensions of the School of Pharmacy clinical teaching program. Senior pharmacy students and preceptors provide service to the pediatric, general medicine, pulmonary care, renal and endocrine units, and to a private medical service. These students also participate in the services on the general medicine and surgery wards. Future plans call for reorganization and further expansion of the clinical pharmacy services throughout H. C. Moffitt Hospital, University of California Hospital, and on an outpatient basis to the new ambulatory clinics building.

## The Survey

For this survey, it was necessary to define the activities involved in clinical pharmacy services. The definition chosen was that clinical pharmacy services are those services performed by a pharmacist exclusive of drug preparation and distribution that assure proper and rational drug therapy relative to the patient's disease and condition.[3] This activity consists mainly of taking admission drug histories, preparation of verbal and written consultations for the medical and nursing staffs, participation in daily ward rounds and medical staff conferences and daily monitoring of patient's drug therapy.

It was felt that the greatest impact the pharmacist has on patient care results from interpersonal relationships and information exchange between the pharmacist and medical staff. Because these relationships are difficult to document, we chose as the basis of our survey the attitude of the medical and surgical staff toward the clinical pharmacy service. A questionnaire was sent to 50 medical and surgical house staff members who had rotated through the areas serviced by pharmacists during the last two years. The physicians were not requested to identify themselves nor were the questionnaires coded in any manner. Thirty-three, or 66%, responded.

## Results

The questions and the results are listed in Table 1.

From these data we can conclude that most physicians, when exposed to clinical pharmacy services, accepted and utilized the pharmacist to provide drug information and continued to utilize the pharmacist after leaving those areas with established clinical services. Most physicians surveyed appeared to prefer the verbal

**Table 1. Results of Survey of Physicians' Attitudes Toward Clinical Pharmacy Services[a]**

1. Did you find it desirable to have a pharmacist available for consultation?
   *Yes:* 33 (100%)   *No:* 0

2. Did you utilize the pharmacist?
   *Yes:* 33 (100%)   *No:* 0

3. How do you rate the overall ability (knowledge of the pharmacist(s) with whom you worked?
   *Excellent:* 23 (71.8%) *Good:* 911 (28.8%) *Fair:* 0
   *Poor:* 0 *No response:* 1

4. Do you see a role for the pharmacist in a setting such as a private practice?
   *Yes:* 27 (87.1%)   *No:* 4 (12.9%)   *No response:* 2
   If yes, would you use the pharmacist in such a setting?
   *Yes:* 26 (100%)   *No:* 0   *No response:* 7

5. Would you have preferred written answers to your questions or did you feel that verbal responses were adequate?
   *Written:* 2 (6%)   *Verbal:* 27 (81.8%)   *Both:* 4 (12.2%)

6. Did you find the information given to you by the pharmacist to be accurate and clinically useful?
   *Yes:* 33 (100%)   *No:* 0

7. Were there any disadvantages (drawbacks) to having the pharmacist located on the wards? If yes, please explain.
   *Yes:* 2 (6.5%)   *No:* 29 (93.5%)

8. Did you utilize the pharmacist after leaving the 9th (surgery) or 10th (medicine) floors?
   *Yes:* 21 (63.6%)   *No:* 12 (26.4%)

9. Do you feel you utilized the pharmacist to a greater extent as a resident than as an intern? (If applicable.)
   *Yes:* 6 (18.2%)   *No:* 8 (24.2%)   *Same:* 1 (8%)   *Not applicable:* 18 (54.6%)

   (Questions 10 and 11 required more than yes or no answers and are discussed in the text.)

10. Please describe a specific instance in which information gained through consultation with the pharmacist helped formulate or change a proposed treatment plan.
    *Instance described:* 21 (63.6%)   *No instance described:* 12 (26.4%)

11. Please briefly describe what you see as the role of the pharmacist on the "health team" that would best meet your needs in caring for your patients. If you do not feel that the pharmacist belongs on the wards, please explain why. (Twelve physicians did not answer question 11.)

[a] Percentages listed do not include those physicians who did not answer the question.

exchange of information that occurs on a personal basis rather than formal consultations.

Two physicians stated that there were minor drawbacks to having the pharmacist on the wards. One felt that the number of personnel on rounds was too great already and that the addition of another person made the group too large for good communications. The other physician stated that because the pharmacist was easily available for consultation, a tendency developed to accept answers to questions without documentation. The first of these problems is difficult to overcome in a teaching institution. The second problem is one of personal preference, and the pharmacist should be prepared to support his recommendations with appropriate literature references, if the physician requests. No physician felt that the pharmacist did not belong on the wards.

The following is an example of a response to question 10 (which asked for a specific instance in which consultation with a pharmacist led to a formulation or change in treatment plan) given by a medical resident:

> A patient was being maintained on hemodialysis and was receiving allopurinol for asymptomatic hyperuricemia. The patient developed a fever, eosinophilia and subsequent rash. Information obtained from the pharmacist allerted the medical team to the parameters of allopurinol allergic reactions, particularly allergic vasculitis and thus helped to diagnose and assist in the management of this patient's particular problem.

Other examples included management of patients on hyperalimentation, control of intractable pain, choice of appropriate antibiotics, drug dosage in renal failure, drug side effects, drug-drug and drug-laboratory test interactions, appropriate use of cancer chemotherapeutic agents, dialyzability of drugs and others. Some physicians answered this question by stating that the situations were too numerous to choose just one.

General comments were attached to a number of questionnaires. Examples of these comments are:

1. I found the information provided by the pharmacist extremely helpful. They have ready access to information that we do not have at hand. A more general application of the ninth floor design would be to our patient's advantage.
2. Frankly, I was impressed with the fund of knowledge the pharmacists had, not only about medication, but also about diseases. I will use their advice more in the future.
3. Helpful in capacity as instant clinical pharmacology consultant. The training of the pharmacist should be more geared toward pharmacology in addition to (traditional) pharmacy. Different programs could be set up for those interested in clinical work vs. dispensing drugs.
4. Very useful and almost essential to perfect all around care of the patient.
5. One of the strong points of the University of California medical internship was the availability and constant review by the pharmacists on the ward service. They taught me a great deal.

Question 11 was included in this survey to determine the expectations of those physicians exposed to clinical pharmacy practice. What did they see as the future role of the pharmacist? Some comments follow:

1. I think that the most appropriate role for the pharmacist would be as a member of the ward team. Many more drugs tend to be used on an inpatient basis and therapy is often much more intense than on an outpatient basis. The pharmacist should (a) make ward rounds with the physicians, (b) be actively critical of all therapeutics, (c) review all charts, and (d) feel free to make suggestions as seen fit.
2. I see the pharmacist as an integral part of a community clinic or city hospital serving as a specialist or consultant advisor.
3. I can see the pharmacist playing an important role in a group practice situation for (a) consulting on problems in clinical pharmacology; (b) helping to educate patients in how to take medications, what to expect, when to report side effects; (c) reviewing, with a group of physicians, the group's total patient records so as to improve prescribing of drugs, look for side effects and compare drug efficacy; and (d) helping the group to keep up on the literature on new drugs.
4. The main role of the pharmacist should be the providing of necessary information about medications. This is no small job considering the number of products on the market and the need for objective information on pharmacokinetics, efficacy, side effects, etc.
5. The most obvious need and use for pharmacists on the "health team" is to review the compatibility of multidrug regimens. Possibly in the future, with sufficiently well-trained pharmacists, it may be feasible for pharmacists to monitor blood levels vs. therapeutic effect.

## Conclusion

In summary, one basic conclusion can be drawn from the study. Physicians realize the need for a drug information specialist, and when exposed to an adequately trained pharmacist, will utilize the pharmacist's knowledge to the benefit of their patients. Physicians will come to expect this type of pharmacy service in the future, and the profession, as it has begun to do, must reorganize its objective to meet this demand.

It is not unusual to hear a pharmacist who is unwilling to attempt development of clinical services say that he does not want to offend or anger the physicians, or that he has attempted to start clinical involvement but the physicians were unreceptive. At least for our hospital, these statements are unsupportable. In many cases, the failure to implement clinical services may be due to the efforts of the pharmacy staff and not to unreceptive medical personnel.

The changes occurring in our profession can be aptly termed a revolution. The opponents to the new direction in pharmacy may not be obvious to many pharmacy practitioners, but they can be described by the quote, "We have met the enemy and he is us."

## References

1. Owyang, E., Miller, R. A. and Brodie, D. C.: The Pharmacist's New Role in Institutional Patient Care, *Amer. J. Hosp. Pharm.* 25:624–633 (Nov.) 1968.
2. Smith, W. E.: The Future Role of the Hospital Pharmacist in the Patient Care Area, *Amer. J. Hosp. Pharm.* 24:228–231 (Apr.) 1967.
3. Plein, J. B.: The Pharmacist's Input in Modern Pharmacotherapy, *Drug Intel. Clin. Pharm.* 5:279–286 (Sept.) 1971.

# Bibliography of Additional Articles on Clinical Pharmacy

This bibliography was prepared through a computer search of the data base of *International Pharmaceutical Abstracts*, a service of the American Society of Hospital Pharmacists. The citations found through this computer search were supplemented manually to add citations that were not yet in the *IPA* data base. While this bibliography is by no means exhaustive, it is a fairly representative selection of articles on clinical pharmacy education and practice. As such, it should serve to suggest additional readings to the users of this book.

The citations are listed in chronological order—the most recent articles appearing first. Because *IPA* initiated its computerization in 1970, only articles covered by the abstracting service since that time are included in the bibliography.

Berquist, S. C. Patient profile card used in clinical pharmacy services. *Am. J. Hosp. Pharm. 32*:597-598 (June) 1975.

Reinders, T. P., Rush, D. R., Baumgartner, R. P., Jr. et al. Pharmacist's role in management of hypertensive patients in an ambulatory care clinic. *Am. J. Hosp. Pharm. 32*: 590-594 (June) 1975.

Reich, J. W. A model for the management of a hospital pharmacy staffed by specialized pharmacists. *Hosp. Pharm. 10*:192-194, 199 (May) 1975.

Gibson, J. T., Alexander, V. L., and Newton, D. S. Influence on medication therapy of increased patient services by pharmacists in a pediatric hospital. *Am. J. Hosp. Pharm. 32*:495-500 (May) 1975.

Ryan, P. B., Johnson, C. A., and Rapp, R. P. Economic justification of pharmacist involvement in patient medication consultation. *Am. J. Hosp. Pharm. 32*:389-392 (Apr.) 1975.

Hunter, R. B. and Osterberger, D. J. Role of the pharmacist in an allergy clinic. *Am. J. Hosp. Pharm. 32*:392-395 (Apr.) 1975.

Beste, D. F., Jr. and Herfindal, E. T. An integrated program of clinical pharmacy. *Hosp. Formul. Manage. 10*: 172-175, 178, 180, 182 (Apr.) 1975.

Perry, P. J. and Hurley, S. C. Activities of the clinical pharmacist in the office of a family practitioner. *Drug Intell. Clin. Pharm. 9*:129-133 (Mar.) 1975.

Gelperin, A. A Supreme Court decision will require clinical pharmacy. *Drug Intell. Clin. Pharm. 9*:124-125 (Mar.) 1975.

Hoffman, R. P. and Moore, L. F. A procedure to formally establish clinical pharmacy services in a hospital. *Hosp. Pharm. 10*:106-108 (Mar.) 1975.

Painter, J. H., Archambault, G. F., and Dodds, A. W. Pharmacist monitoring of prescribed medications. *Hosp. Formul. Manage. 10*:123-125, 129 (Mar.) 1975.

Fong, G. R. The role of the pharmacist in an operant conditioning program for chronic pain patients. *Drug Intell. Clin. Pharm. 9*:68-75 (Feb.) 1975.

McCarron, M. M. A system of inpatient drug monitoring. *Drug Intell. Clin. Pharm. 9*:80-85 (Feb.) 1975.

McCarron, M. M. An approach to clinical pharmacy. *Drug Intell. Clin. Pharm. 9*:12-16 (Jan.) 1975.

McKenzie, M. W., Pevonka, M. P., Stewart, R. B. et al. The pharmacist's involvement in the long-term care facility—monitoring patient drug therapy. *J. Am. Pharm. Assoc. NS15*:16-20 (Jan.) 1975.

Marshall, G. Clinical program may effect savings. *Hospitals 48*:79-80, 102 (Dec. 1) 1974.

Francke, D. E. Directions for clinical pharmacy. *Drug Intell. Clin. Pharm. 8*:631 (Nov.) 1974.

Anon. Report of the Task Force on Specialties in Pharmacy. *J. Am. Pharm. Assoc. NS14*:618-623 (Nov.) 1974.

Penna, R. P. Specialties in pharmacy. *J. Am. Pharm. Assoc. NS14*:607 (Nov.) 1974.

Bergman, H. D., Fletcher, H. P., and Sperandio G. J.

Clinical pharmacy activities in a VA hospital. *Drug Intell. Clin. Pharm.* 8:656–662 (Nov.) 1974.

Cupit, G. C. An approach to pediatric pharmacy practice. *Hosp. Pharm.* 9:399–400, 402 (Oct.) 1974.

Kittel, J. F. and Mann, R. T. The pharmacist's role in a rehabilitation program for cardiac patients. *Hosp. Pharm.* 9:386–387, 390–391 (Oct.) 1974.

Powell, J. R. and Cupit, G. C. Developing the pharmacist's role in monitoring total parenteral nutrition. *Drug Intell. Clin. Pharm.* 8:576–580 (Oct.) 1974.

Juhl, R. P., Perry, P. J., Norwood, G. J. et al. The family practitioner-clinical pharmacist—group practice: a model clinic. *Drug Intell. Clin. Pharm.* 8:572–575 (Oct.) 1974.

Levine, M. E. Pharmacist's clinical role in interdisciplinary care. *Hosp. Formul. Manage.* 9:47–55 (Oct.) 1974.

Elenbaas, R. M. and Jacoby, K. E. Pharmacy resident evaluation using a behavioral rating scale. *Am. J. Hosp. Pharm.* 31:938–942 (Oct.) 1974.

Munden, K. J. Clinical psychiatric training for the pharmacist: a physician's viewpoint. *Hosp. Pharm.* 9:331, 334–336 (Sep.) 1974.

Womble, J. R. Developing and implementing a patient ostomy service managed by a pharmacist. *Hosp. Pharm.* 9:324, 326, 328, 330 (Sep.) 1974.

Zellmer, W. A. ASHP Council on Clinical Pharmacy and Therapeutics. *Am. J. Hosp. Pharm.* 31:831 (Sep.) 1974.

Nona, D. A. and Papovich, N. G. An evaluation of a clinical pharmacy program at the University of Illinois. *Am. J. Pharm. Educ.* 38:402–410 (Aug.) 1974.

Griffin, G. D. The dilemma of clinical pharmacy. *Drug Intell. Clin. Pharm.* 8:483–486 (Aug.) 1974.

Whitney, H. A. K., Jr. Clinical pharmacy education in hospitals. *Hospitals* 48:51–54 (Aug. 16) 1974.

Lipman, A. G. Clinical pharmacy: specialty or norm? *Hosp. Pharm.* 9:257 (July) 1974.

Welk, P. C. III, Burkhard, V., and Lamy, P. P. The technology of patient counselling. *Hosp. Pharm.* 9:224, 226–227, 230–231, 234–235, 238 (June) 1974.

O'Brien, T. E., Vetter, T. G., Sevka, M. J. et al. Introduction to clinical pharmacy. *Hosp. Formul. Manage.* 9:51–52, 54–55, 59 (June) 1974.

Smith, D. L. Teaching communications in the clinical area. *Am. J. Pharm. Educ.* 38:186–195 (May) 1974.

Stimmel, G. L., Katcher, B. S., and Levin, R. H. The emerging role and training program of clinical pharmacy in psychiatry. *Am. J. Pharm. Educ.* 38:179–185 (May) 1974.

Weissman, F. G. and Wynne, G. Functions of a clinically trained pharmacist on an oncology service. *Hosp. Pharm.* 9:203, 206–207 (May) 1974.

Herman, C. M. and Rodowskas, C. A. Development and

testing of a methodology to measure the attitudes of pharmacists toward clinical pharmacy. *Drug Intell. Clin. Pharm.* 8:238–241 (May) 1974.

White, S. J., Toll, M. A., and Godwin, H. N. Teaching patients to administer their own eye, ear and nose medications. *Hosp. Pharm.* 9:149, 151 (Apr.) 1974.

Baumgartner, R. P., Jr. Pharmacist involvement in six levels of health care. *Hosp. Pharm.* 9:141–143, 146, 148 (Apr.) 1974.

Kradjan, W. A. The practice of clinical pharmacy in the Puget Sound area. *J. Am. Pharm. Assoc.* NS14:136–144 (Mar.) 1974.

Griffin, G. D. The pharmacist as primary provider of maintenance health care. *Hosp. Pharm.* 9:84–85, 87–88, 92–94, 100–101 (Mar.) 1974.

Francke, D. E. Specialization in pharmacy. *Drug Intell. Clin. Pharm.* 8:105–108 (Mar.) 1974.

Davis, N. M. First steps toward outpatient counselling. *Hosp. Pharm.* 9:46, 55 (Feb.) 1974.

Canada, A. T. and Iazzetta, S. M. Pharmacy care for ambulatory patients—the consultation concept. *J. Am. Pharm. Assoc.* NS14:18–20 (Jan.) 1974.

Lerario, D. F. and Hanan, Z. I. Educating the diabetic patient. *Hosp. Pharm.* 9:5, 7, 10 (Jan.) 1974.

Miller, W. A. Computer oriented clinical hospital pharmacy services: a conceptual model. *J. Clin. Comput.* 3:276–287 (Jan.) 1974.

Walton, C. A. Clinical pharmacology and clinical pharmacy: a necessary alliance for practical advances in rational drug therapy. *J. Clin. Pharmacol.* 14:1–7 (Jan.) 1974.

Naismith, N. W. Cost effectiveness of a ward pharmacist. *Aust. J. Hosp. Pharm.* 4:161–167 (4) 1974.

Brodie, D. C., Knoben, J. F., and Wertheimer, A. I. Expanded roles for pharmacists. *Am. J. Pharm. Educ.* 37:591–600 (Nov.) 1973.

Gundfest, R. L. and Sandler, A. I. Is clinical pharmacy feasible in an outpatient service? *Pharm. Times* 39:44–49 (Nov.) 1973.

Pitlick, W. H. and Plein, E. M. Scope of undergraduate clinical pharmacy education: the results of a nationwide survey. *Drug Intell. Clin. Pharm.* 7:511–514 (Nov.) 1973.

Kohan, S., Chung, S. Y., and Stone, J. Clinical pharmacy in a psychiatric hospital. *Hosp. Pharm.* 8:290–296 (Sep.) 1973.

Madden, E. E., Jr. Evaluation of outpatient pharmacy patient counselling. *J. Am. Pharm. Assoc.* NS13:437–443 (Aug.) 1973.

Ericson, A. J. and Shainfeld, F. J. Pharmacist in an obstetrical service. *Am. J. Hosp. Pharm.* 30:702–704 (Aug.) 1973.

Jaffee, W. E. and Sisca, R. S. Big-time clinical pharmacy in a small community hospital. *Hosp. Pharm. 8*:244–250 (Aug.) 1973.

Swintosky, J. V. Clinical education and practice in pharmacy. *Am. J. Pharm. 145*:129–134 (Jul.–Aug.) 1973.

Anderson, R. D. Clinical pharmacy in any environment. *Can. J. Hosp. Pharm. 26*:147–151 (Jul.–Aug.) 1973.

Francke, D. E. Establishing a model for clinical practitioners. *Drug Intell. Clin. Pharm. 7*:251 (June) 1973.

Klotz, R. Becoming a pediatric clinical pharmacist. *Hosp. Pharm. 8*:198–199 (June) 1973.

Durgin, Sr. J. M. and Bartilucci, A. J. Learning contracts in clinical pharmacy. *Am. J. Pharm. Educ. 37*:311–319 (May) 1973.

Gever, L. N. Weekly newspaper columns explain to the public clinical pharmacy's value. *Pharm. Times 39*:52–56 (Mar.) 1973.

Weiblen, J. W. Staff attitudes toward clinical pharmacy. *Hospitals 47*:54, 56, 58–59 (Feb. 16) 1973.

Gonzales, Sr. M. and Mattei, T. J. Origin and evolution of a clinical pharmacy program. *Hosp. Formul. Manage. 8*:19–21 (Feb.) 1973.

Francke, D. E. Clinical pharmacy service and education. V. Hospital-based residency programs—redefining the pharmacist. *Drug Intell. Clin. Pharm. 7*:57 (Feb.) 1973.

Feely, J. W. What your administrator needs to know to approve a clinical pharmacy program. *Hosp. Pharm. 8*: 6–7 (Jan.) 1973.

Sisson, M. Student evaluation of a pilot clinical pharmacy course. *Hosp. Pharm. 8*:19–21 (Jan.) 1973.

Francke, D. E. Clinical pharmacy service and education. IV. Objectives of hospital based internships and role of colleges of pharmacy. *Drug Intell. Clin. Pharm. 7*:5 (Jan.) 1973.

Gordon, J. A. Therapeutic pharmacists can help solve the problem of multiple medications. *Pharm. Times 38*:54–59 (Dec.) 1972.

Sumner, E. D. Clinical pharmacy experiences: how a pharmacy educator is closing the gap. *Am. J. Pharm. Educ. 36*: 593–597 (Nov.) 1972.

Wizwer, P. and Deeb, E. N. Experiences with a clinical pharmacy training program in a VA hospital. *Am. J. Pharm. Educ. 36*:575–580 (Nov.) 1972.

Francke, D. E. Clinical pharmacy service and education. II. Pharmacy service—college relationships. *Drug. Intell. Clin. Pharm. 6*:373 (Nov.) 1972.

Smith, G. H. Case studies of a clinical pharmacist. *Am. J. Hosp. Pharm. 29*:958–962 (Nov.) 1972.

Bowles, G. C., Jr. When everyone is a specialist, who will do the work of the hospital pharmacy? *Mod. Hosp. 119*: 126 (Oct.) 1972.

Francke, D. E. Clinical pharmacy service and education.

Drug Intell. Clin. Pharm. 6:341 (Oct.) 1972.

Francke, D. E. Relationship between clinical pharmacology and clinical pharmacy. *J. Clin. Pharmacol. 12*:384–392 (Oct.) 1972.

Heymann, J. Practical approach to the development of a clinical pharmacy program, part 2. *Can. J. Hosp. Pharm. 25*:215–218 (Sep.–Oct.) 1972.

Provost, G. P. Clinical pharmacy—specialty or general direction? *Drug Intell. Clin. Pharm. 6*:285–289 (Aug.) 1972.

Feldmann, E. G. Clinical pharmacology vis-à-vis clinical pharmacy. *J. Pharm. Sci. 61*:I (Aug.) 1972.

Straight, S. P., Ng, K., and Stewart, D. J. Clinical practice of pharmacy: a course and its evaluation. *Can. J. Hosp. Pharm. 25*:169–172 (Jul.–Aug.) 1972.

Von Heymann, J. J. Practical approach to the development of a clinical pharmacy program, part 1. *Can. J. Hosp. Pharm. 25*:161–164 (Jul.–Aug.) 1972.

Zellmer, W. A. Scientific basis for clinical pharmacy practice. *Am. J. Hosp. Pharm. 29*:473 (June) 1972.

Brown, A. A. Clinical pharmacy in a faculty of dentistry. *Can. Pharm. J. 106*:186–187 (June) 1972.

Francke, D. E. Clinical pharmacist and the clinical pharmacologist. *Drug Intell. Clin. Pharm. 6*:207 (June) 1972.

Baumgartner, R. P., Jr., Land, M. J., and Hauser, L. D. Rural health care—opportunity for innovative pharmacy service. *Am. J. Hosp. Pharm. 29*:394–400 (May) 1972.

Bowles, G. C., Jr. Cooperative teaching programs aid hospital pharmacy students. *Mod. Hosp. 118*:131 (May) 1972.

Barker, K. N. and Valentino, J. G. On a political and legal foundation for clinical pharmacy practice. *J. Am. Pharm. Assoc. NS12*:202–206, 237 (May) 1972.

Levin, R. H. Clinical pharmacy practice in a pediatric clinic. *Drug Intell. Clin. Pharm. 6*:171–176 (May) 1972.

Clarke, W. T. W. Hospital pharmacist's participation in the promotion of rational drug therapy. *Can. J. Hosp. Pharm. 25*:65–66 (Mar.–Apr.) 1972.

Mann, J. Clinical pharmacy in drug distribution and therapy. *Hosp. Admin. (Canada) 14*:22 (Feb.) 1972.

Herfindal, E. T. and Levin, R. H. Clinical pharmacy training in an outpatient clinic. *Am. J. Pharm. Educ. 36*:72–87 (Feb.) 1972.

Rosenberg, J. M. Clinical pharmacy methodology concerning drug interactions. *Hosp. Pharm. 7*:39, 42–44 (Feb.) 1972.

Buckley, J. P. Pharmacological therapeutics: objectives and implementation. *Am. J. Pharm. Educ. 35*:803–806 (Dec.) 1971.

Weaver, L. C. Importance of pharmacology and toxicology to the pharmacist in the delivery of improved patient care. *Am. J. Pharm. Educ.* 35:728–734 (Dec.) 1971.

Miller, R. A. Use of pharmacological therapeutics in institutional clinical pharmacy practice. *Am. J. Pharm. Educ.* 35:813–817 (Dec.) 1971.

White, A. M. Short course offers clinical exposure to practicing hospital pharmacists. *Hosp. Top.* 49:51–52 (Dec.) 1971.

Anon. Proceedings of the ASHP-AACP Invitational Workshop on Clinical Pharmaceutical Practice and Education. *Am. J. Hosp. Pharm.* 28:842–906 (Nov.) 1971.

Provost, G. P. Considerations in clinical pharmacy education and practice. *Am. J. Hosp. Pharm.* 28:841 (Nov.) 1971.

Bainbridge, C. V., Jeffery, W. H., and Kabat, H. F. Clinical pharmacy education program benefits mentally retarded. *Hospitals* 45:78, 80 (Nov. 16) 1971.

Calder, G. Light at the end of the dark tunnel: a foreign colleague views clinical pharmacy. *Drug Intell. Clin. Pharm.* 5:368–369 (Nov.) 1971.

Anon. Report of Task Force on the Pharmacist's Clinical Role. *J. Am. Pharm. Assoc.* NS11:482–485 (Sep.) 1971.

Jeffrey, L. P. Pharmacy's challenge: the patient care unit. *Hosp. Top.* 49:57–62 (Sep.) 1971.

Cohen, S. S., Ginsberg, M., and Birmingham, P. Clinical pharmacist in a cardiac-respiratory situation. *Hosp. Pharm.* 6:17–20 (Sep.) 1971.

Plein, J. B. Pharmacist's input in modern pharmacotherapy. *Drug Intell. Clin. Pharm.* 5:279–286 (Sep.) 1971.

McCarron, M. M. Approach to the education of patient-oriented pharmacists. *Am. J. Pharm. Educ.* 35:396–400 (Aug.) 1971.

Barber, S. Development of a clinical pharmacy program at Women's College Hospital. *Can. J. Hosp. Pharm.* 24:138–140 (Jul.–Aug.) 1971.

Hutchinson, R. and Burkholder, D. F. Clinical pharmacy practice—its functional relationship to drug information service. *Drug Intell. Clin. Pharm.* 5:181–185 (June) 1971.

White, A. M. Short course in clinical pharmacy. *Am. J. Pharm. Educ.* 35:196–200 (May) 1971.

American Society of Hospital Pharmacists. Statement on clinical pharmacy and its relationship to the hospital. *Am. J. Hosp. Pharm.* 28:357 (May) 1971.

Baumgart, A. J. Pharmacist in the clinical setting—a nurse's viewpoint. *Can. J. Hosp. Pharm.* 24:83–84 (May–June) 1971.

Sandler, A. I. and Altbach, H. Clinical training for Veterans Administration pharmacy interns. *Am. J. Hosp. Pharm.* 28:260–266 (Apr.) 1971.

Durgin, Sr. J. M. Clinical pharmacy practice: goals and how to attain them. *Hosp. Top.* 48:61–64, 87 (Apr.) 1971.

Emmanuel, S. Patient-oriented pharmacist—a must in today's society. *Hosp. Top.* 49:61–64 (Mar.) 1971.

Liguori, Sr. M. Clinical pharmacy—for all pharmacists? *Can. J. Hosp. Pharm.* 24:54–57 (Mar.–Apr.) 1971.

Tuttle, G. Clinical approach to pharmacy practice in the outpatient department. *Can J. Hosp. Pharm.* 24:51–53, 60 (Mar.–Apr.) 1971.

Whitney, H. A. K., Jr. and Covington, T. R. Future impact of clinical pharmacy on parenteral drugs and the industry. *Bull. Parenter. Drug Assoc.* 25:87–97 (Mar.–Apr.) 1971.

de Leon, R. F. Current trends in the teaching of clinical pharmacy at the University of California. *Am. J. Pharm. Educ.* 35:62–66 (Feb.) 1971.

Tatro, D. S. and Nagata, R., Jr. Clinical atmosphere for pharmacy students and consultants. *Am. J. Pharm. Educ.* 35:71–78 (Feb.) 1971.

Miller, R. A. New courses in the teaching of clinical pharmacy at the University of California. *Am. J. Pharm. Educ.* 35:67–70 (Feb.) 1971.

de Leon, R. F. Clinical pharmacy at the University of California. *J. Am. Pharm. Assoc.* NS11:54–55 (Feb.) 1971.

McLeod, D. C. Clinical pharmacy practice in a community health center. *J. Am. Pharm. Assoc.* NS11:56–59 (Feb.) 1971.

Miller, R. A. Application of clinical pharmacy. *J. Am. Pharm. Assoc.* NS11:46–47 (Feb.) 1971.

Emmanuel, Sr. Community pharmacy practice—its role in the education of clinically oriented pharmacists. *J. Am. Pharm. Assoc.* NS11:49–53, 63 (Feb.) 1971.

Silverman, H. M. Clinical pharmacy training. *Hospitals* 45:67–72 (Jan. 16) 1971.

Kostuk, R. M. Legal aspects of clinical pharmacy. *Can. J. Hosp. Pharm.* 24:11–15 (Jan.–Feb.) 1971.

Provost, G. P. Clinical pharmacy and hospital pharmacy. *Am. J. Hosp. Pharm.* 28:17 (Jan.) 1971.

Kabat, H. F. New dimensions in graduate education: the clinical setting. *Am. J. Pharm. Educ.* 34:812–815 (Dec.) 1970.

Nagata, R. E. and Lerner, C. S. Implementation of clinical pharmacy through training. *Hosp. Pharm.* 5:4–8 (Dec.) 1970.

Smith, W. E., O'Malley, C. D., and Weiblen, J. W. Clinical pharmacy: general hospital. *Hospitals* 44:88–94 (Nov. 1) 1970.

Ginsberg, M. P. and Birmingham, P. H. Clinical pharmacy: long-term care institution. *Hospitals* 44:94, 98–99 (Nov. 1) 1970.

Durgin, Sr. J. M. Paving pathways to clinical practice. *Hosp. Top.* 48:51–52, 56 (Oct.) 1970.

Kabat, H. F. Administrative responsibilities associated

with the development of clinical pharmacy services. *Can. J. Hosp. Pharm. 23*:196-197 (Sep.-Oct.) 1970.

Smith, D. L. Pharmaceutical communications in the clinical environment. *Can. J. Hosp. Pharm. 23*:191-195, 197 (Sep.-Oct.) 1970.

Francke, D. E. Clinical pharmacy in the '70s. *Can. J. Hosp. Pharm. 23*:185-190 (Sep.-Oct.) 1970.

Francke, D. E. Pharmacy's new emphasis. *Drug Intell. Clin. Pharm. 4*:231 (Sep.) 1970.

McLeod, D. C. and Allen, R. J. Hospital and clinical pharmacy principles applied to community health care: student health action committee clinics at the University of North Carolina. *Am. J. Hosp. Pharm. 27*:390-394 (May) 1970.

Emmanuel, Sr. Clinical pharmacist and his relationship to nursing practice. *Hosp. Manage. 109*:44-53 (May) 1970.

Canada, A. T., Jr. Training of a clinical pharmacist. *Am. J. Pharm. Educ. 34*:265-269 (May) 1970.

Stelzer, J. M., Jr. and Wurdack, P. J. Clinical pharmacy course utilizing fourteen selected hospitals. *Am. J. Pharm. Educ. 34*:249-255 (May) 1970.

Smith, D. L. Pharmacist on the ward. *Can J. Hosp. Pharm. 23*:108-112 (May-June) 1970.

Dougherty, F. K. and Ardneser, G. Clinical pharmacy education in the private hospital. *Hosp. Top. 48*:83-90 (Feb.) 1970.

Hlynka, J. N. Clinical pharmacy—myth or must? *Can. Pharm. J. 103*:40-43 (Feb.) 1970.

Cain, R. M. Physician-pharmacist interface in the clinical practice of pharmacy. *Drug Intell. Clin. Pharm. 4*:38-40 (Feb.) 1970.

Whitmore, J. Developing an undergraduate clinical pharmacy course in the community teaching hospital. *Am. J. Pharm. Educ. 34*:69-77 (Feb.) 1970.

Stuart, D. M. A journey to tomorrow. *Am. J. Pharm. Educ. 34*:78-85 (Feb.) 1970.

Sandmann, R. A. Educating the clinical pharmacist. *Hosp. Top. 48*:59-62 (Jan.) 1970.

Canada, A. T. and McHale, M. K. A pharmacy's vital role in clinical drug evaluations. *Hosp. Pharm. 5*:7-9 (Jan.) 1970.

Bouchard, V. E. Toward a clinical practice of pharmacy. *Drug Intell. Clin. Pharm. 3*:342-347 (Dec.) 1969.

Hanan, Z. I. Status quo must go: why pharmacist belongs on patient-care floors. *Hosp. Top. 47*:71-80 (Dec.) 1969.

Francke, G. N. Evolvement of clinical pharmacy. *Drug Intell. Clin. Pharm. 3*:348-354 (Dec.) 1969.

Smith, W. E. Clinical pharmacy. *Drug Intell. Clin. Pharm. 3*:322-323 (Nov.) 1969.

Rosenberg, J. M. and Hanan, Z. I. Clinical pharmacy and drug information at Mercy Hospital. *Hosp. Pharm. 4*:22-24 (Nov.) 1969.

Ellis, M. D. Clinical pharmacist on a pediatric unit. *Hosp. Top. 47*:81-82, 84, 88-89 (Nov.) 1969.

Paoloni, C. U. Medication assistants: a ramification of clinical pharmacy. *Pharm. Times 35*:26-30 (Oct.) 1969.

Knoll, K. R. and Beasley, J. R. Clinical approach to pharmacy education at the University of Arkansas Medical Center. *Hosp. Pharm. 4*:15-20 (Sep.) 1969.

Cheung, A. Students get clinical experience in pharmacy clerkship program. *Hosp. Top. 47*:89-92 (Sep.) 1969.

Smith, W. E. Drugs, the patient and the hospital. *Drug Intell. Clin. Pharm. 3*:244-247 (Sep.) 1969.

Walton, C. A. Clinical pharmacy practice and education—the concept and its implementation. *Am. J. Pharm. 141*:186-197 (Sep.-Oct.) 1969.

White, A. M. Changing role of pharmacy education. *Am. J. Pharm. Educ. 33*:405-410 (Aug.) 1969.

Cacace, L. G. How patient-drug profiles help clinical pharmacist. *Hosp. Top. 47*:53-56, 86 (Aug.) 1969.

McLaughlin, P. P. Clinical pharmacy—the other side of this concept. *Hosp. Manage. 103*:38-40 (July) 1969.

Stewart, D. J., Dancey, J. W., and Straight, S. Clinical pharmacy program as developed at Toronto General Hospital. *Can. J. Hosp. Pharm. 22*:174-177 (July-Aug.) 1969.

Stephenson, J. T. Reevaluating roles. *Hosp. Formul. Manage. 4*:26-27 (July) 1969.

Blake, D. A. Role of pharmacology in the clinically oriented pharmacy curriculum. *Hosp. Pharm. 4*:24-25 (June) 1969.

Paxinos, J. What role can pharmacists play in the clinical environment? *Hosp. Top. 47*:75-78 (May) 1969.

# Index